JRCALC

Clinical Guidelines 2019

JRCALC
Clinical Guidelines 2019

Edited for JRCALC and AACE by

Dr Simon N Brown, Dr Dhushy Surendra Kumar
and Cathryn James

**On behalf of the National Ambulance Service
Medical Directors Group**

Dr Julian Mark and medical director colleagues

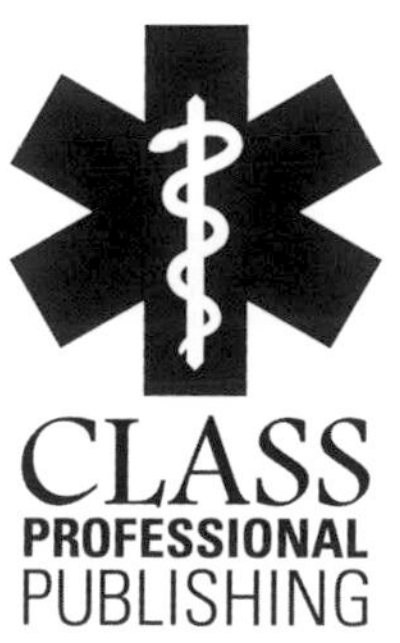

Printing history

This edition published 2019, reprinted 2019.

First edition published 2000, second edition 2004, third edition 2006

Fourth edition published 2013, reprinted 2014, 2015 (twice, Version 1.3)

The content for Reference Edition 1.3 and Pocket Book 1.2 was updated in January 2015

2016 edition published 2016, reprinted 2016 (Version 1.5)

JRCALC Clinical Practice Supplementary Guidelines 2017 published 2017. Reprinted 2018

The authors and publisher welcome feedback from the users of this book.

Please contact the publisher:

Class Professional Publishing,

The Exchange, Express Park, Bristol Road, Bridgwater TA6 4RR

Telephone: 01278 427 800

Email: icpg@class.co.uk

Website: www.classprofessional.co.uk

Class Professional Publishing is an imprint of Class Publishing Ltd

A CIP catalogue record for this book is available from the British Library

This edition: JRCALC Clinical Guidelines 2019 ISBN 9781859596555

ISSN 2514-6084

Also available: JRCALC Clinical Guidelines 2019 (eBook) ISBN 9781859597958

JRCALC Clinical Guidelines 2019 Pocket Book ISBN 9781859596562

JRCALC Clinical Guidelines 2019 Pocket Book (eBook) ISBN 9781859596838

Printed in Slovenia by arrangement with KINT

Contents

Contents

Disclaimer

The Association of Ambulance Chief Executives and the Joint Royal Colleges Ambulance Liaison Committee have made every effort to ensure that the information, tables, drawings and diagrams contained in these guidelines are accurate at the time of publication. However, the guidelines are advisory and have been developed to assist healthcare professionals, and patients, to make decisions about the management of the patient's health, including treatments. This advice is intended to support the decision making process and is not a substitute for sound clinical judgement. The guidelines cannot always contain all the information necessary for determining appropriate care and cannot address all individual situations; therefore, individuals using these guidelines must ensure they have the appropriate knowledge and skills to enable suitable interpretation.

JRCALC has referenced NICE in these guidelines. NICE guidance is prepared for the National Health Service in England and is subject to regular review and may be updated or withdrawn. NICE has not checked the use of its content in these guidelines to confirm that it accurately reflects the NICE publications from which it is taken.

Users of these guidelines must always be aware that alterations after the date of publication cannot be incorporated into the printed edition.

The Association of Ambulance Chief Executives and the Joint Royal Colleges Ambulance Liaison Committee do not guarantee and accepts no legal liability of whatever nature arising from or connected to, the accuracy, reliability, currency or completeness of the content of these guidelines.

Although some modification of the guidelines may be required by individual ambulance services, and approved by the relevant local clinical committees, to ensure they respond to the health requirements of the local community, the majority of the guidance is universally applicable to NHS ambulance services. Modification of the guidelines may also occur when undertaking research sanctioned by a research ethics committee.

Whilst these guidelines cover a range of paramedic treatments available across the UK they will also provide a valuable tool for a range of care providers. Many of the assessment skills and general principles will remain the same. All clinical staff must practise within their level of training and competence.

Updates to these guidelines may be published on the JRCALC apps which will always contain the most current content.

Foreword

Welcome to the JRCALC Clinical Guidelines 2019. It is three years since the last full publication of JRCALC guidelines and two years since the interim supplementary guidelines were published. During this time, many users will have become familiar with accessing guidance and information via the JRCALC apps, iCPG and JRCALC Plus. Take up and use of the digital platforms has been fantastic, but we believe there is still a real need for printed editions to be produced. All the information contained in the earlier 2017 supplementary guidelines is now incorporated into this text along with many new, revised and consolidated guidelines.

New for this edition is a substantial addition to the section on resuscitation where the important influence of human factors on behaviours is acknowledged. A thorough review of all sections of the book has led to updates across medical, trauma and general guidance. Special situations are now detailed in a new major, complex and high risk incidents chapter. The medicines section also sees changes, updates, inclusions and the occasional withdrawal of drugs from our pharmacy.

Maternal and obstetric emergencies can often present challenges and concerns for pre-hospital clinicians. The completely revised and updated guidelines, first published in the 2017 supplementary guidelines provide the detailed knowledge and practical information required for safe, effective practice and decision making.

Caring for an ageing population is of course a growing need, and the section on falls in the older adult provides strategies for dealing with one of the most common calls for pre-hospital clinicians.

Fully revised guidance for convulsions, sepsis, overdose and poisoning, end of life care and medicines, amongst others, will ensure that all paramedics can provide improved care for patients.

All the guidance presented here by JRCALC supports thoughtful delivery of care by professionals rather than the routine following of flowcharts or protocols. Paramedics are developing their practice and we trust that these guidelines support that journey.

On behalf of JRCALC, NASMED and AACE, we would like to thank all those that contributed to this 2019 edition, the committee members who acted as lead authors and the groups of expert and enthusiastic healthcare professionals who all gave so willingly of their time. Our special thanks to two people without whom this project would have taken twice as long: Emma Milman as the lead editor for Class Professional Publishing and Cathryn James of AACE who both provided considerable expertise, knowledge and energy.

DHUSHY SURENDRA KUMAR

Chair, Joint Royal Colleges Ambulance Liaison Committee

SIMON N BROWN

Chair, JRCALC Guideline Development Groups

STEVE IRVING

Executive Officer, Association of Ambulance Chief Executives

Guideline Developers and Contributors

The authors and editors would like to thank everyone who has contributed to the JRCALC guidelines over a number of years. Many people have given freely and generously of their time to help draft, develop and improve the guidelines. In particular, we wish to acknowledge the work of the members of the Joint Royal Colleges Ambulance Liaison Committee, the National Ambulance Service Medical Directors group, the Ambulance Lead Paramedics group and the Ambulance Pharmacists Network. Other contributors have come from multidisciplinary groups and include healthcare professionals, educators and patients.

2019 Guidelines

EDITORIAL LEADS

CATHRYN JAMES, *Clinical Support for NASMeD and JRCALC guidelines editor, AACE*

STEVE IRVING, *Executive Officer, AACE*

DR SIMON N BROWN, *GP and Assistant Medical Director, South Central Ambulance Service, JRCALC member, Royal College of GPs*

DR JULIAN MARK, *Executive Medical Director, Yorkshire Ambulance Service, chair of NASMeD*

FOR JRCALC

DR DHUSHY SURENDRA KUMAR, *Consultant in Critical Care, Prehospital Care and Anaesthesia, University Hospitals Coventry and Warwickshire, chair of JRCALC*

PROFESSOR CHARLES D DEAKIN, *Honorary Professor of Resuscitation & Prehospital Emergency Medicine, University of Southampton and Consultant in Cardiac Anaesthesia & Cardiac Intensive Care at University Hospital Southampton, Executive Committee Member Resuscitation Council (UK)*

DR ED ENGLAND, *Pharmaceutical Advisor, South Central Ambulance Service*

RHYS HANCOCK, *Clinical Lead, South Western Ambulance Service*

MR KIM HINSHAW, *Consultant Obstetrician and Gynaecologist, City Hospitals Sunderland, Royal College of Obstetricians and Gynaecologists*

AMANDA MANSFIELD, *Consultant Midwife, London Ambulance Service, Royal College of Midwives*

DR FIONNA MOORE, *Executive Medical Director, South East Coast Ambulance Service*

PROFESSOR TOM QUINN, *Director for the Centre for Health and Social Care Research, Kingston and St George's*

SUE OAKLEY, *Pharmaceutical Advisor, South Western Ambulance Service*

DR JULIAN SANDELL, *Consultant in Paediatric Emergency Medicine, Poole Hospital*

DR ALISON WALKER, *Consultant in Emergency Medicine at Harrogate and District Hospital*

JRCALC would like to gratefully acknowledge the contribution of South Western Ambulance Service to a number of guidelines, including: abdominal pain, allergic reactions including anaphylaxis, headache, meningococcal meningitis and septicaemia

RESUSCITATION AND CARDIAC ARREST

MARK WHITBREAD, *Consultant Paramedic, London Ambulance Service*

PAUL AITKEN-FELL, *Consultant Paramedic, North East Ambulance Service*

DAVE BYWATER, *Consultant Paramedic, Scottish Ambulance Service*

DR TIM EDWARDS, *Consultant Paramedic, London Ambulance Service*

DAVE HAWKINS, *South East Coast Ambulance Service*

DR MATTHEW HOUSE, *Consultant Paramedic, North West Ambulance Service*

IAN MURSELL, *Consultant Paramedic, East Midlands Ambulance Service*

CHRIS MARTIN, *Advanced Paramedic, East of England Ambulance Service*

JO NEVETT, *Clinical Advisor to the Medical Director, London Ambulance Service*

CARL POWELL, *Clinical Support Officer, Welsh Ambulance Service*

ASHLEY RICHARDSON, *Advanced Paramedic, East of England Ambulance Service*

AMY SAINSBURY, *Paramedic, South Western Ambulance Service*

STEVEN SHORT, *Registered nurse, Scottish Ambulance Service*

MATT WARD, *Consultant Paramedic, West Midlands Ambulance Service*

THOLI WOOD, *Clinical and Quality Lead, Isle of Wight Ambulance Service*

Guideline Developers and Contributors

TRACHEOSTOMY AND LARYNGECTOMY

DOROTHY ANTRIM, *Clinical Tutor, London Ambulance Service*

DR PHILIP O'DONNELL, *Sunderland Royal Hospital & Great North Air Ambulance Service*

DR JONATHAN WHELAN, *Assistant Medical Director, Welsh Ambulance Service*

STROKE AND TRANSIENT ISCHAEMIC ATTACK

Led by Professor TOM QUINN

CHRIS ASHTON, *North West Ambulance Service*

GRAHAM MCCLELLAND, *North East Ambulance Service*

SCOTT MUNRO, *South East Coast Ambulance Service*

LEFT VENTRICULAR ASSIST DEVICE

MR JOHN JM BLACK, *Medical Director, South Central Ambulance Service*

DR CHRISTOPHER BOWLES, *Artificial Heart Specialist, Royal Brompton & Harefield NHS Foundation Trust and Honorary Research Associate, Imperial College London*

The algorithms in the LVAD guidance were first published in the *Emergency Medicine Journal* and are republished with kind permission.

BOWLES CT, HARDS R, WRIGHTSON N, LINCOLN P, KORE S, MARLEY L, DALZELL JR, RAJ B, BAKER TA, GOODWIN D, CARROLL P, PATEMAN J, BLACK JJM, KATTERNHORN P, FAULKNER M, PARAMESHWAR J, BUTCHER C, MASON M, ROSENBERG A, MCGOVERN I, WEYMANN A, GWINNUTT C, BANNER NR, SCHUELER S, SIMON AR and PITCHER DW. Algorithms to guide ambulance clinicians in the management of emergencies in patients with implanted rotary left ventricular assist devices. *Emergency Medicine Journal* 2017, 34:842-850.

TRAUMA EMERGENCIES OVERVIEW IN ADULTS: HAEMORRHAGE FROM RENAL DIALYSIS ARTERIOVENOUS GRAFT AND FISTULA

MR JOHN JM BLACK, *Medical Director, South Central Ambulance Service*

MR PAUL GIBBS, *Consultant Transplant Surgeon and Clinical Director for Transplantation and Renal Surgery, Portsmouth Hospitals*

OVERDOSE AND POISONING

DR MARK ANDERSON, *Consultant Paediatrician, The Newcastle upon Tyne Hospitals*

DR JAMES COULSON, *Consultant Clinical Toxicologist, Cardiff University*

MATTHEW DUNN, *Area Consultant Paramedic, North West Ambulance Service*

JON HARVEY, *Paramedic, West Midlands Ambulance Service*

ANDREW HUMBER, *Paramedic, London Ambulance Service*

CONVULSIONS IN ADULTS

DR JON M DICKSON, *Senior Clinical Lecturer and GP, the University of Sheffield*

DR RICHARD GRUNEWALD, *Consultant Neurologist, Sheffield*

PROFESSOR MARKUS REUBER, *Consultant Neurologist, Sheffield*

PROFESSOR NIRO SIRIWARDENA, *GP, Lincoln and Professor of Primary & Pre-Hospital Health Care, University of Lincoln*

JASON WILES, *Paramedic, West Midlands Ambulance Service*

IAN WILMER, *Advanced Paramedic Practitioner, London Ambulance Service*

END OF LIFE CARE

JOANNE STONEHOUSE, *Macmillan Cancer Care Project Manager, South Western Ambulance Service*

EDWARD O'BRIAN, *End of Life Care Lead and Macmillan Paramedic, Welsh Ambulance Service*

MEMBERS OF THE NATIONAL AMBULANCE END OF LIFE CARE LEADS GROUP

SONIA CHAND, *Pharmaceutical Advisor, West Midlands Ambulance Service*

SHIRMILLA DATTA, *Specialist Paramedic, South East Coast Ambulance Service*

Guideline Developers and Contributors

HEART FAILURE

DR LISA ANDERSON, *Heart Failure Consultant, St George's University Hospitals NHS Foundation Trust*

DR JOHN MCANAW, *Head of Pharmacy, NHS24*

BARRY MURPHY-JONES, *Advanced Paramedic Practitioner, London Ambulance Service*

GLYCAEMIC EMERGENCIES IN ADULTS AND CHILDREN

DR BELINDA ALLAN, *Hull and East Yorkshire Hospital NHS Trust*

DR DAVID FITZPATRICK, *Senior Lecturer, Faculty of Health Sciences and Sport, University of Stirling*

DR PARTHA KAR, *Consultant Endocrinologist, Portsmouth Hospitals NHS Trust and Associate National Clinical Director for diabetes NHS England*

NICKY NICOL, *Paramedic, Welsh Ambulances Service*

PATIENT CONFIDENTIALITY AND CONSENT

CRAIG GARNER, *Information Governance Manager, Welsh Ambulance Service*

MENTAL HEALTH PRESENTATION: CRISIS, DISTRESS AND DISORDERED BEHAVIOUR

Led by DR ALISON WALKER

MEMBERS OF THE AMBULANCE MENTAL HEALTH LEADS GROUP

DR PETER AITKEN, *Director of Research & Development & Medical Education, Devon Partnership*

ROBERT COLE, *Head of Clinical Practice, West Midlands Ambulance Service*

SUE PUTMAN, *Clinical Lead, Mental Health & Learning Disability, South Central Ambulance*

ROBERT TAYLOR, *North West Ambulance Service*

MAJOR, COMPLEX AND HIGH RISK INCIDENTS

Members of the National Ambulance Resilience Unit

CHRISTIAN COOPER, *Head of Compliance, NARU*

JENNA DAVIES, *Quality Assurance Advisor*

DR EDDIE TUNN, *Medical Advisor*

HYPERVENTILATION

CAITLIN WILSON, *North West Ambulance Service*

HYPOTHERMIA

DR LES GORDON, *Consultant Anaesthetist, Royal Lancaster Infirmary, Team Doctor, Langdale & Ambleside Mountain Rescue Team*

HEAD INJURIES

SIMON STANDEN, *Consultant Paramedic, Yorkshire Ambulance Service*

PROFESSOR MARK WILSON, *Consultant Neurosurgeon and Pre-Hospital Care Specialist, Imperial College Healthcare*

2017 Supplementary Guidelines

OBSTETRICS AND GYNAECOLOGY

Led by MR KIM HINSHAW and AMANDA MANSFIELD

SALLY ARNOLD-JONES, *Paramedic, Clinical Development Manager, South Western Ambulance Service*

ANNMARIE BRESLIN, *Midwife and Advanced Life Support Obstetrics faculty*

CLAIRE CAPITO, *Supervisor of Midwives, Support Midwife for London*

PROFESSOR TIM DRAYCOTT, *Consultant Obstetrician, Bristol. Representing PROMPT (PRactical Obstetric Multi-Professional Training) programme*

MR SIMON GRANT, *Consultant in Obstetrics and Fetal Medicine, North Bristol. Representing MOET (Managing Obstetric Emergencies and Trauma) programme*

Guideline Developers and Contributors

CLAIRE HENDERSON, *Paramedic, London Ambulance Service*

SHARON JORDAN, *Midwife, Senior Labour Ward Coordinator*

MICHELLE KNIGHT, *Lead Midwife, Epsom and St Helier Hospital*

PROFESSOR PAUL LEWIS, *OBE, Emeritus Professor, Bournemouth University, Honorary Fellow of the Royal College of Midwives. Representing ALSO (Advanced Life Support in Obstetrics) UK programme*

DENICE MACE, *Senior Clinical Midwife, Sunderland. Representing POET (Prehospital Obstetric Emergency Training) programme*

STEPHANIE MICHAELIDES, *Midwife, Programme Leader, Middlesex University*

ROGER NEUBERG, *retired Consultant in Obstetrics and Gynaecology, Leicester. Representing ALSO (Advanced Life Support in Obstetrics) UK programme*

NICK SILLETT, *Advanced Paramedic Practitioner, London Ambulance Service*

JACQUI TOMKINS, *Chair of Independent Midwives UK*

MRS AARTI ULLAL, *Consultant Obstetrician, City Hospitals Sunderland*

CATHY WINTER, *Research Midwife, Bristol. Representing PROMPT (PRactical Obstetric Multi-Professional Training) programme*

PROFESSOR JONATHAN WYLLIE, *Consultant Neonatologist, James Cook University Hospital*

AIMEE YARRINGTON, *Paramedic and Midwife, West Midlands Ambulance Service*

FALLS IN OLDER ADULTS

Led by DR ALISON WALKER

MARK BAXTER, *Orthogeriatrician, University Hospital Southampton*

DR JAY BANERJEE, *Consultant in Emergency Medicine, University Hospitals of Leicester*

KEITH COLVER, *Paramedic, Clinical Governance Manager, Scottish Ambulance Service*

DAWNE GARRETT, *Professional Lead – Older People and Dementia Care, The Royal College of Nursing*

JOANNA GARRETT, *Paramedic, Clinical Development Officer, South Western Ambulance Service*

JAMES GOUGH, *Paramedic, Welsh Ambulance Service*

TIM JONES, *Advanced Paramedic Practitioner, Clinical Practice Lead, Welsh Ambulance Service*

ANN MURRAY, *Programme Lead, Falls Programme, Active and Independent Living Programme, Scottish Government*

IAN MURSELL, *Consultant Paramedic, East Midlands Ambulance Service*

DUNCAN ROBERTSON, *Consultant Paramedic, North West Ambulance Service*

VICKY KYPTA, *Specialist Paramedic, South East Coast Ambulance Service*

DANIEL HAWORTH, *Advanced Practice Paramedic and Pathway Development Manager, North East Ambulance Service*

JAQUI LINDRIDGE, *Consultant Paramedic, London Ambulance Service*

SAFEGUARDING

SARAH THOMPSON, *Nurse, Head of Safeguarding and Staying Well Service, Designated Officer for Allegations, South Western Ambulance Service*

NIKKI HARVEY, *Nurse and Head of Safeguarding, Welsh Ambulance Service*

SAM THOMPSON, *Forensic Paramedic, Kent Police and Senior Lecturer, St George's, University of London*

SIMON CHASE, *Paramedic, Safeguarding Lead and Freedom to Speak Up Guardian, East of England Ambulance Service*

JANE MITCHELL, *Paramedic and Safeguarding Lead, South East Coast Ambulance Service*

ALAN TAYLOR, *Paramedic and Head of Safeguarding, London Ambulance Service*

SEPSIS

BARRY MURPHY-JONES, *Paramedic, Clinical Watch Manager/Clinical Audit Facilitator, London Ambulance Service*

MIKE SMYTH, *Paramedic, NIHR Clinical Doctoral Research Fellow, University of Warwick*

JAMES WENMAN, *Consultant Paramedic, South Western Ambulance Service*

GRAHAM MCCLELLAND, *Research Paramedic, North East Ambulance Service*

Guideline Developers and Contributors

DR SIMON STOCKLEY, *GP, The Royal College of General Practitioners, JRCALC member*

PAUL KELLY, *Paramedic, Scottish Ambulance Service*

DR MATTHEW INADA-KIM, *Consultant Acute Physician, Hampshire Hospitals, National Clinical Advisor Sepsis, Sepsis Lead for the National Patient Safety Collaborative*

TRACY NICHOLLS, *Paramedic, Head of Clinical Quality, East of England Ambulance Service*

TRAUMA

CHERYLENE CAMPS, *Paramedic, Duty Operations Manager, East Midlands Ambulance Service*

PROFESSOR SIR KEITH PORTER, *Professor of Clinical Traumatology, University Hospitals Birmingham, JRCALC member, Royal College of Surgeons Edinburgh*

DR COLVILLE LAIRD, *GP, JRCALC member, Royal College of Surgeons Edinburgh*

PAIN MANAGEMENT

DR ED ENGLAND, *Medicines and Research Manager, South Central Ambulance Service*

MARTIN PARKINSON, *Paramedic, Yorkshire Ambulance Service*

DR SHYAM BALASUBRAMANIAN, *Consultant in Pain Medicine and Anaesthesia, University Hospitals Coventry*

CONTRIBUTORS

RICHARD BERRY, *Specialist Paramedic, South Central Ambulance Service*

ALICE BRETON, *Education and Research Development Lead, Royal College of Surgeons Edinburgh*

MARK MILLINS, *Associate Director Paramedic Practice, Yorkshire Ambulance Service*

MENAI OWEN-JONES, *Chief Executive Officer, The Pituitary Foundation*

RICHARD PILBERY, *Research Paramedic, Yorkshire Ambulance Service*

PROFESSOR JOHN WASS, *Endocrinologist, Oxford University Hospitals*

KATHERINE WHITE, *Chair, Addison's Disease Self Help Group*

KEVIN WEBB, *Head of Clinical Audit & Effectiveness, Welsh Ambulance Service*

DAVE WHITMORE, *Paramedic and Clinical Advisor, London Ambulance Service*

CHARLES L TILL, *Senior Lecturer in Paramedic Science, Coventry University*

Guideline Development Methodology

The methodology used by JRCALC (Joint Royal Colleges Ambulance Liaison Committee) to develop the UK Ambulance Services Clinical Practice Guidelines is designed to comply with the criteria used by the AGREE II (Appraisal of Guidelines for Research and Evaluation in Europe) instrument. This process is a leading academic tool to identify good quality guidelines: http://www.agreetrust.org/

The purpose of the AGREE II, is to provide a framework to:

- assess the quality of guidelines
- provide a methodological strategy for the development of guidelines
- inform what information and how information ought to be reported in guidelines.

By adopting these principles, guidelines are developed that support safe decision making and high quality patient care.

Guideline Selection

JRCALC, NASMeD (National Ambulance Service Medical Directors) and the ALPG (Ambulance Lead Paramedic Group) will advise on those clinical guidelines which need updating and those clinical conditions which need a new guideline developing. These are then prioritised and assessed with regard to urgency and risk. Clinical topics can be identified through a variety of means including the monitoring of serious incidents within individual UK Ambulance Service Trusts, preventing future death directives issued by coroners and national service reconfiguration e.g. the move to major trauma centres and networks. In addition JRCALC provide extensive clinical expertise and advice on potential new developments to ensure that the guidelines capture latest best practice and future innovations.

Feedback is welcome via JRCALC@AACE.org

Editorial Independence

No external funding has been received for the development of these guidelines and no competing or conflicting interests have been declared by those involved in their development.

Citing the JRCALC Guidelines

The JRCALC Guidelines are cited as:

Joint Royal Colleges Ambulance Liaison Committee, Association of Ambulance Chief Executives (2019) JRCALC Clinical Guidelines 2019. Bridgwater: Class Professional Publishing.

Update Analysis – 'What's changed?'

Note: This table details updates to guidelines made since the 2016 Reference Edition and 2017 Supplementary Guidelines were published.

Note: A number of additional guidelines have had minor changes, relating to consistency and assessment and management tables.

SECTION 1	
General Guidance	
Staff Health and Wellbeing	This guideline has been updated with sources of help and signposting included, and new details on spotting the signs of reduced mental wellness.
Duty of Care	This new guideline covers health and safety, the tort of negligence and the right to life.
Patient Confidentiality	This guideline has been updated with reference to the Data Protection Act 2018 (DPA).
Pain Management in Children	Reference to topical analgesia and tetracaine has been removed.
End of Life Care	We have revised the guideline and made a number of areas clearer with more detail and explanation. ● We mention ReSPECT (Recommended Summary Plan for Emergency Care and Treatment), which has been adopted in a number of areas across the UK. ● There is emphasis placed on shared decision making, and particularly for administering end of life medications. ● There is a new section on recognising patients that may be in the last year of life. ● There is emphasis on liaison with palliative care/nursing teams in line with local pathways, particularly if 'anticipatory' or 'just in case' medicines are prescribed and available. ● There is detail about opioid administration in the last hours of life. ● There is a new section on Naloxone use in end of life care. ● There is new information about transdermal patches and syringe drivers, oxygen considerations and use of fans for breathlessness. ● Finally, it highlights the importance of staff wellbeing as dealing with end of life care can be distressing. (See new monograph for morphine for managing pain in end of life care.)

SECTION 2	
Resuscitation	**This is a fully revised and updated section.**
	● It includes pathophysiology, mechanisms of forward blood flow, CPR-induced consciousness, use of CPR feedback devices and checklists, human factors, the team leader approach to ALS and cardiac arrest downloads. BLS for adults and children has been revised for solo ambulance responders. Foreign body airway obstruction for adult and child has been combined. Special circumstances in cardiac arrest has been updated. ● In advanced life support, more practical ambulance and pre-hospital specific guidance is included, as well as revised guidance on when to stop ALS in cases of 'persistent and continuous asystole for 20 minutes'. ● Principles of defibrillation, fine VF, AED versus manual mode, defibrillator pads, mechanical chest compression devices, use of Naloxone for opiates as a cause of arrest, and bariatric patients are covered.
Emergency Tracheostomy and Laryngectomy	New guidance and management algorithms for confirming tracheostomy patency, emergency management, specific types of equipment used with photographs, suction and oxygen.

Update Analysis – 'What's changed?'

SECTION 3	
Medical Emergencies	**The assessment and management tables have been revised to improve consistency. NEWS2 is included.**
Medical Emergencies in Adults and Children	Revised and improved clinical assessment and management tables.
Acute Coronary Syndrome	This revised guideline includes a new section on the 12-lead ECG.
Abdominal Pain	New common causes have been added and the assessment and management table has been revised.
Allergic Reactions Including Anaphylaxis	The adult and child guidelines have been brought together with new details on the development of symptoms and the management of mild presentations.
Altered Level of Consciousness	Inclusion of NICE red flags and management guidance.
Asthma	The adult and child guidelines have been brought together with new details on personal plans, prednisolone where it is available, and avoiding over ventilation.
Chronic Obstructive Pulmonary Disease	Inclusion of BTS guidance, alert cards, classifications and community management included.
Convulsions in Adults	Fully revised guideline. ● Features of psychogenic non-epileptic seizures (PNES) are described. ● A new section relates to driving. ● New assessment and management tables for ongoing/recurrent seizures and seizures that have stopped. ● Guidance on conveyance decisions. ● Revised treatment algorithm.
Dyspnoea	This update includes more reference to causes with links to other guidelines and better alignment of the management steps. End of life is covered as is reference to the MRC dyspnoea scale.
Febrile Illness in Children	Revised guideline. ● 'Major' and 'minor' illness described. ● Signs and symptoms of specific diseases added. ● Red flags added. ● Points around antipyretics and antibiotics added.
Gastrointestinal Bleeding	TXA is not indicated for gastrointestinal bleeding.
Glycaemic Emergencies in Adults and Children	Adult and child guidelines have been merged. ● New guidance on blood glucose monitors, ketone meters, sick day rules, insulin pumps, driving, impaired awareness, conveyance guidance, mild/moderate hypoglycaemia management have been updated. ● Hyperosmolar hyperglycaemic state (HHS) is detailed.
Headache	A revised and updated guideline. ● Red flags have been revised. ● Types of headache have been added including migraine, cluster, tension and medication overuse headaches, subarachnoid haemorrhage and a detailed management section.
Heart Failure	A revised and updated guideline. ● The indication to give salbutamol for LVF has been removed and the indication for furosemide amended. ● For GTN the systolic blood pressure needs to be 110 mmHg to administer GTN and a new indication to administer for patients with suspected cocaine toxicity presenting with chest pain has been added to bring this in line with the overdose guideline.

Update Analysis – 'What's changed?'

Hyperventilation Syndrome	Revised guideline. ● Differential diagnosis features and signs and symptoms table added.
Hypothermia	This guideline has been updated and aligned to the resuscitation update.
Immersion and Drowning	Updated in line with the resuscitation section.
Management and Resuscitation of Patients with Left Ventricular Assist Devices (LVADs)	A new guideline. ● Detailed diagrams and management algorithms are included.
Meningococcal Meningitis and Septicaemia	This guideline has been updated. ● Assessment and management table and specific clinical features and details about the rash have been added. ● Clarity is added on the administration of benzylpenicillin.
Mental Health Presentation: Crisis, Distress and Disordered Behaviour.	A revised guideline. ● Key assessment skills, communication tips and types of questions to ask, new traffic light tools for common presentations, addition of dementia, pregnancy and mental health, reference to safe-holding.
Respiratory Illness in Children	Revised guideline. ● More information on conveyance/referral pathways/management in the community.
Sickle Cell Crisis	Revised assessment and management table. ● NICE appropriate management pathways are added and there is an update to the tables.
Sepsis	New guideline as part of supplementary guidelines 2017. ● Updated with NEWS2.
Stroke/Transient Ischaemic Attack	This is a revised guideline with the inclusion of childhood stroke and amended signs and symptoms.
Non-traumatic Chest Pain/Discomfort	Revised guideline. ● Features of aneurysm-type pain added. ● Further clarity is added on symptom descriptions. ● An updated management table is included.
Overdose and Poisoning in Adults and Children	A fully updated and revised guideline. Adult and child guidelines merged. ● Inclusion of more details on carbon monoxide poisoning, new signs and symptoms table. ● Revised assessment and management table. ● Revised specific substance management table. ● Inclusion of detail around assessment and management of novel psychoactive substances. ● Awareness and guidance around ingestion of foreign bodies including button battery ingestion. ● Guidance on patients that may not need conveyance to hospital. ● References to use of TOXBASE as per local procedures. ● Naloxone – note very high dose for children, as per BNF, notes around use of Naloxone in end of life care, amended indications. ● Activated charcoal – we are aware that many services are now using activated charcoal, therefore the new monograph has been developed.
Paediatric Gastroenteritis	A traffic light assessment table for clinical dehydration and shock has been added and a decision support tool regarding management in the community.

Update Analysis – 'What's changed?'

SECTION 4	
Trauma	**Revisions made in Supplementary Guidelines 2017.**
Trauma Emergencies in Adults – Overview	Updated to cover haemorrhage from renal dialysis arteriovenous graft and fistulas included.
Head Injury	Revised guideline. ● Includes guidance for mild to moderate head injury, new conveyance decision tool. ● Removal of midazolam for traumatic brain injury – for enhanced care team use only.
Limb Trauma	Additional information on open fractures and re-alignment is included.
Burns and Scalds	The adult and child guidelines have been merged. ● NICE Red Flags are added, as is information on NARU Chemical Burns.

SECTION 5	
Maternity	
Birth Imminent	The description of how to birth the baby's head in the case of malpresentation has changed to: **Head.** If the head does not deliver in the semi-recumbent position (with the baby's body supported on your forearm), *apply pressure to the back of the baby's head with the fingers of your other hand*, to aid flexion while the head delivers. Ectopic pregnancy changes.
Haemorrhage During Pregnancy (including Miscarriage and Ectopic Pregnancy)	There have been some minor amendments to the description of the management of ectopic pregnancy.
Pregnancy-induced Hypertension (including Eclampsia)	'Titrated against effect' removed with reference to diazepam.

SECTION 6	
Special Situations	**This section has been fully reviewed and revised and new guidance re-named: Major, Complex and High-risk incidents. The CBRN medicines ciprofloxacin, dicobalt edetate, doxycycline, obidoxime chloride, potassium iodate, pralidoxime mesylate have been removed.**
Police Incapacitants	The incapacitating agent's guideline has been renamed Police Incapacitants and has been revised.
Atropine	Revised monograph.
Duodote®	New monograph.

Update Analysis – 'What's changed?'

SECTION 7	
Medicines	**Updates include changes to monographs to update them in line with new JRCALC guidance and with the current BNF.** **Reference to the medicines reteplase and tetracaine have been removed.**
Activated Charcoal	A new JRCALC monograph on this medicine is published, in line with the revised overdose and poisoning guideline.
Adrenaline	This has been split into two separate monographs: 1 mg in 1 ml (1 in 1,000) and 1 mg in 10 ml (1 in 10,000). This is due to reported incidents of administration of the wrong route/strength.
Amiodarone	This medicine should not be administered for the birth age group. It has been removed from the birth Page for Age.
Atropine Sulfate	More detail has been added to presentation.
Benzylpenicillin	Concentrations have been updated.
Chlorphenamine	Dosages have been updated. • Dosages for 1 month, 3 months, 6 months and 9 months are now included.
Dexamethasone	Presentations have been updated. • An oral tablet and an oral solution are listed. Dosages have been updated.
Diazepam	Updated in line with adult convulsions update. Addition of indication for symptomatic cocaine toxicity.
Glucose 10%, Glucose 40% and Glucagon	Medicines monographs have been updated in line with glycaemic emergencies guideline.
GTN, Furosemide and Salbutamol	Amended in line with the revised heart failure and overdose guideline. • The indication to give salbutamol for LVF has been removed and the indication for furosemide amended. • For GTN the systolic blood pressure needs to be 110 mmHg to administer GTN for acute heart failure, and a new indication to administer for patients with suspected cocaine toxicity presenting with chest pain has been added to bring this in line with the overdose guideline.
Ibuprofen	Revised monograph, more cautions and contraindications added.
Midazolam	The patient's own buccal midazolam monograph has been merged with the midazolam monograph. The indication for sedation in combative head injury patients has been removed (this is for enhanced care teams only).
Morphine Sulfate for the Management of Pain in Adults at the End of Life	We have created a new separate monograph specifically for morphine administration for pain management in end of life patients with emphasis that the subcutaneous route is the preferred route for administration.
Naloxone	Revised monograph updated in line with the overdose and poisoning guideline. • Dosages for younger children have increased. • Dosage intervals for younger children IV/IO have reduced from 3 minutes to 1 minute. • Indication for use in cardiac arrest where opioids are the likely cause of arrest.
Tranexamic Acid	Brought in line with the development of an England Patient Group Direction.
Page for Age	Dosages are updated according to the medicines guidelines.

List of Abbreviations

The glossary of terms listed below is designed to assist reading ease and is **NOT** provided as a list of short-hand terms. The Joint Royal Colleges Ambulance Liaison Committee reminds the user that abbreviations are not to be used in any clinical documentation.

Term	
AAA	Abdominal Aortic Aneurysm
ABCDE	**A** – Airway
	B – Breathing
	C – Circulation
	D – Disability
	E – Exposure and environment
ABD	Acute behavioural disorder
AC	Alternating Current
ACPO	Association of Chief Police Officers
ACS	Acute Coronary Syndrome
ADHD	Attention Deficit Hyperactivity Disorder
ADRT	Advance Decision to Refuse Treatment
AED	Automated External Defibrillation
AHF	Acute Heart Failure
ALoC	Altered level of consciousness
ALS	Advanced Life Support
AMH	Adult Mental Health Services
AMHP	Approved Mental Health Professional
APC	Antero-Posterior Compression
APGAR	**A** – Appearance
	P – Pulse rate
	G – Grimace or response to stimulation
	A – Activity or muscle tone
	R – Respiration
ARDS	Acute Respiratory Distress Syndrome
ATMIST	**A** – Age
	T – Time of incident
	M – Mechanism
	I – Injuries
	S – Signs and symptoms
	T – Treatment given / immediate needs
ATP	Anti-Tachycardia Pacing
AV	Atrioventricular
AVPU	**A** – Alert
	V – Responds to voice
	P – Responds to pain
	U – Unresponsive

Term	
BBB	Bundle branch block
bd	Twice daily
BG	Blood Glucose
BIA	Best Interest Assessors
BiPAP	Bilevel Positive Pressure Ventilation
BLS	Basic Life Support
BM	Stick Measures blood sugar
BMI	Body mass index
BP	Blood Pressure
bpm	Beats per minute
BR	Breech
BSA	Body Surface Area
BTCS	Bilateral Tonic-Clonic Seizures
BTS	British Thoracic Society
BVM	Bag-Valve-Mask
BMV	Bag-mask ventilation
<C>ABCDE	**<C>** – Catastrophic haemorrhage
	A – Airway
	B – Breathing
	C – Circulation
	D – Disability
	E – Exposure and environment
CA	Cancer
CAMHS	Child and Adolescent Mental Health Services
CBRNE	Chemical, Biological, Radiological, Nuclear and Explosive
CBT	Cognitive Behavioural Therapy
CCF	Congestive cardiac failure
CCS	Central Cord Syndrome
CD	Controlled Drug
CES	Cauda Equina Syndrome
CEW	Controlled Electrical Weapon
CFR	Community first responder
CHD	Coronary Heart Disease
CHF	Congestive Heart Failure
CMHT	Community Mental Health Team
CMI	Combined Mechanical Injury
CNS	Central Nervous System
CO	Carbon monoxide
CO_2	Carbon dioxide

List of Abbreviations

Term	
COP	Code of Practice
COPD	Chronic Obstructive Pulmonary Disease
CPAP	Continuous Positive Airway Pressure
CPN	Community Psychiatric Nurse
CPP	Cerebral Perfusion Pressure
CPP	Coronary perfusion pressure
CPR	Cardiopulmonary Resuscitation
CPR-IC	CPR-induced consciousness
CRT	Capillary Refill Test
CRT	Cardiac Resynchronisation Therapy
CSA	Child Sexual Abuse
CSE	Child Sexual Exploitation
CSE	Convulsive status epilepticus
CT	Computerised Tomography
CVA	Cerebo Vascular Accident
DBS	Disclosure and Barring Service
DC	Direct Current
DIC	Disseminated Intravascular Coagulation
DKA	Diabetic Ketoacidosis
DM	Diabetes Mellitus
DNA	Deoxyribonucleic Acid
DNACPR	Do Not Attempt Cardio-Pulmonary Resuscitation
DoLS	Deprivation of Liberty Safeguards
DPA	Data Protection Act
DVT	Deep Vein Thrombosis
E	Ecstasy
EC	Enteric Coated
ECG	Electrocardiograph
ECT	Electro-convulsive therapy
ECMO	ECMO Extra-corporeal membrane oxygenation
ED	Emergency Department
EDD	Estimated Date of Delivery
EF	Ejection fraction
EMS	Emergency Medical Services
EOC	Emergency Operations Centre
ERC	European Resuscitation Council
ESC	European Society of Cardiology
ET	Endotracheal
ETA	Expected Time of Arrival
$EtCO_2$	Exhaled (end-tidal) carbon dioxide

Term	
EUPD	Emotionally unstable personality disorder
FAST	**F** – Face **A** – Arms **S** – Speech **T** – Test
FBAO	Foreign Body Airway Obstruction
FC	Febrile Convulsions
FEV	Forced Expiratory Volume
FGM	Female genital mutilation
FLACC	**F** – Face **L** – Legs **A** – Activity **C** – Cry **C** – Consolability
FII	Fabricated or Induced Illness
FGM	Female Genital Mutilation
FVC	Forced Vital Capacity
g	Grams
GBS	Group B Strep Infection
GCS	Glasgow Coma Scale
GDPR	General Data Protection Regulations 2018
GI	Gastrointestinal
GP	General Practitioner
GTN	Glyceryl Trinitrate
GUM	Genito-urinary medicine
HART	Hazardous Area Response Team
HCP	Healthcare Professional
HFpEF	Heart failure with preserved ejection fraction
HFrEF	Heart failure with reduced ejection fraction
HIV	Human Immunodeficiency Virus
HME	Heat moisture exchanger
HPV	Human papillomavirus
HNSCC	Head and neck squamous cell carcinoma
HR	Heart Rate
HSE	Health and Safety Executive
HVS	Hyperventilation Syndrome
IA	Impaired awareness
IBS	Irritable Bowel Syndrome
ICD	International Classification of Diseases

List of Abbreviations

Term	
ICD	Implantable Cardioverter Defibrillator
ICE	Infant Cooling Evaluation
ICP	Intracranial Pressure
IGIV	Immunoglobulin Intravenous
IHD	Ischemic Heart Disease
ILCOR	International Liaison Committee on Resuscitation
IM	Intramuscular
IMCA	Independent Mental Capacity Advocates
IO	Intraosseous
IPAP	**I** – Intent **P** – Plans **A** – Actions **P** – Protection
IQ	Intelligence Quotient
ISVA	Independent Sexual Violence Adviser
ITD	Impedance threshold device
ITU	Intensive Care Unit
IV	Intravenous
IVC	Inferior Vena Cava
J	Joule
JESIP	Joint Emergency Services Interoperability Programme
JRCALC	Joint Royal Colleges Ambulance Liaison Committee
JVP	Jugular Venous Pressure
kg	Kilogram
kPa	Kilopascal
kV	Kilovolt
LBBB	Left Bundle Branch Block
LC	Lateral Compression
LMA	Laryngeal Mask Airway
LMP	Last Menstrual Period
LOC	Level of Consciousness
LPA	Lasting Power of Attorney
LSD	Lysergic Acid Diethylamide
LVAD	Left ventricular assist device
LVF	Left Ventricular Failure
LVSD	Left ventricular systolic dysfunction
MAOI	Monoamine Oxidase Inhibitor antidepressant
MAPPA	Multi-Agency Public Protection Arrangements
MAP	Mean Arterial Pressure

Term	
MBRRACE	Mothers and Babies: Reducing Risk through Audits and Confidential Enquiries
MCA	Mental Capacity Act
mcg	Microgram
mCPR	Mechanical chest compression devices
MDMA	Methylene Dioxymethamphetamine
MECC	Making Every Contact Count
mg	Milligram
MH	Mental Health
MHA	Mental Health Act
MHSOP	Mental Health Services for Older People
MI	Myocardial Infarction
MINAP	Myocardial Ischaemia National Audit Project
ml	Millilitre
mmHG	Millimetres of Mercury
mmol	Millimoles
mmol/l	Millimoles per Litre
MOI	Mechanisms of Injury
MSC	**M** – Motor **S** – Sensation **C** – Circulation
msec	Millisecond
MTC	Major Triage Centre
NARU	National Ambulance Resilience Unit
Neb	Nebulisation
NEET	Not in Education, Employment or Training
NEWS	National Early Warning Score
NG	Nasogastric
NHS	National Health Service
NICE	National Institute for Health and Care Excellence
NiPPV	Non-invasive Positive Pressure Ventilation
NLS	Newborn Life Support
NPA	Nasopharyngeal airway
NPIS	National Poisons Information Service
NSAID	Non-Steroidal Anti-inflammatory Drug
NSTEMI	Non-ST Segment Elevation Myocardial Infarction
O_2	Oxygen

List of Abbreviations

Term	
OHCA	Out of Hospital Cardiac Arrest
OOH	Out of Hours
OPA	Oropharyngeal Airway
ORS	Oral Rehydration Salt
P	Parity
PaO_2	Partial pressure of oxygen
PCO_2	Measure of the Partial Pressure of Carbon dioxide
PE	Pulmonary Embolism
PEaRL	Pupils Equal and Reacting to Light
PEA	Pulseless Electrical Activity
PEF	Peak Expiratory Flow
PEFR	Peak Expiratory Flow Rate
PHECG	Pre-hospital 12-lead electrocardiogram
PHTLS	Pre-hospital Trauma Life Support
PIH	Pregnancy Induced Hypertension
PNES	Psychogenic non-epileptic seizures
POM	Prescription Only Medicine
PPCI	Primary Percutaneous Coronary Intervention
PPE	Personal Protective Equipment
PPH	Post-Partum Haemorrhage
pr	Per Rectum
PTSD	Post-traumatic Stress Disorder
PreSep	Prehospital Early Sepsis Detection
PRESS	Prehospital Recognition of Severe Sepsis
PSM	Patient Specific Medication
PSP	Patient specific protocol
prn	When required medication
PV	Per Vaginam
pVT	Pulseless ventricular tachycardia
RAID	Rapid Assessment, Interface and Discharge
RBBB	Right bundle branch block
RCT	Randomised Controlled Trial
ReSPECT	Recommended Summary Plan for Emergency Care and Treatment
ROLE	Recognition Of Life Extinct
ROSC	Return of Spontaneous Circulation
RR	Respiratory Rate
RSV	Respiratory Syncytial Virus
RTC	Road Traffic Collision
RVF	Right Ventricular Failure
RVP	Rendezvous Point(s)

Term	
SAD	Supraglottic Airway Device
SARC	Sexual Assault Referral Centre
SaO_2	Oxygen Saturation Of Arterial Blood
SBAR	**S** – Situation **B** – Situation **A** – Assessment **R** – Recommendation
SBI	Serious Bacterial Infection
SBP	Systolic Blood Pressure
SC	Subcutaneous
SCENE	**S** – Safety **C** – Cause including MOI **E** – Environment **N** – Number of patients **E** – Extra resources needed
SCI	Spinal Cord Injury
SGA	Supraglottic airway
SOB	Shortness of breath
SOBOE	Shortness of breath on exertion
SOCRATES	**S** – Site **O** – Onset **C** – Character **R** – Radiation **A** – Associated symptoms **T** – Time **E** – Exacerbation **S** – Severity
SOP	Standard operating procedure
SORT	Special Operations Response Team
SpO_2	Oxygen Saturation Measured With Pulse Oximeter
SSRIs	Selective Serotonin Re-Uptake Inhibitors
STEMI	ST Segment Elevation Myocardial Infarction
STI	Sexually transmitted infections
SUDEP	Sudden Unexpected Death in Epilepsy
SUDI	Sudden Unexpected Death in Infants
SUDICA	Sudden Unexpected Death in Infants, Children and Adolescents
SVT	Supraventricular Tachycardia
T1DM	Type 1 diabetes mellitus
TARN	Trauma Audit Research Network
TBI	Traumatic Brain injury
TBSA	Total Body Surface Area

List of Abbreviations

Term	
TEP	Tracheoesophageal Puncture
TIA	Transient Ischaemic Attack
TLoC	Transient loss of consciousness
TOBY	Total Body Hypothermia for Neonatal Encephalopathy
URTI	Upper Respiratory Tract Infection
UTI	Urinary Tract Infection
VF	Ventricular Fibrillation
VS	Vertical Shear
VT	Ventricular Tachycardia
VTE	Venous Thromboembolism
WHO	World Health Organisation

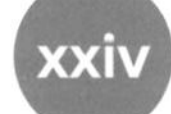

1

General Guidance

Staff Health and Wellbeing

1. Introduction

- The importance of good mental health and wellbeing cannot be underestimated. The World Health Organization defines good mental health as: 'a state of wellbeing in which every individual realizes his or her own potential, can cope with the normal stresses of life, can work productively and fruitfully and is able to make a contribution to her or his community.'[1]
- However, there is evidence to suggest that, for those who work in the emergency services, the risk of experiencing a mental health issue is greater than average.[2] The number and type of significant tragedies and events in the UK in recent years combined with the ever-increasing workload placed upon emergency services has highlighted the difficulties often experienced by staff. As a result, the subject has been looked at from a fresh perspective with many new and useful resources becoming available.
- The blue light scoping survey undertaken by Mind – the mental health charity – suggested that there are a number of areas that are directly attributable to a change in the mental wellbeing of ambulance service workers.[3] Similarly, it highlighted some worrying trends:
  - Emergency service staff are twice as likely to identify work as the cause of their mental health issue, with over 85% of staff experiencing stress, low mood, anxiety or depression at some point of their career.
  - Over 50% of staff are unaware of services they can access to help them with their mental health needs.
  - Despite the Equality Act (2010) offering protection, only 12% would approach a line manager for help and almost 80% said they would never speak to their HR departments.
- But this need not be the case and there is a wealth of resources at hand. The most common issues around ambulance staff mental wellbeing are centred upon several key themes.[3]

2. Anxiety

- Anxiety is a perfectly normal reaction to a stressful situation and is linked closely to the fight or flight response. Anxiety disorders can take several different forms, the most common of which is generalised anxiety disorder and is widely experienced.
- The most commonly experienced symptoms are very much in line with those of PTSD:[3,4]
  - palpitations
  - shortness of breath
  - diarrhoea
  - nausea.
- Once the trigger for the symptoms of anxiety stop, you would expect the anxiety to reduce. However, if the anxiety starts to influence our lives too greatly, we must look for ways to deal with it effectively.

3. Post-traumatic Stress Disorder (PTSD)

- Post-traumatic stress disorder (PTSD) can affect anyone and is closely associated with very intense situations in which someone experiences life-threatening or life-changing events, especially those that involve witnessing death and dying.[5]
- These types of situation are not uncommon for ambulance clinicians, and recognising that you may have been negatively influenced by a single event or accumulation of events should never be considered a weakness. Research points toward the severity, intensity and number of exposures to stressful experiences as being the key reason someone may suffer from PTSD and not because of an individual's personality traits.[6]
- Common symptoms include:
  - flashbacks or reliving traumatic incidents
  - nightmares
  - feeling constantly on edge
  - a numbing of emotions
  - an unwillingness to talk about or visit memories and reminders of an event.
- Other symptoms can include:
  - pain
  - nausea
  - diarrhoea
  - choosing to withdraw and becoming socially isolated
  - increased drug and alcohol use
  - depression
  - low mood
  - anxiety
  - a strong sense of guilt.[7]

4. Low Mood and Depression

- It is estimated one in five people in the UK suffer from depression at some point throughout their lives, making depression amongst the most common of disorders.[8]
- A sense of hopelessness, sadness, loss, and reduced interest in your normal life and activities is felt over an extended period. It can affect appetite, sleep, concentration, self-worth and relationships. At its worst it can lead to feelings and thoughts of self-harm and suicide.[9]
- There are a range of services such as talking therapies, self-help and medication which are available to anyone experiencing symptoms and can be accessed quickly and easily.

5. Spotting the Signs

- The potential for reduced mental wellness is greater throughout the emergency services in all roles. As clinicians we often assist the people we encounter by finding the most appropriate source of help for their current situation. Recognising a need in yourself or a colleague is difficult, but research suggests that ambulance personnel are far more likely to confide in each other rather than their own GP.[3]
- Even when we do recognise the need for help, fear of discrimination and stigma still presents a significant concern for many, despite the protection afforded by the 2010 Equality Act.
- Anyone can experience any number of mental health issues at any point in their lives regardless of their history or circumstance. The cause and nature of any individual's issues can be as unique as the individual and can be cumulative in nature, building over time and for any number and combination of reasons.
- It is not unusual in today's workplace for individuals to see concentrating upon work and careers as vital to maintaining professionalism; however, achieving a healthy work–life balance can have a very positive influence upon the stress and productivity experienced by any individual.[10]
- There is a wealth of independent, confidential and high-quality sources of help. Accessing help in a timely manner can have a significant impact upon the speed and quality of an individual's recovery. The benefits of spending time on relationships outside of work, family, hobbies and interests, volunteering, exercising and continued learning all have a role to play in maintaining and improving wellbeing. This in turn can have benefits not only to ourselves, but also to the many people we encounter in our roles.

6. Sources of Help and Signposting

- Ambulance Hub on NHS Employers website – Head First tool. Available from: https://www.nhsemployers.org/headfirst
- HR/work-related sources
- College of paramedics. Available from: https://www.collegeofparamedics.co.uk
- MIND Blue light. Available from: https://www.mind.org.uk/news-campaigns/campaigns/bluelight/
- TASC. Available from: http://www.theasc.org.uk/
- Samaritans. Available from: https://www.samaritans.org/
- CALM. Available from: https://www.calm.com/
- Step change. Available from: https://www.stepchange.org/
- Alcoholics Anonymous (AA). Available from: https://www.alcoholics-anonymous.org.uk/
- TRiM. Available from http://www.marchonstress.com/page/p/trim
- Education and Training Committee (ETC). Available from: https://www.hcpc-uk.org/news-and-events/news/2018/hcpc-education-and-training-committee-to-consider-proposed-changes-to-the-threshold-level-of-qualification-for-paramedics/

Bibliography

1. World Health Organization. *Mental health: a state of wellbeing*. 2014. Available from: https://www.who.int/features/factfiles/mental_health/en/
2. Fjeldheim CB, Nöthling J, Pretorius K, Basson M, Ganasen K, Heneke R, Cloete KJ, Seedat S. Trauma exposure, post-traumatic stress disorder and the effect of explanatory variables in paramedic trainees. *BMC Emergency Medicine* 2014, 14: 11. Available from: https://www.ncbi.nlm.nih.gov/pubmed/24755358
3. Mind. *Blue Light Scoping Survey*. 2015. Available from: https://www.mind.org.uk/media/4627950/scoping-survey.pdf
4. Rethink Mental Illness. *What are anxiety disorders*? 2018. Available from: https://www.rethink.org/diagnosis-treatment/conditions/anxiety-disorders/about
5. Royal College of Psychiatrists. *Post-traumatic stress disorder*. 2015. Available from: https://www.rcpsych.ac.uk/healthadvice/problemsanddisorders/posttraumaticstressdisorder.aspx
6. Javidi H and Yadollahie M. Post-traumatic stress disorder. *International Journal of Occupational and Environmental Medicine* [online] 2012, 3(1). Available from: http://theijoem.com/ijoem/index.php/ijoem/article/view/127/247
7. National Health Service. *Post-traumatic stress disorder (PTSD)*. 2015. Available from: https://www.nhs.uk/conditions/post-traumatic-stress-disorder-ptsd/symptoms/
8. Royal College of Psychiatrists. *Depression: key facts*. 2014. Available from: https://www.rcpsych.ac.uk/healthadvice/problemsanddisorders/depressionkeyfacts.aspx
9. World Health Organization. *Depression: let's talk*. 2018. Available from: https://www.who.int/mental_health/management/depression/en/
10. Burn SM. *How's your work-life balance? The importance of work-life balance and how to achieve it*. 2015. Available from: https://www.psychologytoday.com/us/blog/presence-mind/201509/hows-your-work-life-balance

Consent in Pre-hospital Care

- The laws and guidance that relate to consent to assessment, treatment, care and other interventions are different in the countries and/or jurisdictions that constitute the United Kingdom.
- Therefore, these guidelines do not offer guidance on obtaining consent beyond the general advice in this statement; the Joint Royal Colleges Ambulance Liaison Committee (JRCALC) advises strongly that readers should seek specific guidance on consent from their ambulance services, Trusts or other relevant employers.
- JRCALC advises that obtaining consent in ways that are lawful in the jurisdiction in which each reader works is fundamental to meeting patients' legal and ethical rights in determining what happens to them and to their own bodies. Therefore, it is important to ensure that you always act in the patient's best interest and that you have legally valid consent to conduct assessments, treatments or interventions, and provide care.
- Consent must be obtained from each patient or their legally valid representative (defined according to the law in the relevant country or jurisdiction) prior to conducting examinations or treatment, or providing care.
- Ensure that you provide patients with the appropriate information to enable them to comprehend the assessment, treatment or interventions being proposed. This means that in order for the patient to provide informed consent, they must be able to understand not only the assessment, treatment and interventions to be carried out, but also the consequences of such actions.
- In pre-hospital situations, it is not uncommon for patients to refuse assessment, care or treatment. Although patients may refuse, there may be, depending on the circumstances, continuing moral duties and legal responsibilities for ambulance clinicians to provide further intervention, particularly if life-threatening risk is involved. Again, ambulance clinicians are advised to obtain advice from their employers about circumstances of this nature so the actions they take are appropriate to the legal jurisdiction in which they are working.
- When communicating with other healthcare professionals, discussion should include information about the patient's ability to consent.

Duty of Care

1. Introduction

It is clear that ambulance clinicians have a duty to provide care to their patients but establishing exactly how that duty applies to various situations can be challenging.

The duty of care represents a moral, professional and legal obligation. The moral obligation to provide care is a matter of individual and social conscience. The professional obligation arises from a clinician's professional registration and organisational procedures or national practice guidelines such as these. The legal obligation arises from several sources which are explained further in this guideline.

It is particularly difficult for ambulance clinicians to discharge their duty of care correctly at incidents where patients need clinical interventions, but circumstances relating to the incident can expose clinicians to varying degrees of risk.

2. Application

The duty of care applies to ambulance clinicians and managers in two key ways:

1 Staff safety: the duty to keep yourself and your team safe.

2 Patient care: the duty to provide a reasonable standard of care to your patient.

The United Kingdom has three separate jurisdictions: England and Wales, Scotland, and Northern Ireland. The duty of care principles are broadly consistent throughout these regions of the UK. The legislation in this guideline applies to English law. Please ensure that you are fully aware of the law in your area of practice and differences if you work across borders.

The aide memoire depicted in Table 1.1 has been developed to assist you in applying the duty of care correctly.

TABLE 1.1 – Duty of Care Aide Memoire

Duty of Care Requirement		**Steps to Take**	**Explanation**
Duty of care to staff	Take all reasonable and practical steps to keep employees safe.	Perform approved activities and apply controls specified in procedures.	These are statutory duties under the *Health and Safety at Work Act 1974* and associated regulatory provisions. These steps will ensure you have a safe system of work.
		Ensure you are trained and competent to undertake the activity.	
		Ensure the minimum equipment mandated by procedures is available and used (including your PPE).	
Duty of care to the patient	Provide a reasonable standard of care without any unreasonable delay.	Undertake a risk assessment and determine the action you need to take as quickly as possible. Continually review the position and deliver care as soon as possible. If you need specialist support, make sure you request it as soon as possible.	This is an established duty at common law. It is a positive duty on the ambulance service to provide a reasonable standard of care without unreasonable delay. This duty is unique to the ambulance service. Police and fire services have duties to the public at large but their duty to individual patients is largely discretionary (*Kent v Griffith* [2001] QB 36).
Article 2 Right to Life	Take steps to protect people from harm which may lead to loss of life.	Balance the two duties set out above.	This is a qualified right. If the correct balance is achieved (duty of care to staff and duty of care to patients) this duty will be discharged. If the rescue is too dangerous for the responders, Article 2 positive duties can be avoided.

Duty of Care

TABLE 1.1 – Duty of Care Aide Memoire *(continued)*

Duty of Care Requirement		Steps to Take	Explanation
Risk assess the activity	Assess the risks for both staff and patients.	Undertake a dynamic risk assessment at the scene based on hazards and what you can do to mitigate them (your available controls). Regularly review the risk assessment.	If the activity is likely to result in death or serious injury to you or a member of your team despite the controls, do not commit. Statutory health and safety obligations provide justification for the delay in care.
Multi-agency Joint Doctrine	Contribute to the joint risk assessment as part of JESIP and ensure a common understanding of the risks.	For complex incidents involving a multi-agency response, ensure there is a joint risk assessment using the JESIP tools. Ensure the ambulance service duty of care is considered as part of this risk assessment.	If the risk of death or serious injury to you or your team can be mitigated by a safe system of work (making the likelihood low) you must avoid delay in committing and providing care or the ambulance service may face liability (Kent v Griffiths [2001] QB 36).

3. Health and Safety Duties

The Health and Safety at Work Act 1974 and associated regulations require ambulance clinicians to have a Safe System of Work. Ambulance services have a legal duty to implement and maintain safe systems of work for staff and volunteers who in turn have a legal duty to comply with these systems.

A safe system of work is usually achieved through:

- Effective procedures, including risk assessments and suitable controls.
- Competence.
- Fit for purpose equipment.

This means you should:

- Ensure you and your colleagues engage in approved activities which have controls to mitigate the risks.
- Ensure that you are competent to perform these activities, i.e. that you have received suitable training and your training is kept up to date.
- Ensure that you have the necessary equipment for that activity and the equipment you are using is fit for purpose and appropriately maintained. This includes personal protective equipment (PPE).

A safe system of work does not necessarily mean one which is completely free of risk. It is one where the risk is being appropriately managed. Given the nature of pre-hospital ambulance work, a level of risk will need to be accepted.

4. The Tort of Negligence

The emergency services do not generally owe a legal duty of care to individual members of the public except in certain, limited circumstances (Hill v Chief Constable of West Yorkshire [1989] AC 53 (HL).

The law will only recognise a breach in the duty by police or fire and rescue services if they have acted in a certain way in certain specific situations. However, the NHS ambulance service has an established legal duty to provide a reasonable standard of care to patients without unreasonable delay. This is a positive duty which engages from the point at which the ambulance service accepts the emergency call and agrees to attend (Kent v Griffiths [2001] QB 36).

A reasonable standard of care is clinical care that conforms to the minimum standards of the profession (Bolam v Friern Hospital Management Committee [1957] 2 All ER 118). These standards are set out in approved clinical practice guidelines, such as these JRCALC Guidelines, and standards set by relevant professional bodies.

Failure to discharge this duty could expose you or your organisation to a charge of clinical negligence.

5. Article 2 – The Right to Life

Article 2 of the Human Rights Act 1998 creates a positive duty on public sector organisations, including the ambulance service, to do all they reasonably can to protect those they know, or ought to know, are at real and immediate risk (Van Colle v CC of Hertfordshire [2007] EWCA Civ 325).

However, Article 2 is a qualified right rather than an absolute one. This means there may be occasions where it is justifiable not to act to save someone's life. For example, ambulance clinicians are not expected to risk sacrificing their own life to save a patient.

If you manage to effectively balance your two main duty of care obligations by putting a safe system of work in place and avoiding any unreasonable delay in providing care to patients, then you will invariably discharge your obligations under Article 2.

Duty of Care

KEY POINTS!

- **The duty of care requires you to achieve a careful balance. You must ensure you and your colleagues are safe. You must also be prepared to take some risk in order to deliver effective care to patients in the pre-hospital setting.**
- **To do this you must:**
  - **Have a safe system of work.**
  - **Avoid any unreasonable delays in providing emergency care to patients that require it.**

Patient Confidentiality

1. Introduction

Health professionals have a duty of confidentiality regarding patient information. They also have a priority, which is to ensure that all relevant information about their patients, their assessments, examinations and advice is recorded clearly and accurately, and passed to other staff whenever it is necessary for provision of ongoing care.

Sometimes, aspects of legislation relating to these issues appear to conflict with each other. This guideline provides a brief overview of the relevant legislation under the following headings:

- Patient Identifiable Information.
- Data Protection Act 2018 (DPA).
- General Data Protection Regulations 2018 (GDPR)
- NHS Policy.
- Protecting Patient Information.
- Patients' Rights of Access to Personal Health Records.
- Disclosure to Other Bodies and Organisations.
- Research.
- Consent.

2. Patient Identifiable Information

Patient Identifiable Information is any information that may be used to identify a patient directly or indirectly. It may include:

- Patient's name, address, postcode or date of birth.
- Any image or audio/digital recording of the patient.
- Any other data or information that has the potential, however remote, to identify a patient (e.g. rare diseases, drug regimes, statistical analysis of small groups, IP addresses or biometric data).
- Patients' record numbers.
- Combinations of any of the items here that may increase the risk of a breach of confidentiality, that include all verbal, written and electronic disclosure, whether formal or incidental.

3. Data Protection Act 2018

The main principles of the GDPR should be read in conjunction with this guideline. GDPR describes processes for obtaining, recording, holding, using and sharing information, and forms part of the data protection regime in the UK, together with the DPA 2018.

- Patients must be informed and give explicit consent to any sharing of their personal information.
- Only the minimum amount of data should be collected and used to achieve the agreed purpose.
- Information can only be retained for as long as it is needed to achieve its originally intended purpose.
- Strict rules apply to sharing information and with whom it may be shared.

4. NHS Policy

All NHS employees must be aware of and respect a patient's right to confidentiality and protect their personal information. A disciplinary offence may have been committed for any behaviour contrary to their organisation's policy or the *NHS Code of Practice: Confidentiality* (in Scotland, the *NHS COP on Protecting Patient Confidentiality*). Ambulance clinicians should be aware of how to gain access to training, support or information, which they may need, and be able to show that they are making every reasonable effort to comply with the relevant standards.

5. Protecting Patient Information

There are five essential steps that all ambulance clinicians should take to ensure that they comply with the relevant standards of confidentiality. They are listed below:

5.1 Record information given by, and about, patients concisely and accurately

- Inaccurate clinical records about patients may contain false information that has been created by, for example, omissions, errors, unfounded comments or speculation. This breaches DPA standards. It also brings the professional integrity of ambulance clinicians and their employing organisations into question. Any comments and opinions, whether verbal, written or electronic, must be justifiable and accurate.

5.2 Keep patient information physically secure

- Ambulance services have particular difficulties in ensuring that information is not shared accidentally with the public. Not only must patients be treated confidentially, but the information gained must not be disclosed to anyone else unless to do so genuinely promotes patient care. (Comments to the public must be guarded.) Information given to other clinicians when handing over patients' care should not be overheard or shared with people who are not directly involved in each patient's care. Patients' records, either electronic or written, must be protected against unwarranted viewing: thus, patients' clinical records must be shielded from the view of other people, stored securely after case closure, and only handed over to staff who are entrusted with ongoing care of particular patients or other authorised personnel who have legitimate reasons for possessing the information. Personal health data must be destroyed in an approved manner and according to each

SECTION 1 General Guidance

organisation's policies when they have served their function. Discussions of each patient must not disclose personal information unless there is genuine and provable health benefit.

- Leaders of healthcare and health information systems believe that electronic health information systems, which include computer-based patient records, can improve healthcare. Achieving this goal requires systems to be in place that: protect the privacy of individual persons and data about patients; provide appropriate access; and use data security measures that are adequate. Sound policies and practices relating to handling confidential information must be in place prior to deploying health information systems. Strong and enforceable policies on privacy and security of confidential and patient identifiable information must shape the development and implementation of these systems.

5.3 Follow guidance before disclosing any patient information

- It is not sufficient for ambulance clinicians to understand the basic principles of confidentiality alone. They must also understand and comply with their employing organisations' requirements for information-sharing. Similarly, it is the responsibility of each service to ensure that policies for data-sharing are produced, communicated, monitored, updated and reviewed. Each ambulance service will have a senior advisor available. There must be a Data Protection Officer, Information Governance Manager, and/or a Caldicott Guardian available to advise ambulance clinicians if they have any doubts about sharing information.

5.4 Conform to best practice

- All grades of ambulance clinicians come into contact with the public and other NHS clinicians. Any temptation for ambulance clinicians to share information unnecessarily with other people who are known to them must be avoided, and the responsibility lies firmly with the holder of the data, both personally and in respect of employing organisations. Commitment to best practice should be applied to all information in any form about patients (e.g. patients' records, electronic data, surface mail, email, faxes, telephone calls, conversations that may be overheard, and private comments to friends or colleagues).
- If, for any reason, ambulance staff discover that personal data has been lost or has the potential for being viewed by anyone not authorised to view it, they have a duty to immediately:
  - take every action possible to recover the data and/or protect it, and
  - to inform immediately an officer in their employing organisation who has responsibility for data (or their immediate supervisor) that such an event has occurred
  - record the event.

5.5 Anonymise information where possible

- Information about patients is said to be anonymised when items such as those listed in section 2 are removed. It means that patients cannot be identified by any receiver of the information and any possibility of recognition is extremely small.
- Ambulance clinicians are advised to anonymise confidential data about patients wherever possible and reasonable. If information is recorded, retained or transmitted in any way, it should be anonymised unless to do so would frustrate any genuine reasons for its collection/storage that create identifiable benefits to patients' health.

6. Patients' Rights of Access to Personal Health Records

- Patients have a right to see, and obtain a copy of, personal health information held about them. This right in law includes any legally appointed representative and those persons who have parental responsibility for children who are patients. Children also have this right provided they have the capability to understand the information. Services have the right to charge for this information; and there are guidelines on the processes that are to be followed.
- There are exceptions to the rights of patients to see their personal health information. The information is subject to legal restrictions if it could identify someone else and if that information cannot be removed from the record. Also, a request can be refused if there is substantial opinion that access to the information could cause serious harm to a particular patient or to someone else's physical or mental well-being. These instances are extremely rare in ambulance service operations. If there were to be doubt about whether exceptions such as these do exist, staff should consult the Caldicott Guardian, Information Governance Manager or Data Protection Officer and agreement should be reached with each patient's lead clinician.
- Notwithstanding the exceptions noted here, clinicians should make every effort to support each patient's right to gain access to their personal health information. It is a requirement that this information should be received by a patient who requests it within 30 days of their request. Services should have clear written procedures in place to deal with these requests.

7. Disclosure to Other Bodies and Organisations

7.1 Police

- The police have the right of access via ambulance service systems to personal information (name, address, etc.) in their investigation, detection and prevention of any crime. They also have the right of access to confidential health information (type of illness or injury, etc.) in their investigation, detection or prevention of a serious crime (e.g. rape, arson, terrorism, murder, etc.). This information must go through an ambulance service system, as per local pathways.
- They have no right to expect to receive information when criminality, crew safety or public safety are not involved. Generalised information regarding attendance at an incident may be passed to the police through locally agreed procedures, when details of the location of an incident and what is involved **may** be disclosed – but passage of personal or confidential health data **may not**.

7.2 Local authorities

- A local authority officer may require any person holding health, financial or other records relating to a person whom the officer knows or believes to be an adult at risk to give the records, or copies of them, to the officer, for the purposes of enabling or assisting the authority to decide whether it needs to do anything in order to protect an adult at risk from harm.

7.3 Secretary of State (by proxy)

- The Secretary of State's '***security management functions***' in relation to the health service mean that his or her powers to take action for the purpose of protecting and improving the security of health service providers (and persons employed by them) includes releasing documents for the purpose of preventing, detecting or investigating fraud, corruption or other unlawful activities.

7.4 Fire service and other emergency services

There is no right of access for emergency service personnel, other than the police, to patients' personal health information. Situations may occur in which ambulance clinicians feel that such disclosure would be in the best interests of a particular patient, or that, by not disclosing it, other emergency workers could be put at risk. Ambulance clinicians should be fully aware of their obligations towards their patients' confidentiality. Avoidable breaches of confidentiality occur when colleagues and authorities (such as the police and persons in a judicial context) ask for information. On these occasions ambulance clinicians should follow the best practice advice given in the relevant section of the NHS Code of Practice; otherwise, access to information should be governed by formal documented requests and consideration by the Data Protection Officer, Information Governance Manager and/or the Caldicott Guardian.

7.5 The media

- There is no basis for disclosure of confidential or patient identifiable information to the media. Services may receive requests for information in special circumstances (e.g. requests for updates on celebrity patients or following large incidents, and when responding to press statements – public interest exemption). In instances such as these the explicit consent of the persons about whom information is sought should be gained and recorded prior to any disclosure. Occasionally, services or ambulance clinicians can be criticised in the press by patients or by someone else with whom a patient has a relationship. Criticism of this nature may contain inaccurate or misleading details of behaviour, diagnosis, or treatment. Services or ambulance clinicians should always seek advice from professional bodies on how to respond (if at all) to press criticism and about any legal redress that may be available. Although these instances may cause frustration or distress, they do not relieve anyone of their duty to respect the confidentiality of any patient.

7.6 For commercial purposes

- Ambulance services are not registered to use information for primarily commercial purposes. If such use was permitted, each patient would have to give explicit consent for information given by, or about them to be used within the express commercial setting and each patient should be given an opt-out facility. This includes all intended purposes of all parties to the agreement and lists of all persons/groups who would have access to the data. Due to the nature of commercial enterprise, this consent must be explicit (expressly and actively given) as opposed to implied (acceptance without voicing an objection).

8. Research

All data for research should be anonymised wherever possible. If anonymisation would be contrary to the aims of the research, prior consent must be gained. Formal research guidelines exist for the use of health-related data and they must be adhered to.

9. Consent

Consent and patients' confidentiality are inextricably linked. In essence, each patient is said to be the owner of their own personal, non-anonymised patient information and/or data. Therefore, each patient should give approval before information provided by, or about them, is used by other people. There are exceptions to this general rule:

Patient Confidentiality

- There may be legal requirements to disclose data without consent (e.g. due to persons having **notifiable diseases**). Even then, however, each patient must be informed that this situation has arisen.
- When there is a risk to a patient's well-being by not informing other professionals without consent (e.g. where a child or vulnerable adult, an adult without capacity, or a patient who is being treated using powers given by the Mental Health Act, may be in need of protection) and informing the relevant authorities would appear to be to the patient's wider benefit.
- Inability to consent (e.g. some children, adults who lack capacity or patients who are seriously ill or injured and who could reasonably be expected to give consent if it were otherwise possible to do so). Even in circumstances such as these, information must be used cautiously and anonymised when possible. A proxy, guardian or parent should be consulted if such a person is available.
- Use of personal information without consent may be justified if it is in the **public interest** to do so. This may occur to prevent or detect a serious crime, for example.
- In all of the instances that are described here, the advice of the service's Caldicott Guardian, Information Governance Manager and/or Data Protection Officer should be sought prior to using or releasing any personal health information or data. Each service must advise their own ambulance clinicians in relation to consent, and this advice must be studied by ambulance clinicians.

KEY POINTS!

Patient Confidentiality

- **Health professionals have a duty of confidentiality regarding information about, or that may identify, patients. They also have a priority to ensure that all relevant information is recorded clearly and accurately, and passed to others when this is necessary for providing ongoing care.**
- **Inaccurate clinical records may contain false information about patients, which is created by, for example, omissions, errors, unfounded comments or speculation. Any comments or opinions, whether verbal, written or electronic, must be justifiable and accurate.**
- **Data Protection Officers, Information Governance Managers and Caldicott Guardians are available to advise and assist ambulance clinicians of the ambulance services.**
- **Consent and confidentiality of information that is held about patients are inextricably linked. In essence, patients are the owners of personal, non-anonymised information that is provided by, or about them, and they, therefore, are required to give approval before it is used by other people.**
- **Ensure you are aware of the rules in your service regarding patients' confidentiality and follow them – but remember that ongoing care of patients should never be compromised in their application.**

SECTION 1 General Guidance

Bibliography

1. Health and Care Professions Council. *Standards of Conduct, Performance and Ethics: Your duties as a registrant.* London: Health Professions Council, 2016. Available from: https://www.hcpc-uk.org/standards/standards-of-conduct-performance-and-ethics/
2. Gold M, Philip J, McIver S, Komesaroff PA. Between a rock and a hard place: exploring the conflict between respecting the privacy of patients and informing their carers. *Internal Medicine Journal* 2009, 39(9): 582–7.
3. Department of Health. *Confidentiality: NHS Code of Practice.* London: Stationery Office, 2003. Available from: https://www.gov.uk/government/publications/confidentiality-nhs-code-of-practice
4. NHS Scotland. *NHS Code of Practice on Protecting Patient Confidentiality.* Available from: https://www2.gov.scot/Publications/2010/04/20142935/0, 2010.
5. Department of Health. *Confidentiality: NHS Code of Practice – supplementary guidance: public interest disclosures.* Available from: https://www.gov.uk/government/publications/confidentiality-nhs-code-of-practice-supplementary-guidance-public-interest-disclosures, 2010.
6. General Medical Council. *Confidentiality: good practice in handling patient information* London: General Medical Council, 2018. Available from: https://www.gmc-uk.org/ethical-guidance/ethical-guidance-for-doctors/confidentiality
7. Thomas MG. Team learning: the issue of patient confidentiality. *Work Based Learning in Primary Care* 2004, 2(4): 377–80.
8. Department of Health. *The Caldicott Committee Report on the Review of Patient-Identifiable Information.* London: Stationery Office, 1997. Available from: https://webarchive.nationalarchives.gov.uk/20130123204013/http://www.dh.gov.uk/en/Publicationsandstatistics/Publications/PublicationsPolicyAndGuidance/DH_4068403
9. Woodward B. The computer-based patient record and confidentiality. *The New England Journal of Medicine* 1995, 333(21): 1419–22.

10. Gostin LO. Health information privacy. *Cornell Law Review* 1995, 80(3): 451–528.

11. Brooks J. Caldicott Guardians: driving the confidentiality agenda. *British Journal of Healthcare Computing and Information Management* 2004, 21(3): 20–1.

12. White C, Hardy J. What do palliative care patients and their relatives think about research in palliative care? A systematic review. *Support Care Cancer* 2010, 18(8): 905–11.

13. Department of Health. *The Data Protection Act 2018*. London: HMSO, 2018. Available from: http://www.legislation.gov.uk/ukpga/2018/12/contents/enacted

14. Griffith R, Tengnah C. Access to health records: the rights of the patient. *British Journal of Community Nursing* 2010, 15(7): 344–7.

15. Wougare J. Patient rights to privacy and dignity in the NHS. *Nursing Standard* 2005, 19(18): 33–7.

16. Ministry of Justice. *The Mental Capacity Act 2005 Code of Practice 2007.* London: The Stationery Office, 2005. Available from: https://www.gov.uk/government/publications/mental-capacity-act-code-of-practice

17. British Medical Association. *The Mental Capacity Act 2005: Guidance for health professionals.* Available from: https://egret.psychol.cam.ac.uk/medicine/legal/BMA_MCA_2005_guidance_March2007.pdf, 2007.

18. Information Commissioner's Office. *Guide to the General Data Protection Regulation (GDPR).* Cheshire: Information Commissioner's Office. Available from: https://ico.org.uk/for-organisations/guide-to-the-general-data-protection-regulation-gdpr/, 2018.

19. NHS Digital. *General Data Protection Regulation (GDPR) guidance*. Leeds: NHS Digital. Available from: https://digital.nhs.uk/data-and-information/looking-after-information/data-security-and-information-governance/information-governance-alliance-iga/general-data-protection-regulation-gdpr-guidance, 2018.

Pain Management in Adults

1. Introduction

- Relief of pain is one of the most important clinical outcomes in paramedic practice. Often, pain is the chief complaint that has resulted in seeking assistance. Apart from the humanitarian dimension, managing pain has several clinical benefits. Analgesia should be swiftly initiated as soon as clinically possible after arriving on scene. There is no reason to delay pain relief because of uncertainty with the definitive diagnosis. It does not affect later diagnostic efficacy, but may potentially aid in arriving at a prompt diagnosis, as patients are more cooperative when comfortable. Intense pain can modify the nervous system leading to chronic persistent pain – a troublesome long-term problem with huge health and socioeconomic impact.
- Barriers to effective pain management include:
  - patient factors (general condition, communication, cooperation)
  - knowledge and experience of the clinician
  - environment and available resources.

2. Assessment

- Pain is a complex and dynamic experience and all clinicians should place the requirements and needs of the individual at the forefront of all assessments. Ideally, multidisciplinary assessment ascertains the most appropriate and efficient course of treatment in both acute and chronic pain conditions, but limited resources in the pre-hospital environment can make comprehensive assessment a challenging task.
- The pain experience of individuals is influenced by bio-psycho-social factors, such as:
  - the nature of any underlying medical condition
  - age, gender, genetics
  - prior pain experience, culture, beliefs
  - environment and social conditions.

2.1 Measuring Pain

- Although different scoring systems are used to gauge the intensity of pain, patients' experiences cannot be objectively validated in the same way as other vital signs. JRCALC recommend the 0–10-point verbal numerical scale in which 0 refers to no pain and 10 is the worst imaginable pain. In most pre-hospital situations, this score is suitable to assess severity of pain and the response to treatment. As there is inter-individual variability, the trend in the scores is more important than the absolute value in assessing efficacy of treatment. Apart from initial assessment and scoring, subsequent periodic measurement after each intervention is a recommended practice. However, no pain assessment tool is set in stone and the patient's needs should always be considered above the findings of the assessment tool.
- Scoring can be difficult in patients with dementia, cognitive impairment, altered level of consciousness or communication difficulties. In these scenarios, pain is assessed through behavioural cues. Remember: no behaviour is unique to pain; behaviour is unique to individuals.[1]
- The prevalence of persistent pain in older adults is high, with the main causes originating as a result of degenerative changes. In both sexes, incidence of arthritis increases with age. Both osteoarthritis and osteoporosis are more common in women. Due to unmet healthcare needs, other concurrent medical conditions or poor compliance with medications, managing pain in older adults is often suboptimal. This has adverse effects on mood, sleep and activity. Ageing-related alteration to pharmacokinetics, pharmacodynamics and polypharmacy also contribute to poorly controlled pain. Older adults may not complain or effectively communicate their needs. In addition, they may also be living with dementia. The process of assessing older adults should be the same as for younger people, utilising numerical or pictorial pain assessment scales. The Abbey Pain Scale can used to measure pain (refer to Figure 1.1).

2.2 Clinical Evaluation of Acute Pain

- Assessment and treatment of acute pain has to be immediate with minimal interruption to other aspects of the patient's life. Poorly managed acute pain can result in certain changes in the nervous system, commonly described as 'plasticity', which predispose to development of chronic pain. Knowledge of exacerbating and relieving factors can complement pain management.
- A commonly used mnemonic in acute pain assessment is SOCRATES:
  - **Site** (e.g. calf pain due to deep venous thrombosis; associated chest pain may be due to pulmonary embolism).
  - **Onset** (acute onset or progressive worsening of an underlying condition).
  - **Character** (aching pain with movements can be musculoskeletal; burning pain, pins and needles can be neuropathic).
  - **Radiation** (back pain radiating to legs can be due to nerve root irritation; chest pain with radiation to the left arm can be due to angina).
  - **Associated symptoms** (fever, chills, nausea may be due to infectious cause).
  - **Time**/duration.
  - **Exacerbation** and relieving factors (pain with movement may be musculoskeletal, pain associated with bowel and bladder disturbance may be due to abdominal problems).
  - **Severity** (scoring tools to assess baseline intensity and monitor progress).

The Abbey Pain Scale

For measurement of pain in people who cannot verbalise.

How to use scale: While observing the patient, score questions 1 to 6.

Q1. Vocalisation
e.g. whimpering, groaning, crying
Absent 0 Mild 1 Moderate 2 Severe 3 Q1 ☐

Q2. Facial expression
e.g. looking tense, frowning, grimacing, looking frightened
Absent 0 Mild 1 Moderate 2 Severe 3 Q2 ☐

Q3. Change in body language
e.g. fidgeting, rocking, guarding part of body withdrawn
Absent 0 Mild 1 Moderate 2 Severe 3 Q3 ☐

Q4. Behavioural change
e.g. increased confusion, refusing to eat, alteration in usual patterns
Absent 0 Mild 1 Moderate 2 Severe 3 Q4 ☐

Q5. Physiological change
e.g. temperature, pulse or blood pressure outside normal limits, perspiring, flushing or pallor
Absent 0 Mild 1 Moderate 2 Severe 3 Q5 ☐

Q6. Physical changes
e.g. skin tears, pressure areas, arthritis, contractures, previous injuries
Absent 0 Mild 1 Moderate 2 Severe 3 Q6 ☐

Add scores for Q1 to Q6 and record here → Total pain score ☐

Now tick the box that matches the Total Pain Score →

0–2 No pain	3–7 Mild	8–13 Moderate	14+ Severe

Finally, tick the box which matches the type of pain →

Chronic	Acute	Acute on chronic

Abbey J, De Bellis A, Piller N, Esterman A, Gilles L, Parker D, Lowcay B. The Abbey Pain Scale. Funded by the JH & JD Gunn Medical Research Foundation 1998–2002.
(This document may be reproduced with this reference retained.)

Figure 1.1 – The Abbey Pain Scale.

- All patients with pain should have at least two pain scores taken, the first one before the treatment and the subsequent measurements after the treatment is commenced. Scoring and systematic assessment increases awareness of pain management, reveals previously unrecognised pain and improves analgesic administration.

2.3 Clinical Evaluation of Chronic Pain

- Chronic pain is not prolonged acute pain. The experience of pain is influenced by 'bio-psycho-social' factors, such as medical condition, mood, sleep, beliefs and behaviour, cultural and social factors.
- Patients with chronic pain may have heightened sensitivity of the nervous system and are prone to develop exacerbation episodes necessitating a call for urgent help.
- The fundamental principles of assessing these patients are the same as described above, but consideration should be given to psychological and social factors. The challenges for paramedics include seeing these patients for the first time and hence difficulty in obtaining a global picture, and limited resources/time to conduct a comprehensive assessment. This may result in disbelief of the patient's report of pain. Without precise knowledge of patient's background medical history, malingering may be suspected and this impression may negatively affect the quality of care. A safer approach is to seek and accept the patient's self report of their pain.

Examples of questions to assess patients with chronic pain

- How would you rate your pain on a 0 to 10 scale at the **present**, where 0 is 'no pain' and 10 is 'worst imaginable pain'?
- In the past six months, how intense was your **worst** pain, rated on a 0 to 10 scale?
- In the past six months, on **average**, how intense was your pain, rated on a 0 to 10 scale?
- In the past six months, how much has the pain interfered with your daily activities, rated on a 0 to 10 scale where 0 is 'no interference' and 10 is 'unable to carry on any activities'?
- In the past six months, how much has the pain changed your ability to take part in recreational, social and family activities where 0 is 'no change' and 10 is 'extreme change'?
- In the past six months, how much has the pain changed your ability to do housework where 0 is 'no change' and 10 is 'extreme change'?
- About how many days in the past six months have you been kept from your usual activities (work, school or housework) because of pain?

3. Management

- Whenever possible, treat the cause (for example, glyceryl trinitrate sublingual spray for angina and oxygen for sickle cell crisis). When the cause is not readily treatable or if it is not apparent, then other analgesic interventions are necessary.
- The pain relief options are:
  - psychological (e.g. reassurance, distraction)
  - physical (e.g. dressing burns wound, splinting fracture)
  - pharmacological (e.g. paracetamol, NSAID, morphine).
- 'Balanced analgesia' with a multimodal pain plan is recommended by JRCALC in pre-hospital pain management and involves administration of analgesics with different mechanisms of action. The synergistic effects should improve effectiveness while limiting the side effects. An example is the combination of paracetamol and morphine. Studies show that the dose of morphine can be reduced by 40–50% when administered alongside paracetamol or ibuprofen. This complementary effect not only offers a more effective pain solution for the patient, but will also improve safety when paramedics administer morphine. Often, a combination of pharmacological and non pharmacological methods may be necessary, for example, Entonox, morphine or ketamine may be required to enable the application of a splint for fractures.
- Treatment of acute pain may not follow the WHO analgesic ladder as closely as in other elective clinical scenarios. Initially, effective pain control is facilitated with stronger opioids and, wherever appropriate, local anaesthetic techniques. Entonox can be judiciously used for a short period until the other analgesics have had time to take effect. Once controlled, enteral options, such as regular oral opioid analgesics (codeine) and then simple analgesics (paracetamol, NSAID) are introduced.
- Any pain relief must be accompanied by careful explanation of the patient's condition and the pain relief methods being used. Understanding the basic sites of action of different analgesics will aid in choosing the optimal combinations.

3.1 Choice of Analgesics

Refer to Figure 1.3.

- Simple analgesics:
  - paracetamol, non-steroidal anti-inflammatory drugs (NSAID), e.g. ibuprofen, Diclofenac, Naproxen.
- Opioids:
  - codeine, morphine.
- Miscellaneous:
  - Entonox, Methoxyflurane, ketamine, local anaesthetic blocks.

Pain Management in Adults

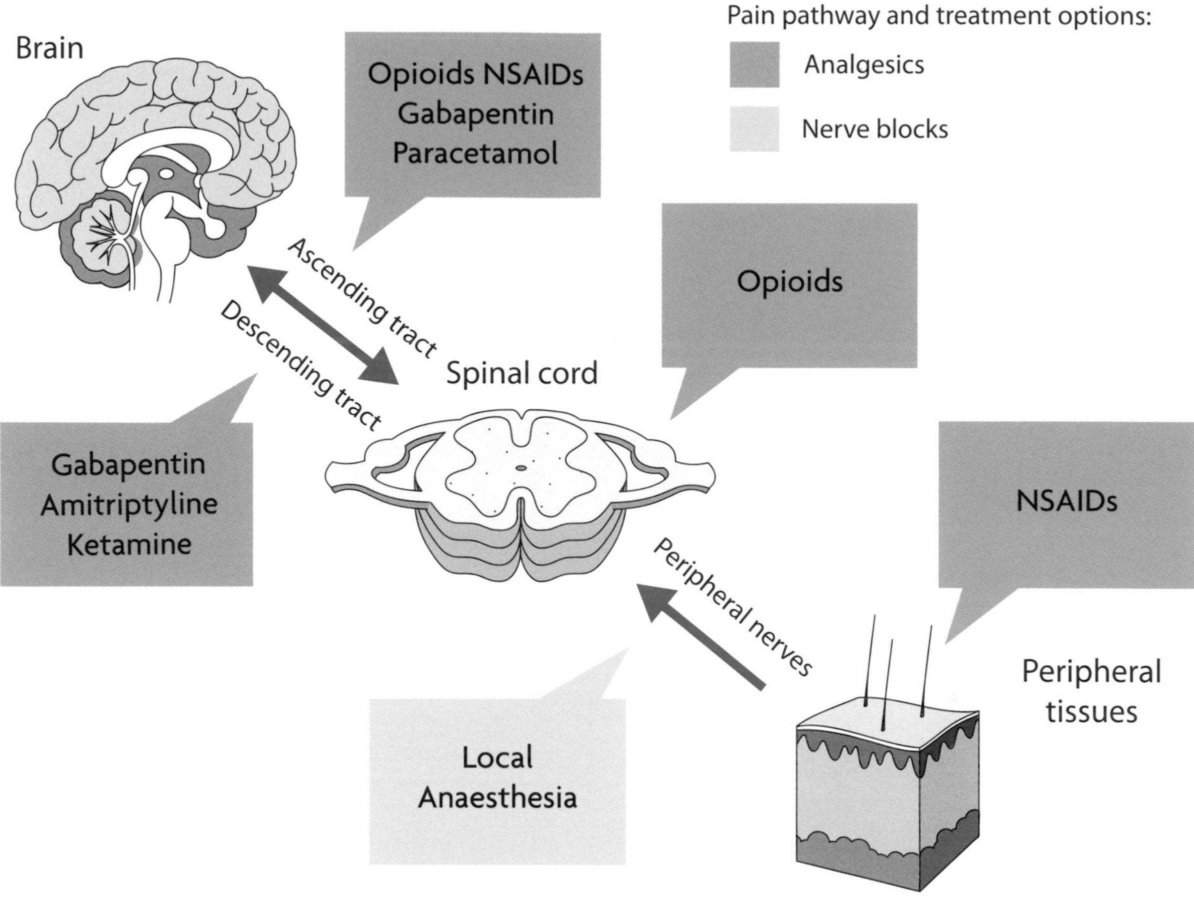

Figure 1.2 – Pain pathway and treatment options.

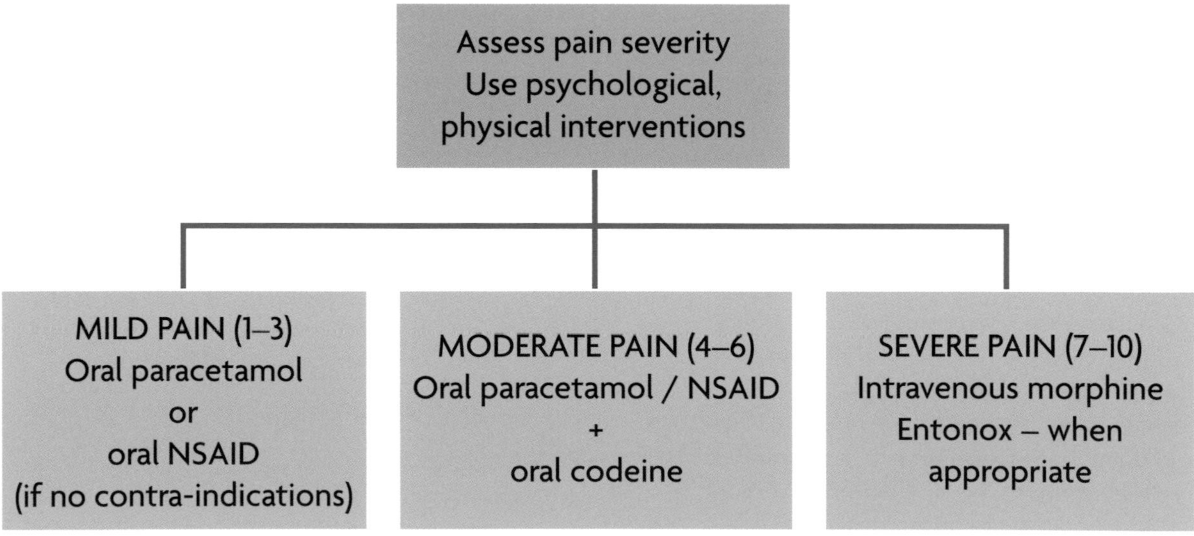

Figure 1.3 – Choice of analgesics.

3.2 Routes of Administration

- The oral route is mostly sufficient for mild to moderate pain. In severe pain, the intravenous route has the advantage of rapid onset and the dose can be titrated against analgesic effect. In a subgroup of patients, such as those suffering from sickle cell disease or requiring end of life care, intramuscular or subcutaneous injections are appropriate and local Trust guidelines should be followed. In specific circumstances, the intraosseous route may be considered.

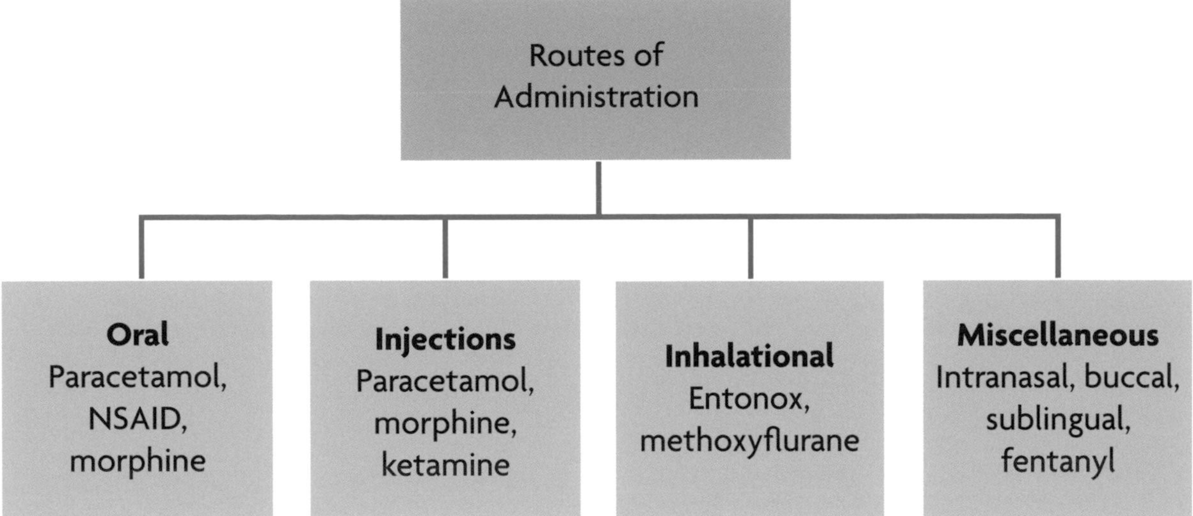

Figure 1.4 – Routes of administration.

- The intranasal route of offering pain relief has many advantages over the traditional routes. It overcomes the cannulation barrier associated with the administration of opioid analgesia that has been shown to be a major problem in the young, the elderly, the shocked patient and the cognitively impaired. Studies looking at pain management in children have found that the intranasal route offers a kinder and less intrusive mechanism for drug delivery while at the same time offering the same level of analgesia as the intravenous route.
- Inhalational analgesia is particularly useful when venous access is not readily secured or when there is a need for immediate relief of severe pain. It can be used as the first analgesic while other pain relief is instituted, or in conjunction with other medications until satisfactory control is achieved. Inhalational analgesia is only for short-term use.

3.3 Chronic Pain[2,3]

- These patients are commonly on pain medications, such as gabapentin, pregabalin, amitriptyline, duloxetine, and a significant dose of opioids. Unlike acute pain management, complete resolution of symptoms can be challenging in 'acute on chronic' pain management. Understanding the complexity of chronic pain helps in handling the situation. Ensuring compliance to the prescribed chronic pain medications can help to avoid adding more medicines. Patients may be on a significant dose of opioids such as morphine, oxycodone, Fentanyl or buprenorphine patches. Recent evidence throws light on the limitations of using stronger opioids in chronic pain management.
- If patients require intravenous morphine or inhalation of Entonox to help break the pain-spasm cycle and enable assessment, it is prudent to reiterate that this is only a short-term intervention for temporary relief; long-term exposure to opioids or Entonox can be potentially harmful.
- In general, the treatment plan for patients with chronic pain runs closely alongside the principle of 'start low and go slow' with regards to the analgesics. If clinical assessment did not identify any fresh cause for exacerbation of pain, reassurance, compliance with prescribed medicines, simple non-pharmacological interventions, such as a TENS machine, may minimise the need for transportation to the emergency department and instead facilitate elective review with the general practitioner or the pain clinic.
- Modern medicine has heavily relied on the 'biomedical model', where clinicians regarded diseases as derangement in normal body structure and function that can be fixed with a drug or a procedure. We now recognise that the brain does not work in isolation, especially in pain. When managing chronic illnesses, the major shortcoming is lack of emphasis placed on the person as a whole. The bio-psycho-social model encompasses all the three important facets that influence pain experience, i.e. biological, psychological and social factors (refer to Table 1.2).

Pain Management in Adults

TABLE 1.2 – The Bio-Psycho-Social Model
Biological Concerns itself with the biological aspects of the illness and is usually managed within the biomedical model. Although alleviating pain with good analgesics is still the main aim, it is equally important that clinicians do not reduce the problem of pain to simply labeling it as a broken or dysfunctional part of the body in isolation and apply a specific treatment for that cause.
Psychological Explores the emotional aspect of the person and behaviour, or indeed the change in the behaviour that accompanies pain. Commonly, patients with persistent pain also have mental health issues such as anxiety and depression, either as a cause or as an association. Timely recognition of mental health difficulties and facilitating appropriate psychological support can avoid escalation into other complex long-term problems.
Social Pain-related beliefs and behaviour could have social repercussions at home, work and in the wider society. Patients will rationalise what is happening to them within a social model, which will have impacts on their relationships, family, employment etc. In chronic pain, a social constructionist approach will help to develop a holistic treatment plan.

TABLE 1.3 – Non-Pharmacological Methods of Pain Relief	
• **Physical**	• Cooling of burns can reduce the pain. Burns should not be cooled for longer than 20 minutes total time and care should be taken with large burns to avoid hypothermia. • Splintage and immobilisation of fractures provides pain relief as well as minimising ongoing tissue damage, bleeding and other complications. • Warm blankets can help to keep the patient comfortable and avoid hypothermia.
• **Psychological**	• Fear and anxiety worsen pain; reassurance and explanation can go a long way towards alleviation of pain. • Distraction makes pain easier to tolerate; simple conversation is the simplest form of distraction.

TABLE 1.4 – Pharmacological Methods of Pain Relief (Refer to Specific Drug Protocols)	
• **Oral analgesia**	• Paracetamol and ibuprofen may be used in isolation or together for the management of mild to moderate pain when used in appropriate dosages. It is important to assess the presence of contra-indications to all drugs, including simple analgesics. Non-steroidal anti-inflammatory drugs are responsible for large numbers of adverse events, because of their gastrointestinal and renal side effects and their effects on asthmatics. Some ambulance services may also choose to add a paracetamol/codeine combination and/or other opioid-based oral analgesics to their formulary. • Oral morphine is useful for less severe pain but has the disadvantage of delayed onset, some unpredictability of absorption and having to be given in a set dose. It has the advantage of avoiding the need for intravenous access. It is widely used for patients with mild/moderate pain from injuries such as fractures.
• **Parenteral analgesia (intravenous, intramuscular, subcutaneous, intraosseous)**	• Morphine is approved for administration by paramedics. Intravenous morphine is a potent analgesic to manage acute pain, but has significant side effects. For satisfactory relief, in presentations such as severe musculoskeletal pain, co-administration of intravenous paracetamol should be considered. This will improve effectiveness while keeping the dose of morphine to a minimum. As with other opioids, effects of morphine are reversed with the opioid-antagonist, naloxone. The person administering opioids should have the expertise and

TABLE 1.4 – Pharmacological Methods of Pain Relief (Refer to Specific Drug Protocols) *(continued)*	
	resources for maintaining airway, breathing and circulation, and have ready access to naloxone. Decisions to reverse the opioid's effect using naloxone should be made cautiously as this will return the patient to their pre-treatment pain level. Another common unpleasant side effect of opioids is nausea and vomiting, which may require administration of an antiemetic, such as ondansetron. ● Intramuscular and subcutaneous injections are offered in special circumstances, such as patients with sickle cell disease or end-of-life care pathways as per pre-agreed local Trust guidelines. Occasionally, when the only available vascular access is the intraosseous route and the patient is in severe pain, intraosseous morphine can safely be administered with good effect.
● **Inhalational analgesia**	● Entonox (50% nitrous oxide, 50% oxygen) is a good analgesic for adults who are able to self-administer and who can rapidly be taught to operate the demand valve. It is fast acting but has a very short half-life, so the analgesic effect wears off rapidly when inhalation is stopped. It can be used as the first analgesic while other pain relief is instituted. It can also be used as part of a balanced analgesic approach, particularly during painful procedures such as splint application and patient movement. It is safest to avoid its use in situations such as head injuries (as it can raise intracranial pressure) and pneumothorax (or any other condition where air is trapped in the body). ● Methoxyflurane (Penthrox) is an inhaled analgesic designed for self-administration. It can be used as a non-opioid alternative to morphine or in conjunction with morphine for very severe pain. Evidence has shown that methoxyflurane works well when combined with morphine and, therefore, morphine administration is encouraged at the earliest possible opportunity (as with Entonox) to work alongside methoxyflurane as part of a multi-modal approach to pain management.[4] If methoxyflurane treatment has been initiated prior to the arrival of clinicians on scene, this should be continued providing the treatment is helping to manage pain and the clinician is confident in using methoxyflurane. It is particularly useful when venepuncture cannot be achieved or when there is a need for immediate relief of severe pain. It also has advantage over Entonox in patients with chest injuries/pneumothorax. ● Methoxyflurane is presented in 3 ml doses, which will provide analgesia for approximately 30 minutes with continuous inhalation, or up to 60 minutes with intermittent inhalation. Intermittent inhalation is recommended. A maximum dose of 6 ml per day is considered safe.

TABLE 1.5 – Methods that Require Appropriately Trained Practitioners	
● **Ketamine analgesia**	● Ketamine is a NMDA receptor antagonist with some action on opioid receptors. Depending upon the dose, it can produce analgesia, sedation or anaesthesia. It is particularly useful in serious trauma because it is less likely to significantly depress blood pressure or respiration compared to other agents. Ketamine is also useful in entrapments, where a person can be extricated with combined analgesic and sedative effects. ● When used in moderate to higher dosages, adults may experience unpleasant side effects, such as hallucinations and agitation. Ketamine produces salivation so careful airway management is important, although unnecessary interference should be avoided as laryngospasm may occasionally occur. Concurrent use of atropine may minimise excessive salivation.

(continued)

TABLE 1.5 – Methods that Require Appropriately Trained Practitioners *(continued)*	
• **Intranasal opioids (e.g. Fentanyl)**	• Evidence of its effectiveness in the emergency department has highlighted the potential of intranasal Fentanyl for helping paramedics treat severe pain where venous access is compromised. Studies have shown that intranasal Fentanyl compares with the analgesic standard set by intravenous administration. Also, due to the lack of significant histamine release with Fentanyl, the risk of hypotension is less; this is especially useful in trauma situations. The combined lung surface area of around 50–75 m^2 offers a large capillary-rich environment for absorption. In addition, the duration of action of 30 minutes offers greater control for the clinician. Intranasal Fentanyl at a dose of 1.5 mcg/kg, to a maximum of 100 mcg divided evenly between nares, appears to be a safe and effective analgesic in the pre-hospital management of acute severe pain and may be an attractive alternative to both oral and intravenous opiates.
• **Local anaesthetic techniques**	• There is limited room for regional nerve blocks because of the environment and the need to transport the patient to hospital in a timely manner. However, they can be effective in certain circumstances of severe pain and do not induce drowsiness or disorientation. Examples include femoral nerve/fascia iliaca block for lower limb injuries such as a fractured femur. Clinicians undertaking regional analgesia techniques must be able to manage local anaesthetic toxicity.

KEY POINTS!

Pain Management in Adults

- **Timely management of pain has clinical benefits.**
- **Pain relief does not affect later diagnosis.**
- **Multimodal analgesia is effective and has to be tailored to both patient and practitioner variables.**
- **Pain measurements and re-assessments will help to monitor progress.**

Further Reading

Further important information and evidence in support of this guideline can be found in the Bibliography.[5,6,7,8]

Bibliography

1. Alzheimer's Australia. *Pain and Dementia*. Available from: https://www.fightdementia.org.au/files/helpsheets/Helpsheet-DementiaQandA16-PainAndDementia_english.pdf, 2011.
2. Von Korff M, Ormel J, Keefe FJ, Dworkin SF. Grading the severity of chronic pain. *Pain* 1992, 50: 133–149.
3. Scottish Intercollegiate Guidelines Network. *Management of Chronic Pain* (SIGN 136). Edinburgh: SIGN, 2013.
4. Bendall JC, Simpson PM, Middleton PM. Effectiveness of prehospital morphine, fentanyl, and methoxyflurane in pediatric patients. *Prehospital Emergency Care* 2011, 15(2).
5. Lo JC, Kaye DA. Benzodiazepines and muscle relaxants. *Essentials of Pharmacology for Anesthesia, Pain Medicine, and Critical Care*. New York: Springer, 2015: 167–178.
6. National Institute for Health and Care Excellence. *Diazepam*. Available from: https://bnf.nice.org.uk/drug/diazepam.html.
7. Lord B, Deveson M. Assessment and management of chronic pain in adults: implications for paramedics. *Journal of Paramedic Practice* 2011, 3(4): 166–172.
8. Pak SC, Micalos PS, Maria SJ, Lord B. Nonpharmacological interventions for pain management in paramedicine and the emergency setting: a review of the literature. *Evidence-Based Complementary and Alternative Medicine* 2015 (2015).

Pain Management in Children

1. Introduction

All children in pain need analgesia, regardless of age or situation, and when appropriate, analgesia should be administered as soon as clinically possible after arriving on scene although this can be done en-route so as not to delay time-critical patients. There is no reason to delay relief of pain because of uncertainty with the definitive diagnosis.

Pain is one of the commonest symptoms in patients presenting to ambulance services.

Control of pain is important not only for humanitarian reasons but also because it may prevent deterioration of the child and allow better assessment.

There is no excuse for leaving a child in pain because of lack of necessary skills in the clinician. If necessary, suitable expertise should be sought to provide pain relief.

Pain is a multi-dimensional construct (see below).

Pain consists of several elements:

- Treatment of the underlying condition.
- Non-pharmacological methods including:
  - psychological support and explanation
  - physical methods e.g. splinting
- Pharmacological treatment.

Pain relief will depend on:

- Cause, site, severity and nature of the pain.
- Age of child.
- Experience/knowledge of the clinician.
- Distance from receiving unit.
- Available resources.

2. Assessment

An assessment should be made of the requirements of the child. Pain is a complex experience that is shaped by gender, cultural, environmental, social and personal factors, as well as prior pain experience. Thus the experience of pain is unique to the individual.

It is important to remember that the pain a child experiences cannot be objectively validated in the same way as other vital signs. Attempts to estimate the child's pain should be resisted, as this may lead to an underestimation of the child's experience. Several studies have shown that there is a poor correlation between the patient's pain rating and that of the health professionals, with the latter often underestimating the patient's pain.

Instead, ambulance clinicians need to seek and accept the child's self-report of their pain. This is reinforced by a popular and useful definition of pain: 'pain is whatever the experiencing person says it is, existing whenever they say it does'.

All children in pain should have their pain assessed for its location, nature, severity and duration. Any factors related to, or that exacerbate or improve, the pain should also be assessed.

Pain scoring

There is no validated method of pain scoring for children in the pre-hospital environment. It is suggested that, pending this, a method that has been validated in the paediatric emergency department (ED) setting is used. The Wong–Baker 'faces' (scoring 0 = no hurt, 1–2 = hurts little bit, 3–4 = hurts little more, 5–6 = hurts even more, 7–8 = hurts whole lot, 9–10 = hurts worst) (refer to Appendix 1) are useful for younger children. The FLACC scale is useful for preverbal children and may also be used for older children if needed (refer to Appendix 2).

The trend in the scores is more important than the absolute value in assessing efficacy of treatment. Scoring will not be possible in all circumstances (e.g. cognitively impaired individuals, and those with communication difficulties or altered level of consciousness) and in these circumstances behavioural cues will be more important in assessing pain.

3. Management

Analgesia should normally be introduced in an incremental way with each agent being titrated to effect, considering timeliness, effectiveness and potential adverse events. Utilising a balanced analgesic approach will often allow improved efficacy with reduced side effects. Generally this should always include the non-pharmacological methods of treatment as a starting point and background to all pharmacological therapy (refer to Tables 1.6–1.9).

However, it may be apparent from the assessment that it is appropriate to start with stronger analgesia because of the child's condition; for example, a child with bilateral fractured femurs is likely to require vascular access to provide circulatory replacement and will be in severe pain. It would, therefore, be inappropriate to only try paracetamol and ibuprofen and wait for them to work. Other agents including inhaled (entonox) and intravenous/transmucosal agents as part of a balanced analgesic approach would be indicated at an early stage (this may include paracetamol, opioids and ketamine when appropriate). This along with non-pharmacological methods of pain control would provide the best possible analgesia with a lower risk of side effects. However, in a child with a small superficial burn one might try paracetamol with or without ibuprofen and along with non-pharmacological methods, this may be adequate. The child will still require regular re-assessment and a change of approach if needed.

Entonox should be given using an appropriate technique until the other drugs have had time to take effect, and if the child is still in pain. Administering analgesia in this step-wise, incremental way minimises the amount of potent analgesia that is required while still achieving adequate analgesia with fewer side effects.

Any pain relief must be accompanied by careful explanation, involving the child, where possible, and the carer. Include details of the child's condition, the pain relief methods being used, and any possible side effects.

TABLE 1.6 – Non-Pharmacological Methods of Pain Relief
Psychological Fear and anxiety worsen pain and a child-friendly environment (e.g. removing equipment which may cause fear and having toys or child-friendly pictures around) may go a long way towards alleviation of pain as may keeping the patient comfortable (e.g. warm). The presence of a parent has been shown to reduce the unpleasantness of hospital emergency procedures more than any other single factor and there is no reason why this should not be true in the pre-hospital setting. Distraction (toys, stories, games etc.) is a potent analgesic – whatever is to hand may be used, but there is no substitute for forward planning.
Dressings Burns dressings that may cool, such as those specifically designed for the task or cling film, can alleviate the pain in the burnt or scalded child. Burns should not be cooled for more than 20 minutes total time and care should be taken with large burns to prevent the development of hypothermia.
Splintage Simple splintage of fractures provides pain relief as well as minimising ongoing tissue trauma, bleeding and other complications. **NB** These should be part of all other methods of pain relief.

TABLE 1.7 – Pharmacological Methods of Pain Relief (Refer to Specific Drug Protocols)
Oral analgesia Initially administer either **paracetamol** or **ibuprofen** alone. Both are suitable first-line choices for treating mild to moderate pain in children. If the child does not respond to the first analgesic, recommend switching to the alternative alone. If the child has not responded sufficiently to appropriate doses of either drug alone, consider alternating paracetamol and ibuprofen. Care needs to be taken not to exceed the maximum dose of each drug in a 24-hour period. Evidence shows that the simultaneous use for the treatment of fever is not beneficial and does not reduce the fever duration over ibuprofen use alone. Alternating these agents may be suggested to carers to manage longer term pain in accordance with any pain plan.[2,3] **Oral morphine solution** may also prove very effective in the child with moderate to severe pain such as a fractured forearm (although in isolation this is not the ideal class of drug for musculoskeletal pain), but has the disadvantage of delayed onset, some unpredictability of absorption and having to be given in a set dose. It has the advantage of avoiding the need for intravenous access. Those with severe pain are best treated with an intravenous preparation, augmented with entonox if required.
Inhalational analgesia **Entonox (50% nitrous oxide, 50% oxygen)** is a good analgesic for children who are able to self-administer and who can rapidly be taught to operate the demand valve. It is rapid acting but has a very short half-life, so the analgesic effect wears off rapidly when inhalation is stopped. It can be used as the first analgesic whilst other pain relief is instituted. It can also be used in conjunction with morphine, particularly during painful procedures such as splint application and patient movement. Quite young children can use the system providing they can be taught to operate the demand valve, and the child's fear of the noise of the gas flow and the mask can be overcome. Flavoured (e.g. bubblegum) clear masks may help the child overcome the fear.

Pain Management in Children

TABLE 1.7 – Pharmacological Methods of Pain Relief (Refer to Specific Drug Protocols) *(continued)*
Parenteral and enteral analgesia
Morphine remains an important component for balanced analgesia and can be administered intravenously, intraosseously, and orally (refer to **Morphine Sulfate**). Opioid analgesics should be given intravenously rather than intramuscularly to avoid erratic absorption when possible. When used in isolation for musculoskeletal pain, there may be an increased risk of side effects before achieving adequate analgesia, emphasising the need for a balanced analgesic approach. Therefore other agents such as IV paracetamol should be considered. As with the other opioids, morphine is reversed by naloxone. When administering opioids to children, ability to maintain airway/breathing/circulation and naloxone **MUST** be available and the required dose calculated in case urgent reversal is necessary. If clinically significant sedation or respiratory depression occurs following the administration of opioids, the child's ventilation should be assisted. Decisions to reverse the opioid effects using an opioid antagonist such as naloxone should be made cautiously as this may return the child to their pre-opioid pain level depending on dosage of naloxone given, which should therefore be titrated to desired effect. Intranasal opioids (morphine, diamorphine and fentanyl) are not currently approved for paramedic administration. Intranasal opioid analgesia is becoming used more frequently in hospital and has the advantage of potent, rapid action without needing parenteral administration. However, it is fairly difficult to prepare the appropriate dose and concentration in the pre-hospital context. In certain patients the subcutaneous routes may be used effectively, and these may be most appropriate for patient specific protocols for groups of patients such as end of life and sickle cell disease. In the event of break-through pain with palliative care, advice should be sought from the patient's care team whenever possible. There is no evidence that metoclopramide is effective in relieving nausea induced by opioids. Children have a significant risk of dystonic reactions with metoclopramide and therefore it is not advised in these circumstances. Other anti-emetics (e.g. ondansetron) can be used for opioid-induced nausea and vomiting.

TABLE 1.8 – Pain Relief Which Requires Appropriately Trained Practitioners
Ketamine analgesia/anaesthesia
Ketamine is particularly useful in entrapments where a child can be extricated with combined analgesic and sedative effects. At present only appropriately trained practitioners may carry ketamine. Ketamine has a predominantly non-opioid mechanism of action. At higher doses it can be used as a general anaesthetic agent. It is particularly useful in serious trauma because it may not significantly depress blood pressure or respiration depending on the particular patient (acute and chronic co-morbidity) and the time since injury. Older children in particular may experience unpleasant emergence phenomena but these tend to be less common in the young especially if appropriate analgesic doses are utilised and titrated to effect. Ketamine in higher doses (not often a problem with appropriate analgesic doses titrated to effect) produces salivation so careful airway management is important, although unnecessary interference should be avoided as laryngospasm may occasionally occur. Atropine may be used with care concurrently to minimise hypersalivation.
Regional anaesthesia
There is very limited room for regional nerve blocks because of the environment and the need to transport the child to hospital in a timely manner. However, they can be effective in certain circumstances of severe pain and do not induce drowsiness or disorientation. Femoral nerve blocks may be useful and provide good analgesia for a fractured femur. Clinicians undertaking regional anaesthesia must be suitably trained, prepared, experienced and fully understand and have the mechanism to treat local anaesthetic toxicity in the pre-hospital environment.

Pain Management in Children

TABLE 1.9 – Pre-Hospital Analgesic Drugs Used in Children

Drug	Route	Pain severity	Advantages	Disadvantages
Paracetamol	Oral (the rectal route is no longer recommended for analgesia) Intravenous	Mild–moderate (may be opioid sparing when used for more severe pain as better efficacy for musculoskeletal pain than opioids alone)	Readily accessable and well tolerated orally. Well accepted antipyretic	Slow action when given orally. Inadequate and unpredictable plasma levels if given rectally
Ibuprofen	Oral (other IV NSAIDs are available but currently not available for paramedic use)	Mild–moderate (may be opioid sparing when used for more severe pain as better efficacy for musculoskeletal pain than opioids alone)	Moderately good analgesic, antipyretic and anti-inflammatory	Slow action. May cause bronchospasm in asthmatics. Caution in trauma and patients with regards to platelet and renal function
Entonox	Inhaled	Mild–moderate (may be opioid sparing when used for more severe pain as better efficacy for musculoskeletal pain than opioids alone)	Quick, dose self-regulating. Relative contra-indications are important	Fear of mask. Understanding, coordination and cooperation required. (Demand valves for younger children becoming more available. Cannot use free-flow if not scavenging in confined space, e.g. ambulance.)
Oral morphine	Oral	Moderate	Good analgesic for minor/moderate pain particularly of a visceral nature	May need to adjust dose of IV morphine if given subsequently. Reduced oral bioavailability. Slow action
Morphine	Intravenous Intraosseous Intramuscular Subcutaneous	Severe	Rapid onset. Reversed with naloxone (although requires care). Some euphoria	Not ideal as solo agent when used for musculoskeletal pain. Need access. Respiratory depression, vomiting. Controlled drug
Diamorphine[a]	Intranasal Intravenous Intraosseous	Moderate–severe pain particularly of visceral nature	Intranasal – quick and effective although logistically difficult in pre-hospital practice. Best efficacy if used with other agents (e.g. paracetamol)	As for morphine if given IV. More euphoria. Intranasal not currently approved for paramedics

SECTION **1** General Guidance

Pain Management in Children

TABLE 1.9 – Pre-Hospital Analgesic Drugs Used in Children *(continued)*				
Drug	**Route**	**Pain severity**	**Advantages**	**Disadvantages**
Ketamine[b]	Intravenous Intramuscular Oral	Severe pain from either musculoskeletal or visceral aetiologies (excluding acute coronary syndromes)	Can be increased to general anaesthesia in experienced hands. Less respiratory and cardiovascular depression than other strong analgesic/ anaesthetic drugs. Concerns re-raised ICP less clinically relevant than previously thought	Emergence phenomena, salivation, occasional laryngospasm (usually with higher doses, therefore small doses 0.1 mg/kg/dose for analgesia and titrate to effect). Comes in three different concentrations which may lead to confusion

4. Pain Relief which Requires Appropriately Trained Practitioners

These methods are included because it is necessary to know what can be done to reduce pain in children before hospital, if time and logistics allow. A suitably licensed and trained pre-hospital practitioner should be called early to the scene if it is thought that such assistance may be necessary. Hospital personnel may not all have these skills.

KEY POINTS!

Pain Management in Children

- **All children in pain need analgesia.**
- **The method of pain relief used will depend on the cause, site, severity, nature of the pain and age of child.**
- **Analgesia should be introduced incrementally and titrated to effect.**
- **Pain scoring faces and the FLACC scale are useful for use with young children.**
- **A balanced analgesic approach to pain management consists of treating the cause wherever possible, and analgesia involving psychological, physical and pharmacological interventions (more than one agent, when possible, in smaller and titrated doses to achieve better analgesia with fewer side effects by acting at different areas involving the pain pathways).**
- **Balanced analgesia remains the objective and should be tailored according to both patient and practitioner variables.**

a Currently not approved for general paramedic administration; doctor and suitably trained and authorised paramedic administration only.

b Currently not approved for general paramedic administration; doctor and suitably trained and authorised paramedic administration only.

APPENDIX 1 – The Wong-Baker FACES Pain Rating Scale

The Wong Baker Faces Scale is available at: http://wongbakerfaces.org/instructions-use

This rating scale is recommended for persons aged three years and older.

Instructions: Point to each face using the words to describe the pain intensity. Ask the child to choose the face that best describes their own pain and record the appropriate number.

Explain to the child that each face is for a person who feels happy because he has no pain (hurt) or sad because he has some or a lot of pain.

Face 0 is very happy because he doesn't hurt at all.

Face 2 hurts just a little bit.

Face 4 hurts a little more.

Face 6 hurts even more.

Face 8 hurts a whole lot.

Face 10 hurts as much as you can imagine, although you don't have to be crying to feel this bad.

From Hockenberry MJ, Wilson D, Winkelstein ML: Wong's Essentials of Pediatric Nursing, ed. 7, St. Louis, 2005, p. 1259. Copyright, Mosby.

APPENDIX 2 – The FLACC Scale

The **Face, Legs, Activity, Cry, Consolability scale** or **FLACC scale** is a measurement used to assess pain for children up to the age of seven years or individuals who are unable to communicate their pain. The scale is scored on a range of 0–10 with 0 representing no pain. The scale has five criteria which are each assigned a score of 0, 1 or 2.

TABLE 1.10 – The FLACC Scale

Criteria	Score - 0	Score - 1	Score - 2
Face	No particular expression or smile	Occasional grimace or frown, withdrawn, uninterested	Frequent to constant quivering chin, clenched jaw
Legs	Normal position or relaxed	Uneasy, restless, tense	Kicking, or legs drawn up
Activity	Lying quietly, normal position, moves easily	Squirming, shifting back and forth, tense	Arched, rigid or jerking
Cry	No cry (awake or asleep)	Moans or whimpers, occasional complaint	Crying steadily, screams or sobs, frequent complaints
Consolability	Content, relaxed	Reassured by occasional touching, hugging or being talked to, distractible	Difficult to console or comfort

Bibliography

1. Malviya S, Voepel-Lewis T, Burke C, Merkel S, Tait AR. The revised FLACC observational pain tool: improved reliability and validity for pain assessment in children with cognitive impairment. *Pediatric Anesthesia* 2006, 16(3): 258–65.
2. National Institute for Health and Clinical Excellence. *Analgesia - mild-to-moderate pain.* London: NICE, 2015. Available from: https://cks.nice.org.uk/analgesia-mild-to-moderate-pain#!scenario.
3. National Institute for Health and Clinical Excellence. *When using paracetamol or ibuprofen in children with fever, do not give both agents simultaneously.* London: NICE, 2013. Available from: https://www.nice.org.uk/donotdo/when-using-paracetamol-or-ibuprofen-in-children-with-fever-do-not-give-both-agents-simultaneously.

Safeguarding Children

1. Introduction

- Safeguarding is everyone's responsibility and a statutory duty under the Children Act.[1] Ambulance clinicians must be aware of the signs, symptoms and indicators of abuse and neglect that constitute harm. This applies to staff who have direct contact, either face-to-face or on the telephone.
- Throughout this section, reference to a child equates to someone who is not yet 18 years of age.
- Members of staff in an ambulance trust have a **duty of care to report abuse or neglect**. If the abuse is not reported, the victim may be at greater risk. They may also feel discouraged from disclosing again, as they may feel they were not believed. This may put other people at risk.
- All partners who work with children, including local authorities, police, the health service, courts, professionals, the private and voluntary sectors and individual members of local communities, share the responsibility for safeguarding and promoting the welfare of children and young people. It is vital that all partners are aware of, and appreciate, the role that each of them plays in this area.[2]
- Healthcare professionals have a statutory duty to report, while social care and the police have statutory authority to investigate allegations or suspicions of child abuse.
- Ambulance clinicians are often the first professionals on scene and, therefore, may identify initial concerns regarding a child's welfare and alert social care, the police, the GP, or other appropriate health professional, in line with locally agreed procedures. Accurate recording of events/actions may be crucial to subsequent enquiries.
- The role of the ambulance service is not to investigate suspicions but to ensure that any suspicion is passed to the appropriate agency (e.g. social care or the police). Ambulance clinicians need to be aware of child abuse issues and the aim of this guideline is to:
  - ensure all staff are aware of, and can recognise, cases of suspected child abuse or children at risk of significant harm, and provide guidance enabling operational and control staff to assess and report cases of suspected child abuse
  - where appropriate, ensure that all staff involved in a case of suspected abuse are aware of the possible outcome and of any subsequent actions.
- Further information on local procedures can be obtained from the safeguarding services within individual ambulance trusts.

2. Significant Harm

- All children have the right:
  - to be protected from significant harm/ill-treatment
  - to be protected from impairment of their health[a] and development
  - to grow up in circumstances consistent with the provision of safe and effective care.
- The maltreatment of children, physically, emotionally, sexually or through neglect, can have a major impact on their health, well-being and development.
- There are no absolute criteria on which to rely when judging what constitutes significant harm. In some cases, a single traumatic event may constitute significant harm, but more generally it is a compilation of significant events, both acute and long-standing, which interrupt, change or damage the child's physical and psychological development. Considerations include:
  - the degree and extent of physical harm
  - the duration and frequency of abuse and neglect
  - the extent of premeditation
  - the degree of threat, coercion, sadism and bizarre or unusual elements.
- In order to understand and identify significant harm, consider:
  - the nature of harm, in terms of maltreatment or failure to provide adequate care
  - the impact on the child's health and development
  - the child's development within the context of the family and wider environment
  - any special needs, such as a medical condition, communication impairment or disability, that may affect the child's development and care within the family and the capacity of parents/carers to meet adequately the child's needs.
- Consideration is needed towards other siblings and/or vulnerable people living in the household/establishment.
- Abuse and neglect are forms of maltreatment, and children may suffer as a result of a deliberate act or failure on the part of a parent, legal guardian or carer to act to prevent harm (descriptions of abuse and neglect are detailed in Table 1.11).
- Children can be abused in any care or community setting, and abuse can be perpetrated by those known to them or by a stranger.

a Health means physical or mental health.

TABLE 1.11 – Examples of Types of Abuse and Neglect

Emotional abuse

The persistent emotional maltreatment of a child so as to cause severe and persistent adverse effects on the child's emotional development, which may:

- involve conveying to the child(ren) that they are worthless or unloved, inadequate, or valued only insofar as they meet the needs of another person
- involve not giving the child opportunities to express their views, deliberately silencing them or 'making fun' of what they say or how they communicate
- feature age or developmentally inappropriate expectations being imposed on children (e.g. interactions that are beyond the child's developmental capability), as well as overprotection and limitation of exploration and learning, or preventing the child from participating in normal social interaction
- involve seeing or hearing the ill-treatment of another
- involve serious bullying (including cyberbullying), causing children frequently to feel frightened or in danger, or the exploitation or corruption of children.

Some level of emotional abuse is involved in all types of maltreatment of a child, though it may occur alone.

Emotional abuse alone can be difficult to recognise as the child may be physically well cared-for and the home in good condition. Some common factors that may indicate emotional abuse are:

- if the child is constantly denigrated/humiliated before others
- if the child is constantly given the impression that the parents are disappointed in them
- if the child is blamed for things that go wrong or is told they may be unloved/sent away
- if the parent does not offer any love or attention (e.g. leaves them alone for a long time)
- if the child is obsessive about cleanliness, tidiness etc.
- if the parent has unrealistic expectations of the child (e.g. educational achievement/toilet training)
- if the child is either bullying others or being bullied themselves
- if there is an atmosphere of domestic abuse, adults or parents with mental health problems or a history of drug or alcohol abuse (toxic trio)
- if there is evidence of self-harm, intentional overdose or the excessive use of alcohol on the part of either the parent(s) or child
- unusual behaviour of the parents/carers towards the child(ren) in an emergency situation (e.g. are they comforting a distressed child? What is the interaction like between the child and care giver?).

Sexual abuse

Sexual abuse involves forcing or enticing a child or young person to take part in sexual activities. Both girls and boys of all age groups are at risk.

The sexual abuse of a child is often planned and chronic. A large proportion of sexually abused children have no physical signs, and it is therefore necessary to be alert to behavioural and emotional factors that may indicate abuse.

The activities may involve physical contact, including assault by penetration (e.g. rape or oral sex) or non-penetrative acts, such as masturbation, kissing, rubbing and touching outside of clothing. They may include non-contact activities, such as involving children in looking at, or in the production of, sexual images, watching sexual activities, encouraging children to behave in sexually inappropriate ways, or grooming a child in preparation for abuse (including via the internet).

Men, women and children perpetrate sexual abuse. However, most abuse is perpetrated by someone known to the child.

Child sexual exploitation/abuse (CSE/CSA)

Sexual exploitation/abuse of children and young people under 18 can involve gangs or individuals. It is defined when children and young people receive something (such as food, accommodation, drugs, alcohol, cigarettes, affection, gifts or money) as a result of performing, and/or others performing on them, sexual acts. It can occur through direct contact or the use of the internet or mobile phones. Perpetrators have power over the child(ren) because of their age, gender, intellect, physical strength and/or resources. Both girls and boys of all age groups are at risk.

TABLE 1.11 – Examples of Types of Abuse and Neglect *(continued)*
There are four models used to describe CSE: 1 **Peer on peer exploitation**: outlines instances when children are sexually exploited by their own peers who could be known to them at school, through mutual friends or in the neighbourhood. 2 **Boyfriend model**: targets children by posing as boyfriends and showers the child(ren) with attention, which results in them becoming infatuated. The perpetrator then initiates a sexual relationship with the child, who is then expected to return it as 'proof of their love', or they are told they owe money for the gifts, and sexual activities are a way of paying back. 3 **Party model**: organised by groups who lure young people by offering drinks, drugs and car rides often for free and an introduction to an exciting environment. This often results in incriminating evidence being obtained at the party, such as photos or videos of sexual acts, that is then used to exploit through fear. 4 **Exploitation through befriending and grooming**: befriending directly by the perpetrator, either in person, or online, or through other children or young people. Children who are most vulnerable and at higher risk of CSE/CSA are: ● missing or runaway children ● children in care ● those with experience of sexual abuse or violence in the home ● neglected children ● children who are homeless/sofa surfing ● children who are misusing substances ● children with mental health issues ● those with a learning disability ● children not in education, employment or training (NEET).
Physical abuse
Physical abuse may involve hitting, shaking, throwing, poisoning, burning (including cigarette burns or scalding), suffocating, use of restraint, spitting, force feeding or otherwise causing physical harm. Physical harm may also be caused when a parent or carer fabricates the symptoms of, or deliberately induces, ill-health; this situation is commonly described as 'fabricated or induced illness' (FII).
Neglect
Neglect is the persistent failure to meet a child's basic physical and/or psychological needs, and is likely to result in the serious impairment of the child's health or development. Neglect may occur during pregnancy as a result of maternal substance abuse. A neglected or abused infant may show signs of poor attachment. They may lack the sense of security to explore, and appear unhappy and whining. There may be little sign of attachment behaviour, and the child may move aimlessly around a room or creep quietly into corners. Signs of potential neglect include: ● poor weight gain ● failure to use prescribed medication or medication withheld by parent/carer ● severe nappy rash ● tooth decay ● failure to immunise ● poor hygiene and dirty clothes ● obesity ● poor growth ● delayed development ● failure to attend appointments ● delayed presentation ● poor physical condition ● child not at school ● child not registered with a GP ● clothes not consistent with the climate.

Safeguarding Children

2.1 Children in Need

- Children are defined as being 'in need' when:
  - they are unlikely to reach or maintain a satisfactory level of health or development
  - their health and development will be significantly impaired without the provision of services (section 17 (10) of the Children Act 1989)
  - they have a disability.
- Local authorities have a duty to safeguard and promote the welfare of children in need.

3. Recognition of Abuse

Ambulance clinicians may receive information or make observations that suggest that a child has been abused or is at risk of harm, for example:

- the nature of the illness/injury
- the account given for the illness/injury may be inconsistent with what is observed: this is known as 'disguised compliance'
- observation of hazards in the home (e.g. alcohol or drug paraphernalia, home conditions such as lack of bedding)
- child(ren) has/have been locked in a room
- signs of distress shown by other children in the home
- observations regarding the condition of other children or adults in the household (e.g. an environment where domestic abuse has taken place). In the case of domestic dispute between adults, the presence of children in the household creates a need to notify even if the child(ren) was/were not injured
- parents or carers who seek medical care from a number of sources.

3.1 Non-accidental/Deliberate Injury

- When assessing an injury in any child, you should be aware of the possibility of the injury being non-accidental/deliberate and you should consider this possibility in every case, even if you promptly dismiss the idea.
- For an injury to be accidental it should have a clear, credible and acceptable history and the findings should be consistent with the history and with the development and abilities of the child.

3.2 Suspicion of Abuse

Suspicions should be raised by:

- any injury in a non-mobile (non-independent) baby
- accidents/injuries in unusual places (e.g. the buttocks, trunk, inner thighs)
- extensive injuries or signs of both recent and old injuries
- small deep burns in unusual places
- repeated burns and scalds
- 'glove and stocking' burns
- poor state of clothing, cleanliness and/or nutrition
- delayed reporting of the injury
- inappropriate sexual knowledge for the child's age
- overt sexual approaches to other children or adults
- fear of particular people or situations (e.g. bath time or bedtime)
- drug and alcohol abuse
- suicide attempts and self-injury
- running away and fire-setting
- environmental factors and family situations (e.g. domestic abuse, drug or alcohol abuse, learning disabilities that affect parents, carers and/or child).

The following symptoms should give cause for concern and further assessment:

- soreness, discharge or unexplained bleeding in the genital area (including anal area and severe nappy rash)
- chronic vaginal/anal infections
- bruising, grazes or bites to the genital/anal or breast area
- sexually transmitted infections
- pregnancy, especially when the identity of the father is vague or if it is a concealed or denied pregnancy.

When assessing an injured child, you should use your clinical knowledge regarding what level of accidental injury would be appropriate for their stage of development. Although stages of development vary (e.g. children may crawl or walk at different ages), injuries can broadly be divided between mobile and non-mobile children.

4. Non-mobile (Non-independent) Babies

- Babies aged under 1 year are the most vulnerable group of children as they cannot speak for themselves and are dependent on their parents/carers. Any injury in a non-mobile baby requires review by a clinician. If there is any doubt, the clinician should speak with the on-call paediatrician in the acute trust and/or the child should be conveyed.
- Healthy babies do not bruise or break their bones easily. They do not bruise themselves with their fists or toys, bruise themselves by lying against the bars of a cot, or acquire bruises on the legs when they are held for a nappy change. When in an environment, checks can be made for safety equipment, such as stair gates etc.

- Bruising on the ears, face, neck, trunk and buttocks is particularly suspicious. A torn frenulum (behind the upper lip) is rarely accidental in babies, and bleeding from the mouth of a baby should always be regarded as suspicious.

4.1 Fractures

- Fractures may not be obvious on observation and the baby may present only with crying on handling. Often a fracture will not be diagnosed until an X-ray is performed. Fractures in babies are seldom caused by 'rough handling' or putting their legs through the bars of the cot. Babies rarely fracture their skull after a fall from a bed or a chair. Fractures in non-mobile infants should be assessed by an experienced paediatrician to exclude non-accidental injury (refer to Table 1.12 for types of fractures).
- Children's bones tend to bend rather than break and require considerable force to damage them. There are various kinds of fractures (refer to Table 1.12), depending on the direction and strength of the force that caused them.
- Unless there is an obvious bony deformity, bone injuries may not be apparent on initial clinical assessment. A clear history and appreciation of the mechanism of injury are crucial parts of the initial assessment and must be clearly documented.

4.2 Shaking Injuries

- When small babies are shaken violently their head and limb movements cannot be controlled, causing brain damage and haemorrhage within the skull. This can also be caused by being thrown.
- Finger bruising on the chest may indicate that a baby has been held tightly and shaken. These babies usually present with collapse or respiratory problems and the diagnosis is only made on further detailed assessment.

5. Mobile Babies and Toddlers

5.1 Bruising

- It is normal for toddlers to have accidental bruises on the shins, elbows and forehead. Bruises in unusual areas such as the back, upper arms and abdomen do not tend to occur accidentally. Defensive wounds commonly occur on the forearm, upper arm, back of the legs, hands or feet. You may see clusters of bruises on the upper arm, outside of the thigh or on the body. You may see bruises with dots of blood under the skin. A bruised scalp and swollen eyes may suggest that hair has been pulled violently.
- Bruising caused by a hand slap leaves a characteristic pattern of 'stripes' representing the imprint of fingers. Forceful gripping leaves small round bruises corresponding to the position of the fingertips. 'Tramline' bruising is caused by a belt or stick, and shows as lines of bruising with a white patch in between.

5.2 Burns and Scalds

- Burns and scalds can result from hot liquids, hot objects, flames, chemicals or electricity.
- Burns are caused by the application to the skin of dry heat, and the depth of the burn will depend on the temperature of the object and the length of time it is in contact with the skin.

TABLE 1.12 – Types of Bone Fractures
Greenstick
The bones bend rather than break. This is a very common accidental injury in children.
Transverse
The break goes across the bone and occurs when there is a direct blow or a direct force on the end of the bone (e.g. a fall on the hand may break the forearm bones or the distal humerus).
Spiral or oblique
A fracture line that goes right around the bone or obliquely across it is due to a twisting force, which may be a feature in non-accidental injuries.
Metaphyseal
These fractures occur at the extreme ends of the bone and are usually only confirmed radiologically. These are caused by a strong twisting force.
Skull
These must be consistent with the history and explanation given. Complex (branched), depressed or fractures at the back of the skull are suspect of abuse.
Rib
These do not occur accidentally, except in a severe crushing injury. Any other cause is highly suspicious of non-accidental injury.

- Abusive burns are frequently small and deep, and may show the outline of the object (e.g. the soleplate of an iron), whereas accidental burns rarely do so because the child will pull away in response to pain.
- Cigarette burns are not common. They are round, deep and have a red flare around a flat brown crust. These burns usually leave a scar.
- Scalds are caused by steam or hot liquids. Accidental scalds may be extensive but show splash marks unlike the sharp edges of damage done when the child is dunked in hot water (although splash marks may also feature in a non-accidental burn indicating that the child had tried to escape hot water). The glove and stocking pattern of burns on the arms and legs is typical of non-accidental injury. The head, face, neck, shoulders and front of the chest are the areas affected when a child pulls over a kettle accidentally.

5.3 Bite Marks

Bites result in small bruises forming part or all of a circle. They are usually oval or circular in shape. There may be visible wounds, indentations or bruising from individual teeth.

5.4 Deliberate Poisoning and Attempted Suffocation

These are very difficult to assess and may need a period of close observation in hospital. Deliberate poisoning, such as might be found in a child in whom illness is fabricated or induced by carers with parenting responsibilities (fictitious or induced illness), may be suspected when a child has repeated puzzling illnesses, usually of sudden onset. The signs include unusual drowsiness, apnoeic attacks, vomiting, diarrhoea and fits. There may be respiratory problems due to suffocation.

6. Older Children and Adolescents

- If the injury is accidental, older children will give a very clear and detailed account of how it happened. The detail will be missing if they have been told what to say.
- Overdosing and other self-harm injuries must be taken seriously in this age group, as they may indicate sexual or other abuse (such as exploitation).

6.1 Parental Factors

Parental unavailability for whatever reason increases the risk to the child of all forms of abuse, especially neglect and emotional abuse. Specific consideration of the effects of the parent's problem on the children must be made, whatever the circumstances of presentation. Sources of stress within families may have a negative impact on a child's health, development or well-being, either directly or because they affect the capacity of parents to respond to their child's needs. Sources of stress may include social exclusion, domestic abuse, unstable mental illness of a parent or carer, or drug and alcohol misuse. Parents who appear overanxious about their child when there is no sign of illness or injury may be signalling their inability to cope.

Parental factors that might have a negative impact on parenting capacity include:

- learning difficulties
- mental health problems
- substance abuse
- domestic abuse
- chronic ill health
- physical disability
- unemployment or poverty
- homelessness/frequent moves
- social isolation
- young, unsupported parents
- parents with poor role models of their own
- lack of, or poor, education
- criminality
- unwanted or unplanned pregnancy.

7. Special Circumstances

7.1 Individuals Who Pose a Risk to Children

- Once an individual has been sentenced and identified as presenting a risk of harm to children, agencies have a responsibility to work collaboratively to monitor and manage the risk of harm to others.
- Where an offender is given a community sentence, Offender Managers or Youth Offending Team workers will monitor the individual's risk of harm to others and their behaviour, and liaise with partner agencies as appropriate.
- Multi-Agency Public Protection Arrangements (MAPPA) should be in place to enable agencies to work together within a statutory framework for managing risk of harm to the public.
- There are certain work forces that are exempt from the Rehabilitation of Offenders Act 1974. Patient-facing roles within the ambulance service are part of this. Safer recruitment checks will be undertaken including an enhanced DBS (Disclosure and Barring Service).

7.2 Disabled Children

Abuse may be difficult to separate from symptoms of disability (e.g. increase in seizures in a child with epilepsy if anticonvulsants are withheld). Induced and fabricated illness may be even more difficult to recognise because the child may have coexistent diagnoses.

Important points to remember about abuse of disabled children are:

- It may be more common than abuse of non-disabled children, but evidence for this is poor.
- It may be under-reported.
- Children may have difficulty communicating their abuse.
- Abuse may compound pre-existing disability, or be the cause of the disability.
- All forms of abuse are seen, including neglect and sexual abuse.
- It is easy to fail to recognise abuse in disabled children by making too many allowances for the disability as a cause of problems.
- Be aware that professionals can be drawn into collusion with families; this is a term known as 'disguised compliance'.

These children are at risk of achieving poor outcomes. Ambulance clinicians need to be aware of the role they can play in recognition of these children, identifying their particular needs and preventing significant harm. In the current multicultural society of the United Kingdom, it is important to recognise that there may be children and families in need of skilled interpreters, and that differences may exist in child-rearing practices in minority groups.

7.3 Special Circumstances for Consideration

- **Children and young people living away from home** – many looked-after children and young people that live independently have been abused or neglected prior to going into care. This is a particular group where assessment may be made more difficult, because of pre-existing symptoms and behaviour. There should be a low threshold for seeking advice from experienced professionals in these circumstances (e.g. designated/named professional).
- **Asylum-seeking children or refugees, both with families and unaccompanied** – the importance of having skilled interpreters in assessment of these children cannot be over-emphasised. The children's behaviour on entering the country may already have been influenced by previous experience. It is important to remember their general health needs and that families will need help in accessing services. It is also important to refer children who are victims of human trafficking.
- **Children with maladjusted parent(s)/carers** (see also Parental Factors) – these include children of substance-misusing parents/carers, children living with domestic abuse, children whose parents/carers have chronic mental or physical health problems, children whose parents/carers have a learning disability, children with a parent/carer in prison, and children living in flexi-families. Effects on the child/ren can be profound and include fearfulness, withdrawal, anxious behaviour, lack of self-confidence and social skills, difficulties in forming relationships, sleep disturbance, non-attendance at school, aggression, bullying, post-traumatic stress disorder, and behaviour suggestive of ADHD.

The following children may also have unmet health needs (low immunisation levels, poor dental health and either poor or non-attendance at clinic appointments).

- **Children in the armed forces** – extra strains are placed upon the families engendered by frequent moves, frequent changes of school, separation of parents by the nature of the job, and separation from immediate support from family and friends.
- **Children of travelling families** – these children are subjected to the same problems because of frequent moves. They may also suffer from poor health, poor access to primary healthcare and vaccinations, in addition to poor living conditions.
- **Runaway children and exploitation** – many runaway children may already have been the subject of abuse and are at risk of exploitation. They are also at risk of child trafficking for sexual exploitation.
- **Children as young carers** – neglect and emotional abuse may be part of the difficulties of taking on parental responsibilities and a caring role at a young age. Young carers lose out on normal childhood experiences and should be considered at higher risk of abuse whether intentional or unintentional (e.g. school attendance, peer groups).

8. Mandatory Reporting of Female Genital Mutilation (FGM)

On 31st October 2015 the FGM Act introduced a mandatory reporting duty that requires health and social care professionals as well as teachers to report known cases of FGM in those under 18 years of age to the police.

FGM is child abuse and the current procedure is set out below:

- **Children and vulnerable adults** – if any child (under 18) or vulnerable adult has symptoms or signs of FGM, or if there is good reason to suspect they are at risk of FGM on consideration of their family history or other relevant factors, they **must** be referred using existing safeguarding procedures as with all instances of child abuse. This will involve referral to police and social care in the usual way.
- In all cases where staff are unsure of their actions, they should seek the advice of the Trust Safeguarding Service.

9. Assessment and Management

If physical, sexual, or emotional abuse or neglect is suspected, follow local procedures; information can be obtained from the named professional for safeguarding within individual ambulance Trusts. Ambulance clinicians may obtain contact information from ambulance control.

9.1 If the Child is the Patient

- The first priority is the health and safety of the child. Ambulance clinicians should follow the usual **ABCDE** and **<C>ABCDE** assessment (refer to **Medical Emergencies in Children – Overview** and **Trauma Emergencies in Children – Overview**). Children with significant injury should be transferred to further care without delay.
- Where a child is thought to be at immediate risk, they should be referred to the police as an emergency by contacting ambulance control for a 999 response.

In all circumstances:

- Limit questions to those of routine history taking, asking questions only in relation to the injury or for clarification of what is being said. It is important to stop questioning when suspicions are clarified. Unnecessary questioning or probing may affect the credibility of subsequent evidence.
- Accept the explanations given and do not make any suggestions to the child as to how an injury or incident may have happened.
- Care must be taken not to directly accuse parents or carers of abuse as this may result in a refusal to transfer to further care and place the child at further risk. Always work in partnership with parents or carers as far as possible, and inform them of concerns and the need to share these with the statutory agencies, unless to do so would put the child or others at greater risk of harm. Professional curiosity and judgement is crucial as to what information should be shared with parents.
- Any allegation of abuse made by a child is an important indicator and should always be taken seriously – it is important to listen to the 'voice of the child' and what they are saying. Do not ask probing questions. Consider what is a 'safe space' for them to talk.
- Adult responses can influence how able a child feels to reveal the full extent of the abuse. Listen and react appropriately to instil confidence. It is important to note that children may only tell a small part of their experience initially.
- It is important to make an accurate record of events and actions. Write down exactly what the child says. Their first language may not be English and care must be taken not to use family members or carers as interpreters in cases of suspected abuse. Take note of any inconsistency in history and any delay in calling for assistance.
- On arrival at hospital inform the receiving staff and the most senior member of nursing staff on duty of any concerns or suspicions. When reporting suspected abuse, the emphasis must be on shared professional responsibility and immediate communication.
- Complete safeguarding documentation/report as per local procedures; complete in private if possible. Follow local/Trust protocols/guidelines.
- Ambulance clinicians must report suspected child abuse to the relevant statutory bodies (e.g. social care and the police), but they do not have a statutory duty to investigate it.
- Where a practitioner feels that their concerns have not been taken up (commonly known as professional challenge), they have a duty to escalate their concerns to a higher level by discussing this with their line manager, a more experienced colleague or named/designated doctor or nurse.

9.2 If the Child is Not the Patient

- If the circumstances are suspicious, the ambulance clinician(s) should consider the implications of leaving the child.
- If the child is accompanying another person (e.g. a parent/carer) who is being conveyed, the ambulance clinician(s) should inform ED staff of their concerns and remember to report through their own safeguarding services as required.
- If no one is transferred to hospital, follow local/Trust protocols/guidelines and inform safeguarding services of the incident/concerns at the earliest opportunity.
- Complete safeguarding documentation/report as per local procedures; complete in private if possible. Follow local/Trust protocols/guidelines.

9.3 Allegations Against Ambulance Clinicians

- An allegation made by a child against an ambulance clinician is no different from an allegation made against any other healthcare professional, and the appropriate procedures should be followed, that is a referral to social care or the police. In other words, a child protection inquiry must follow such allegations.
- No staff, regardless of their position, volunteer, commissioned service or person associated with delivering services on behalf of an NHS Trust, must act in any way that constitutes any of the following:
  - Behaviour that harms, or may harm, a child, young person or adult.
  - Behaviour that results in a criminal offence against, or related to, a child, young person or adult.

  - Behaviour towards a child, young person or adult that indicates s/he is unsuitable to work in a position of trust.
- The member of staff who is alleged to have abused the child must report the allegation to his/her line manager/named professional, who should follow employment procedures, that is a possible restriction of practice or suspension while investigations are conducted. There should be close liaison between the police carrying out the investigation and the line manager/named professional, who should be guided by the police as to how much information about the inquiry should be relayed to the member of staff. There will also need to be a support system in place for the member of staff.

KEY POINTS!

Safeguarding children

- **The safety and welfare of the child is paramount.**
- **There is a duty to report concerns. Staff should not investigate suspicions themselves.**
- **Be aware of any special circumstances that the child is in which may increase the risk of abuse.**
- **Police should be involved where there may be an immediate risk to the child.**
- **Staff should document the circumstances giving rise to their concern as soon as possible.**

Further Reading

Further important information and evidence in support of this guideline can be found in the Bibliography.[3,4,5,6,7,8,9,10]

Other useful resources include:

Barnado's – http://www.barnados.org.uk/

Child Exploitation and Online Protection Command – http://www.ceop.gov.uk

Childline – http://www.childline.org.uk/

Children's Legal Centre – http://www.childrenslegalcentre.com

Every Child Matters – http://www.everychildmatters.co.uk/

Family Lives – http://www.familylives.org.uk/

Kidscape – http://www.kidscape.org.uk

National Service Framework for Children, Young People and Maternity Services – https://www.gov.uk/government/publications/national-service-framework-children-young-people-and-maternity-services

NSPCC – http://www.nspcc.org.uk

Samaritans – http://www.samaritans.org.uk

Think You Know – http://www.thinkuknow.co.uk/

Victim Support – http://www.victimsupport.org.uk

Victoria Climbié Inquiry – https://www.gov.uk/government/uploads/system/uploads/attachment_data/file/273183/5730.pdf

Bibliography

1. Department of Health. *The Children Act 1989*. London: HMSO, 1989. Available from: https://www.gov.uk/government/uploads/system/uploads/attachment_data/file/441643/Children_Act_Guidance_2015.pdf.
2. Department for Children, Schools and Families. *Working Together to Safeguard Children: A guide to interagency working to safeguard and promote the welfare of children*. London: HMSO, 2015. Available from: https://www.gov.uk/government/publications/working-together-to-safeguard-children--2.
3. National Institute for Health and Clinical Excellence. *When to Suspect Child Maltreatment* (CG89). London: NICE, 2009. Available from: https://www.nice.org.uk/guidance/cg89.
4. Department of Children, Schools and Families. *Safeguarding Disabled Children – Practice guidance*. London: HMSO, 2009. Available from: https://www.gov.uk/government/uploads/system/uploads/attachment_data/file/190544/00374-2009DOM-EN.pdf.
5. Department of Health. *The Data Protection Act 2018*. London: HMSO, 2018. Available from: http://www.legislation.gov.uk/ukpga/2018/12/contents/enacted.
6. Department of Health. *Responding to Domestic Abuse: A handbook for health professionals*. London: HMSO, 2005.
7. Department of Health. *Women's Mental Health: Into the mainstream*. London: HMSO, 2002.
8. Department of Health. *Improving Safety, Reducing Harm – Children, young people and domestic violence*. London: HMSO, 2009.
9. Home Office. *Adoption and Children Act 2002*. London: HMSO, 2002. Available from: http://www.legislation.gov.uk/ukpga/2002/38/contents.
10. Home Office. *Female Genital Mutilation Act 2003*. London: HMSO, 2003. Available from: http://www.legislation.gov.uk/ukpga/2003/31/pdfs/ukpga_20030031_en.pdf.

11. Krug E, Dahlberg L, Mercy J, Zwi A. Lozano R. *World Report on Violence and Health*. Geneva: World Health Organisation, 2002.

12. O'Keefe M. Predictors of child abuse in martially violent homes. *Journal of Interpersonal Violence* 1995, 10: 3–25.

13. Royal College of Paediatrics and Child Health. *Safeguarding Children and Young People: Roles and competences for health care staff.* Available from: http://www.rcpch.ac.uk/sites/default/files/asset_library/Education%20Department/Safeguarding/Safeguarding%20Children%20and%20Young%20people%202010G.pdf. 2010.

14. Scottish Parliament. *Prohibition of Female Genital Mutilation (Scotland) Act 2005*. Edinburgh: HMSO, 2005. Available from: http://www.refworld.org/pdfid/47d159902.pdf.

15. Sullivan PM, Knutson JF. Maltreatment and Disabilities: A population-based epidemiological study. *Child Abuse and Neglect* 2000, 24(10): 1257–1273.

16. Taskforce on the Health Aspects of Violence Against Women and Children Improving Safety. *Responding to Violence Against Women and Children – the role of the NHS.* Available from: http://www.fflm.ac.uk/wp-content/uploads/documentstore/1268669895.pdf, 2010.

17. Walby S, Allen J. *Domestic Violence, Sexual Assault and Stalking: Findings from the British Crime Survey*. Home Office Research Study 276. Available from: http://womensaidorkney.org.uk/wp-content/uploads/2014/08/Home-office-research.pdf, 2004.

18. WHO/UNICEF/UNFPA. *Female Genital Mutilation: A joint statement*. Geneva: WHO. Available from: http://apps.who.int/iris/bitstream/10665/41903/1/9241561866.pdf, 1997.

19. World Health Organization. *Eliminating Female Genital Mutilation: An interagency statement*. Geneva: WHO. Available from: http://www.un.org/womenwatch/daw/csw/csw52/statements_missions/Interagency_Statement_on_Eliminating_FGM.pdf, 2008.

Sexual Assault

1. Introduction

- Sexual assault is extremely distressing, causing a broad spectrum of psychological, emotional and physical effects on patients. They may be agitated or hysterical, in shock or disbelief, or calm and extremely controlled. Clinicians should understand there is no 'normal' response and have no expectation of the patient exhibiting a prescribed pattern of behaviour.[1]
- It may be appropriate for the patient to be accompanied by another person. The patient may be anxious when left alone with a person of the same sex as the assailant. On the other hand, they may be reassured by the presence of a professional person. The wishes of the patient must be considered and attempts made to reassure them and make them feel safe.
- The patient has just experienced a major psychological and potentially physical trauma, often committed by someone they believed in and trusted. The clinician must not only manage their physical, medical and psychological needs, but must absolutely act as the patient's advocate, facilitating their wishes wherever possible.
- Patients experiencing sexual assault may believe they are responsible for the assault and need reassuring that they are victims and what has happened was not their fault.[2]
- A sensitive and kind approach by those providing an initial response is known to be beneficial in facilitating recovery and decreasing long-term use of health services post rape. In contrast, health professionals inexperienced in dealing with survivors, who use insensitive language, subscribe to rape myths and stereotypes, who are judgemental, inconsiderate or critical, are known to increase the risk of revictimising the survivor, delaying recovery, sometimes forever.[3]
- Importantly, victims of sexual violence must be treated with respect and dignity irrespective of either the victim's or the clinician's social status, race, religion, culture, sexual orientation, lifestyle, sex or occupation.[1]
- It is not the role of the clinician to determine if the assault has occurred; that is the job of the courts. Instead they must provide a sensitive, non-judgemental, holistic approach that is neither moralistic nor opinionated. Victims who blame themselves, or fear being blamed or doubted, are less likely to report sexual assault. Recovery may also be hampered by the blame or disbelief of others, whether real or perceived. Body language, gestures and facial expressions all contribute to conveying an atmosphere of believing the patient's account, which is known to be critical to recovery.[4]
- The intimate nature of sexual assault, combined with the inevitable feelings of guilt and shame these patients experience, complicates their care. During the assault, they may have seen, experienced and been forced to do things that are outside their normal moral or ethical code. They may believe it to be unspeakable.
- Many victims cite fear of not being believed as a reason for not reporting sexual assault and recovery may be hindered when others disbelieve or blame the patient for the assault. Validation of the patient's feelings is thus critical to recovery.[3] Body language, gestures and facial expressions all contribute to conveying an atmosphere of believing the patient's account.

2. Disclosure to Police

- Some patients will refuse care or transfer to hospital because they believe police may be informed without their consent and fear perceived catastrophic consequences. Historically, reporting without patient consent has been common practice amongst both control room and operational staff of all levels.
- The decision to report a sexual assault on an adult is entirely the decision of the victim. There is no statutory obligation for victims of sexual violence to report to police and many victims elect not to report to protect their safety, privacy or both.[5]
- Similarly, no statutory obligation mandates the reporting by healthcare professionals of cases involving rape or sexual assault.[5] Where the patient is an adult with full capacity to consent, and is not classed as 'vulnerable', there is no requirement for clinicians to breach confidentiality and report to police without consent. Control room staff should not routinely inform police and request their attendance unless this is the specific wish of the patient, and no attempt to persuade or coerce the patient to agree to police attendance should be made by anyone involved in their care pathway at any time.[6,7]
- The only exception to this would be where disclosing the information is necessary to prevent a serious crime or serious harm to others. Generally, if the ambulance service is involved, the serious crime has already occurred. Unless there are reasonable grounds to assume there is imminent risk to either the patient or the public, the patient's decision, as an autonomous adult, should be fully respected.[8]
- Where it is perceived there is a clear and present immediate danger to the patient or others if disclosure to police is not made, and that risk is greater than the possible consequences to the patient of disclosure, then it would be appropriate to breach that confidentiality.

3. Forensic Requirements

- Where the victim requests police involvement, forensic awareness is essential. Within the limits of any immediate care needs, there is a responsibility to preserve evidence. Where police are on scene and injuries do not require emergent care, the police will normally take responsibility for the patient.[9]
- While awaiting police arrival patients should be kept within the environment in which they present, unless this is unsafe or increasing the patient's distress; if so, they can be moved to the ambulance, seated on a clean sheet and wherever possible discouraged from any activities that jeopardise collection of evidence. This will include cutting, removing or changing clothing, eating or drinking, passing urine or opening bowels or washing.[9]
- Where the patient cannot be dissuaded from the natural need to clean themselves, they should be encouraged to place any tissues or towels along with any bloodstained clothes into paper (not plastic) bags, which do not destroy biological evidence.[9]
- Where patients are transported to hospital and police action is requested, all blankets, sheets, towels and associated paraphernalia should be passed to police for forensic retrieval.[9]

Additional forensic information:

- Where patients have not presented for immediate care following rape, clinicians should be aware of how long forensic material may be preserved within the patient. The approximate times after contact for which evidentially relevant material has been identified – the 'forensic window' - is detailed in Table 1.13.
- Differences exist between pre- and post-pubescent patients; this is because the vaginal area is hostile to semen in the pre-pubescent patient.

4. Care Pathways

As primary caregiver and advocate, clinicians should inform the patient of their options without judgement, bias or coercion. Any physical examination should allow identification of life-threatening injuries and those requiring emergent care only. Genital areas should only be exposed and examined if there is evidence of bleeding requiring immediate treatment.

Allow the patient space and as much choice about options for their treatment as possible. Options for the care of sexual assault victims may be summarised as:

- **Accident and Emergency**:
  - if the victim has injuries requiring emergent care
  - if the level of distress makes it impossible for the patient to consent or coherently express their wishes.
- **Police**:
  - only where the patient gives express and informed consent as discussed above.
- **Sexual Assault Referral Centres (SARC)**:
  - SARCs provide recent victims of sexual assault with immediate care and crisis support from specialist staff trained to allow patients to make informed decisions. They also provide access to acute physical assessment with testing for STIs, provision of post-infection prophylaxis and emergency contraception.[10]
  - SARCs also facilitate access to the criminal justice system. Forensic retrieval may be undertaken regardless of whether the patient reports to police or not. Where the patient decides not to report, forensic samples may be stored, allowing patients time to consider their options until after the immediate 'crisis period'.[10]
  - SARCs provide direct access to Independent Sexual Violence Advisers (ISVAs) who provide advice, support and access to follow-up services addressing the patient's medical, safeguarding, psychosocial and ongoing needs.
  - ISVAs will also support patients through the judicial process; importantly, patients supported by ISVAs are more likely to go through the full course of criminal justice

TABLE 1.13 – Preservation of Forensic Material[9]

Type of Incident	Type of Sample	Forensic Window
Digital penetration	Vulval, vaginal, peri-anal and anal swabs	Up to 12 hours
Oral penetration	Mouth swabs and oral rinse	Up to 48 hours – even where the patient has eaten, drunk or brushed their teeth
Anal penetration	Peri-anal, perineal, internal anal and rectal swabs Penile swabs	Up to 72 hours
Vaginal penetration	Vulval, vaginal and endocervical swabs	Pre-pubescent: Up to 72 hours Post-pubescent: Up to 120 hours

SECTION 1 General Guidance

proceedings, which highlights the importance of encouraging patients to access SARCs wherever possible.[11]

4.1. Access to SARCs

- **Self-referral** – patients may self-refer to SARCs by telephone; clinicians may also call on the patient's behalf. Patients have a brief conversation with a crisis worker who helps them decide on an immediate plan and makes an appointment for them to attend. Where this appointment is immediate, subject to time constraints and local protocols, ambulance crews may transport the patient directly to the SARC or alternatively make certain the patient will be able to be taken safely by a third party.
- Local SARC contact details should be held centrally by ambulance control rooms; they are also available on NHS Choices.
- **Police referral** – the patient reports to police, who contact the SARC and arrange for the patient to be transferred.

4.2. Refusal of Care

- Patients refusing referral to support services place a duty of care on clinicians to ensure their immediate safety. Encouraging patients to call a friend or relative for support is a priority. In these cases, patients should be given details of their nearest GUM clinic and rape crisis services. These conversations require tact and sensitivity as patients may not have considered risks of STIs or pregnancy, and this alone may create another crisis.
- In cases of sexual assault in vulnerable adults and children refer to **Safeguarding Adults at Risk** and **Safeguarding Children**.

5. Incidence

- Approximately 11 adults are raped every hour in England and Wales. That amounts to 85,000 women and 12,000 men becoming victims of rape every year, while nearly half a million adults are sexually assaulted.
- Of these, 90% know the perpetrator prior to the offence, and only around 15% of these will choose to report to police.[12]
- In 2012–13, 23,663 sexual offences against children were reported to police in England and Wales including 6,296 rapes, with 80% of these involving girls.[13]
- Given this incidence, as a profession, paramedics should be well versed in the care of this most vulnerable group and have a comprehensive understanding of the care pathways and services available to them.

6. Severity and Outcome

- The severity of the assault can vary from sexual touching to sustaining life-threatening injuries. The outcome of the assault can lead to long-term psychological and physical effects.

7. Pathophysiology

The Sexual Offences Act (2003) defines four offences:[14]

- Rape – penetration of the vagina, anus or mouth with a penis without consent.
- Assault by penetration – non-consensual, intentional insertion of an object (other than a penis) into the vagina or anus.
- Sexual assault – non-consensual violation of the victim's sexual anatomy, e.g. touching another person in a sexual way without consent.
- Causing a person to engage in sexual activity without consent.

8. Assessment and Management

For the assessment and management of sexual assault refer to Table 1.14.

TABLE 1.14 – ASSESSMENT and MANAGEMENT of: Sexual Assault

ASSESSMENT	MANAGEMENT
● Assess **<C>ABCD**	If any TIME CRITICAL features present major ABCD problems: ● start correcting <C>ABCD problems ● undertake a TIME CRITICAL transfer to nearest receiving hospital ● continue patient management en-route ● provide an ATMIST information call.
● Assess	● Limit questions to those identifying the need for medical treatment, but allow the patient to talk and document what is said. **NB** It is not appropriate to probe for details of the assault and could affect the outcome of criminal investigations.

(continued)

TABLE 1.14 – Assessment and Management of: Sexual Assault *(continued)*	
ASSESSMENT	**MANAGEMENT**
	• Manage according to condition: – Acute injury – refer to **Trauma Emergencies in Adults – Overview** and **Trauma Emergencies in Children – Overview** – Acute illness – refer to **Medical Emergencies in Adults – Overview** and **Medical Emergencies in Children – Overview**. • It may be appropriate to delay assessment for non-urgent injuries until transfer to a Sexual Assault Referral Centre to avoid further distress and disturbing the evidence.
• Approach	• Rape is about power and control, not the sexual act. Listen to the patient with a sensitive and respectful manner and return control to them. • Establish the patient's safety. • Let the patient know you believe them. • If possible, ensure privacy. • Consider cultural/religious issues. • Where possible accommodate patient's requests. • Where possible avoid disturbing the scene. • Where possible avoid being alone with the patient. • Patients are not required by law to report sexual violence to police. • Healthcare professionals are not required by law to report cases of sexual violence to police unless: – the patient does not have capacity to consent – the patient is classed as 'vulnerable' – there is a clear and present danger of immediate risk to the patient or public. • No attempt should be made to persuade the patient to agree to police attendance; decision making should be facilitated by presenting available options. • Where this is requested, police should be called promptly so the scene may be secured. • Where patients decline any support or referral, they should be encouraged to obtain community support ensuring their ongoing safety is secured. These patients should be encouraged to contact their nearest GUM clinic or local rape crisis services with tact and care.
• Forensic examination	• Forensic examination will focus specifically on the areas affected, including wounds, mouth, anus and vagina and other areas where the patient has been kissed, licked or bitten, as these areas may well be contaminated with the assailant's DNA. • Clinicians should be aware of forensic windows, and where this is relevant patients should be encouraged **not** to: – wash (shower/bathe) or brush their teeth – change clothes, throw away or destroy clothes – urinate – the police will want to collect early evidence samples including a urine sample to screen for the presence of drugs, as some drugs have a very short half-life – smoke, eat or drink – a mouth swab and mouth wash may also be requested by the police – defecate. • If a blanket is required for modesty or warmth, a single-use blanket should be used and kept with the patient – the blanket needs to be retained in order to analyse cross-contamination.

TABLE 1.14 – Assessment and Management of: Sexual Assault *(continued)*	
ASSESSMENT	**MANAGEMENT**
	● If the patient is not wrapped in a single-use blanket, place a sterile sheet or single-use blanket under the patient where they sit or lie and retain for forensic examination. ● Avoid cleaning any wounds unless clinically absolutely necessary – if possible keep 'washings'. ● If required, lightly apply dry dressings – retain any used dressing and swabs for forensic examination; also keep the sterile packets in which they were contained in order to examine for cross-contamination. **NB** All of these recommendations are vital to conserve evidence for a successful prosecution of the offender; BUT the need for this approach must be conveyed with great sensitivity to the patient, who may well want to wash and change.
● Care pathways	**Accident and Emergency is appropriate:** ● if the patient has injuries requiring emergency care ● if the level of distress makes it impossible for them to consent or coherently express their wishes. **Sexual Assault Referral Centres can provide:** ● immediate care and crisis support ● acute physical assessment ● testing for STIs ● post-infection prophylaxis ● emergency contraception ● access to the criminal justice system ● forensic retrieval with storage where police involvement is declined ● access to ISVA services ● access to follow-up services addressing medical, safeguarding, psychosocial and ongoing needs. Access to SARCs, where the patient consents, is either by: ● **Self referral** – the patient telephones the SARC themselves (this can easily be initiated by the ambulance crew), who give them an appointment normally within a few hours unless they are busy. There is no reason why ambulance crews – subject to local protocols and time restraints, should not transport the patient directly to the SARC or alternatively make certain the patient will be able to be taken safely by a third party. ● **Police referral** – the patient reports to police, who make contact with the SARC and arrange for the patient to be transferred. **Sexual Health Clinics provide treatment for:** ● sexually transmitted infections ● emergency contraception ● post-exposure prophylaxis. **Rape Crisis Centres provide:** ● confidential telephone helpline and support ● face-to-face counselling for survivors of rape or sexual assault ● ISVA services ● handover to an appropriate member of staff and not in a public area. Where a patient is competent and refuses hospital treatment, advise them to seek further medical attention. They may need post-exposure prophylaxis, vaccination and/or contraception, all of which can be provided confidentially.

(continued)

Sexual Assault

TABLE 1.14 – Assessment and Management of: Sexual Assault *(continued)*	
ASSESSMENT	**MANAGEMENT**
• Documentation	• Complete the clinical record in great detail contemporaneously and document: – only facts, not personal opinion – what the patient says – clinical findings with relevant timings – the ambulance identification number. • A police statement may be required later.

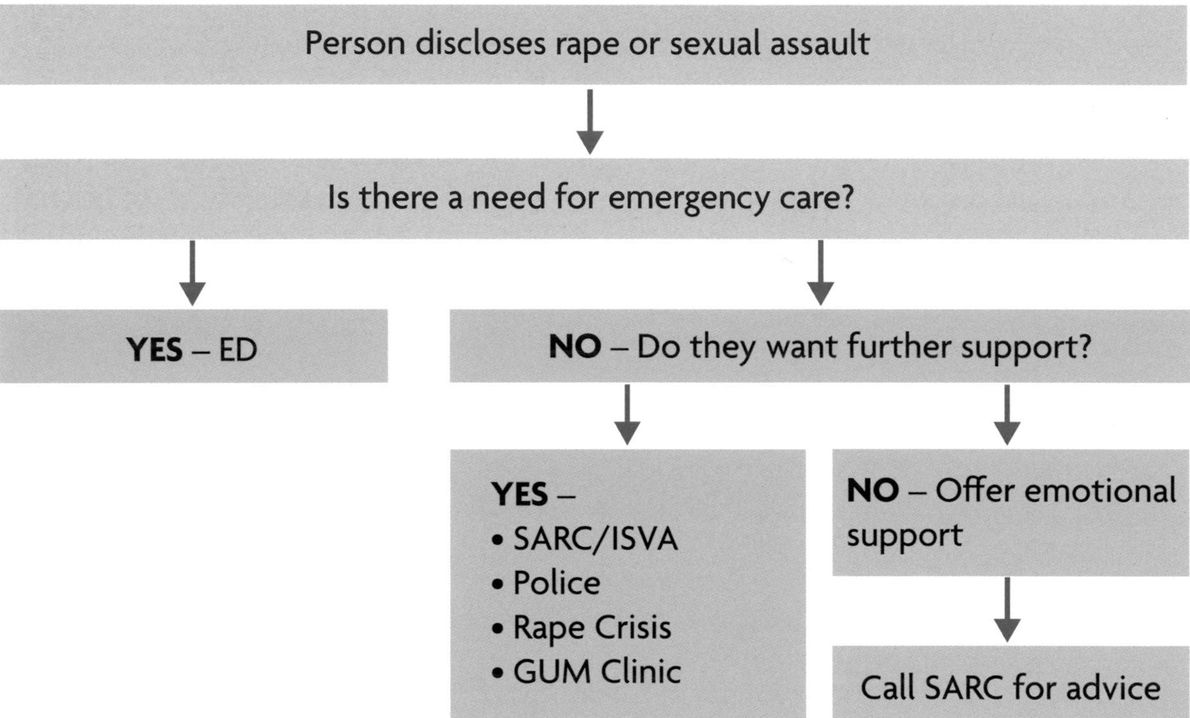

Figure 1.5 – Assessment and management of sexual assault.

KEY POINTS!

Sexual Assault

- **Sexual assault may be concurrent with other injuries that will need treating.**
- **Treatment should avoid disturbing evidence where possible.**
- **The patient's rights to autonomy should be respected unless they do not have capacity to consent or are 'vulnerable'.**
- **Leave the investigation to the police.**
- **Accommodate the patient's wishes where possible.**
- **Police may have special facilities for managing patients.**

Further Reading

Further important information and evidence in support of this guideline can be found in the Bibliography.[15,16,17,18,19,20,21,22,23]

Sexual Assault

Bibliography

1. World Health Organization. *Guidelines for Medico-legal Care for Victims of Sexual Violence*. Geneva: WHO, 2003. Available from: http://apps.who.int/iris/bitstream/10665/42788/1/924154628X.pdf.
2. Beckmann CR, Groetzinger LL. Treating sexual assault victims. A protocol for health professionals. *Female Patient* 1989, 14(5): 78–83.
3. Ranibar V, Speer SA. Revictimization and recovery from sexual assault: implications for health professionals. *Violence and Victims* 2013, 28(2): 274–287.
4. Dunn S, Gilchrist V. Sexual Assault. Primary Care 1993, 20: 359–373.
5. Department of Health. *Public Health Functions to be exercised by NHS England - Service Specification No 30, Sexual Assault Services*. London: HMSO, 2013. Available from: https://www.gov.uk/government/uploads/system/uploads/attachment_data/file/256501/30_sexual_assault_services.pdf.
6. British Association for Sexual Health and HIV. *UK National Guidelines on the Management of Adult and Adolescent Complainants of Sexual Assault 2011. Macclesfield: BASHH, 2011*. Available from: http://www.nordhaven.co.uk/BASHH.PDF.
7. Department of Health. *Confidentiality: NHS Code of Practice*. London: HMSO, 2003.
8. Department of Health. Confidentiality: *NHS Code of Practice Supplementary Guidance on Public Interest Disclosures*. London: HMSO, 2010.
9. Crown Prosecution Service. *Prosecution Policy and Guidance; Legal Guidance; Rape and Sexual offences: Forensic, Scientific and Medical Evidence*. Available from: https://www.cps.gov.uk/legal-guidance/rape-and-sexual-offences-chapter-9-forensic-scientific-and-medical-evidence.
10. Department of Health, Home Office, Association of Chief Police Officers. *Revised National Service Guide – A Resource for Developing Sexual Assault Referral Centres*. London: HMSO, 2009. Available from: https://www.sericc.org.uk/pdfs/4313_sacentres.pdf.
11. Robinson AL. *Independent Sexual Violence Advisers: A process evaluation*. University of Cardiff funded by the Home Office, 2009. Available from: http://library.college.police.uk/docs/horr/horr20.pdf.
12. Ministry of Justice, Home Office and Office of National Statistics. *An Overview of Sexual Offending in England and Wales*. London: HMSO, 2013. Available from: https://www.gov.uk/government/statistics/an-overview-of-sexual-offending-in-england-and-wales.
13. Jutte S. et al. *How Safe Are Our Children?* London: NSPCC, 2014.
14. Legislation.gov.uk. Sexual Offences Act (2003). Available from: http://www.legislation.gov.uk/ukpga/2003/42/part/1.
15. Avegno J, Mills TJ, Mills LD. Sexual assault victims in the emergency department: analysis by demographic and event characteristics. *Journal of Emergency Medicine* 2009, 37(3): 328–334.
16. Dalton M. *Forensic Gynaecology: Towards better care of the female victim of sexual assault.* London: Royal College of Obstetricians and Gynaecologists Press, 2004.
17. Department of Health. *Improving Services for Women and Child Victims of Violence: The Department of Health Action Plan.* Available from: http://www.dh.gov.uk/prod_consum_dh/groups/dh_digitalassets/@dh/@en/@ps/documents/digitalasset/dh_122094.pdf, 2010.
18. Du Mont J, White D, McGregor MJ. Investigating the medical forensic examination from the perspectives of sexually assaulted women. *Social Science and Medicine* 2009, 68(4): 774–780.
19. Martin EK, Taft CT, Resick PA. A review of marital rape. *Aggression and Violent Behavior* 2007, 12(3): 329–347.
20. Mein JK, Palmer CM, Shand MC, Templeton DJ, Parekh V, Mobbs M et al. Management of acute adult sexual assault. *Medical Journal of Australia* 2003, 178(5): 226–230.
21. Pesola GR, Westfal RE, Kuffner CA. Emergency department characteristics of male sexual assault. *Academic Emergency Medicine* 1999, 6(8): 792–798.
22. Regan L, Lovett J, Kelly L. *Forensic Nursing: An option for improving responses to reported rape and sexual assault.* London: Home Office, 2004.
23. Taskforce on the Health Aspects of Violence Against Women and Children Improving Safety. *Responding to Violence Against Women and Children – the role of the NHS.* Available from: http://www.fflm.ac.uk/wp-content/uploads/documentstore/1268669895.pdf, 2010.

Safeguarding Adults at Risk

1. Introduction

- Everyone has the right to live their life free from harm. Safeguarding adults at risk from significant harm is reliant on effective joint working and communication between agencies and professionals.
- This guidance is for the management of people aged 18 years and over; for those under 18 years, refer to **Safeguarding Children**.
- Ambulance clinicians are often the first professionals to make contact with an adult at risk and may identify initial concerns regarding abuse. The role of the ambulance service is not to investigate suspicions but to ensure that any suspicion is passed, with the consent of the adult (where no consent, state why), to the appropriate agency (e.g. social care or the police) in line with locally agreed procedures.
- Ambulance clinicians need to be aware of local policies and procedures relating to the abuse of vulnerable adults. The aim of this guideline is to assist ambulance clinicians to recognise and report cases (with consent) of suspected abuse of adults at risk.
- The principles of adult protection differ from those of child protection in that adults have the right to take risks and may choose to live at risk if they have the capacity to make such a decision (refer to **Mental Capacity Act 2005**).
- Anyone can be a victim of abuse.
- An abuser may be anyone, including a friend or family member, carer or professional involved in delivering care to the adult.

The introduction of the Care Act 2014[1] provides a statutory framework to safeguard adults at risk of abuse or neglect. The Care Act puts the wishes and experience of the adult at the centre of safeguarding and is a move away from the previous process-led culture.

2. Making Safeguarding Personal

2.1 'No decision about me without me'[2]

Under the Care Act 2014 there has been a move away from process-led practice to a person-centred approach that works in partnership with the adult to achieve the outcomes that they need to make them feel safe. In the words of Lord Justice Munby, 'What good is it making someone safer if it merely makes them miserable?'[3]

2.2 Six key principles

There are six key principles underpinning the Care Act guidance that put the patient at the heart of decision making:

1 **Empowerment** 'I am asked what I want as the outcome from the safeguarding process, and this directly informs what happens.'

2 **Prevention** 'I receive clear and simple information about what abuse is, how to recognise the signs and what I can do to seek help.'

3 **Proportionality** 'I am sure that the professionals will work in my interest, as I see them, and they will only get involved, as much as needed.'

4 **Protection** 'I get help and support to report abuse and neglect. I get help so that I am able to take part in the safeguarding process to the extent that I want.'

5 **Partnership** 'I know that staff treat any personal and sensitive information in confidence, only sharing what is helpful and necessary. I am confident that professionals will work together and with me to get the best result for me.'

6 **Accountability** 'I understand the role of everyone involved in my life and so do they.'

The aim of safeguarding is to:

- stop abuse or neglect wherever possible
- prevent harm and reduce the risk of abuse or neglect to adults with care and support needs
- safeguard adults in a way that supports them in making choices and having control about how they want to live
- promote an approach that concentrates on improving life for the adult concerned.

3. Definition of Adult at Risk

Not every adult will require safeguarding. To meet the criteria set out in the Care Act 2014 the adult must meet the following criteria:

- demonstrates a need for care and support (whether or not the local authority is meeting any of those needs) **and**
- is experiencing, or at risk of, abuse or neglect **and**
- as a result of those care and support needs, is unable to protect themselves from either the risk or the experience of abuse or neglect.

An adult's needs meet the eligibility criteria for care and support if:

1 the adult's needs arise from, or are related to, a physical or mental impairment or illness

2 as a result of the adult's needs, the adult is unable to achieve two or more of the outcomes

3 as a consequence there is, or is likely to be, a significant impact on the adult's well-being.

The specified outcomes are:

1 managing and maintaining nutrition

2 maintaining personal hygiene

3 managing toilet needs

4 being appropriately clothed

5 being able to make use of the adult's home safely

6 maintaining a habitable home environment
7 developing and maintaining family or other personal relationships
8 accessing and engaging in work, training, education or volunteering
9 making use of necessary facilities or services in the local community including public transport, and recreational facilities or services
10 carrying out any caring responsibilities the adult has for a child.

TABLE 1.15 – Types and Signs of Abuse

Types of Abuse	Signs of Abuse
• **Physical**: hitting, slapping, misuse of medication, restraint.	• Multiple bruising. • Fractures. • Burns. • Bed sores. • Fear. • Depression. • Unexplained weight loss. • Assault (can be intentional or reckless).
• **Domestic violence**: incidents, or pattern of incidents, of controlling, coercive or threatening behaviour, violence or abuse by someone who is, or has been, an intimate partner or family member, regardless of gender or sexuality.	Includes: psychological, physical, sexual, financial, emotional abuse; so-called 'honour' based violence; female genital mutilation; forced marriage. Note: the age range extended down to 16 (for the purpose of the safeguarding adult arrangements, safeguarding children arrangements would be applied to a person under 18).
• **Sexual abuse**: rape, indecent exposure, subjection to pornography, not consented or pressured to consent.	• Loss of sleep. • Unexpected or unexplained change in behaviour. • Bruising. • Soreness around the genitals. • Torn, stained or bloody underwear. • Preoccupation with anything sexual. • Sexually transmitted diseases. • Pregnancy. • Rape – e.g. a male member of staff having sex with a mental health client (see Mental Health Act 1983). • Indecent assault.
• **Psychological abuse:** emotional abuse, threat of harm or abandonment, blaming, humiliation, isolation.	• Fear. • Depression. • Confusion. • Loss of sleep. • Unexpected or unexplained change in behaviour. • Deprivation of liberty could be false imprisonment. • Aggressive shouting causing fear of violence in a public place may be an offence against the Public Order Act 1986, or harassment under the Protection from Harassment Act 1997.

(continued)

TABLE 1.15 – Types and Signs of Abuse *(continued)*	
Types of Abuse	**Signs of Abuse**
• **Financial or material abuse:** internet scamming, will issues, inheritance, financial transactions, theft.	• Unexplained withdrawals from the bank. • Unusual activity in bank accounts. • Unpaid bills. • Unexplained shortage of money. • Reluctance on the part of the person with responsibility for the funds to provide basic food and clothes etc. • Fraud, theft.
• **Modern slavery:** human trafficking, forced labour, domestic servitude, coerce, deceive and force individual into life of abuse.	Modern slavery is an international crime, it can include victims that have been brought from overseas, and vulnerable people in the UK. Slave masters and traffickers will deceive, coerce and force adults into a life of abuse, callous treatment and slavery.
• **Discriminatory abuse:** slurs, issues of race, gender, disability etc.	Abuse can be experienced as harassment, insults or similar actions due to race, religion, gender, gender identity, age, disability or sexual orientation.
• **Organisational abuse:** neglect or poor care within an institution or care setting. Neglect or poor professional practice as a result of policies and processes.	• Inflexible and non-negotiable systems and routines. • Lack of consideration of dietary requirements. • Name calling; inappropriate ways of addressing people. • Lack of adequate physical care – an unkempt appearance.
• **Neglect and acts of omission:** ignoring medical, emotional or physical care needs. Failure to provide access to appropriate health care.	• Malnutrition. • Untreated medical problems. • Bed sores. • Confusion. • Over-sedation. • Deprivation of meals may constitute 'wilful neglect'.
• **Self-neglect:** wide-ranging neglect for one's personal hygiene, health or surroundings and includes behaviour such as hoarding.	This includes various behaviours: disregarding one's personal hygiene, health or surroundings, resulting in a risk that impacts on the adult's wellbeing – this could consist of behaviours such as hoarding.
Incidents can be a one-off or multiple and may affect one person or more.	

4. Wellbeing

Ambulance clinicians often come across adults who have an unmet or increasing care need. Whilst these are unlikely to meet the threshold for safeguarding, raising an alert is still possible with the patient's consent. Please follow your local reporting procedures.

5. Consent

Adults at risk should, where possible, be given full information about any concerns for their safety to enable them to give informed consent to the ambulance service raising a safeguarding alert with the local authority or other appropriate agency. Where the adult does not have capacity (refer to **Mental Capacity Act 2005**), or having a discussion may increase the risk to the adult, ambulance clinicians can raise an alert in the patient's best interest.

If there is a risk to others (i.e. other residents in a care setting or an identified fire or public health risk), ambulance clinicians can share information without consent (refer to **Mental Capacity Act 2005**).

6. Mandatory reporting of Female Genital Mutilation (FGM)

From 31st October 2015 the FGM Act introduces a mandatory reporting duty which requires health and social care professionals as well as teachers to report known cases of FGM in those under 18 years of age to the police.

FGM is child abuse and the current procedure is set out below:

- **Children and vulnerable adults**: if any child (under 18) or vulnerable adult in your care has symptoms or signs of FGM, or if you have good reason to suspect they are at risk of FGM having considered their family history or other relevant factors, they **must** be referred using existing safeguarding procedures as with all instances of child abuse. This will involve referral to police and social care in the usual way.
- **Adults**: there is no requirement for automatic referral of adult women with FGM to adult services or the police. Ambulance clinicians should be aware that a disclosure may be the first time that a woman has discussed her FGM with anyone. Referral to police must not be introduced as an automatic response when identifying adult women with FGM, and each case must be individually assessed. Ambulance clinicians should seek to assist women by offering referral to community groups for support, clinical intervention or other services as appropriate, for example through an NHS FGM clinic. The wishes of the woman must be respected at all times. If she is pregnant, the welfare of the unborn child or others in her extended family must be considered at this point as they are potentially at risk, and action taken accordingly.
- In all cases where staff are unsure of their actions, they should seek the advice of the Trust Safeguarding Service.

7. Prevent

7.1 Introduction

- The NHS, including the ambulance service, has a statutory responsibility to comply and engage with *Prevent*.[a]
- This involves the formulation of policy and procedures, the training of staff and, importantly, having appropriate mechanisms in place to ensure that concerns are noted and shared.

The three key objectives of the national *Prevent* strategy are to:

1 Challenge the **ideology** that supports terrorism and those who promote it.

2 Prevent vulnerable **individuals** from being drawn into terrorism, and ensure that they are given appropriate advice and support.

3 Work with sectors and **institutions** where there are risks of radicalisation.

It remains clear that while the focus is an imminent threat from Al-Qaida or Islamic State (IS), it should be noted that radicalisation of vulnerable individuals can be undertaken by any extremist group. These forms of terrorism include (but are not limited to):

- far-right extremists, e.g. English Defence League
- Al-Qaida-influenced groups
- environmental extremists
- animal rights extremists.

7.2 Definitions

The following examples of vulnerability are included within 'Building Partnerships, Staying Safe' (DoH 2011).

Identity crisis Adolescents/vulnerable adults who are exploring issues of identity can feel both distant from their parents/family and cultural and religious heritage, and uncomfortable with their place in the society around them. Radicalisers can exploit this by providing a sense of purpose or feelings of belonging. Where this occurs, it can often manifest itself in a change in a person's behaviour, their circle of friends, and the ways in which they interact with others and spend their time.

Personal crisis This may, for example, include significant tensions within the family, which produce a sense of isolation in the vulnerable individual from the traditional certainties of family life.

Personal circumstances The experiences of migration, local tensions or events affecting families in countries of origin may contribute to alienation from UK values and a decision to cause harm to symbols of the community or state.

Unemployment or under-employment Individuals may perceive their aspirations for career and lifestyle to be undermined by limited achievements or employment prospects. This can translate into a generalised rejection of civic life and the adoption of violence as a symbolic act.

Criminality In some cases, a vulnerable individual may have been involved in a group that engages in criminal activity or, on occasion, a group that has links to organised crime, and be further drawn to engagement in terrorist-related activity.

An additional vulnerability is around young people moving from childhood into adulthood,

a Section 26 of the Counter-Terrorism and Security Act 2015 places a duty on certain bodies (including the NHS) in the exercise of their functions to have 'due regard to the need to prevent people from being drawn into terrorism'.

and, in particular, those children known to children's services as they transition into adult services.

7.3 Duties/Responsibility

- Any member of staff identifying concerns that vulnerable people may be radicalised, should report to the safeguarding service, their *Prevent* lead or their line manager in the Trust.
- If the incident occurs outside of office hours, staff should contact police for advice.

8. Assessment and Management

- Identify an adult(s) at risk.
- Report concerns following local guidelines:
  - Ascertain the patient's wishes wherever possible.
  - Gain consent if it is safe and appropriate to do so.
  - Consider the use of the Mental Capacity Act (MCA) if needed.
- Ensure concerns are clearly and concisely documented and jargon free.

KEY POINTS!

Safeguarding Adults at Risk

- **Stop abuse and neglect wherever possible.**
- **Respect the adults wishes wherever possible.**
- **Concerns of suspected abuse must be reported as soon as possible following trust policy and procedures.**
- **Ambulance clinicians must document fully the reasons for concern and any action taken.**
- **Documentation of consent or the reason it has not been obtained must be clearly recorded.**
- **Ambulance clinicians should not investigate concerns, but should identify and report appropriately.**

SECTION 1 General Guidance

Further Reading

Further important information and evidence in support of this guideline can be found in the Bibliography.[4,5,6,7,8,9,10,11]

Bibliography

1. Department of Health. *Care Act 2014*. London: HMSO, 2014. Available from: http://www.legislation.gov.uk/ukpga/2014/23/pdfs/ukpga_20140023_en.pdf.
2. Department of Health. *Liberating the NHS: No decision about me without me*. London: HMSO, 2012.
3. Munby J. *Safeguarding Adults: Advice and guidance to directors of adult social services*, March 2013. Available from: https://www.adass.org.uk/safeguarding-adults/public-content/advice-and-guidance-to-directors-of-adults-social-services-march-2013.
4. Office of the Public Guardian. *Office of the Public Guardian and Local Authorities: A protocol for working together to safeguard vulnerable adults*. London: HMSO, 2008.
5. Office of the Public Guardian. *Safeguarding Policy: Protecting vulnerable adults*. Available from: https://www.gov.uk/government/publications/safeguarding-policy-protecting-vulnerable-adults, 2015.
6. Lord Chancellor's Department. *Who Decides? Making decisions on behalf of mentally incapacitated adults*. London: HMSO, 1997.
7. Department of Health. *Clinical Governance and Adult Safeguarding: An integrated process*. London: HMSO, 2010. Available from: http://webarchive.nationalarchives.gov.uk/20130107105354/http:/www.dh.gov.uk/en/Publicationsandstatistics/Publications/PublicationsPolicyAndGuidance/DH_112361.
8. Department of Health. *Safeguarding Adults: Report on the consultation on the review of No Secrets*. London: HMSO, 2009. Available from: http://webarchive.nationalarchives.gov.uk/20130107105354/http:/www.dh.gov.uk/prod_consum_dh/groups/dh_digitalassets/documents/digitalasset/dh_102981.pdf.
9. Department of Health. *No Secrets: Guidance on developing and implementing multi-agency policies and procedures to protect vulnerable adults from abuse*. London: HMSO, 2000. Available from: https://www.gov.uk/government/uploads/system/uploads/attachment_data/file/194272/No_secrets__guidance_on_developing_and_implementing_multi-agency_policies_and_procedures_to_protect_vulnerable_adults_from_abuse.pdf.
10. Department of Health. *Safeguarding Adults: The role of health services*. London: HMSO, 2011. Available from: http://www.dh.gov.uk/en/Publicationsandstatistics/Publications/PublicationsPolicyAndGuidance/DH_124882.
11. Biarent D, Bingham R, Eich C, López-Herce J, Maconochie I, Rodriguez-Nunez A, et al. European Resuscitation Council Guidelines for Resuscitation 2010 Section 6: Paediatric life support. *Resuscitation* 2010, 81(10): 1364–88.

Domestic Abuse

1. Introduction

- Domestic abuse includes any threatening behaviour, violence or abuse between adults, young people, intimate partners, family members or extended family members, regardless of gender or sexuality.
- Domestic abuse is extremely distressing; managing such cases demands sensitive, non-judgemental medical and emotional care and an awareness of the forensic requirements.
- In December 2015 a new criminal offence of domestic abuse, 'coercive and controlling behaviour', came into force, making all domestic abuse a reportable crime.
- Patients are likely to be very distressed about the events surrounding domestic abuse. They may not want to involve anybody else, and may not consent to disclosure of information to other parties such as the police. Do not judge, or give the appearance of judging the patient. Be kind and considerate, and allow the patient space, and as much choice about options for their treatment as possible.
- Alcohol and drugs may also be involved.
- **Further care** – it is important to encourage all victims of domestic abuse to seek medical help, and inform the police. Both will be able to provide physical, medical and emotional support.
- In cases of domestic abuse in vulnerable adults and children refer to **Safeguarding Adults at Risk** and **Safeguarding Children**.

2. Incidence

- Domestic abuse affects approximately 28% of women and 13% of men. 52% of child protection cases involve domestic abuse. Each week, 2–3 women or men are killed by their current or former partner. Disabled women are raped twice as often as non-disabled women, and 50% have experienced domestic abuse. Of teenagers, 1 in 5 have been physically abused by their boyfriend or girlfriend.
- The average length of time someone is in an abusive relationship before leaving is 8 years.
- The number of women convicted of perpetrating domestic abuse has more than quadrupled in the past ten years.
- A third of all domestic abuse starts or escalates during pregnancy.
- In 90% of domestic abuse cases, children are in the same or the next room.

3. Severity and Outcome

- The severity of the abuse can vary from verbal abuse to sustaining life-threatening injuries or death. The outcome of the abuse can lead to long-term psychological and physical effects.

4. Pathophysiology

- Domestic abuse is an incident or pattern of incidents of controlling, coercive or threatening behaviour, violence or abuse to those aged 16 or over. These types of abuse include: psychological, physical, sexual, financial and emotional.
- Domestic abuse also includes 'honour' based violence, forced marriage and female genital mutilation (for FGM also refer to **Safeguarding Adults at Risk** and **Safeguarding Children**).

5. Assessment and Management

For the assessment and management of domestic abuse refer to Table 1.16.

TABLE 1.16 – Assessment and Management of: Domestic Abuse

ASSESSMENT	MANAGEMENT
• Assess **<C>ABCD**	If any **TIME CRITICAL** features present major **ABCD** problems: • start correcting <C>ABCD problems • undertake a **TIME CRITICAL** transfer to nearest receiving hospital • continue patient management en-route • provide an ATMIST information call.
• Assess	• Limit questions to those identifying the need for medical treatment, but allow the patient to talk and document what is said. **NB** It is not appropriate to probe for details of the abuse and could affect the outcome of criminal investigations. • Manage according to condition: – Acute injury – refer to **Trauma Emergencies in Adults – Overview** and **Trauma Emergencies in Children – Overview**. – Acute illness – refer to **Medical Emergencies in Adults – Overview** and **Medical Emergencies in Children – Overview**.

(continued)

Domestic Abuse

TABLE 1.16 – Assessment and Management of: Domestic Abuse *(continued)*	
	Indicators in the patient: ● Seem afraid or anxious to please their partner. ● Agreeing with everything their partner says. ● Checking everything first with their partner. ● Talk about their partner's temper or jealousy. ● Have frequent injuries, often described as 'accidents'. ● Dress in clothing designed to hide bruises or scars. ● Restricted from seeing family and friends. ● Have limited access to money, credit cards etc. ● Have low self-esteem. ● Depressed, anxious or have suicidal thoughts/action.
● Approach	● Use a sensitive and respectful manner. ● Focus on your care but be mindful of your surroundings and the information that is being passed to you, both verbal and non-verbal. ● If possible, ensure privacy. ● Consider cultural/religious issues. ● Where possible accommodate the patient's requests. ● Where possible avoid disturbing the scene. ● Where possible try to get the patient on their own so that they can be open and honest with you.
● Criminal offence/ forensic examination	● Many forms of domestic violence are criminal offences and staff must report all serious crimes to the police, particularly if: – the patient has suffered from abuse involving a weapon/strangulation/ smothering or has sustained a significant injury – the patient is in fear of the perpetrator – the abuse is escalating – the alleged perpetrator is stalking the patient – there is an immediate risk to the patient or any children in the household. ● Forensic examination may be required if a physical assault has taken place. Domestic abuse is a criminal offence and the police must be informed immediately (refer to **Sexual Assault**).
● Transfer[a]	● Encourage all patients to attend further care and to inform the police. ● Transfer patients to further care according to local guidelines. ● Where a patient is competent and refuses hospital treatment, advise them to seek further medical attention. ● If safe to do so, provide information on where the patient may seek further support in relation to domestic abuse. ● If children are involved, a safeguarding notification of concern must be made using local ambulance procedures. ● If the patient is transported to hospital, do not leave children in the care of the alleged perpetrator. ● Always try to speak to the patient alone. ● Remember consent is not always required from the patient to report the crime, particularly if the patient remains at risk. ● Share concerns at the receiving hospital.

a In some areas arrangements exist for patients to be examined and interviewed in police or other facilities.

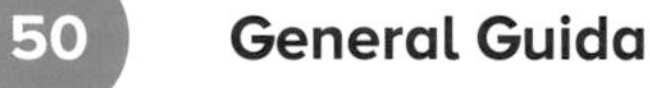

Domestic Abuse

TABLE 1.16 – Assessment and Management of: Domestic Abuse *(continued)*

• Documentation	• Complete the clinical record in great detail contemporaneously and document: – only facts, not personal opinion – what the patient says – clinical findings with relevant timings – the ambulance identification number. • A police statement may be required later. • Consideration must be given with regard to leaving any documentation (such as a clinical record) with a victim, which could potentially increase the risk of harm.

KEY POINTS!

Domestic Abuse

- **If staff suspect a crime has been committed resulting in harm to the patient, the police must be called.**
- **Listen closely to the patient for disclosure, and document this on the patient record.**
- **If possible, take the patient away from the scene.**
- **Treatment should avoid disturbing evidence where possible.**
- **Take into account any information that is disclosed by children.**
- **Never leave a child with an alleged perpetrator if transporting the patient to hospital.**
- **Accommodate patient wishes where possible.**

Further Reading

Other useful resources include:

Department of Health: Domestic violence and abuse. Professional guidance – https://www.gov.uk/government/uploads/system/uploads/attachment_data/file/211018/9576-TSO-Health_Visiting_Domestic_Violence_A3_Posters_WEB.pdf.

Mankind Initiative: information and support for male victims of domestic abuse or violence – https://www.mankind.org.uk.

Broken Rainbow: Support for lesbians, gay men, bisexuals and transgender people suffering domestic violence throughout UK – 0300 999 5428, www.broken-rainbow.co.uk.

Refuge – National helpline: 0808 2000 247, email: helpline@refuge.org.uk.

Every Child Matters – https://www.gov.uk/government/publications/every-child-matters.

Foreign and Commonwealth Office: Forced marriage – www.fco.gov.uk/en/travel-and-living-abroad/when-things-go-wrong/forced-marriage.

Bibliography

1. Department of Health. *Improving Services for Women and Child Victims of Violence: The Department of Health Action Plan*. Available from: http://www.dh.gov.uk/prod_consum_dh/groups/dh_digitalassets/@dh/@en/@ps/documents/digitalasset/dh_122094.pdf, 2010.
2. Taskforce on the Health Aspects of Violence Against Women and Children Improving Safety. *Responding to Violence Against Women and Children – the role of the NHS*. Available from: http://www.fflm.ac.uk/wp-content/uploads/documentstore/1268669895.pdf, 2010.
3. Department of Health. *Guidance for Health Professionals on Domestic Violence*. Available from: https://www.gov.uk/government/publications/guidance-for-health-professionals-on-domestic-violence, 2013.
4. National Institute for Health and Clinical Excellence. *Domestic Violence and Abuse: Multi-agency working* (PH50). London: NICE, 2014. Available from: https://www.nice.org.uk/guidance/ph50/chapter/introduction.
5. National Institute for Health and Clinical Excellence. *Domestic Violence and Abuse Overview Pathways*. Available from: http://pathways.nice.org.uk/pathways/domestic-violence-and-abuse, 2014.
6. British Crime Survey (2008–2009). Available from: www.crimereduction.homeoffice.gov.uk/dv/dv01.htm.

7. Department of Health. *Responding to Domestic Abuse: A handbook for professionals*. London: HMSO, 2005.

8. Department of Health. *Improving Safety, Reducing Harm – A practical toolkit for front-line practitioners*. London: HMSO, 2009.

9. Department of Health. *Multi–Agency Practice Guidelines – Handling cases of forced marriage*. London: HMSO, 2009.

10. Edelson JL. The overlap between child maltreatment and women battering. *Violence Against Women* 1999, 5(2): 134–154.

11. Home Office. *Female Genital Mutilation Act 2003*. London: HMSO, 2003. Available from: http://www.legislation.gov.uk/ukpga/2003/31/pdfs/ukpga_20030031_en.pdf.

12. Home Office, *Domestic Violence: A National Report*. Available from: http://webarchive.nationalarchives.gov.uk/+/http:/www.crimereduction.homeoffice.gov.uk/domesticviolence/domesticviolence51.pdf, 2004.

13. McAfee RE. *Domestic Abuse as a Woman's Health Issue*. Chicago: Elservier Science Inc, 2001.

14. McWilliams M, McKiernan S. *Bringing It Out in the Open*. Belfast: HMSO, 1999.

15. Department of Health. *National Service Framework for Children, Young People and Maternity Services*. London: HMSO, 2004.

End of Life Care

1. Introduction

Approximately 1% of the population of the UK die each year, which is about half a million people, and around 75% of these deaths are expected. This presents an opportunity to plan for an individual's death, to improve the quality of life remaining, to support those close to the patient, to provide symptom control and to establish preferences for care as an illness progresses.

End of life care is considered for those who have advanced, progressive or incurable illnesses. In addition to cancers this encompasses organ failure and conditions such as COPD, renal failure, advanced dementia, heart failure and motor neurone disease.

End of life care applies to those who are expected to be in their last year of life but, as illness trajectories differ for each condition, this can refer to the last few years, months, weeks or days of life.

Ambulance clinicians frequently come into contact with patients who are approaching their end of life, facilitating planned transfers or providing an emergency response to a sudden crisis.

Due to an ageing population and an expected 17% increase in annual deaths by 2030, there will be an increasing demand for high quality end of life care. This will be reflected in the workload of ambulance services.

Unlike conventional areas of pre-hospital care, such as cardiac arrest and trauma, which aim to save life and rely on algorithms and clear parameters, end of life care seeks to provide supportive care using a holistic approach tailored to each individual. This presents unique challenges to ambulance clinicians. Most commonly there is no pre-existing relationship with the patient, no knowledge of their condition or treatment preferences and, based on limited information, time critical decisions have to be made.

People at the end of life may have contact with ambulance services on several occasions, for example, when a complication occurs, which creates a sudden health crisis, or for an unrelated event such as a fall. Be aware of the underlying condition(s) and any advance care planning decisions that may be in place when administering care.

Increasingly, calls to ambulance services may indicate that a person's condition is deteriorating, for example, in a person with COPD who is experiencing more difficulty breathing. Here, ambulance clinicians may be the first point of contact for the person. They need to be able to recognise signs, signals and clues that suggest that it may be time to initiate discussions about end of life care and relay this information onto the person's GP, hospital, other health professionals or organisations so that appropriate action can be taken.

2. Severity and Outcome

The focus in managing end of life care situations should always be to enable a person to achieve care according to their needs and wishes.

For those who are nearing the terminal phase of illness, the aspirational outcome would be for that person to have a 'good death'; to die in a place of their choosing, with dignity and respect, without pain, in a calm and familiar atmosphere, surrounded by loved ones.

Not all clinical presentations are during the end stages of disease or should be managed with supportive care alone.

Several acute presentations are reversible and require urgent treatment and transfer to the Emergency Department in order to improve an individual's prognosis or quality of life.

3. Management – Patients Who Are Not Expected to Die Within 72 Hours

- Establish the patient's wishes for their care, including their desire for interventions and place of care.
- If the patient does not have the capacity for decision making, establish if an advance care plan, a Recommended Summary Plan for Emergency Care and Treatment (ReSPECT) or an Advanced Decision to Refuse Treatment (ADRT) exists.
- Consult with family members and carers but remember the patient's best interests take precedence.
- Access personalised care plans and follow directions where appropriate.

If not in the active stage of dying determine:

- if there is a reversible cause for symptoms and manage as per guidance below
- if the patient's symptoms can be managed in their home environment or if hospital/hospice admission is required
- if the patient has psychological, emotional or spiritual needs that would benefit from specialist support
- if the patient requires additional social support at home or if hospital admission is necessary: Are family members exhausted? Can they manage to provide care? Is physical equipment required to support care at home?

3.1 Care Pathways

Unless the patient clearly requires urgent hospital conveyance for a reversible condition, seek specialist advice to support decision making.

- Be aware of any advance care plans, especially for patients receiving palliative care and those with long term conditions, such as COPD and dementia.

- Be prepared to ask the person/carer about possible end of life care planning and related issues.
- Contact the palliative care team using contact details in a personalised care plan.
- Contact the patient's GP or District Nurse.
- Contact local palliative care pathways (e.g. rapid response teams or hospice at home services).
- Consider contacting a religious leader if appropriate.
- Consider referral to social services if appropriate.

3.2 Shared Decision Making

Ambulance clinicians often become involved in the complex care of patients with whom they have had no prior contact. In managing end of life situations, where there may be a need to administer medicines for symptom control or facilitate the patient's preference with regard to the place of care, remember that the patient's existing care team will hold more information about them and have met them in person in the past. Shared decision making by contacting and discussing cases with the patient's GP, an out of hours GP or local palliative care teams is invaluable.

3.3 Palliative Emergencies

Metastatic Spinal Cord Compression

Background

- Spinal cord compression due to direct pressure or collapse of a vertebral body due to spinal metastases can result in vascular injury, cord necrosis and neurological disability.

Signs and Symptoms

- Pain in thoracic or cervical spine and/or progressive, severe lumbar spinal pain.
- Pain aggravated by straining (passing stools, coughing or sneezing) or nocturnal pain preventing sleep.
- Limb weakness.
- Difficulty walking.
- Sensory loss or bladder or bowel dysfunction.
- Localised spinal tenderness.

Management

1. If any of the following time critical features are present:
   - major ABCD problems
   - neurological deficit in lower limbs

   Undertake a time critical transfer to nearest Emergency Department.

   Provide patient management en-route.

   Provide an alert/information call.
2. Measure and record a pain score.

Offer analgesia, refer to **Pain Management in Adults**.

3. Position supine with neutral spine alignment for patients with severe pain, neurological symptoms or signs of compression. Exceptions to this would be patients with severe COPD or heart failure who, due to co-morbidity, are unable to tolerate lying supine. In these cases the patient should be transferred in the most comfortable position for them.

   (**Note** – there are no clear guidelines and a lack of evidence to advise the correct position for patients – adopt NICE guidelines as in the pre-hospital phase it seems prudent to manage as if the spine is unstable until an MRI can confirm this.)
4. Transfer to the nearest Emergency Department or to a specialist unit if advised by expert team.

Superior Vena Cava Compression

Background

- Occlusion of the superior vena cava due to either external compression or internal obstruction. This is most commonly caused by a tumour of the bronchus or lymphomas, or cancers of the breast, colon or oesophagus. Patients with lung, prostate and breast cancer are at the greatest risk, with the thoracic spine most commonly affected.
- Severity of symptoms varies depending on the degree of obstruction but reflects the underlying venous congestion, laryngeal and cerebral oedema.

Signs and Symptoms

- Facial, neck or arm swelling, worse on lying or bending over.
- Dilated veins on neck, chest and arms.
- Dyspnoea.
- Cough or hoarseness.
- Headache.
- Dizziness, confusion or lethargy.

Management

1. If any of the following time critical features are present:
   - major ABC problems
   - stridor or severe difficulty in breathing

   Start correcting A and B problems.

   Undertake a time critical transfer to the nearest Emergency Department.

   Provide patient management en-route.

   Provide an alert/information call.
2. Sit the patient upright or elevate the head.
3. If the patient is hypoxaemic, administer supplemental oxygen and aim for a target

saturation within the range of 94.–98.% – refer to **Oxygen**.

(**Note** – Points 2 and 3 provide symptomatic relief.)

4. Transfer to the nearest Emergency Department or to a specialist unit if advised by an expert team.

Neutropenic Sepsis

Background

- Neutropenic sepsis is a potentially fatal complication of treatments for cancer, such as chemotherapy or radiotherapy. Such treatments can suppress the ability of bone marrow to respond to infection.
- Patients that have received chemotherapy and anti-cancer treatments in the past 6 weeks are at particular risk (the highest risk is within the first 10 days after treatment).

Signs and Symptoms

- Classic signs of sepsis may be absent. A neutropenic patient at risk of sepsis can look deceptively well but deteriorate rapidly. A high index of suspicion is necessary, particularly in a patient who has recently undergone chemotherapy and has an increased temperature.
- Neutropenic patients are unable to produce the pus normally associated with skin infections.
- Minor illness or feels unwell.
- Vomiting and/or diarrhoea.
- Raised temperature. Fever may be absent in some infected patients who are dehydrated, severely shocked, taking steroids or NSAIDs.

Management

1. Treat suspected neutropenic sepsis as an acute medical emergency.
2. Manage as per sepsis guidelines.
3. Identify a patient alert card and contact an oncology unit.
4. Consider the patient's advanced care plan, ReSPECT plan or ADRT. They may wish to remain at home. Otherwise transfer to the nearest Emergency Department or to a specialist unit if advised by an expert team.

3.4 Recognising the Last Year of Life

End of life care is defined as care of a patient with any disease process who is thought to be in their last year of life.

The Gold Standards Framework outlines a process to help clinicians decide whether or not their patient may be in the last year of life. This process can be useful for ambulance clinicians who attend patients and feel they are approaching the end of life. The GSF is a tool useful for flagging people who may have increasing care needs and clinicians may wish to engage the patient with the health care team to help prevent unnecessary suffering or admissions during the approach to death, wherever possible.

The process begins with asking the surprise question: Would you be surprised if this patient were to die in the coming Months, Weeks or Days? It goes on to provide both general indicator of decline and disease specific indications that a patient may be in the last year of life.

General indications of the last year of life may include:

- Decreasing activity: functional performance status declining, limited self-care, in bed or a chair for half of the day and increasing dependence during most activities of daily living
- Co-morbidity: this is regarded as the biggest predictive indicator of mortality and morbidity
- General physical decline and increasing need for support
- Advanced disease: unstable, deteriorating and complex symptom burden
- Decreasing response to treatments and decreasing reversibility
- Choice of no further active treatment
- Progressive weight loss >10% in the past six months
- Repeated unplanned and crisis admissions
- Sentinel event, for example a serious fall, bereavement or transfer to nursing home

Specific indicators may include:

- Cancer: metastatic disease. The Gold Standard Framework explains that 'the single most important predictive factor in cancer is performance status and functional ability'
- COPD: disease is severe, recurrent hospital admissions i.e. at least three in the last twelve months due to COPD, fulfils long term oxygen therapy criteria, Medical Research Council (MRC) Dyspnoea Scale grade 4/5, shortness of breath after 100 metres and confined to house
- Dementia: unable to walk without assistance, urinary and faecal incontinence, no consistently meaningful conversation and unable to undertake Activities of Daily Living (ADL)

3.5 Care in the Last Few Days of Life

A point comes when the person enters the 'dying phase'. Ambulance services are frequently called upon at this stage. This may be for planned transport, such as the rapid transfer of a person from hospital or hospice to their preferred place of death.

Ambulance services are also frequently called during the dying phase because of an unexpected complication, or a sudden deterioration in condition. Good call-handling procedures can help ascertain and pass on to ambulance clinicians what outcome the person or carer wants and expects from ambulance services – to make the person comfortable, for example, and avoid unwanted hospital admission or attempts at resuscitation.

Families and carers may sometimes wish for ambulance services to be called even where the person themselves has indicated a preference to die at home or in their usual care setting, such as a care home.

At the scene, the focus must at all times be on providing the patient with the care and treatment that is in their best interests. Families and carers can be valuable sources of knowledge and expertise on this and should be kept informed. Ambulance clinicians must at the same time be alert to the possibility of differing views and/or resistance to following an agreed care plan or stated preference among families and carers, including GPs, and be prepared to deal with these. Be aware that relatives and carers may be distressed by the situation, especially in the case of unexpected complications or sudden deterioration.

- Focus on care and treatment that is in the patient's best interests.
- Try and establish the wishes of the patient but be aware of differing views or resistance to follow an agreed care plan among families and carers.
- Seek clinical decision support, i.e. shared decision making with medical colleagues, e.g. GP or palliative medicine consultant; or follow the patients care plan (if appropriate).
- Recognise the signs that a patient is at the end of life and that lifesaving skills, interventions and clinical observations may not be appropriate.

3.6 Signs That a Patient is at the Very End of Life

It can sometimes be difficult to decide when someone is in the last few days or hours. However, some of the signs below may become noticeable.

- Abnormal clinical observations.
- Breathing may become irregular (shallow with deep sighs), with pauses (apnoeic episodes).
- Reduced conscious levels; sleeping more and at times being difficult to waken.
- Impaired vision and may develop a fixed stare.
- Confusion about time or may not recognise familiar persons.
- Restlessness, pulling at the bed linen and having visions of persons or things that are not present.
- Loss of appetite.
- Loss of control of urine or bowels. The amount of urine may decrease or stop as death approaches.
- Occasionally after death there may be a 'last sigh' or gurgling sound. There is no need to become alarmed about this, as it is the normal pattern.
- Secretions collect at the back of the throat that sound like a rattle.
- Cool arms and legs as the circulation slows down. The face may become pale, and the feet and legs take on a purple-blue mottled appearance.

3.7 Care at and After Death

Ambulance clinicians will often be on the scene at or shortly after the point of death. There may be occasions where it is clear that the patient is in the final stages of dying. If all reversible causes have been considered, then supportive care for the patient and the relatives/carers may be all that is required. Refer to **Verification of Death and Termination of Resuscitation by Paramedics**.

4. Pain Management in End of Life Care

4.1 Introduction

Adequate pain management at the end of life is a right of the dying patient and the duty of all clinicians. This provides one of the most challenging tasks that the clinician will face and requires a treatment of the 'whole person' as well as the pain by adopting a biopsychosocial approach.

Pain is present in approximately 70% of patients with advanced cancer, and 65% in patients with a nonmalignant disease. However, due to the longevity and nature of the dying process it is likely that most patients nearing the end of life will feel pain at some stage. In 10% of patients the pain is described as 'difficult' and may require a more in-depth investigation and pain management programme.

Most of these patients who are suffering with complex pain have input/support from a palliative care team/clinic who, along with the patient's GP, have the responsibility of monitoring for changes in pain intensity and character, and adjusting the management strategy accordingly. For those not under the guidance of a pain specialist/clinic, it is advisable for the clinician to make a referral or to make contact with a doctor so that a long term plan to manage the pain can be sought.

Of patients in the last week of life, 35% describe their pain as 'severe' or 'intolerable', and should be treated as a medical emergency where the challenge is to provide comprehensive pain management in order to alleviate suffering.

Be aware that not all people in the last days of life experience pain. If pain is identified, manage it promptly and effectively, and identify and treat any reversible causes of pain, such as urinary retention.

End of Life Care

4.2 Aims

The aim of a good pain management programme is to keep patients pain-free when both resting at home and performing everyday activities. This is achieved through good pharmacological and non-pharmacological treatments, as well as providing advice and education to the patient, their family, and their carers.

Many patients nearing the end of life live with a degree of persistent pain for which they may already be receiving treatment. This is termed 'background pain'. If a new pain or an increase in the severity of the background pain occurs, then this should be treated as a new condition and assessed as such. An increase in severity of background pain or a new pain is termed as 'breakthrough' or 'breakout' pain.

The three principles in providing end of life pain relief:

1 Pain can be controlled in most patients by using the WHO step-care approach.

2 Acute or escalating pain is a medical emergency requiring a prompt response.

3 Addiction is not an issue in patients with a terminal illness.

4.3 Assessment

Pain is a complex, subjective and dynamic phenomenon, which is affected by the emotional context in which it is endured. In line with current JRCALC guidelines set out in the guidelines **Pain Management in Adults** and **Pain Management in Children**, clinicians should pay particular attention to any psychological and sociological factors. Wherever possible a patient self-assessment strategy should be used and only substituted when the patient is unable to do so. A patient-centred approach should take into account the patient's needs and preferences so that they may be able to make an informed decision about their care. For this, good communication and understanding is essential.

Medical assessment: It is important to be more thorough when assessing end of life patients as there may be other underlying issues that need addressing.

As well as the usual assessments carried out in line with clinical training and local protocols, it is advisable to also check for pressure sores and dressings as these may be in need of attention. If the patient is catheterised, it may be worth asking if it is fitted comfortably or causing any issues. If possible advise the patient to maintain a degree of movement as this helps to prevent muscle atrophy and joint stiffness.

Sociological assessment: A sociological assessment builds upon the premise that no illness is suffered in isolation; in fact, the assumption is that people will rationalise what is happening to them within a social model and create a social construction that is based on their relationships, past experience and language. The sociological assessment should look at how the individual makes sense of the illness and the physical and social interactions that are affected as a result. This 'individualism' of the disease combined with the social factors cannot, and does not, fit into the biomedical model which lends its intellect mainly to the giving of drugs to treat a specific dysfunction. If left untreated, the sociological aspect of dying will affect both the medical and psychological states of the patient.

Psychological assessment: For many patients nearing the end of life the dying process will lead to various psychological problems, especially disorders such as depression and anxiety. These have long since been known to accompany chronic pain and long-term illness, with research showing that increased pain perception contributes to the variables seen in the development of the symptomatology of psychological disorders.

The general assumption is that pain perception, alongside cognitive behavioural traits, plays an important part in the symptomatology of chronic pain, and therefore patients suffering from more intense, more frequent, and longer lasting painful episodes are more likely to suffer severe depression.

A lack of treatment will only serve to increase the level of depression, which acts as a vicious circle that is degenerative in nature and contributes, or even exacerbates, the psychological problems encountered.

4.4 Patient-Centred Approach

A patient-centred approach places the patient in charge of their care and offers them more powers to choose and make decisions for themselves. This should provide them with a greater sense of comfort and self-control but also reduce the amount of calls made to the emergency services. A patient-centred approach should educate and inform the patient on how best to manage their pain. Good advice includes:

- Where pain is continuous, take pain relief on a regular basis, not 'as required'.
- Pain is easier to prevent than to relieve.
- Where additional pain is felt through everyday activities, then additional pain medication should be taken prior to such activities.

- Recommend that 'anticipatory' or 'just in case' medication be available and that these pain medications are adequate for the patient's needs.
- Take pain relief medications as often as prescribed as for other medications (poor compliance is common in pain management).

4.5 Pharmacological Treatment

Where pain is intense and opioids are already prescribed, morphine should be the first line treatment for breakthrough pain. This should be administered in line with local protocols and as part of a multi-modal pain management strategy (i.e. to be administered alongside other analgesics like NSAIDs or paracetamol). Where the new pain is not intense, the WHO analgesic ladder should be followed. It is important that the baseline medication is checked FIRST before administering any medication. If morphine is not the baseline medication then it should not be used as a breakthrough; there may be a reason why another opioid has been chosen and morphine should be avoided. Use the opioid of choice for breakthrough.

Step 1 – (<3/10) non opioid +/- adjuvant

Step 2 – (3–6/10) opioid for mild to moderate pain +/- non opioid +/- adjuvant

Step 3 – (>6/10) opioid for moderate to severe pain +/- non opioid +/- adjuvant

The use of subcutaneous morphine is often used in end of life patients not wishing to attend hospital. It is important to administer morphine cautiously so as to achieve a stable and satisfactory level of pain relief without the unwanted adverse effects. The use of intravenous paracetamol may also be used by the clinician and has shown to be good at relieving symptoms of bone pain (a pain which is often difficult to fully control using morphine alone).

Note:

- Do not dilute the morphine, as more than 1 ml of fluid injected into the site of administration is not recommended.
- The effects of IM/SC morphine are evident after 15–20 minutes.
- For pain in the last days or hours of life when the patient is in the dying phase, morphine may be given with caution for patients with a systolic blood pressure of 90mmHg or less.
- It is important to check for prior paracetamol and opioid use before administration to avoid overdosing the patient. The minimum dose of paracetamol should not be less than 4 hours apart (6 hours in renal impairment).
- Paracetamol should be administered over a 15 minute period.
- Check that if the patient has a syringe driver in situ:
  - it is connected to the patient
  - where it is infusing into the patient the infusion site is not red/inflamed and therefore likely to be affecting the absorption and effect of the morphine
  - that the syringe driver or tubing is not leaking
  - that it is 'running to time' as if the delivery of medication is slow then breakthrough symptoms may become evident e.g. an increase in pain if a morphine syringe driver is leaking or running slow.
- After any drug has been administered, it is good practice to inform the patient's own GP or palliative team.
- Be cautious if the patient is on a syringe driver. In such cases contact the patient's doctor prior to the administration of any analgesic.

Naloxone use in end of life care

The use of Naloxone in palliative care is not routinely practiced and is only indicated in circumstances where a clinician suspect's opioid induced toxicity, from intentional or unintentional overdose. The aim is to reverse life threatening respiratory depression only i.e. If the respiratory rate is <8 breaths per minute and the patient is unconscious and or cyanosed.

Do not give Naloxone for opioid induced drowsiness or reduced level of conscious level if the respiratory rate is satisfactory or if the patient is in the final dying stage.

If the respiratory rate is ≥8 breathes per minute and the patient is easily rousable/not cyanosed adopt a wait & see approach; consider reducing or omitting the next regular dose or discontinuing continuous parenteral administration.

Patients on regular opioids for pain and symptom control can be physically dependant; naloxone given in too large a dose or too quickly can cause an acute withdrawal reaction and an abrupt return of pain that is difficult to control, this is also extremely distressing for patients with cancer or advanced progressive illness.

It is important, in the management of patients in pain that the signs of advanced progressive disease are not confused with those of opioid overdose.

Management of opioid overdose in end of life patients

Opioid reversal in end of life patients is a specialist skill and should never be undertaken without advice and guidance from specialist palliative care teams.

If the patient is opioid naïve (not on regular opioids) then it is safe to reverse the opioid effect immediately – refer to **Naloxone Hydrochloride**. This is unlikely in end of life patients.

End of Life Care

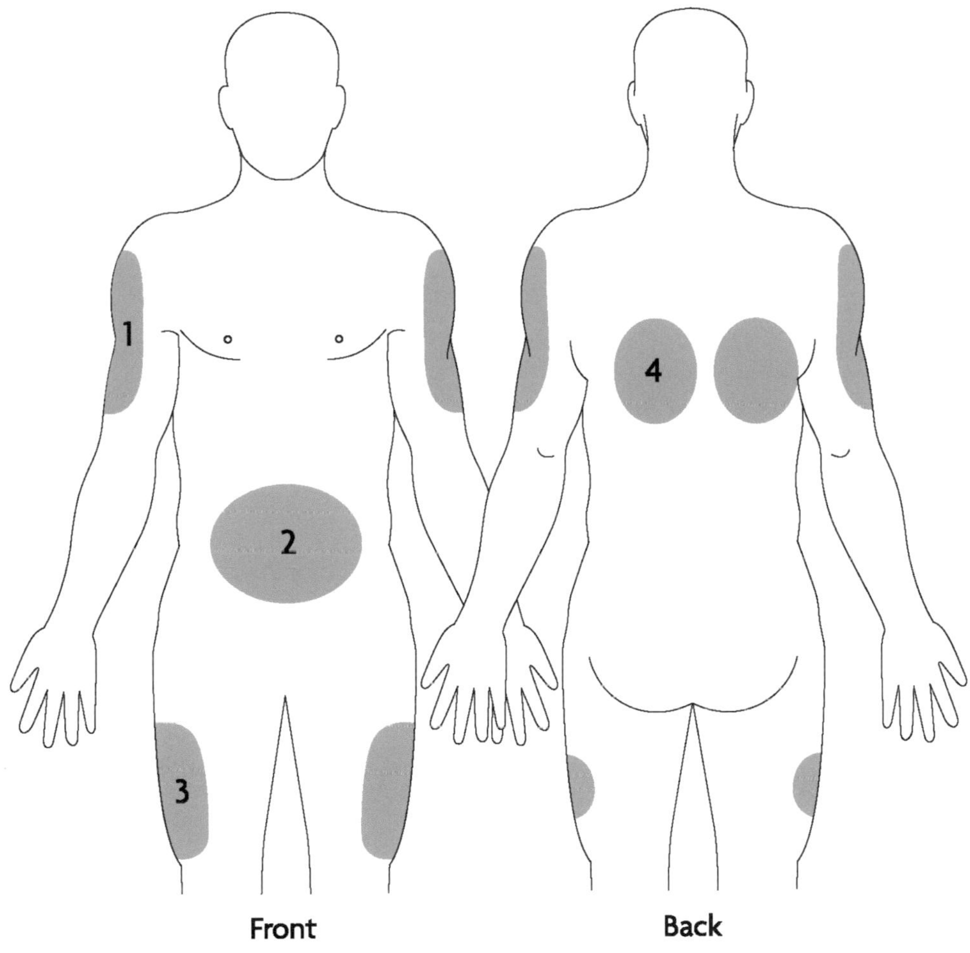

1. The deltoid (upper arm)
2. The abdomen (avoid the umbilicus)
3. The thigh
4. The scapula

Figure 1.6 – Sites for injection of intramuscular and subcutaneous administrations.

If the patient is taking regular opioids, the aim is to reverse the respiratory depression only:

- Stop the opioid
- Administer oxygen if saturations <94%
- Give Naloxone until the respiratory status is satisfactory (>8 respirations per minute) – ensure the cannula is flushed after each administration. Refer to **Naloxone Hydrochloride**.
- The aim is for slow administration of the drug to avoid a surge of pain from complete antagonism of opioid.
- If there is no response consider other causes.

4.6 Non-Pharmacological Treatment

- Non-pharmacological treatment of end of life pain involves addressing many different issues.
- *Patient position* – As many palliative care patients spend considerable lengths of time in the same position it may be possible to help reduce levels of pain through movement and pillow placement. Always be aware of pressure areas and treat if required.
- *Psychological, social and spiritual concerns* – Although the clinicians' time with the patient is limited, studies have shown that addressing these areas will help to provide comfort for the patient. The mental state is very important and will impact on pain levels if left untreated.
- *A good bed-side manner* – Calm and reassurance may be all that the patient needs in some circumstances, and this plays a big role in caring for end of life patients.

4.7 Patients' Own Medications

Many more patients nearing the end of life are being cared for at home in their final days/ weeks with the express wish to remain at home. As part of their end of life care plan they may have 'anticipatory' or 'just in case' medications.

End of Life Care

Clinicians are permitted to administer these medications provided:

- The clinician is competent in the method of administration. A person who administers a prescribed medicine is accountable for their own practice.
- A signed Medication Administration Record (MAR) chart is present and authorised by an independent prescriber.
- The clinician has access to the relevant paperwork supplied with the 'just in case' medication providing the necessary information of each drugs indication, dosage, adverse effects, signs and treatments for overdose.
- In law anyone may follow a Patient Specific Direction (PSD), but some organisations may extend or limit those who are authorised to administer medicines under a PSD within their local medicines policies and governance arrangements. Therefore check local policy.

Follow this best practice advice when working with 'just in case' medications:

- Establish what medication the patient has already received including the drug name, dosage and time of administration.
- Use shared decision making if appropriate, see section 3.2.
- Only administer via the prescribed route and the prescribed dose.
- Consider reversible causes.
- Consider if the patient is opioid naïve. Start on the lowest dose prescribed.
- Leave transdermal patches in situ.
- Do not alter syringe driver settings.
- Talk to the patient, family and caregivers. Ask what helps ease their discomfort and what does not.

Documentation

The administration chart MUST be filled out so that the specialist palliative team or GP can see what Medications have been used. This will also help them decide if an increase in medications is required, or a syringe driver needs addition or alteration. There are some selfexplanatory pages at the back of the administration chart, which should be filled in and signed to show the use of certain controlled medications, and also the current stock level. Always be mindful of the stock balance; fill out on the form when a medication is administered and arrange a GP follow up if the stock is sufficiently depleted. Be particularly mindful of this when approaching a weekend or bank holiday when medication prescriptions can be harder to source. Proactive care ensures crisis management is minimised and makes a great deal of difference in the patient's experience in their last days or hours of life.

Renal Failure

Prescribing at the end of life for patients with renal failure is complex and advice should always be sought from the renal and palliative care specialists. Many of the medicines used for symptom control in end of life care are eliminated by the kidney to a greater or lesser degree. Morphine and diamorphine accumulate in even modest degrees of renal impairment, great care is needed to avoid toxicity.

Syringe Drivers and Transdermal Patches

If the patient has a syringe driver or transdermal patch in situ and suddenly experiences an increase in pain then some problem solving is required.

Assess:

- When was the patch (Fentanyl or Buprenophine) last changed and when should it have been changed? Some patches need to be changed every 7 days, whereas others require changing every 3 days.
- Is the patch fully attached to the skin? The dose of the drug depends on the surface area. If the patch is falling off the dose of drug administered/ absorbed will be reduced. Sometimes the patch can become dislodged due to body hair, sweating or movement. Take advice if the patch has been dislodged. Ensure safe disposal of any patches.
- Is the syringe driver running properly? Is the battery light flashing? Is the battery still in? If not, take advice.
- Is the syringe driver site (subcutaneous butterfly cannula) intact? Is there any evidence of it becoming dislodged or a significant amount of unabsorbed fluid being present around the cannula site? If so, take advice.

Opioid Administration in the Last Hours of Life

The BMA Medical Ethics Today (2012) explains the use of opioids and sedatives in end of life care and the principle of double effect as follows: the principle of double effect allows doctors to provide medical treatment that has both good and bad effects, as long as the intention is to provide an overall good effect. They can give sedatives and analgesics with the intention of and in proportion to the relief of suffering, even if as a consequence the patient's life risks being shortened. The moral distinction is between intending and foreseeing harm. The intention of giving the drugs is to relieve pain and distress; the harmful but unintended effect is the risk of shortening life, which the doctor may foresee but not intend.

Death After Medicine Administration

It must be recognised that the prognosis for patients receiving palliative care is poor and death is an expected consequence of their condition. It is entirely possible that a patient may die whilst in our care or shortly after an intervention we have provided. As ambulance clinicians we should be prepared for this, but it's also important to explain to any relatives or carers present that the purpose of any intervention, whether pharmacological or not, is to relieve symptoms, not advance death.

If an ambulance clinician has followed the correct process for administration of a patient's own 'just in case' medication set out by their Ambulance Service, then it would be entirely unreasonable to conclude that any subsequent death was attributable to the treatment provided. It is far more reasonable to conclude that the administration of a 'just in case' drug made their last few days or hours more comfortable.

4.8 Managing Breathlessness

- Identify and if appropriate, treat reversible causes of breathlessness in the dying person, for example, pulmonary oedema or pleural effusion.
- Consider patient positioning.
- Consider non-pharmacological management of breathlessness in a person in the last days of life. Do not routinely start oxygen to manage breathlessness. Only offer oxygen therapy to people known or clinically suspected to have symptomatic hypoxaemia.
- Medications to manage breathlessness may include:
  - an opioid
  - a benzodiazepine
  - a combination of an opioid and benzodiazepine.

Oxygen Administration

There is no evidence that oxygen therapy relieves breathlessness, unless the patient suffers hypoxaemia. Considering its disadvantages, namely an invasive intervention requiring tubing and tanks, the risk of nosebleeds, and the patient's psychological addiction to this 'umbilical cord', it cannot be recommended for routine use.[1] The British Thoracic Society (2017) has published guidelines on the use of oxygen in adults which includes a review of oxygen use for the patient with breathlessness associated with palliative illness in the emergency care setting.[2]

'Oxygen therapy for the symptomatic relief of breathlessness in palliative care patients is more complex than the simple correction of hypoxaemia.

Consider the following issues:

- Consider early involvement of palliative care specialists and physiotherapists.
- As breathlessness is a multifactorial sensation—a comprehensive assessment of contributing factors (such as anxiety) should be carried out.
- Low-dose opioids should be considered because they are effective for the relief of breathlessness in palliative care patients.
- A trial of a hand held fan to help relieve breathlessness is recommended prior to trial of oxygen.
- Oxygen use has to be tailored to the individual and a formal assessment made of its efficacy for reducing breathlessness and improving quality of life for that person.
- Oxygen therapy should not be continued in the absence of patient benefit or where its disadvantages (e.g. discomfort of masks or nasal cannulae, drying of mucous membranes) outweigh any likely symptomatic benefit.' (BTS, 2017)[3]

From a pre-hospital care perspective, as an ambulance clinician it is vital that you are mindful of the evidence which concludes that the use of a fan and low dose opiates is as effective, if not more effective, than the administration of oxygen. The disadvantages often outweigh the benefit of administering oxygen in that if a patient feels that they cannot breathe and a paramedic attends and administers oxygen, the patient may believe that they need oxygen therapy each time thereafter that they feel breathlessness. Even worse, the patient may fear that the thing they need to breathe is being taken away when you leave the house. This may result in the person feeling that they need an emergency response whenever they feel breathless.

4.9 Managing Nausea and Vomiting

- Consider likely causes of nausea or vomiting in the dying person. These may include:
  - certain medicines that can cause or contribute to nausea and vomiting
  - recent chemotherapy or radiotherapy
  - psychological causes
  - biochemical causes, for example hypercalcaemia
  - raised intracranial pressure
  - gastrointestinal motility disorder
  - ileus or bowel obstruction.
- If the patient had previous well controlled nausea and vomiting using medicines via a syringe driver, consider reviewing the syringe driver to confirm it is not leaking and the infusion site is not inflamed (inflammation at the infusion site which might reduce absorption and therefore effectiveness of medication).
- Discuss the options for treating nausea and vomiting with the dying person and those important to them.
- Consider non-pharmacological methods for treating nausea and vomiting. For people in the last days of life with obstructive bowel disorders who have nausea or vomiting, medications used include:
  - hyoscine butylbromide
  - octreotide

- cyclizine
- Haloperidol
- Levomepromazine.

See 4.7 Patient's Own Medication.

4.10 Managing Anxiety, Delirium and Agitation

- Explore the possible causes of anxiety or delirium, with or without agitation, with the dying person and those important to them. Be aware that agitation in isolation is sometimes associated with other unrelieved symptoms or bodily needs, such as unrelieved pain, their positioning, medications, a full bladder or rectum, organ failure or infection.
- Consider non-pharmacological management of agitation, anxiety and delirium in a person in the last days of life.
- Consider any reversible causes of agitation, anxiety or delirium, for example, psychological causes or certain metabolic disorders, such as renal failure or hyponatraemia.
- Medications used include:
  - benzodiazepine to manage anxiety or agitation, e.g. lorazepam and midazolam
  - an antipsychotic medicine to manage delirium or agitation.
- Seek specialist advice if the diagnosis of agitation or delirium is uncertain, if the agitation or delirium does not respond to antipsychotic treatment or if treatment causes unwanted sedation.

See 4.7 Patient's Own Medication.

4.11 Managing Noisy Respiratory Secretions

- These can be associated with the disease process, or a result of excessive weakness in the patient and an inability to maintain their own airway through normal physiological procedures, such as coughing.
- Assess for the likely causes of noisy respiratory secretions in people in the last days of life. Establish whether the noise has an impact on the dying person or those important to them. The noise associated with respiratory secretions can be a source of distress for carers. Ambulance clinicians may need to provide additional explanation and reassurance that although the noise can be distressing, it is unlikely to cause discomfort. Repositioning the patient can be effective in managing secretions. Suctioning is not usually used or recommended.
- Be prepared to talk about any fears or concerns the patient or carers may have.
- Consider non-pharmacological measures to manage noisy respiratory or pharyngeal secretions, to reduce any distress in people at the end of life.
- Medications include:
  - glycopyrronium bromide
  - hyoscine butylbromide
  - hyoscine hydrobromide.

See 4.7 Patient's Own Medication.

5. Staff Wellbeing and End of Life Care

Managing a patient at the end of their life and supporting their families and carers is very distressing for all those involved. Opportunities for debriefing and/or counselling should be available for ambulance clinicians. Follow local procedures for post critical incident debriefing and refer to **Staff Wellbeing and Health** for more guidance.

KEY POINTS!

- **Providing adequate pain management at the end of life is a right of the dying patient and the duty of all clinicians.**
- **Acute or escalating pain is a medical emergency requiring a prompt response.**
- **Wherever possible a patient self-assessment strategy should be used and only substituted when the patient is unable to do so.**
- **Pain is easier to prevent than to relieve.**
- **Where pain is intense and opioids are already prescribed, morphine should be the first line treatment for breakthrough pain.**
- **The presence (or absence) of a DNACPR type form should not direct treatment options or discussion in a patient who is actively dying. In the absence of a valid DNACPR form, any ambulance clinician who has diagnosed a patient as dying is not obliged to commence CPR should the patient suffer a cardiac arrest.**
- **Patients' own medication and/or medicines carried on the ambulance vehicles may be administered by a trained clinician via a valid Patient Specific Direction.**

End of Life Care

Further Resources

Visit https://www.respectprocess.org.uk for more information on caring for people when they do not have capacity to make or express choices.

Further important information and evidence in support of this guideline can be found in the Bibliography.[4,5,6,7,8,9,10,11,12,13,14,15,16,17,18,19,20,21,22,23,24,25,26,27,28,29,30,31,32,33,34,35,36,37,38,39,40,41,42,43,44,45,46,47,48,49,50,51]

Bibliography

1. Kloke M, Cherny N. Treatment of dyspnoea in advanced cancer patients: ESMO Clinical Practice Guidelines, *Annals of Oncology* 2015, 26:5
2. British Thoracic Society. Guidelines. 2017. Available from: www.brit-thoracic.org.uk/standards-of-care/guidelines
3. British Thoracic Society Emergency Oxygen Guideline Development Group. BTS guideline for oxygen use in adults and healthcare and emergency settings. *Thorax* 2017, 72(1): 1–90. Available from: https://www.brit-thoracic.org.uk/document-library/clinical-information/oxygen/2017-emergency-oxygen-guideline/bts-guideline-for-oxygen-use-in-adults-in-healthcare-and-emergency-settings/, 2017
4. Colvin L, Forbes K, Fallon M. ABC of palliative care: difficult pain. *British Medical Journal* 2006, 332(7549): 1081–1083.
5. Vantafridda V, Ripamonti C, DeConno F, et al. Symptom prevalence and control during cancer patients' last day of life. *Journal of Palliative Care* 1990, 6: 7.
6. McCaffery M, Pasero CL. Assessment: underlying complexities, misconceptions, and practical tools. *Pain Clinical Manual*, 2nd Edition. St Louis: Mosby, 1999, 35–102.
7. World Health Organization. *Cancer Pain Relief: with a guide to opioid availability*, 2nd Edition. Geneva, 1996.
8. Freidman DP. Perspectives on the medical use of drugs of abuse. *Journal of Pain Symptom Management* 1990, 51 suppl: S2–5.
9. Scottish Intercollegiate Guidelines Network, *Control of Pain in Adults with Cancer*. SIGN, 2008. Available from: https://www.sign.ac.uk/assets/sign106.pdf.
10. Quill TE, Brady RV. "You promised me I wouldn't die like this." A bad death as a medical emergency. *Arch Interim Med* 1995, 155: 1250.
11. Rudy TE, Kerns RD, Tuerk DC. Chronic pain and depression: Toward a cognitive-behavioural medication model. *Pain* 1988, 35: 129–140.
12. Tan G, Jensen MP, Robinson-Whelen S, Thornby JI, Monga TN. Measuring control appraisals in chronic pain. *The Journal of Pain* 2002, 3(5): 385–393.
13. Turner JA, Dworkin SF, Manel LL, Huggins KH, Truelove EL. The roles of beliefs, catastrophizing, and coping in the functioning of patients with temporomandibular disorders. *Pain* 2001, 92:41–51.
14. Fishbain DA, Cutler R, Rosomoff HL, Rosomoff RS. Chronic pain-associated depression: Antecedent of consequence of chronic pain? A review. *Clinical Journal of Pain* 1979, 13(2): 116–137.
15. Poole H, White S, Blake C, Murphy P, Bramwell R. Depression in chronic pain patients: Prevalence and measurement. *World Institute of Pain* 2009, Vol 9.3: 173–180.
16. Morley S, Williams AC, Black S, A confirmatory factor analysis of the Beck Depression Inventory in chronic pain. *Pain* 2009, 99: 289–298.
17. Leeds-Hurwitz W. Social construction of reality. In Littlejohn S, Foss, K. *Encyclopedia of Communication Theory*. Thousand Oaks, CA: SAGE Publications, 2009.
18. Bury M. Chronic illness as biographical disruption. *Sociology of Health and Illness* 1982, 4: 167–182.
19. Gonzales MJ, Pantilat SZ. Pain at the end of life. *Hospital Medicine Clinics* 2012, 1 (1): 109–123.
20. National Institute for Health and Clinical Excellence. *Supportive and Palliative Care: the manual*. NICE, 2004. Available from: http://guidance.nice.org.uk/CSGSP/Guidance/pdf/English.
21. Patient UK, *Palliative Care*. Available from: http://patient.info/doctor/palliative-care.
22. Department of Health. *End of Life Care Strategy – promoting high quality care for all adults*. DOH, 2008. Available from: https://www.gov.uk/government/publications/end-of-life-care-strategy-promoting-high-quality-care-for-adults-at-the-end-of-their-life.
23. Beauchamp TL, Childress JF. *Principles of Biomedical Ethics*, 6th Edition. Oxford University Press, 2008.
24. European Court of Human Rights. *Convention for the Protection of Human Rights and Fundamental Freedoms (European Convention on Human Rights, as amended)* (ECHR), Article 2.
25. European Court of Human Rights. *Convention for the Protection of Human Rights and Fundamental Freedoms (European Convention on Human Rights, as amended)* (ECHR), Article 3.
26. European Court of Human Rights. *Convention for the Protection of Human Rights and Fundamental Freedoms (European Convention on Human Rights, as amended)* (ECHR), Article 8.
27. South Western Ambulance Service Trust. *Palliative Care Clinical Guideline,* 2014.
28. South Western Ambulance Service Trust. Palliative Care Clinical Guideline. Available from: http://www. swast.nhs.uk/.../Clinical%20Guidelines%20SWASFT%20staff/CG29, 2014.
29. Scottish Palliative Care Guidelines. Palliative Emergencies. 2014; Scotland: NHS Scotland View website https://www.palliativecareguidelines.scot.nhs.uk
30. Health and Care Professions Council. *Standards of Conduct, Performance and Ethics: Your duties as a registrant*. London: Health Professions Council, 2003.
31. Blackmore S, Pring A, Verne J. *Predicting death: Estimating the proportion of deaths that are 'unexpected'*. London: National End of Life Intelligence Network, 2011.
32. Department of Health. *End of Life Care Strategy. Promoting high quality care for all adults at the end of life*. London: HMSO, 2008.
33. Office for National Statistics. *Mortality in the United Kingdom*, 2010. London: Crown Copyright, 2012.
34. NHS England. *Actions for End of Life Care: 2014–16*. London: NHS England, 2014.

SECTION 1 General Guidance

35. Gomes B, Higginson I. Where people die (1974–2030): past trends, future projections and implications for care. *Palliative Medicine* 2008, 22: 33–41.

36. National End of Life Care Programme. *The Route to Success in End of Life Care – achieving quality in ambulance services*. London, 2012.

37. Leadership Alliance for the Care of Dying People. *One Chance to Get it Right. Improving people's experience of care in the last few days and hours of life*. London: Leadership Alliance for the Care of Dying People, 2014.

38. Robson P. Metastatic spinal cord compression: a rare but important complication of cancer. *Clinical Medicine* 2014, 14(5): 542–545.

39. Sui J, Fleming JS, Kehoe M. An audit of current practice and management of metastatic spinal cord compression at a regional cancer centre. *The Irish Medical Journal* 2011, 104(4): 111–114.

40. McLinton A, Hutchison C. Malignant spinal cord compression: a retrospective audit of clinical practice at a UK regional cancer centre. *British Journal of Cancer* 2006, 94: 486–491.

41. National Institute for Health and Care Excellence. *Metastatic Spinal Cord Compression. Diagnosis and management of adults at risk of and with metastatic spinal cord compression*. Manchester, 2008.

42. Watson M, Lucas C, Hoy A, et al., (eds) *Palliative Adult Network Guidelines*: Anglia, Kent and Medway, Mount Vernon, Northern Ireland, South East London, Surrey, West Sussex and Hampshire, Sussex Cancer Networks and Palliative Care Cymru Implementation Board, 2011.

43. McCurdy M, Shanholtz CB. Oncological emergencies. *Critical Care Medicine* 2012, 40(7): 2212–2222.

44. Samphao S, Eremin JM, Eremin O. Oncological emergencies: clinical importance and principles of management. *European Journal of Cancer Care* 2010, 19: 707–713.

45. Walji N, Chan AK, Peake DR. Common acute oncological emergencies: diagnosis, investigation and man. *Postgraduate Medical Journal* 2008, 84: 418–427.

46. Abner A. Approach to the patient who presents with superior vena cava obstruction. *Chest* 1993, 103: 394–397.

47. National Institute for Health and Care Excellence. *Neutropenic Sepsis: prevention and management of neutropenic sepsis in cancer patients*. Manchester, 2012.

48. Royal College of General Practitioners. *The National GSF Centre's guidance for clinicians to support earlier recognition of patients nearing the end of life*. Available from: https://www.goldstandardsframework.org.uk/cd-content/uploads/files/General%20Files/Prognostic%20Indicator%20Guidance%20October%202011.pdf, 2011.

49. BMA. Medical Ethics Today. Available from: https://www.bma.org.uk/advice/employment/ethics/medical-ethics-today, 2012

50. Kloke M, Cherny N. Treatment of dyspnoea in advanced cancer patients: ESMO Clinical Practice Guidelines, *Annals of Oncology* 2015, 26:5

51. British Thoracic Society Emergency Oxygen Guideline Development Group. BTS Guideline for Oxygen Use in Adults in Healthcare and Emergency Settings. *Thorax: An International Journal of Respiratory Medicine*. 2017, 72:1

2

Resuscitation

Out of Hospital Cardiac Arrest – Overview

Every five years, the International Liaison Committee on Resuscitation (ILCOR) reviews current resuscitation science from which the European Resuscitation Council (ERC) then draws up evidence-based guidelines. These guidelines then form the basis from which the Resuscitation Council (UK) provides national, NICE-accredited guidelines for both hospital and pre-hospital UK practice.

JRCALC guidelines are based directly on these RC(UK) guidelines, currently the 2015 iteration (https://www.resus.org.uk/resuscitation-guidelines).

1. Incidence of Cardiac Arrest and Epidemiology

- NHS England data indicates that ambulance services respond to approximately 59,000 cardiac arrest calls and attempt to resuscitate approximately 28,000 people from out-of-hospital cardiac arrest (OHCA) each year. This is in addition to the annual 3,500 resuscitation attempts reported by Scotland, 2,800 cardiac arrests reported by Wales and 1,400 resuscitation attempts reported by Northern Ireland.
- Table 2.1 shows the rate of return of spontaneous circulation (ROSC) on arrival at hospital and survival to hospital discharge when resuscitation is attempted.
- The Utstein group is defined as those with witnessed cardiac arrests where the initial rhythm is found to be ventricular fibrillation (VF).

TABLE 2.1 – Current Resuscitation Outcomes

	ROSC on arrival at hospital	**Survival to Discharge**
All Patients	27%	7–8%
Utstein Patients	45%	22%

- 2% of cases were children; of the remainder, one third were less than 64 years of age.
- The incidence of bystander cardiopulmonary resuscitation (CPR) rates before ambulance arrival is approximately 55%.
- The initial rhythm is VF in approximately 20% and asystole in 50% of cases. The remainder present in pulseless electrical activity (PEA).
- Unless in a specialist role, most paramedics attend cardiac arrests relatively infrequently.
- Anyone involved in the resuscitation of patients in cardiac arrest (including those involved in the training) should have annual competency assessments and regular training to include high-quality CPR and associated skills, such as airway management, aligned to their scope of practice.
- This guideline makes reference to enhanced care. This includes specialist and advanced practice roles above the paramedic skill set. Refer to local procedures and definitions.

2. Chain of Survival

The Chain of Survival, Figure 2.1, links the critical actions required to treat cardiac arrest, recognising that all links need to be intact and functioning to achieve neurologically intact survival. The links are:

1 Early recognition and call for help.

2 Early CPR to support circulation to the heart and brain until normal heart activity is restored;

3 Early defibrillation to treat cardiac arrest caused by shockable rhythms.

4 Post-resuscitation care to improve survival rates.

The earlier links contribute far more to survival that the later links, because rapid recognition and good quality BLS with defibrillation are the key factors influencing a good outcome.

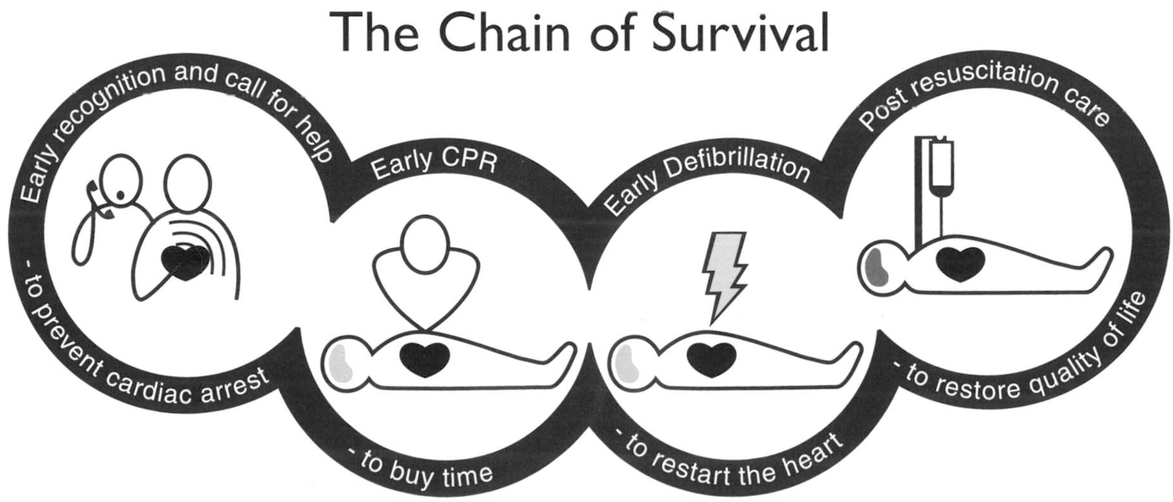

Figure 2.1 – The chain of survival

3. Pathophysiology of Cardiac Arrest and Resuscitation

- The pathophysiology of cardiac arrest, due to a primary cardiac cause resulting in ventricular fibrillation, consists of three phases:
  1. **Electrical phase** Constitutes the initial 4–5 minutes during which tissue metabolism is relatively normal and restoration of a perfusing rhythm can lead to a good chance of neurologically intact survival. Early defibrillation in the electrical phase can achieve survival rates in excess of 50%.
  2. **Circulatory phase** From 4–5 minutes to approximately 10–15 minutes after cardiac arrest. Worsening tissue hypoxia and accumulating metabolites reduce the likelihood of successful defibrillation. The most important treatment is to initiate high-quality CPR to optimise tissue oxygenation and to deliver defibrillation. Restoration of a spontaneous circulation requires a coronary perfusion pressure (CPP) > 15–20 mmHg, which may require the administration of adrenaline.
  3. **Metabolic phase** Extends beyond approximately 10–15 minutes after cardiac arrest. Survival becomes less likely due to myocardial and cerebral ischaemia. Reperfusion injury is more likely to occur if ROSC is achieved. Defibrillation and drug therapy become less effective in this phase.
- CPR aims to circulate adequate amounts of oxygen to vital organs (particularly the heart and brain) to maintain tissue viability until ROSC is achieved. In the immediate few minutes after cardiac arrest, reserves in the arterial circulation can provide adequate tissue oxygenation through compression-only CPR, although they are rapidly depleted and rescue breaths are then needed to oxygenate the blood.

4. Mechanisms of Forward Blood Flow

- There are three main mechanisms thought to generate forward blood flow:
  - **Cardiac pump theory** Direct compression of the cardiac chambers between the sternum and vertebral column increases intracardiac pressure. This ejects blood from the heart into the pulmonary artery and aorta. Recoil of the sternum generates a negative pressure, which contributes to the passive filling of the ventricles before the subsequent compression.
  - **Thoracic pump theory** Chest compressions increase the pressure in the thorax which raises the pressure in the great vessels. The thinner-walled veins tend to collapse, while the arteries remain patent, and blood flows from the arterial to venous circulation due to the resulting pressure gradient.
  - **Lung pump theory** It has been suggested that neither the heart compression nor thoracic pump hypotheses fully explain blood flow resulting from cardiac compressions. The 'lung pump' model suggests that chest compressions causes a cyclical rise in intrathoracic pressure which acts to compress the pulmonary vasculature and eject blood from the lungs with each compression.
- Chest compressions must generate a coronary perfusion pressure of >15–20 mmHg to create sufficient coronary blood flow for the heart to be re-oxygenated and start contracting. Achieving this coronary perfusion pressure requires high-quality chest compressions. When chest compressions are interrupted, coronary perfusion pressure drops very quickly but takes some time to increase again after compressions are restarted – this may contribute to worse survival and hence the importance of minimising interruptions to chest compressions
- Cerebral blood flow is also dependent on high-quality chest compressions.

5. Rate and Depth of Chest Compressions

- Chest compressions hold the key to survival. Even when chest compressions are performed optimally, cardiac output is no more than 25–40% of pre-arrest values.
- Every effort must be made to ensure that compressions are carried out correctly and effectively. Rescuer fatigue is well described with an onset time between one and three minutes. Ideally no-one should perform chest compressions for greater than two minutes wherever practicable.
- Interruptions to CPR are associated with a reduced chance of survival and must be avoided wherever possible.
- Too slow a compression rate fails to generate sufficient circulatory pressure, resulting in inadequate coronary blood flows. An excessive rate reduces the time for passive ventricular filling between compressions and also reduces coronary blood flow.
- Inadequate compression depth fails to generate adequate circulatory pressures, but excessive depth does not increase cardiac ejection and may risk myocardial and other organ damage.
- Allowing complete recoil of the sternum between each chest compression optimises the negative pressures generated inside the thorax during passive chest recoil and draws some blood back into the heart. This assists the passive refilling of the heart and increases the amount of blood ejected with the subsequent compression.

Inadvertent leaning on the chest, preventing it from fully recoiling after each compression, reduces the above mechanisms.

- Where a patient presents in a shockable rhythm, chest compressions and defibrillation is the most effective treatment. Do not allow any advanced life support intervention to compromise delivery of high-quality BLS and defibrillation in these patients.
- For the solo responder, over-the-head CPR may be considered until other help arrives.
- Delivering good chest compression means:
  - Interruptions are minimised.
  - Proper depth is ensured (5–6 cm).
  - Full recoil is ensured between compressions.
  - Appropriate rate is maintained (100–120 per minute); metronome use is recommended.
  - CPR compressions provider is swapped every two minutes.
  - When changing the compressions provider, work as a team, communicate with each other and plan to minimise the time spent with hands off the chest.
  - Be ready to charge the defibrillator after the rhythm check and deliver a shock with no more than a 5 sec interruption to CPR (Charging the defibrillator five seconds before rhythm check, and either delivering the shock or dumping the charge as required is an acceptable alternative).
  - Recommencing CPR as soon as rhythm check/shock is complete.
  - Minimal interruptions to CPR for airway manoeuvres.
  - No interruptions for IV/IO placement.

6. Ventilation

- Ventilation aims not only to deliver oxygen, but also to remove CO_2 from the blood.
- Each positive pressure breath inflates the lungs, enabling oxygenation of pulmonary blood and CO_2 excretion. The ventilation tidal volume should be approximately 6 7 ml/kg (about 600 ml for most adults), delivered as either two breaths after 30 compressions or at a rate of 10/min as asynchronous breaths. Inadequate ventilation rates and/or tidal volumes will not provide sufficient blood oxygenation/CO_2 removal.
- Positive pressure breaths increase intrathoracic pressure, which has the adverse effect of reducing venous return to the heart and therefore reducing cardiac filling. Too much ventilation (excessive rates and/or tidal volumes) has a significant adverse impact on cardiac output.
- Each positive pressure breath also increases intracranial pressure (ICP), thus reducing cerebral blood flow. Optimising cerebral and myocardial oxygen delivery therefore requires no more than gentle ventilation that is sufficient to inflate the lungs and remove CO_2.

6.1 Gasping

- Gasping occurs in about 40% of patients in the first few minutes after cardiac arrest and may also be seen during CPR that is sufficiently effective to oxygenate the brainstem. Gasping during CPR creates negative intrathoracic pressure. This causes inhalation of air, increases venous return to the heart, and decreases ICP, facilitating increased cerebral and coronary perfusion. It is this mechanism that is thought to be responsible for the more favourable outcomes that result in patients who have been gasping.
- Do not mistake gasping (slow, deep, irregular breaths) for normal breathing. An unresponsive patient who is gasping requires CPR.

7. Drug Therapy

- **Adrenaline**: Adrenaline acts to stimulate beta-adrenergic receptors to increase the force and rate of contraction, and stimulate alpha-adrenergic receptors to cause vasoconstriction.
- Following the publication of the PARAMEDIC-2 trial, the use of adrenaline in cardiac arrest is being reviewed, but continues to be unchanged at present.
- **Amiodarone**: Ischaemic myocardial cells may spontaneously depolarise as they lose the ability to control their internal metabolism. Cumulatively, this may result in wave fronts of depolarisation that spread across the myocardium to cause ventricular ectopic beats, ventricular tachycardia or ventricular fibrillation.
- Antiarrhythmic medicines, primarily amiodarone, are used to:
  - decrease conduction velocity
  - reduce myocyte excitability
  - suppress abnormal automaticity

which assists in terminating shockable rhythms in conjunction with defibrillation.

- **Atropine**: Vagal (parasympathetic) stimulation is not thought to be the cause of cardiac arrest in sustained asystole. That is why atropine is not recommended in the mangament of asystolic cardiac arrest. However, it may be a mechanism that causes peri-arrest bradycardia by slowing the sinoatrial node. Vagal tone may be blocked by atropine in patients where bradycardia is contributing to hypotension.

7.1 Acid-base Balance

- The acid–base balance of the body is carefully regulated to optimise cellular metabolism. During cardiac arrest, the build-up of metabolites and CO_2 may cause an acidosis, which acts to reduce oxygen delivery to cells, reduce myocardial contractility and cause myocardial irritability. This makes ROSC more difficult to achieve. The longer the duration of cardiac arrest, the more severe the acidosis.
- CO_2 build-up that causes respiratory acidosis can be limited by ventilating with the correct rate and tidal volume. The use of sodium bicarbonate is not routinely indicated unless blood gas measurements are available on scene.

8. Ambulance Services Response to Out-of-Hospital Cardiac Arrest

8.1 Checklist Use in Resuscitation

- Cardiac arrest checklists should be used by all responders.
- The out-of-hospital paramedic does not usually function as an individual – they are part of a team, and members usually have varying levels of expertise.
- The checklist may help compensate to some degree for this.
- The purpose of a checklist is to help ensure efficient and effective treatment delivery by individuals and teams, to minimise the risk of elements of care and avoid treatment being omitted, delayed or delivered inappropriately in a stressful situation, as a result of human factors.
- The European Resuscitation Council (ERC) states that the use of checklists may improve adherence to guidelines as long as they do not cause delays in starting CPR.

8.2 Cardiac Arrest Downloads

- Data downloads should be used to review each cardiac arrest to understand the quality of care and chest compressions for future and real-time improvement.
- Hot debriefs after cardiac arrest incidents should be provided wherever possible.
- There is evidence to suggest that where these downloads are reviewed and an appropriate debriefing session is held, rescuer performance improves.
- Where download summaries are available, paramedics should take advantage of this opportunity to reflect on the resuscitation attempt, critically analysing their performance and planning how they could improve on their next attempt.

8.3 Use of CPR Feedback Devices

- The use of CPR feedback and coaching devices is strongly recommended on all occasions where resuscitation is taking place.
- A number of studies have shown that the quality of CPR during training and in clinical practice is often sub-optimal, with inadequate compression depth, interruptions in chest compression, prolonged pre- and post-shock pauses and hyperventilation occurring frequently.
- CPR feedback and prompt devices (e.g. voice prompts, metronomes, visual dials, numerical displays, waveforms, verbal prompts, and visual alarms) aim to improve the performance of resuscitation skills.
- These devices enable the CPR provider to receive real-time objective feedback on the quality of CPR and have been evaluated in several clinical studies that support their use to improve the quality of CPR delivered.
- Devices on the market give prompts (i.e. signal to perform an action e.g. metronome for compression rate or voice feedback), give feedback (i.e. after-event information based on effect of an action such as visual display of compression depth), or give a combination of prompts and feedback.

8.4 Clinical Handover

- Clinical handover begins with a pre-alert. Concise and appropriate information should be passed to the Emergency Department using the ATMIST format (or a format as per local protocol).
- The clinical handover with the patient can be challenging to deliver succinctly. Standardised tools such as ATMIST should be used as per locally agreed protocols (refer to Table 2.2).
- Useful information includes the time of collapse, whether bystander CPR was being performed, the time of arrival of the first crew, the initial rhythm and the patient's pre-arrest co-morbidities.
- Try to speak loudly and clearly, being concise, and use the template headings before communicating the information for each heading.

TABLE 2.2 – ATMIST

A	Age
T	Time of incident
M	Mechanism of injury
I	Injuries
S	Signs and symptoms
T	Treatment given and immediate needs

Out of Hospital Cardiac Arrest – Overview

Bibliography

1. Resuscitation Council (UK). *Resuscitation guidelines 2015*. London: Resuscitation Council (UK), 2015. Available at: https://www.resus.org.uk/resuscitation-guidelines

2. NHS England. *Resuscitation to Recovery: A national framework to improve care of people with out-of-hospital cardiac arrest (OHCA) in England.* London: NHS England, 2015. Available from: https://aace.org.uk/wp-content/uploads/2017/03/FINAL_Resuscitation-to-Recovery_A-National-Framework-to-Improve-Care-of-People-with-Out-of-Hospital-Cardiac-Arrest-in-England_March-2017.pdf.

3. Scottish Government. *Scottish Out-of-Hospital Cardiac Arrest data linkage project: initial results.* Edinburgh: Scottish Government, 2017. Available from: https://www.gov.scot/publications/initial-results-scottish-out-hospital-cardiac-arrest-data-linkage-project/.

4. Perkins GD, Brace-McDonnell SJ. The UK Out of Hospital Cardiac Arrest Outcome (OHCAO) project. *BMJ Open* 2015; 5:e008736. Available from: https://bmjopen.bmj.com/content/5/10/e008736.

5. Weisfeldt ML, Becker LB. Resuscitation after cardiac arrest: a 3-phase time-sensitive model. *JAMA* 2002, 288: 3035–3038. Available from: https://www.researchgate.net/publication/10992588_Resuscitation_after_cardiac_arrest_A_3-phase_time-sensitive_model.

6. Georgiou M, Papathanassoglou E, Xanthos T. Systematic review of the mechanisms driving effective blood flow during adult CPR. *Resuscitation* 2014, 85: 1586–1593. Available from: https://www.sciencedirect.com/science/article/abs/pii/S0300957214007400

7. Lurie, K. G., Nemergut, E. C., Yannopoulos, D., & Sweeney, M. The Physiology of Cardiopulmonary Resuscitation. *Anesthesia & Analgesia* 2016: 122(3), 767–783. Available from: http://umanitoba.ca/faculties/health_sciences/medicine/units/anesthesia/media/The_Physiology_of_Cardiopulmonary_Resuscitation.pdf

8. Perkins GD, Ji C, Deakin CD, et al, on behalf of PARAMEDIC2 collaborators. A Randomized Trial of Epinephrine in Out-of-Hospital Cardiac Arrest. *New England Journal of Medicine* 2018; 379: 711-721. Available from: https://www.nejm.org/doi/full/10.1056/NEJMoa1806842

9. Soar J, Callaway CW, Abiki M, et al.; on behalf of the Advanced Life Support Chapter Collaborators. Part 4: Advanced Life Support. 2015 International Consensus on Cardiopulmonary Resuscitation and Emergency Cardiovascular Care Science With Treatment Recommendations. *Circulation* 2015;132 [suppl 1]:S84-S145. Available from: https://www.ahajournals.org/doi/pdf/10.1161/CIR.0000000000000273

10. Perkins GD, Travers AH, Berg RA, et al; on behalf of the Advanced Life Support Chapter Collaborators. Part 3: Basic Life Support and automated external defibrillation. 2015 International Consensus on Cardiopulmonary Resuscitation and Emergency Cardiovascular Care Science with Treatment Recommendations. *Circulation*. 2015;132[suppl 1]: e43-e69. Available from: https://www.ahajournals.org/doi/pdf/10.1161/CIR.0000000000000272

Human Factors in Out-of-Hospital Cardiac Arrest

1. Team Resource Management – Human Factors in OHCA

- A coordinated, well-rehearsed resuscitation attempt, with a team leader and all team members effectively delivering specific roles will improve the effectiveness of CPR and the overall resuscitation.
- Four people with a minimum skillset of basic life support (BLS) and defibrillation should attend patients in cardiac arrest where possible. This should include at least one registered healthcare professional with ALS competencies. One person with clinical decision making and leadership skills should form part of the team. Some members of the team could be non-ambulance staff, for example a community first responder (CFR) or other emergency service personnel trained in BLS.
- An effective resuscitation attempt requires a series of actions, skills and decisions to be delivered quickly and efficiently, including:
  - scene management
  - clinical assessment
  - effective delivery of interventions
  - teamwork
  - communication.
- These often-simultaneous tasks can have a cumulative effect on workload and potentially compromise the overall effectiveness of the resuscitation attempt.
- Team resource management, a component of human factors, is a discipline that seeks to understand the interaction of humans, their work, and the systems and environment they inhabit in order to utilise **ALL** available resources, both human and technological, to achieve safe and efficient clinical best practice.
- Effective leadership skills are vital when it comes to ensuring maximal efficiency of a cardiac arrest team; but most of the errors occur when there is a failure to establish leadership in the first place (refer to Table 2.3).

2. Situational Awareness

- Situational awareness is made up of three elements:
  1. **Perception** – the understanding of where you and your team are in the environment around you.
  2. **Comprehension** – how this will impact on your ability to undertake the task at hand.
  3. **Projection** – what is likely to happen next.
- Although effective team resource management requires that everyone is situationally aware, the team leader will be best placed to focus on these three elements, sharing and implementing this mental model with the team.
- Failure to appreciate and act on any one of those elements within a critical situation may lead to situational awareness errors occurring.

3. Communication

- As well as strong leadership, and shared situational awareness, an important indicator of team function is the extent and quality of communication. Effective leaders will utilise and encourage those around them, fostering an environment of respectful communications.
- In the early stages of the resuscitation, team members' bandwidth may be predominantly utilised for technical tasks. As the team grows, its capacity for simultaneous activity increases. So too does the need for the team leader to

TABLE 2.3 – Leadership Skills

Good Practice	Poor Practice
• Advocates own position and acknowledges lead role	• Lacks team awareness
• Coordinates and drives the scene	• Unable to hear or acknowledge team suggestions
• Motivates and coaches	• Passive and unapproachable
• Guidelines and standard operating procedure (SOP) compliant	• Fails to adhere to or ignores evidence base and SOP
• Challenges deviation	• Blinded to errors
• Encourages and utilises team around them	• Self-reliant and task focused
• Uses clear and inclusive communications	• Changes plans without involving the team
• Maintains situational awareness	• Fails to recognise failure in own capacity
• Maintains team focus and role allocation	• Unable to oversee task completion

establish a shared mental model of what the team must achieve, and how it will go about doing so.

- This is where the need for clear and concise communications is vital. Effective communications should have clarity, brevity, empathy and an element of feedback for confirmation of instructions passed or decisions being made.

4. Clinical Decision Making

- Clinical decision making involves the assimilation of information leading to an appropriate course of action.
- There are many barriers to effective decision making, including time, incomplete facts, stress or seniority barriers. These barriers can be overcome by utilising tools such as checklists and SOPs. Using the 'page-for-age', for example, will save time and reduce workload when calculating drug doses, and ensure accurate calculations.
- Trying to do too much yourself will only lead to cognitive overload; a high risk during resuscitation.
- Stress can have positive and negative effects on our performance and, ultimately, some level of stress is necessary to achieve an ideal mental state for performance. However, very high levels of stress are associated with disordered thinking and reduced motor control, which will hinder performance.
- Human factors can greatly influence the clinical effectiveness and efficiency of cardiac arrest management. Only by understanding these factors and applying principles of their management can the efficiency and effectiveness of resuscitation be optimised, leading to improved patient outcomes.

Bibliography

1. Resuscitation Council UK. *Acute Care – Quality Standards for CPR (2010).* London: Resuscitation Council UK, 2010. Available from: https://www.resus.org.uk/quality-standards/acute-care-quality-standards-for-cpr/#team.
2. Resuscitation Council (UK). *ALS Course. Chapter 2: Human factors and Quality in Resuscitation.* Available from: https://lms.resus.org.uk/modules/m40-v2-decisions/10346/resources/chapter_2.pdf.

Basic Life Support in Adults

1. Introduction

- When there is only one person on scene, resuscitation is limited to providing basic life support (BLS) and defibrillation.
- When available, the first priority is to attach defibrillation pads to reduce the time to first shock and then begin BLS with minimal delay.
- If a bystander is willing and able to provide good quality chest compressions, utilise their skills until further trained assistance arrives. This is particularly helpful in ensuring immediate uninterrupted chest compressions are delivered while the defibrillator is attached.
- Once other providers are in attendance, BLS and defibrillation should continue, while advanced life support (ALS) interventions are provided.

2. Assessment and Management

- The assessment and management of a collapsed patient is detailed in Table 2.4. The adult BLS sequence is detailed in Figure 2.2.

TABLE 2.4 – Basic Life Support in Adults: ASSESSMENT and MANAGEMENT

This sequence is for a single ambulance paramedic; however, when more than one person is present, tasks can be shared and undertaken simultaneously.

ASSESSMENT	MANAGEMENT
● Assess safety	● Ensure that you are safe.
● Check responsiveness	● Check the responsiveness of the patient. ● If there are no signs of life (and the patient is not breathing normally) and it is in the best interest of the patient, begin CPR. ● A pulse check is often inaccurate and may lead to an erroneous diagnosis, delaying CPR. ● Agonal breathing (occasional irregular gasps; slow, laboured, noisy breathing) is common in the early stages of cardiac arrest and should not be confused with signs of life/circulation.
● Next steps	● As a solo responder, the first priority is to attach defibrillation pads to reduce the time to first shock, but commence BLS as quickly as possible with minimal delay. (With two or more responders, chest compressions/ventilations should be commenced immediately while the defibrillator is applied by the second responder). ● Ensure further/enhanced resources are en-route. ● BLS should be commenced while obtaining details to inform a best-interest decision. ● Every effort should be made to gain 360° access to the patient. ● Start chest compressions at a rate of 100–120 per minute. ● Compression depth should be 5–6 cm. ● Allow the chest to recoil completely after each compression. ● Take approximately the same amount of time for each compression and recoil. ● Minimise interruptions to chest compressions. ● A palpable pulse (carotid, femoral or radial) during CPR is not a gauge of effective blood flow.
● Combine chest compressions with ventilations	Refer to **Airway and Breathing Management**. ● Maintain patency of the airway during CPR: ● Consider the use of a laryngoscope and forceps if foreign body airway obstruction (FBAO) is suspected. Refer to **Foreign Body Airway Obstruction**. ● Establishing a patent airway takes priority over concerns about a potential spinal injury. After 30 compressions: ● Open and inspect the airway. ● Provide two ventilations with the most appropriate equipment available.

(continued)

Basic Life Support in Adults

TABLE 2.4 – Basic Life Support in Adults: ASSESSMENT and MANAGEMENT *(continued)*	
	• Use an inspiratory time of one second with adequate volume to produce a visual rise of the chest. • Resume chest compressions without delay. • Add high flow oxygen as soon as possible; refer to **Oxygen**. • Continue chest compressions and ventilation in a ratio of 30:2. • Stop to recheck only if the patient starts breathing normally; otherwise do not interrupt chest compressions and ventilation. • Performing chest compressions is tiring; try to change the person doing chest compressions every two minutes; ensure the minimum of delay during the changeover. • Ventilate gently 10 times per minute. Hyperventilation and hyperinflation must be avoided. Refer to **Airway and Breathing Management**. • Do not attempt more than two breaths each time before returning to chest compressions.

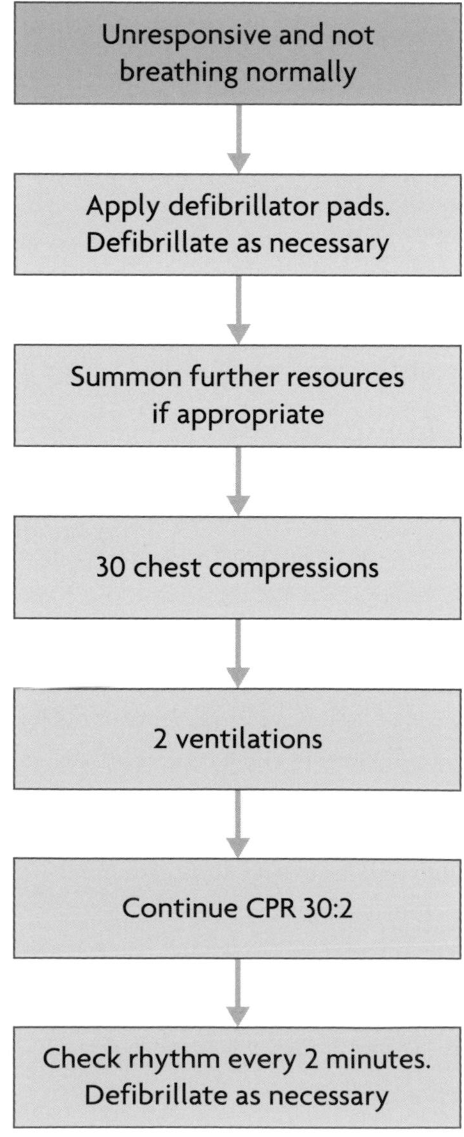

Figure 2.2 – Adult Basic Life Support Sequence

Reproduced with permission from the Resuscitation Council (UK) Guidelines 2015 (www.resus.org.uk).

SECTION 2 Resuscitation

Basic Life Support in Adults

KEY POINTS!

Basic Life Support in Adults

- **High-quality basic life support is a key determinant of survival from OHCA. Begin and maintain chest compressions and ventilations without interuption.**
- **Chest compressions should be provided at a rate of 100–120 per minute and a depth of 5-6 cm using a ratio of 30:2 compressions to ventilations.**
- **Attach defibrillator pads as soon as available, to identify and treat shockable rhythms.**
- **Agonal breathing is common in the early stages of cardiac arrest and should not be confused as a sign of life or spontaneous circulation.**

Bibliography

1. Perkins GD, Handley AJ, Koster RW, Castrén M, Smyth MA, Olasveengen T et al. European Resuscitation Council Guidelines for Resuscitation 2015: Section 2. Adult basic life support. *Resuscitation* 2015:95, 81–99. Available from: https://cprguidelines.eu/sites/573c777f5e61585a053d7ba5/content_entry573c77e35e61585a053d7baf/573c781e5e61585a053d7bd1/files/S0300-9572_15_00327-5_main.pdf.
2. Resuscitation Council (UK). Adult basic life support and automated external defibrillation 2015. London: Resuscitation Council (UK), 2015. Available from: https://www.resus.org.uk/resuscitation-guidelines/adult-basic-life-support-and-automated-external-defibrillation.

Basic Life Support in Children

1. Introduction

- Cardiac arrest in children is different from that of the adult patient in its aetiology and early pathophysiology, with the vast majority of cases being caused by hypoxia.
- It is a rare phenomenon, with an incidence of 9 per 100,000 children. Paramedics are less likely to encounter a paediatric than adult cardiac arrest.
- Proactive dispatch of enhanced care, where available, should be considered.
- Due to the prevalence of hypoxia as a cause of paediatric cardiac arrest, paediatric resuscitation focusses primarily on ensuring a patent airway and adequate oxygenation/ventilation.
- A small number of paediatric patients will experience cardiac arrest without warning, often during exertion, and present in a shockable rhythm as a result of an often undiagnosed cardiac abnormality. The possibility of a successful outcome is high if appropriate action is taken promptly in these cases, i.e. rapid defibrillation.

2. Age Definitions

- This guideline covers:
  - infants (defined as under one year old)
  - children (defined as between one year and puberty).
- In this guideline, the term 'child' includes infants, unless specified otherwise.
- Newborn life support is not covered in this guideline. For newborn babies, refer to **Newborn Life Support**.

3. General Principles

- The priorities should include:
  - effective airway management
  - effective ventilations
  - effective chest compressions
  - early defibrillation, if appropriate.
- Do not delay on scene once these interventions have been attempted.
- Consider conveyance to the most appropriate hospital with early pre-alert.
- In the event of a life-threatening episode for any child, consideration must be given to the need for clinical assessment of other siblings in the property if the cause of illness is unknown.
- In the event of a life-threatening episode for any child, consideration must be given to safeguarding concerns for that child and siblings.

4. Airway Management

- Bag-mask ventilation (BMV) is the recommended first-line method for achieving airway control and ventilation in children.
- Appropriate padding behind the shoulder blades which also supports the head in children, may aid airway management.
- Gastric insufflation is a complication of paediatric resuscitation, leading to splinting of the diaphragm, vomiting and compression of the vena cava causing diminished venous return.
- This is best avoided by delivering gentle ventilations over one second, just sufficient to cause chest rise.
- Basic airway adjuncts may assist in maintaining an open airway.
- Although bag-mask ventilation remains the recommended first line method for achieving airway control and ventilation in children, a supraglottic airway is an acceptable airway device for providers trained in its use. It is particularly helpful in airway obstruction caused by supraglottic airway abnormalities or if bag-mask ventilation is not possible.

TABLE 2.5 – Basic Life Support in Children: ASSESSMENT and MANAGEMENT

This sequence is for a lone paramedic; however, when more than one person is present, tasks can be shared and undertaken simultaneously.

ASSESSMENT	MANAGEMENT
• Assess safety	• Ensure that you are safe.
• Check responsiveness	• Check the responsiveness of the patient. • Agonal breathing (occasional irregular gasps; slow, laboured, noisy breathing) is common in the early stages of cardiac arrest and should not be confused with signs of life/circulation. • It may be difficult to be certain that there is no pulse. If there is any doubt and it is in the best interest of the patient, begin CPR.

SECTION 2 Resuscitation

Basic Life Support in Children

TABLE 2.5 – Basic Life Support in Children: ASSESSMENT and MANAGEMENT *(continued)*		
● Next steps	● Every effort should be made to gain 360° access to the patient. ● The first priority is to open, inspect and clear the airway and begin effective ventilations using BMV with high-flow oxygen. ● Open the child's airway by tilting the head and lifting the chin: – Place your hand on the forehead and gently tilt the head back. Be careful not to hyperextend the neck. – At the same time, lift the point of the chin with your fingertip(s). Do not push on the soft tissues under the chin as this may block the airway. – If you still have difficulty in opening the airway, try a jaw thrust: place the first two fingers of each hand behind each side of the child's mandible (jaw bone) and push the jaw forward. ● Maintain patency of the airway during CPR: – Refer to **Airway and Breathing Management**. ● There is a high incidence of choking in children. – Consider the use of a laryngoscope and forceps if FBAO is suspected. Refer to **Foreign Body Airway Obstruction.** – Establishing a patent airway takes priority over concerns about a potential spinal injury. ● Give five ventilations.	
● Ventilations	**Child** ● Ensure head tilt and chin lift. ● Use paediatric BMV (with a mask appropriate to the size of the child) and inflate the chest steadily over 1 second, watching for chest rise. ● Maintaining head tilt and chin lift, watch the chest fall. ● Repeat this sequence 5 times. ● Identify effectiveness by observing the child's chest rise and fall in a similar fashion to the movement produced by a normal breath.	**Infant** ● Ensure a neutral position of the head and apply a chin lift. ● Use paediatric BMV (with a mask appropriate to the size of the child) and inflate the chest steadily over 1 second, watching for chest rise. ● Maintaining the chin lift, watch the chest fall. ● Repeat this sequence 5 times. ● Identify effectiveness by observing the child's chest rise and fall in a similar fashion to the movement produced by a normal breath.
● If there is difficulty achieving an effective breath, the airway may be obstructed	● Open the child's mouth and remove any visible obstruction. ● **DO NOT** perform a blind finger sweep. ● Ensure that there is adequate head tilt and chin lift but also that the neck is not over-extended. ● If head tilt and chin lift has not opened the airway, try the jaw thrust method. ● Make up to 5 attempts to achieve effective breaths. ● If still unsuccessful, examine the oropharynx with a laryngoscope and remove any obstruction. If an obstruction is removed, make 5 further attempts at ventilations. ● If still unsuccessful move on to chest compressions.	
● Assess the child's circulation	● Look for signs of life. This includes checking for a pulse, any movement, coughing or normal breathing (not agonal gasps – these are infrequent, irregular breaths). ● **NB If you are not sure if there is a pulse, assume there is no pulse.**	

(continued)

Basic Life Support in Children

<table>
<tr><th colspan="3">TABLE 2.5 – Basic Life Support in Children: ASSESSMENT and MANAGEMENT (continued)</th></tr>
<tr><td>• Pulse Check</td><td>Child
• Feel for the carotid pulse in the neck.</td><td>Infant
• Feel for the brachial pulse on the inner aspect of the upper arm.</td></tr>
<tr><td>• Where a pulse is present and breaths are absent:</td><td colspan="2">• Continue ventilating, until the child starts breathing effectively on their own.
• Re-assess the child frequently.</td></tr>
<tr><td>• If there are no signs of a circulation – OR there is any doubt:</td><td colspan="2">• Start chest compressions.
• Combine ventilations and chest compressions.
• NB – for paediatric patients in a collapsed state, with no signs of life and a heart rate < 60 beats per minute, compressions must be commenced.</td></tr>
<tr><td>• For all children, compress the lower half of the sternum</td><td colspan="2">• Avoid compressing the upper abdomen by locating the xiphisternum (i.e. find the angle where the lowest ribs join in the midline) and compressing the sternum one finger's breadth above this point.
• Compressions should be sufficient to depress the sternum by at least one third of the depth of the chest (approximately 4 cm for an infant and 5 cm for a child).
• Release the pressure, and repeat at a rate of 100–120 per minute.
• After 15 compressions, give two ventilations.
• Continue compressions and ventilations in a ratio of 15:2.
• Lone rescuers may use a ratio of 30:2, particularly if they are having difficulty with the transition between compressions and ventilations.
• The best method for compression varies slightly between infants and children (see below).</td></tr>
<tr><td>• Compressions</td><td>Child
• Place the heel of one hand over the lower half of the sternum (as above).
• Lift the fingers to ensure that pressure is not applied over the child's ribs.
• Position yourself vertically above the child's chest and, with your arm straight, compress the sternum to depress it by approximately 5 cm.
• In larger children or for small rescuers, this may be achieved most easily by using both hands with the fingers interlocked.
• Ensure complete recoil following each compression.</td><td>Infant
• The lone rescuer should compress the sternum with the tips of two fingers.
• If there are two or more rescuers, an alternative method would be to use the encircling technique:
– Place both thumbs flat, side by side on the lower half of the sternum (as above) with the tips pointing towards the infant's head.
– Spread the rest of both hands with the fingers together to encircle the lower part of the infant's rib cage with the tips of the fingers supporting the infant's back.
– Press down on the lower sternum with the two thumbs to depress it by approximately 4 cm.
• Ensure complete recoil following each compression.</td></tr>
</table>

Basic Life Support in Children

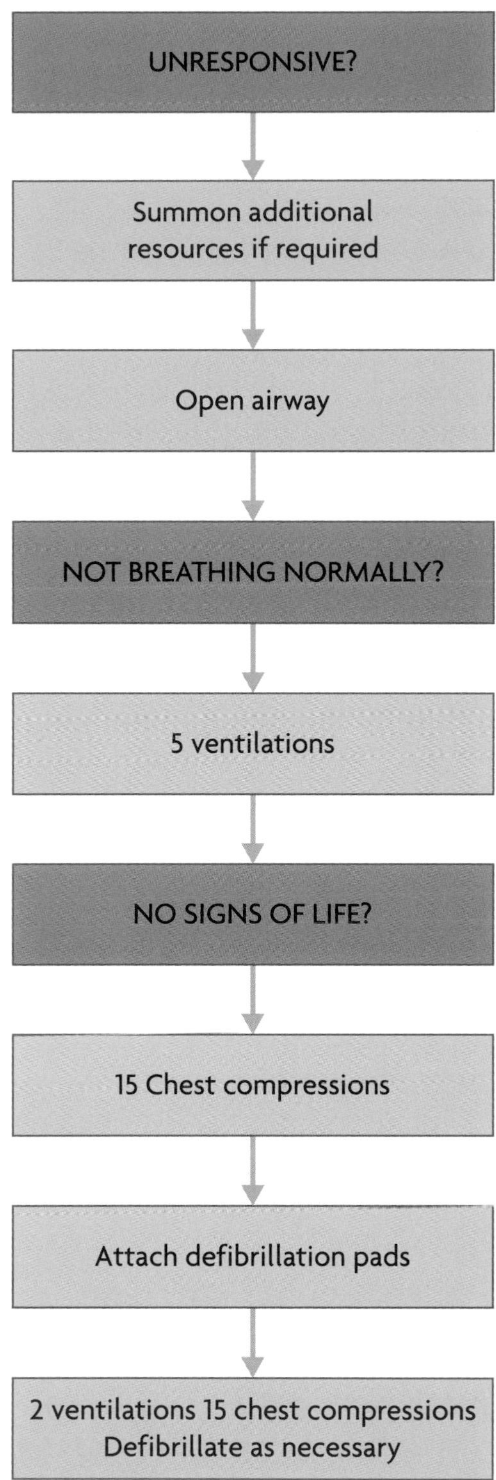

Figure 2.3 – Child basic life support sequence algorithm – Reproduced with permission from the Resuscitation Council (UK) Guidelines 2015 algorithm (www.resus.org.uk).

Basic Life Support in Children

KEY POINTS!

Basic Life Support in Children

- **Hypoxia is the most common cause of cardiac arrest.**
- **Some children may present in a shockable rhythm as a result of an often undiagnosed cardiac abnormality.**
- **Treatment should focus on rapidly correcting the cause where possible.**
- **If the child is not breathing, carefully remove any obvious airway obstruction but DO NOT perform blind finger sweeps.**
- **Give five initial ventilations using a BVM, watching for chest rise.**
- **Adopt a high index of suspicion of airway obstruction and treat accordingly.**
- **The duration of ventilations is about one second (comparable with adult practice).**
- **If there are:**
  - **no signs of life**
  - **or an absent or slow pulse (<60 bpm with poor perfusion)**
  - **or you are not sure**

  start chest compressions at a rate of 100–120 per minute.
- **Continue alternating compressions and breaths at a ratio of 15:2.**

Bibliography

1. Maconochie IK, Bingham R, Eich C et al. European Resuscitation Council Guidelines for Resuscitation 2015: Section 6. Paediatric life support. *Resuscitation* 2015:95, 223–248. Available from: http://doi.org/10.1016/j.resuscitation.2015.07.028.
2. Resuscitation Council (UK). Paediatric resuscitation guidelines 2015. London: Resuscitation Council (UK), 2015. Available from: https://www.resus.org.uk/resuscitation-guidelines/paediatric-basic-life-support/

Foreign Body Airway Obstruction

1. Introduction

- Foreign body airway obstruction (FBAO) is an uncommon but potentially treatable cause of accidental death.
- Most cases occur when eating or playing (in children) and are consequently witnessed. Therefore, interventions are usually initiated when the patient is conscious.
- The signs and symptoms vary, depending on the degree of airway obstruction (refer to Table 2.6).
- FBAO is characterised by the sudden onset of respiratory distress associated with coughing, gagging or stridor.
- Similar signs and symptoms may also be associated with other causes of airway obstruction such as laryngitis or epiglottitis, which tend to be of slower onset and require different management.
- This guideline covers:
  - infants (defined as under one year old)
  - children (defined as between one year and puberty)
  - adults (defined as after puberty, generally > 12 years of age).
- In this guideline, the term 'child' includes infants, unless specified otherwise.

2. General Management Principles

- When a foreign body enters the airway, the patient will usually react immediately by coughing in an attempt to expel it.
- A spontaneous cough is likely to be more effective and safer than any manoeuvre a rescuer might perform.
- If coughing is absent or ineffective and the object completely obstructs the airway, the patient will rapidly become asphyxiated.
- Active interventions to remove FBAO are only required when coughing becomes ineffective; but when required, these should be commenced confidently and rapidly.
- A high index of suspicion of airway obstruction must be maintained where airway compromise is noted and paramedics should examine the oropharynx with a laryngoscope at an early stage if chest rise is not witnessed.
- Finger sweeps are not recommended, particularly when paramedics have the benefit of McGill forceps and suction, as they may drive any foreign body deeper into the airway. If an obstruction is seen and it can be grasped easily, make an attempt to remove it with forceps and/or suction

TABLE 2.6 – General Signs of Foreign Body Airway Obstruction

Mild airway obstruction	**Severe airway obstruction**
• The patient is able to: – speak – cough – breathe.	• The patient is unable to: – speak – breathe. • Attempts at coughing are silent. • The patient may be unconscious.
Other indicators • The episode was witnessed. • The patient may clutch their neck. • The patient may appear panicked or anxious. • Coughing or choking may be present: – Cough may be ineffective, silent, quiet or loud. • A stridor or wheeze may be present. • Onset is sudden. • There is recent history of playing with, or eating, small objects. • The patient is cyanosed. • The patient has a decreasing level of consciousness. • The patient may be crying. • The patient was able to breathe before coughing.	

Foreign Body Airway Obstruction

3. Assessment and Management

For the assessment and management of foreign body airway obstruction, refer to Table 2.7.

<table>
<tr><th colspan="4">TABLE 2.7 – Foreign Body Airway Obstruction (FBAO)</th></tr>
<tr><th>ASSESSMENT</th><th>MANAGEMENT – Adult</th><th>MANAGEMENT – Child > 1 year</th><th>MANAGEMENT – Infant < 1 year</th></tr>
<tr><td>• Assess for severity of obstruction</td><td colspan="3">• Consider enhanced care.
• Determine the patient's level of consciousness.
• Refer to Table 2.6.
• Consider severe allergic reaction which can cause airway obstruction, refer to Allergic Reactions including Anaphylaxis.</td></tr>
<tr><td>• Mild airway obstruction</td><td colspan="2">Adult and Child > 1 year
• Encourage the patient to cough but do nothing else.
• Monitor carefully and re-asses frequently.
• Rapid transport to hospital.</td><td>Infant < 1 year
• Monitor carefully and re-asses frequently.
• Rapid transport to hospital.</td></tr>
<tr><td>• Severe airway obstruction – conscious patient</td><td colspan="2">Adult and Child > 1 year
• Give up to 5 back blows – after each back blow, check to see if the obstruction has been relieved.
• If 5 back blows do not relieve the airway obstruction, give up to 5 abdominal thrusts.
• These manoeuvres increase intrathoracic pressure and may dislodge the foreign body.
• Alternate these until the obstruction is relieved or the patient loses consciousness.</td><td>Infant < 1 year
• Give up to 5 back blows – after each back blow, check to see if the obstruction has been relieved.
• If 5 back blows do not relieve the airway obstruction, give up to 5 CHEST thrusts.
• These manoeuvres increase intrathoracic pressure and may dislodge the foreign body.
• Alternate these until the obstruction is relieved or the infant loses consciousness.</td></tr>
<tr><td>• Severe airway obstruction – unconscious patient</td><td colspan="3">Adult, Child > 1 year and Infant < 1 year
• Open the mouth and look for any obvious obstruction.
• Attempt to visualise the vocal cords with a laryngoscope.
• If an obstruction is seen and it can be grasped easily, make an attempt to remove it with forceps, or suction.
• DO NOT attempt finger sweeps – these can cause injury and force the object more deeply into the pharynx.
• If the patient is unconscious or becomes unconscious, begin basic life support – refer to Basic Life Support in Adults and Basic Life Support in Children
• If all other measures fail and airway remains obstructed, also consider cricothyroidotomy or surgical airway (<u>not</u> infants) where trained and authorised.
• During CPR, the patient's mouth should be checked for any foreign body that has been partly expelled each time the airway is opened.</td></tr>
</table>

Foreign Body Airway Obstruction

<table>
<tr><th colspan="4">TABLE 2.7 – Foreign Body Airway Obstruction (FBAO) (continued)</th></tr>
<tr><th>ASSESSMENT</th><th>MANAGEMENT – Adult</th><th>MANAGEMENT – Child > 1 year</th><th>MANAGEMENT – Infant < 1 year</th></tr>
<tr><td>● Additional information</td><td colspan="3">Adult, Child and Infant
● Chest thrusts/compressions generate a higher airway pressure than back blows.
● Following successful treatment for FBAO, foreign material may remain in the upper or lower respiratory tract and cause complications later.
● Patients with a persistent cough, difficulty swallowing or the sensation of an object being stuck in the throat must be assessed further.
● Abdominal thrusts can cause serious internal injuries and all patients who receive them must be assessed for injury in hospital.
● Infants (< 1 year of age): 5 back blows, alternating with 5 chest thrusts.
Child (> 1 year of age): 5 back blows, alternating with 5 abdominal thrusts.</td></tr>
<tr><td>Back blows</td><td colspan="2">Child > 1 year
● Back blows are more effective if the child is positioned head down.
● A small child may be placed across the rescuer's lap.
● If this is not possible, support the child in a forward-leaning position and deliver the back blows from behind.</td><td>Infant < 1 year
● Support the infant in a head-down, prone position, to allow gravity to assist the removal of the foreign body.
● Support the infant's head by placing the thumb of one hand at the angle of the lower jaw, with one or two fingers from the same hand at the same point on the other side of the jaw.
● Do not compress the soft tissues under the infant's jaw, as this will exacerbate the airway obstruction.
● Deliver up to 5 sharp back blows with the heel of one hand in the middle of the back between the shoulder blades, aiming to relieve the obstruction with each blow.</td></tr>
<tr><td>Chest/abdominal thrusts</td><td colspan="2">Abdominal thrusts – children
● Stand or kneel behind the child. Place your arms under the child's arms and encircle their torso.
● Clench your fist and place it between the umbilicus and the xiphisternum. Grasp this hand with the other hand and pull sharply inwards and upwards.
● Repeat up to 5 times (if required).
● Ensure that pressure is not applied to xiphoid process or lower rib cage (as this may result in abdominal trauma).</td><td>Chest thrusts – infants
● Turn the infant into a head-down, supine position (this can be safely achieved by placing the paramedic's arm along the infant's back and encircling the occiput with the hand). Rest this arm against a solid surface or the paramedic's thigh.
● Identify the landmark for chest compression (lower sternum, approximately a finger's breadth above the xiphisternum).
● Deliver 5 chest thrusts (if required).
● These are similar to external chest compressions but sharper in nature and delivered at a slower rate.</td></tr>
</table>

Foreign Body Airway Obstruction

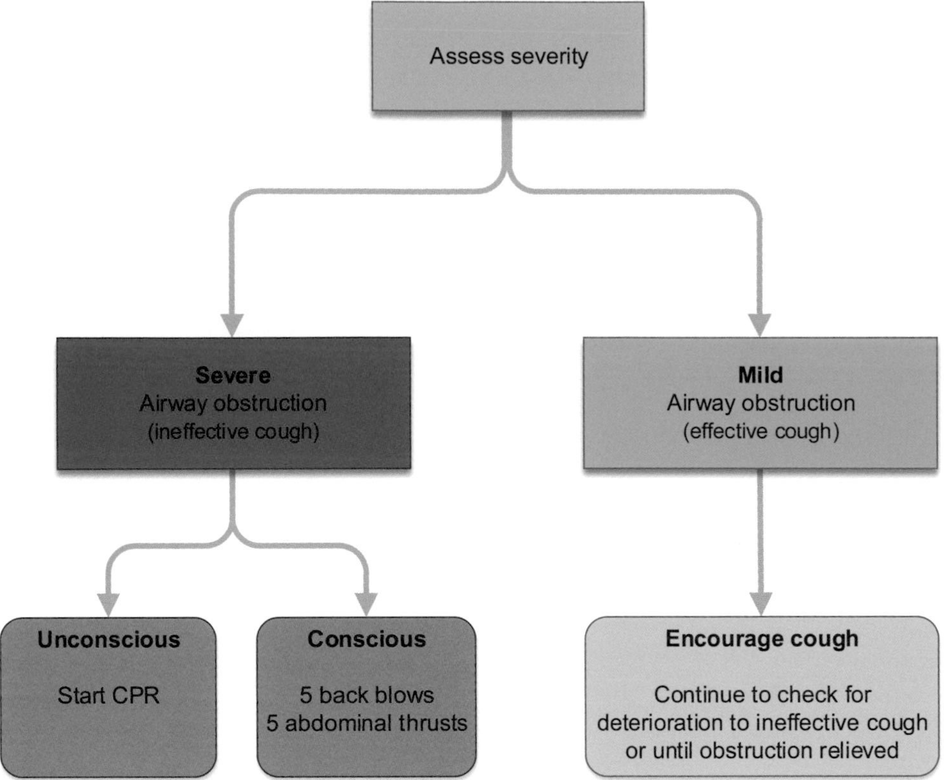

Figure 2.4 – Foreign body airway obstruction in adults – Reproduced with permission from the Resuscitation Council (UK) Guidelines 2015 algorithm (www.resus.org.uk).

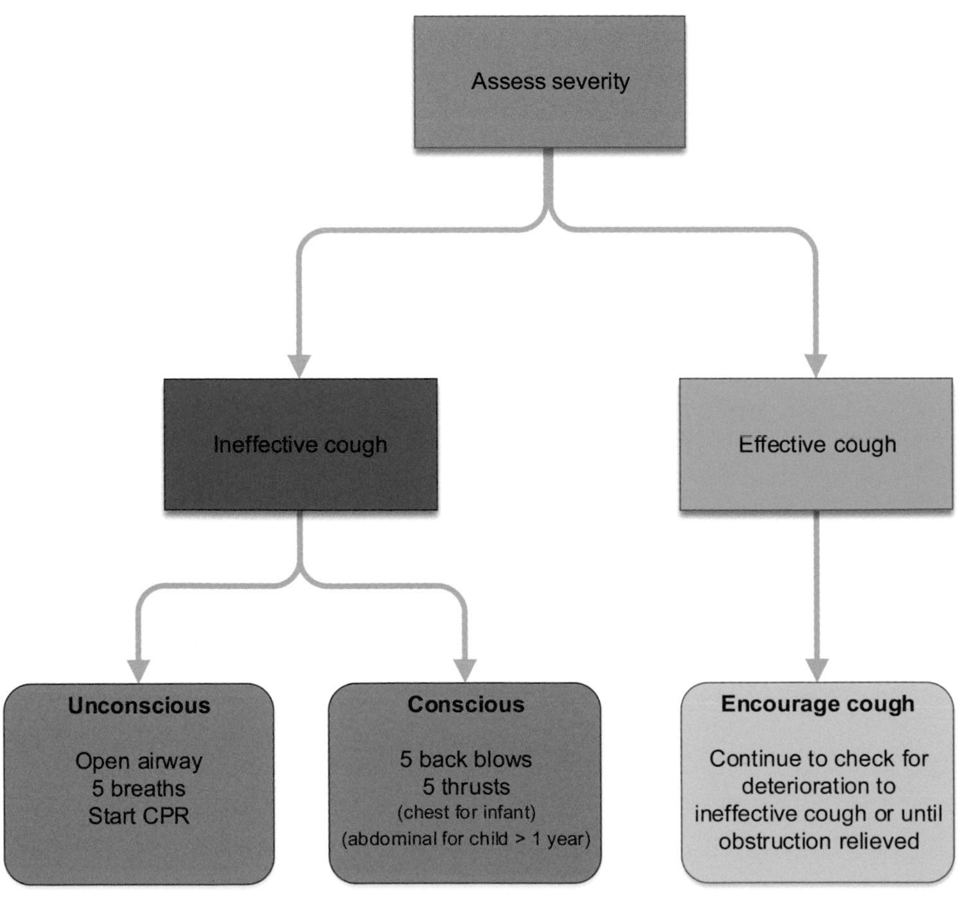

Figure 2.5 – Foreign body airway obstruction in children – Reproduced with permission from the Resuscitation Council (UK) Guidelines 2015 algorithm (www.resus.org.uk).

Foreign Body Airway Obstruction

KEY POINTS!

Foreign body airway obstruction

- **FBAO is a potentially treatable cause of death that often occurs while playing or eating. It is more common in children.**
- **It is characterised by the sudden onset of respiratory distress.**
- **If the patient is coughing effectively, encourage them to cough.**
- **If coughing is ineffective, back blows should initially be given.**
- **If the patient becomes unconscious, use chest thrusts in infants and abdominal thrusts in children and adults.**
- **Avoid finger sweeps; use suction and/or McGill forceps.**
- **Check after each manoeuvre to see if the obstruction is removed.**
- **If the object is expelled successfully, assess the patient's clinical condition. It is possible that part of the object may remain in the respiratory tract and cause complications.**
- **Abdominal thrusts may cause internal injury – patients who have received abdominal thrusts require further hospital assessment.**

Bibliography

1. Perkins GD, Handley AJ, Koster RW, Castrén M, Smyth MA, Olasveengen T et al. European Resuscitation Council Guidelines for Resuscitation 2015: Section 2. Adult basic life support. *Resuscitation* 2015:95, 81–99. Available from: https://cprguidelines.eu/sites/573c777f5e61585a053d7ba5/content_entry573c77e35e61585a053d7baf/573c781e5e61585a053d7bd1/ files/S0300-9572_15_00327-5_main.pdf.

2. Maconochie I, Bingham R, Eich C, López-Herce J, Rodriguez-Nunez A, Rajka T, Van de Voorde P, Zideman D, Biarent D. European Resuscitation Council Guidelines for Resuscitation 2015 Section 6: Paediatric life support. *Resuscitation* 2015, 95: 223–248. Available from: https://www.resuscitationjournal.com/article/S0300-9572(15)00340-8/fulltext.

3. Resuscitation Council (UK). Adult basic life support and automated external defibrillation 2015. London: Resuscitation Council (UK), 2015. Available from: https://www.resus.org.uk/resuscitation-guidelines/adult-basic-life-support-and-automated-external-defibrillation.

4. Resuscitation Council (UK). Paediatric resuscitation guidelines 2015. London: Resuscitation Council (UK), 2015. Available from: https://www.resus.org.uk/resuscitation-guidelines/paediatric-basic-life-support/

Advanced Life Support

1. Advanced Life Support Overview

1.1 Introduction

- Advanced life support (ALS) may be defined as the use of resuscitation drugs and interventions above and beyond basic life support and AED use. However, if a trained ALS provider attends as a solo responder, they are limited to basic life support (BLS) and defibrillation until other responders arrive.
- The availability of ALS, must not affect the provision of high-quality cardiopulmonary resuscitation (CPR) and appropriate defibrillation.
- Out-of-hospital cardiac arrest (OHCA) management follows similar principles for ALS as in-hospital treatment. It is recognised, however, that the environment, equipment, resources, access to the patient, extrication and transportation of the patient play a pivotal part in the overall clinical management decisions.
- A team approach should be adopted as early as possible and a team leader appointed (resources allowing), who can use cardiac arrest checklists for the overall management of the cardiac arrest and for specific clinical skills, e.g. intubation checklists.

1.2 Stages of Assessment and Management

- The assessment and management of an out-of-hospital medical cardiac arrest includes:
  - Confirmation of the cardiac arrest.
  - Early implementation and continuation of effective BLS and defibrillation.
  - The addition of ALS, including IV/IO access, the administration of medicines, advanced airway management and clinical decision making, where appropriate.
  - Early identification and management of reversible causes.
  - Early decision making on:
    - the appropriateness of the resuscitation attempt (ReSPECT, recognition of life extinct, futility and best interests)
    - an early transportation plan if a reversible cause is identified that cannot be treated on-scene or if admission to a cath lab is considered appropriate (according to local protocols).
    - requesting enhanced care resources to attend the scene to help with clinical decision making, enhanced assessments (e.g. ultra-sound) and interventions (e.g. blood products)
    - seeking senior remote advice where available through a structured and governed system.

2. Advanced Life Support in Adults

Refer to ALS algorithm, Figure 2.6.

Additional Information

- Once adrenaline has been administered, further doses should be given every 3–5 minutes, irrespective of rhythm, while the patient remains in cardiac arrest.
- Peripheral IV access should be established as soon as possible. However, paramedics could consider external jugular vein access if appropriately trained.
- If IV access is too difficult or not possible, consider intraosseous access.
- If a patient who is being **monitored** has a **witnessed** arrest:
  - Confirm cardiac arrest.
  - Request further resources if appropriate.
  - If the rhythm is ventricular fibrillation/pulseless ventricular tachycardia (VF/pVT) and a defibrillator is not immediately available, consider a precordial thump.
  - If the rhythm is VF/pVT and a defibrillator is immediately available, give a shock first and immediately commence CPR; treat any recurrence of VF/pVT following the shockable rhythm algorithm.
  - Where the arrest is witnessed but unmonitored, defibrillation pads must be applied immediately.
  - Three stacked shocks may be considered as per local protocols in a witnessed and monitored cardiac arrest only when the patient is already connected to a manual defibrillator. For the purposes of medicine administration, these three shocks should be treated as the first shock in the ALS algorithm.
  - If VF persists, refer to **Defibrillation**.

ADULT ALS - SUMMARY

- During ALS, the priority remains to deliver high quality chest compressions and effective ventilations with high flow oxygen.
- When indicated, defibrillate and resume chest compressions for two minutes without reassessing the rhythm or feeling for a pulse.
- Defibrillation energy levels should be at least 150J for the first shock. Consider escalating energy for subsequent shocks.
- Give amiodarone 300mg IV/IO after three shocks for VF/pVT, irrespective of whether these are sequential or intermittent shockable rhythms.
- A further 150 mg may be administered after a total of five shocks.
- Promptly identify and treat reversible causes (4H's and 4 T's).

Advanced Life Support

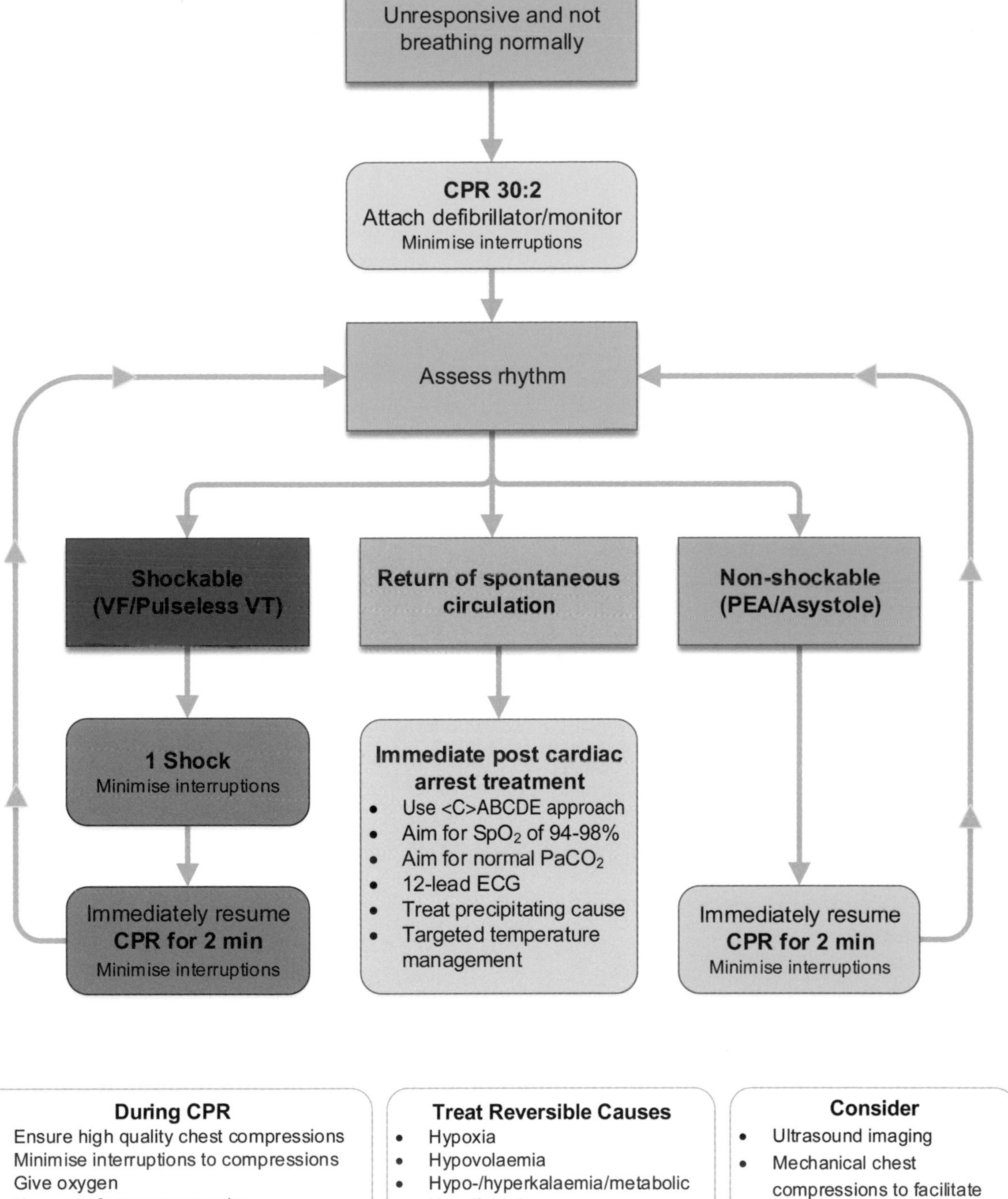

During CPR

- Ensure high quality chest compressions
- Minimise interruptions to compressions
- Give oxygen
- Use waveform capnography
- Continuous compressions when advanced airway in place
- Vascular access (intravenous or intraosseous)
- Give adrenaline every 3-5 min
- Give amiodarone after 3 shocks, consider half dose after 5th shock

Treat Reversible Causes

- Hypoxia
- Hypovolaemia
- Hypo-/hyperkalaemia/metabolic
- Hypothermia
- Thrombosis - coronary or pulmonary
- Tension pneumothorax
- Tamponade – cardiac
- Toxins

Consider

- Ultrasound imaging
- Mechanical chest compressions to facilitate transfer/treatment
- Coronary angiography and percutaneous coronary intervention
- Extracorporeal CPR

Figure 2.6 – Advanced life support in adults algorithm – reproduced with permission from the Resuscitation Council (UK) Guidelines 2015 algorithm (www.resus.org.uk).

- In most patients where ROSC is not achieved on scene, despite appropriate ALS and treatment of any reversible causes, there is little to be gained from transferring these patients to hospital. The exceptions are:
  - Children - aim for minimum scene time.
  - Refractory/recurrent VF (or pVT) - consider early departure from scene for PPCI, according to local protocols.
  - Cardiac arrest in pregnancy - Make plans to undertake a time critical transfer to hospital – this should be commenced within 5 minutes of arrival at the cardiac arrest (seek senior advice early).
  - Penetrating traumatic cardiac arrest - Make plans to undertake a time critical transfer to hospital – this should be commenced within 5 minutes of arrival at the cardiac arrest. These patients are absolutely time critical if they are to survive.
  - Possible electrolyte disturbances (e.g. renal dialysis patients, anorexic patients, dehydration, excessive fluid intake, chronic diarrhoea and vomiting etc).
  - Hypothermia as a contributory factor.
- In cases of **persistent** and **continuous** asystole for 20 mins in adults, despite ALS and where all reversible causes have been identified and treated, the chances of survival are so unlikely that resuscitation can be ceased.

3. Advanced Life Support in Children

3.1 Introduction

- Paediatric ALS resuscitation broadly follows adult protocols.
- This guideline covers:
  - infants (defined as under one year old)
  - children (defined as between one year and puberty).
- In this guideline, the term 'child' includes infants, unless specified otherwise.
- Newborn life support is not covered in this guideline. For newborn babies, refer to **Newborn Life Support**.
- ALS procedures (e.g. establishing vascular access) must not delay the transfer of the child to hospital – start and continue good quality BLS on scene as the priority. Attempt ALS procedures en-route, if practical.
- Paediatric defibrillation (4 J/kg) should be carried out using paediatric defibrillation pads. However, if these are not available, use adult defibrillation pads. Ensure that the defibrillation pads are not in contact with each other; usually a front to back (anterior-posterior) pad placement ensures adequate pad separation.

PAEDIATRIC ALS - SUMMARY

- During ALS, the priority remains to deliver high quality chest compressions and effective ventilations with high flow oxygen. Particular focus should be to ensure reversal of any hypoxia.
- Supraglottic airways (SGAs) may be considered if BMV ventilation is ineffective.
- Intubation is rarely indicated and should only be undertaken by those with appropriate skills, according to local protocols and only when waveform capnography is available.
- Defibrillation should be delivered at 4 J/kg, rounded up to the energy level the defibrillator can deliver.
- As with adults, give amiodarone IV/IO after three shocks and a further half dose after five shocks. Refer to **Amiodarone**, **Page for Age** for children.
- Do not delay on scene to deliver ALS interventions. Early extrication and transport to hospital is mandatory; aim to deliver ALS on route.

4. Defibrillation

4.1 Principles of Defibrillation

- The purpose of defibrillation is to terminate VF/pVT by passing an electrical current across the heart to depolarise a critical mass of myocardial cells.
- Defibrillation is more likely to be successful if:
  - Time from collapse to shock is minimised.
  - The collapse has been witnessed and the patient has received bystander CPR.
  - BLS is of good quality (correct rate and depth, complete chest recoil, minimal interruptions and maximal chest compression fraction).
  - The pre-shock pause is as short as possible (< 5 secs).
  - The defibrillation pads are placed correctly (refer to Figure 2.8).
- Minimise pre-shock pauses, by resuming chest compressions immediately after the rhythm check while the defibrillator charges. It is also acceptable to charge the defibrillator at the end of the two minutes of CPR approaches while continuing chest compressions. All team members should stand clear for the rhythm check so that the shock can be delivered without delay if appropriate, before immediately resuming CPR.
- Current guidelines for biphasic waveforms recommend commencing with an initial shock of at least 150 joules if using a manual defibrillator. Consider increasing the energy for second and subsequent shocks if using a manual defibrillator.

Advanced Life Support

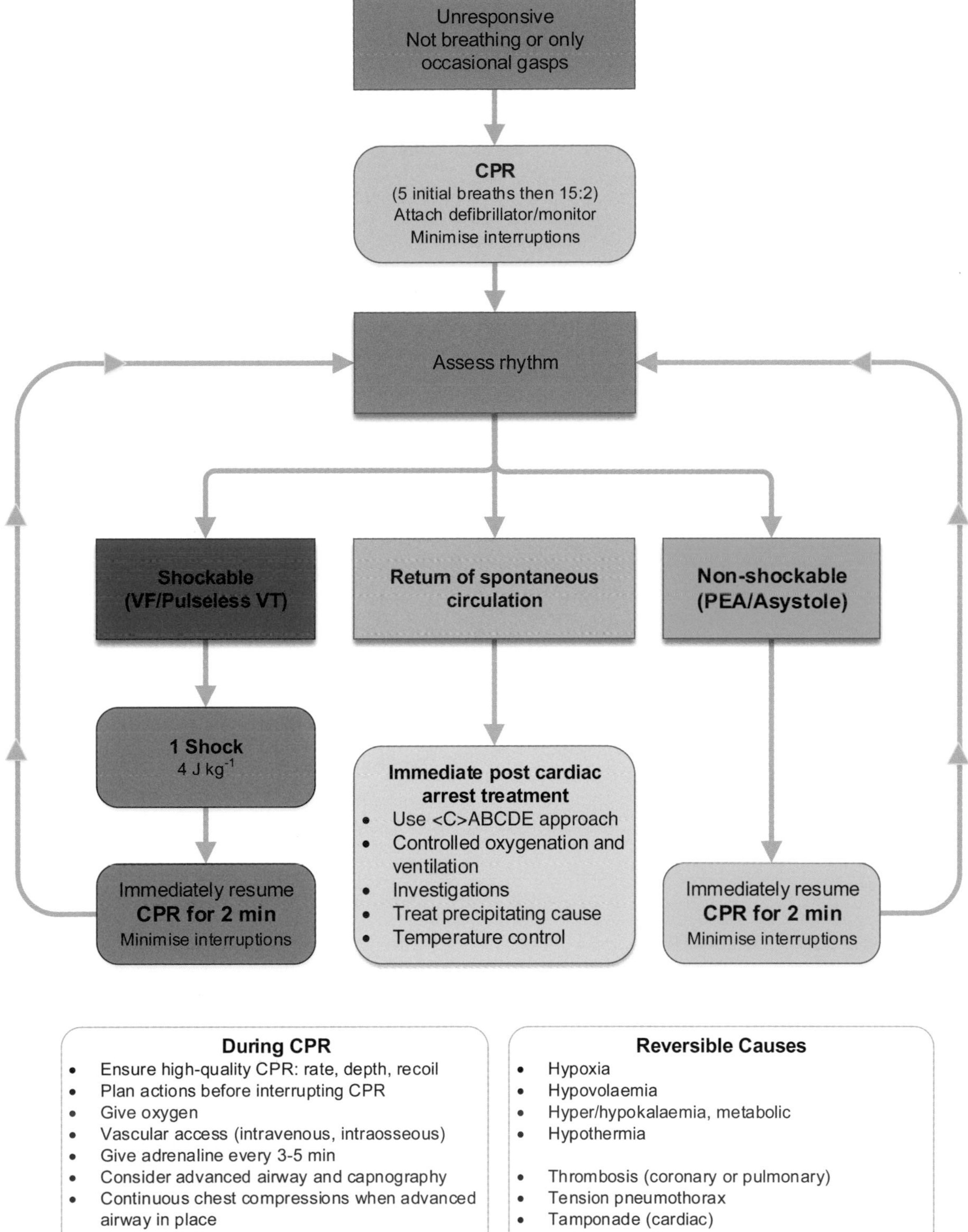

Figure 2.7 – Advanced life support in children algorithm – Reproduced with permission from the Resuscitation Council (UK) Guidelines 2015 (www.resus.org.uk).

- Paediatric defibrillation should be delivered at 4 J/kg, rounded up to the nearest energy level the defibrillator can deliver. (N.B. Defibrillators that deliver a maximum output of 200J at least match the current delivered by defibrillators with a 360J output).
- When using a monitor that filters out ECG movement artefact and the underlying rhythm can be clearly seen without having to pause for a rhythm check, charge the defibrillator with ongoing CPR. If using manual chest compressions, stand clear to then deliver the shock. If using mechanical chest compression, there is no need to stop this when the shock is delivered. Note that the mechanical chest compression device may move when the shock is delivered, therefore, it is important to ensure the device remains correctly positioned.

4.2 Priorities in Delivery of Defibrillation

- Delivering the first shock as soon as possible is the priority. Therefore, when attending as a solo responder equipped with a defibrillator, immediate assessment of the rhythm and defibrillation (when indicated), should take precedence over airway or breathing interventions. If possible use a bystander to start and continue chest compressions while the defibrillator is attached. Although defibrillation is an initial priority, it is important to minimise delays and interruptions in delivering chest compressions.

4.3 Fine VF

- Immediate defibrillation should always be performed in patients where a shockable rhythm is identified on the ECG, irrespective of the amplitude. Automated defibrillators use a low threshold for the recognition of fine VF.

4.4 AED vs Manual Modes

- Most manual defibrillators carried in ambulances can also be used in an AED mode where they analyse the ECG and recommend delivery of a shock when appropriate. There are advantages and disadvantages of each mode. Although AED mode may improve the time to first shock, manual mode may reduce pre-shock pauses and increase chest compression fraction which is associated with increased ROSC. Therefore, although manual defibrillation should be the preferred option for appropriately trained paramedics it should be recognised that solo responders are potentially in a stressful environment, and are attempting to manage multiple complex factors. Therefore, the initial use of the AED function is acceptable until additional help arrives.

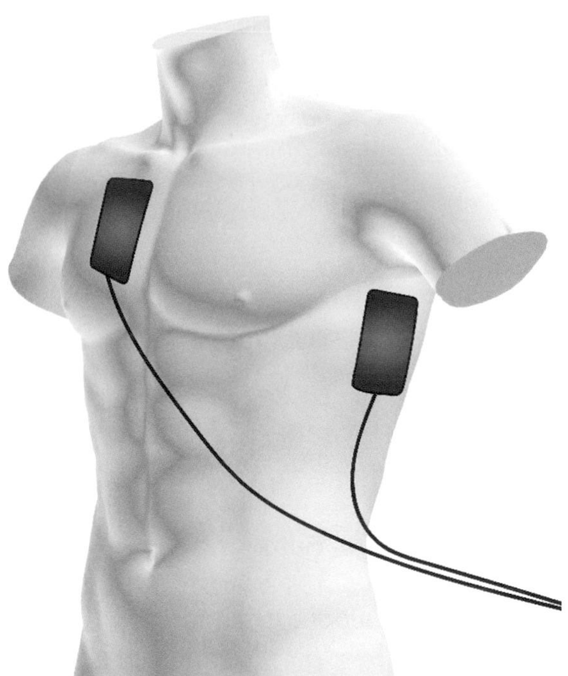

Figure 2.8 – Correct placement of defibrillation pads in the antero-lateral position. Note the relatively high and lateral positioning of the lateral pad (just below the armpit).

4.5 Defibrillator Pads

- It is important to ensure correct pad positioning so that adequate current traverses the myocardium in order to optimise defibrillation success. In the conventional sternal–apical position the right (sternal) pad is placed to the right of the sternum, below the clavicle. The apical pad is placed in the left mid-axillary line, approximately level with the V6 ECG electrode. This pad must be placed sufficiently laterally, as shown in Figure 2.8.
- Other acceptable pad positions include:
  - Anterior posterior – one pad anteriorly, over the left precordium, and the other pad posteriorly to the heart just inferior to the left scapula.
  - Bi-axillary – one pad placed just below each axilla, in the mid-axillary line (for example in patients with burns or where a subcutaneous pacing box may preclude standard pad placement).
- When paediatric defibrillation pads are not available, adult pads can be used as an alternative for children. Ensure that the pads are not in contact with each other; usually a front to back (anterior-posterior) pad placement ensures adequate pad separation.
- Self-adhesive defibrillation pads have a water/electrolyte-based matrix to improve conductivity

with the skin. Defibrillation pads do not need to be changed during a resuscitation attempt unless visibly damaged, although they may be replaced if the pads need to be moved for an alternative position.

4.6 Hands-on Defibrillation

- Delivering continuous chest compressions during defibrillation, can minimise pre-shock pause and prevent interruption of chest compressions. However, the benefits of hands-on defibrillation are not proven and further studies are required to assess the safety and efficacy of this technique. Standard clinical examination gloves (or bare hands) do not provide a safe level of electrical insulation.

4.7 Recurrent and Refractory VF

- Recurrent VF refers to VF that is cardioverted following each shock but returns before the next rhythm check. Recurrence of VF after a successful shock is common.
- By contrast, refractory VF refers to VF that persists despite defibrillation attempts. In the out-of-hospital environment, it may be difficult to determine whether persistent VF is recurrent or refractory, as CPR is resumed immediately post-shock.
- Administer 300 mg amiodarone IV after the third shock and give a further 150 mg IV dose after the fifth shock.
- Optimise oxygenation and ventilation and ensure high-quality CPR.
- Ensure that the defibrillation pads are placed correctly and that electrical contact is not impaired by moisture or a hairy chest. If using antero-lateral defibrillation pad placement, ensure that the lateral pad is placed sufficiently laterally, as shown in Figure 2.8.
- Consider early transport to a primary percutaneous coronary intervention (PPCI) centre. Consider requesting enhanced care support.

4.8 Dual Sequential Defibrillation (DSD)

- DSD involves the use of two separate manual defibrillators, delivering shocks at the same time or in rapid succession.
- This is not recommended practice and it is not licenced or recommended by the defibrillator manufacturers.
- Delivering twice as much defibrillation energy carries with it the risk of myocardial stunning and conversion to asystole rather than a perfusing rhythm.
- No cohort studies or meta-analysis have demonstrated any benefits over conventional defibrillation.
- Without a well-designed prospective study, the true benefit (or harm) of DSD remains unknown.

4.9 Pacemakers

- Pacemakers (and internal defibrillators) are generally positioned below the left clavicle, although on occasion they may be placed on the right side. They appear as a subcutaneous firm mass, approximately 5 x 5 cm, over which is a scar from the insertion. Check the patient for a MedicAlert bracelet.
- In relation to resuscitation, pacemakers may have several different functions:
  - **Pacing only** – to keep the heart rate above a set level (may be ventricular pacing only, but may be set to deliver both atrial and ventricular pacing).
  - **Defibrillation only** (implantable cardioverter-defibrillator – ICD) – to monitor the heart continually and deliver a shock when a shockable arrhythmia is detected. They give no warning when firing and are programmed to give repeated shocks if indicated.
  - **Pacing and defibrillation** – a combination of both functions.
- These devices may be damaged during defibrillation if current is discharged through pads placed directly over the device.
- Place the pad away from the device (at least 8 cm) or use an alternative pad position (anterior–lateral, anterior–posterior, bi-axillary).
- Pacemakers will continue to discharge even in a patient who is deceased. This appears as very narrow pacing spikes on the ECG and the monitor may even display a heart rate. However, an ECG showing pacing spikes not followed by any ventricular (or atrial) complex is effectively an asystolic trace.
- Placing a magnet over a pacing device will generally result in it pacing at a fixed (asynchronous mode) rate of 50–100/min and does not stop pacemaker function.
- Placing a magnet over an ICD will result in disabling of the defibrillation function and shocks will not be delivered. This may be necessary in some cases of fast atrial arrhythmias, or if the pacing (sensing) lead is faulty, when the ICD may repeatedly discharge erroneously which is distressing for the patient.

4.10 Safe Use of Oxygen

- Use oxygen safely during defibrillation by:
  - removing any oxygen mask or nasal cannulae and placing them at least 1 metre away from the patient's chest during defibrillation
  - leaving the ventilation bag connected to the tracheal tube or SGA.

- Oxygen-powered LUCAS devices discharge large amounts of oxygen over and around the defibrillation pads which may be a significant hazard, particularly in a closed environment (e.g. the back of an ambulance).

5. Airway and Breathing Management

5.1 Introduction

- The Airways2 trial found that the initial approach to airway management is bag- mask ventilation (BMV) for approximately half of all cardiac arrest patients, with the remainder managed with a supraglottic airway (SGA) (20%) or tracheal intubation (25%).
- The most common reason cited by paramedics for changing from BMV was to carry out ALS, followed by regurgitation and inadequate ventilation.
- Inadequate ventilation was the most common reason cited for removing an SGA.
- A stepwise approach to airway management is recommended. This should include a strategy on how and when to progress from one airway technique to another.
- It should be noted that the stepwise approach is not one-way. If a technique is failing, then it is sometimes appropriate to move to a less advanced technique, than to attempt techniques that are more advanced.
- However, in the context of out-of-hospital cardiac arrest, it might also be appropriate to move directly to more advanced techniques, depending on the circumstances. For example, the early application of an SGA may be beneficial, rather than attempting oropharyngeal, or nasopharyngeal airways. Tracheal intubation as the initial airway is not recommended; use of a BMV or supraglottic airway should proceed any attempt at tracheal intubation.
- Spinal precautions must be started at the same time as airway management, but these do not take priority. Refer to **Spinal Injury and Spinal Cord Injury**.

5.2 Bag-mask ventilation (BMV)

- The initial approach to airway management should usually be BMV. An oropharyngeal airway (OPA) or nasopharyngeal airway (NPA) may be used to improve the efficacy of ventilations via the BMV.
- A complication of ventilation (with a BMV) is gastric inflation, resulting in impaired ventilation and regurgitation, especially where forceful ventilations are delivered. This risk is reduced where gentle ventilations are delivered over one second or where a SGA is used. As such, it is reasonable to place a suitable SGA as part of BLS, when trained in its use.

5.3 Airway Sizes

- Table 2.8 provides a guide for airway sizes in children and adults.

5.4 Supraglottic Airways

- There are several SGAs (e.g. iGel and laryngeal mask airway); all sit above the larynx, and are simpler and quicker to insert than a tracheal tube. They can be inserted with minimal interruption to chest compressions.
- A number of case reports exist describing patients who have been found to have foreign bodies deep within their oropharynx. It is recommended that if there is a high degree of suspicion of foreign body airway obstruction, inspection of the oropharynx should be undertaken with a laryngoscope before inserting any SGA.
- Once an SGA has been placed, continuous chest compressions with 10 ventilations per minute are preferred. However, 30 compressions to 2 ventilations are acceptable if ventilation is inadequate when delivering continuous compressions.
- Air leaks from around the SGA are common. If the chest wall can be seen to be moving, ventilation is generally adequate. However, repositioning of replacement of the airway with a more suitable size may be necessary if the air leak is of sufficient magnitude to prevent the chest rising and falling with each breath.

5.5 Tracheal Intubation

- The tracheal tube is a challenging airway device to insert successfully and requires both adequate initial training and ongoing practice. Paramedics must ensure that they have appropriate competence to undertake it safely and that this skill has been regularly updated and evidenced through maintaining an airway skills log.
- There is no evidence that patient outcome is any better following tracheal intubation compared with any other type of airway.
- When tracheal intubation is undertaken, the availability of a bougie and use of waveform capnography is mandatory.
- Visualisation of the tube entering the trachea, auscultation over both axillae and epigastrium

and observation of chest wall movement should all aid confirmation but are not in themselves 100% diagnostic of correct tube placement. This can only be achieved by using waveform capnography.

- If the capnography trace is flat, then it must be assumed that the tracheal tube is sited incorrectly and must be removed.
- Once a tracheal tube is in place, continue continuous chest compressions with 10 ventilations per minute. It is important to avoid hyperventilation when continuous chest compressions are delivered.
- It is important to remember the following for tracheal intubation:
  - Ensure 360° access around the patient where possible (This may involve rapidly moving the patient to give better access).
  - Prepare a kit dump of all the necessary equipment close to the patient before starting the process of intubation. This must include a bougie and immediate access to capnography monitoring and any additional airway equipment necessary for a failed intubation.
  - Do not routinely use cricoid pressure for tracheal intubation during CPR.
  - If during laryngoscopy the paramedic needs a better view, use external laryngeal manipulation. Pressure directed to move the trachea backwards, upwards and to the right (BURP maneouvre) may improve visualisation of the vocal cords.
  - Secure the tracheal tube immediately after insertion, noting length at incisors. This is approximately:
    - adult males: 22–24 cm
    - adult females: 21–23 cm.
  - Listen to any team member who suggests that the attempt has become a 'Can't intubate, can't ventilate scenario', irrespective of clinical grade.
  - Avoid hypoxaemia during intubation: pre-oxygenate the lungs before and between intubation attempts.
  - Where possible, use two team members to attempt intubation, and ensure a failed intubation plan has been communicated to all the team.

5.6 Capnography

- Capnography (measurement of exhaled (end-tidal) carbon dioxide – $EtCO_2$) assists in confirmation and continuous monitoring of tracheal tube placement, can provide feedback on the quality of CPR, and can provide an early indication of return of spontaneous circulation (ROSC).
- Waveform capnography is a real-time waveform display of $EtCO_2$ and is more accurate and reliable than a paper indicator.
- The use of waveform capnography is mandatory in paramedic intubation. Tracheal intubation and subsequent monitoring must only be performed with the assistance of waveform capnography monitoring. Recorded values must be documented on the patient record. In the absence of waveform capnography, an alternative airway technique or device should be employed.
- Any decision to terminate resuscitation should not be based on either the presence or absence of $EtCO_2$ alone.
- Waveform capnography is recommended where an SGA has been placed as it is useful in providing positive feedback on the quality of CPR.

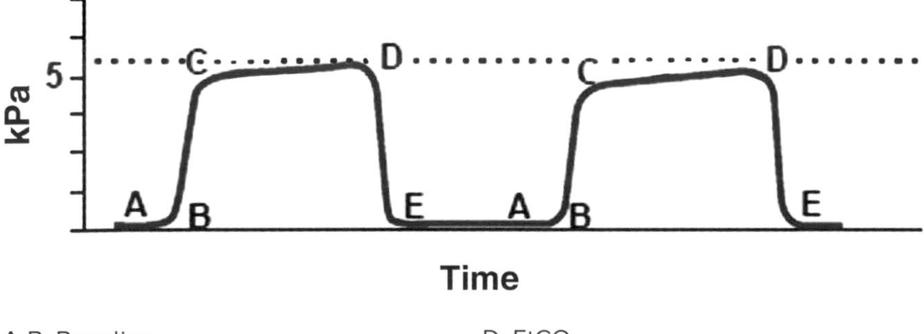

A-B: Baseline
B-C: Expiratory upstroke
C-D: Expiratory plateau
D: $EtCO_2$
D-E: Inspiration

Figure 2.9 – Capnography

TABLE 2.8 – Airway Sizes by Type

Age	Airway Size by Device Type		
	Oropharyngeal	**SGA**	**Tracheal tube** Internal diameter Length at the lips
Birth	000	1.0	Diameter: 3.0 mm Length: 10 cm
1 month	00	1.0	Diameter: 3.0 mm Length: 10 cm
3 months	00	1.5	Diameter: 3.5 mm Length: 11 cm
6 months	00	1.5	Diameter: 4.0 mm Length: 12 cm
9 months	00	1.5	Diameter: 4.0 mm Length: 12 cm
12 months	00 OR 0	1.5 OR 2.0	Diameter: 4.5 mm Length: 13 cm
18 months	00 OR 0	1.5 OR 2.0	Diameter: 4.5 mm Length: 13 cm
2 years	0 OR 1	1.5 OR 2.0	Diameter: 5.0 mm Length: 14 cm
3 years	1	2.0	Diameter: 5.0 mm Length: 14 cm
4 years	1	2.0	Diameter: 5.0 mm Length: 15 cm
5 years	1	2.0	Diameter: 5.5 mm Length: 15 cm
6 years	1	2.0	Diameter: 6.0 mm Length: 16 cm
7 years	1 OR 2	2.0	Diameter: 6.0 mm Length: 16 cm
8 years	1 OR 2	2.5	Diameter: 6.5 mm Length: 17 cm
9 years	1 OR 2	2.5	Diameter: 6.5 mm Length: 17 cm
10 years	2 OR 3	2.5 OR 3.0	Diameter: 7.0 mm Length: 18 cm
11 years	2 OR 3	2.5 OR 3.0	Diameter: 7.0 mm Length: 18 cm
Adult >70kg	4 OR 5	4.0 OR 5.0	Female diameter: 7.0–8.0 mm length: 21–23 cm Male diameter: 8.0–9.0 mm length: 22–24 cm

Advanced Life Support

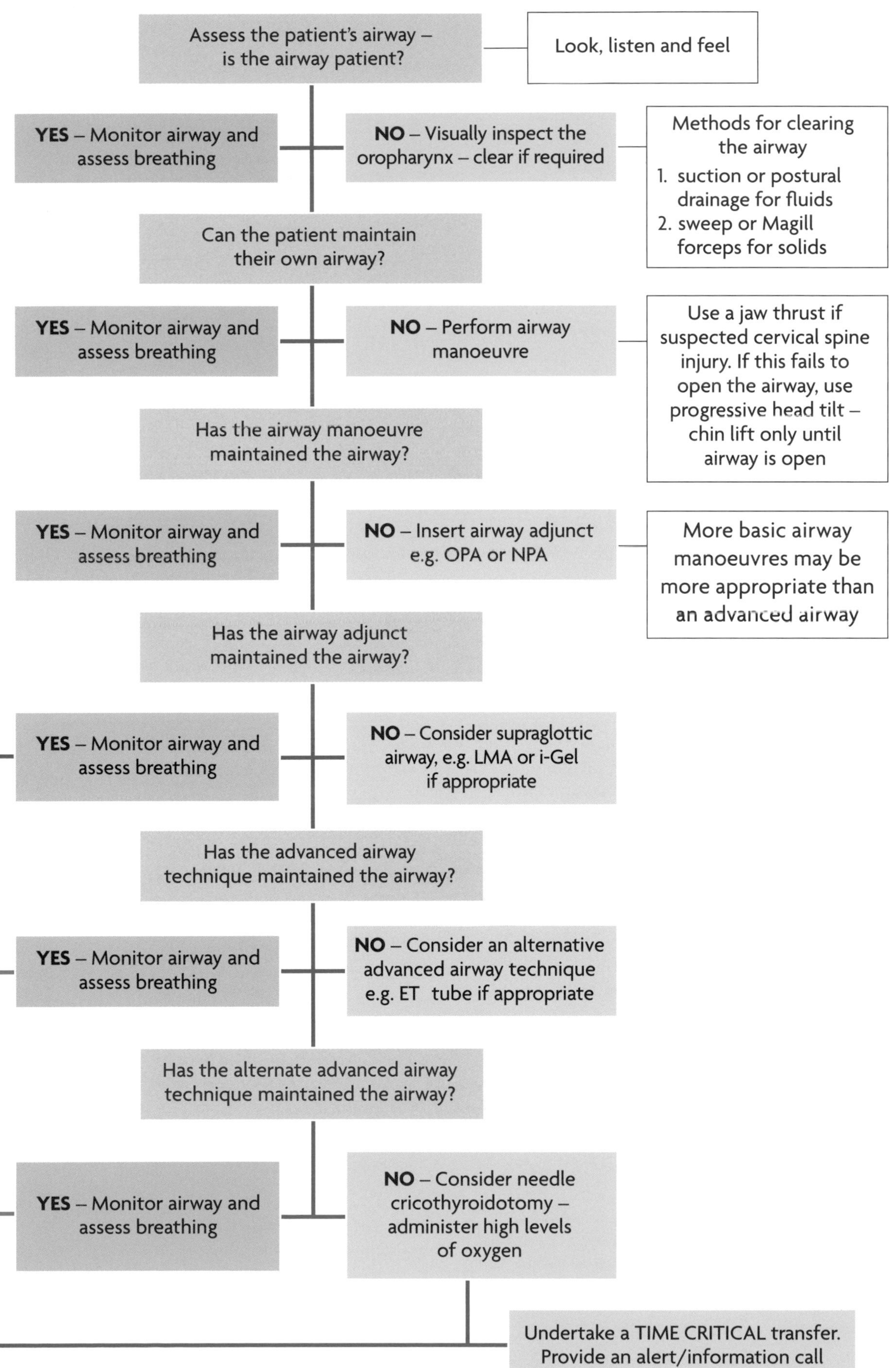

Figure 2.10 – Breathing assessment and management overview.

SECTION 2 Resuscitation

6. Mechanical Chest Compression Devices (mCPR)

- Delivery of manual chest compressions are often inconsistent and subject to fatigue. Mechanical chest compression (mCPR) devices are designed to provide consistent high-quality chest compressions to the required depth and frequency for prolonged periods of time.
- However, large randomised controlled trials of the routine use of mCPR in the out-of-hospital setting have found no evidence of improved patient outcome compared with manual CPR. Routine use of mCPR it is therefore not indicated.
- However, mCPR can be considered during the extrication and transportation of a patient in cardiac arrest, when prolonged CPR is indicated (e.g. ECMO, hypothermia, refractory VF etc) or for patients being taken to the cath lab for PCI where manual chest compression during the procedure is not possible.
- mCPR should be deployed by dedicated teams that are regularly drilled, practiced and signed off in its deployment to ensure effective use and minimal interruption to CPR during its placement.

6.1 Impedance Threshold Valve

- In the same way that gasping generates negative intrathoracic pressure, mechanical devices that enhance negative intrathoracic pressure during CPR may also increase venous return and enhance forward blood flow.
- Some, but not all, studies have shown that impedance threshold devices (ITDs) may improve outcome; but where they are effective, they appear to be so only in the context of CPR that delivers correct compression rate and depth.
- In the absence of evidence for the benefits of this device, the routine use of an ITD is not recommended.

7. Head-Up CPR

- Animal and human cadaver studies have suggested that gradual head and thorax elevation to an angle of 30° while performing CPR, when combined with an ITD, improves cerebral perfusion pressures
- A head-up position improves cerebral venous return by facilitating cerebral venous drainage. It also lowers intracranial pressure, which together results in an increase in cerebral perfusion pressure.
- In the absence of any clinical studies, the use of head-up CPR must only be undertaken in the context of a closely monitored trial or evaluation, with regular review of neurological outcome in survivors.

8. Extra-Corporeal Membrane Oxygenation (ECMO) and Possible Out-of-Hospital Applications

- One area of growing interest is the use of ECMO in refractory cardiac arrest where survival is poor.
- Conventional cardiopulmonary resuscitation involves chest compressions, which produce a 'low flow' cardiac output. The longer the period of chest compressions, the greater the likelihood of irreversible organ damage, and the less the chance of a return of spontaneous circulation (ROSC).
- Because ECMO can match a normal native cardiac output (5.0 litres/min), it is very effective in perfusing the heart and the brain, and preventing on-going damage despite a patient being in cardiac arrest.
- When used in this way, it is referred to as extracorporeal cardiopulmonary resuscitation (ECPR). It is normally achieved by placing a large cannula in the femoral vein to drain venous blood, and pumping oxygenated blood through another large cannula placed in the femoral artery.
- Some ambulance services in Europe and North America have begun trials of pre-hospital ECPR for out-of-hospital cardiac arrest. Trials are shortly planned for the UK.

9. CPR-Induced Consciousness

- In some patients, the application of CPR may produce sufficient cerebral perfusion for signs of consciousness in the absence of ROSC.

9.1 Characteristics

- Patients may display a variety of signs including:
  - eye opening
  - increased jaw tone
  - incomprehensible sounds
  - recognisable words or speech
  - limb movement
  - purposeful movements, e.g. localising to pain
  - combative movements, e.g. pushing rescuers away.

9.2 Key Points for CPR-Induced Consciousness

- Even if a patient is displaying any of these features, frequent rhythm checks are not recommended and paramedics should limit rhythm checks to once every 2 minutes, as per conventional guidance.
- CPR-induced consciousness (CPR-IC) should be recognised at the earliest opportunity. Signs that

may help paramedics distinguish CPR-IC from ROSC may include:

- an absence of palpable pulses
- a rapid deterioration in consciousness when chest compressions are stopped
- a cardiac rhythm considered incompatible with life.

- In patients with symptoms that create difficulty in delivering high quality CPR or when the patient may be distressed, paramedics may wish to consider requesting enhanced care support or advice as per local procedures/pathways or rapid conveyance to hospital to facilitate ongoing treatment.

10. Reversible Causes and Specialist Circumstances in Cardiac Arrest (4Hs and 4Ts)

10.1 Hypoxia

- All patients in cardiac arrest should be ventilated with high concentration oxygen to minimise the risk of hypoxia. Ensure regular checks of the oxygen cylinder and replace it if needed before the cylinder runs empty.

10.2 Hypovolaemia

- Hypovolaemia may be due to blood loss or a depleted intravascular volume as may occur in sepsis or severe dehydration. Prevent further hypovolaemia by controlling any catastrophic haemorrhage. Where hypovolaemia is suspected, intravascular volume should be restored rapidly with IV fluid. Up to 2 litres of normal saline should be rapidly infused. Early transportation of these patients should be considered.

10.3 Hypo/Hyperkalaemia

- Diagnosing this in the pre-hospital setting is challenging. The patient's medical history or identification of a dialysis fistula may give an indication of dialysis history and potential hyperkalaemia. Patients with a history of diabetic ketoacidosis (DKA) will often also have a high serum potassium. Frail elderly patients, or those with eating disorders, who have a recent history of gastric disease, may have low serum potassium. On suspicion or identification of any potential reversible metabolic disorder, a time critical transfer to hospital should be considered. Blood sugar should remain an important consideration during cardiac arrest.

10.4 Hypothermia

- Accidental hypothermia is often under-diagnosed in temperate climates. Generally, hypothermia can develop during exposure to cold environments and in people who have been immobilised or immersed in cold water. In the older/frail person and the very young, where thermoregulation is impaired, hypothermia can follow a very mild insult. The risk of hypothermia is also increased by exhaustion, illness, injury, neglect, reduced level of consciousness or when drugs or alcohol have been ingested.

- Severe hypothermia is associated with the depression of cerebral blood flow and oxygen requirement, reduced cardiac output and decreased arterial pressure. Patients can appear to be clinically dead because of significant depression of brain and cardiovascular function, but the threshold for full resuscitation should remain low as recovery with intact neurology is possible.

- The patient's peripheral pulses and respiratory effort may be difficult to detect. Therefore, resuscitation should not be withheld based on clinical presentation. Consider whether on the basis of history, hypothermia is believed to be the primary cause of the cardiac arrest. If hypothermia is believed to be the primary cause, follow the guidance below.

- Pre-hospital core temperature measurement can be inaccurate and so should not always be relied upon to confirm hypothermia. In a hypothermic patient, resuscitation should not be withheld unless the cause of the cardiac arrest is clearly attributable to fatal illness, prolonged asphyxia, lethal injury or if the chest is incompressible.

- Because hypothermia itself may produce a very slow, small-volume, irregular pulse and un-recordable blood pressure, signs of life may be so minimal that it is easy to overlook them. Palpate a major artery, obtain an ECG and look for signs of life (pulse, chest rise, breathing efforts, movements, eye opening or shockable rhythm) for up to one minute before concluding that there is no cardiac output. Hypothermia can cause stiffness of the chest wall, making chest compressions and ventilations difficult; however, if the patient is pulseless, start chest compressions and ventilations at the same rate as for normothermic patients.

- It is important to prevent further heat loss from the patient's body core, by removing wet garments (providing this does not result in additional exposure), protecting against heat loss and wind chill by using blankets/heated blankets, head coverings and insulating equipment.

- The hypothermic heart may be unresponsive to cardioactive drugs and defibrillation; therefore, when the core temperature is between 30 – 35°C, double intervals between medicines should be used, e.g. adrenaline every 6–10 minutes.

- Where the core temperature is < 30°C, no drugs should be administered until the temperature reaches 30°C, at which point double intervals should be used. A maximum of 3 shocks should be delivered to a patient in a shockable rhythm below 30°C. **NB** consideration should be given where Trusts do not have equipment to differentiate between <35°C and <30°C. In these cases, double intervals between medicines should be used.
- Consider hospital bypass to a centre that can provide extracorporeal rewarming and phone ahead to discuss the case, as per local procedures.

10.5 Hyperthermia

- Hyperthermia occurs when the body's ability to thermoregulate fails and core temperature exceeds that normally maintained by homeostatic mechanisms. Either the body's metabolic heat production or environmental heat load exceeds the body's normal heat loss capacity, or heat loss is impaired.
- In addition to heat stroke, patients with acute behavioural disorder (ABD) often present with hyperthermia. Both groups are at risk of hyperthermia contributing to metabolic disturbance and an ensuing cardiac arrest.
- When managing the hyperthermic patient in cardiac arrest, follow standard procedures for basic and advanced life support and cool the patient by removing excess clothing and adjusting the surrounding environmental temperature if possible.
- Prognosis is poor when compared to normothermic cardiac arrests. High body temperature is capable of producing irreversible brain damage and the risk of unfavourable neurological outcome increases for each degree of body temperature above 37°C.

10.6 Toxins

- Patients who may have ingested a deliberate or accidental amount of toxin before their cardiac arrest should be transported to the ED, with effective resuscitation delivered en-route. Consider mechanical CPR if resuscitation attempts are likely to be prolonged. If possible, communication regarding the suspected ingestion substance should be made with the ED as early as possible. Crew safety regarding cross contamination must always be a high priority in these situations.
- Where there is suspicion of poisoning of unknown origin, e.g. snake or animal bites etc., the antidote is required rapidly and will rarely be available in the pre-hospital setting. Paramedics should therefore aim for rapid conveyance.
- Refer to **Overdose and Poisoning in Adults and Children**.

10.7 Tension Pneumothorax

- The diagnosis of a tension pneumothorax in the pre-hospital environment can be challenging. If there is suspicion of tension pneumothorax, supported by clinical findings, the chest should be decompressed using needle thoracentesis. This procedure may not always relieve the tension and even in patients where it does, a tension pneumothorax may recur as the cannula becomes blocked or dislodged. A high index of suspicion should be applied to any re-occurrence of tension pneumothorax.
- Consider enhanced care for insertion of a more definitive thoracostomy incision.

10.8 Thrombosis – Coronary or Pulmonary

- **Coronary** Where the rhythm is shockable, this should be managed as outlined in the ALS algorithm.
- **Pulmonary** This will be challenging to diagnose in the cardiac arrest situation. If available, the patient's history before cardiac arrest may give some indication. If pulmonary thrombosis is suspected, a time-critical transfer to hospital is indicated. In situations where thrombolysis is administered, CPR for as long as 90 mins may be required to break up the clot. In these circumstances, consider mechanical CPR.

10.9 Cardiac Tamponade

- Diagnosis of this in the pre-hospital environment is challenging due to its occult nature. Cardiac tamponade compresses the heart, prevents adequate filling and ejection and leads to cardiac arrest; it requires urgent decompression. Therefore, if suspected, a time-critical transfer to hospital is indicated. Consider enhanced care support where available.
- In patients presenting in PEA, evaluation of the ECG waveform may assist in identifying any reversible causes. Figure 2.11 shows a classification of Pulseless Electrical Activity (PEA) according to the reversible cause.

11. Special Considerations in Cardiac Arrest

11.1 Pregnancy

- Refer to **Maternal Resuscitation**.
- Establishing effective resuscitation, focussing on delivering ALS to the mother, is the first priority. Specific modifications include:
  - The hand position for chest compressions may need to be slightly higher on the sternum for patients in the third trimester.
  - Hypoxia and hypovolaemia are common causes of maternal cardiac arrest and should be considered early.
  - Tracheal intubation may be considerably more difficult. A tracheal tube may need to

PEA – EVALUATION

QRS NARROW MECHANICAL (RV) PROBLEM	QRS WIDE METABOLIC (LV) PROBLEM
• Cardiac tamponade • Tension PTX • Mechanical hyperinflation • Pulmonary embolism	• Severe hyperkalemia • Sodium-channel blocker toxicity
	AGONAL RHYTHM
ACUTE MI Myocardial rupture	ACUTE MI Pump failure

Figure 2.11 – Classification of PEA based on its initial electrocardiographic manifestation. LV = Left ventricular; PTX = pneumothorax; US = ultrasound; RV = right ventricular. Source: Littmann L et al. Med Princ Pract 2014. Simplified and Structured Teaching Tool for the Evaluation and Management of Pulseless Electrical Activity.

Republished with permission.

be 0.5–1.0 mm smaller than that for a non-pregnant woman of the same size.

- Manually displace the uterus to the left to ensure that there is adequate venous return to the heart. Add left lateral tilt (ideally 15-30° but even a small amount of tilt may be better than no tilt).
- Make plans to undertake a time critical transfer to hospital – this should be commenced within 5 minutes of arrival at the cardiac arrest.

- Advanced life support intervention can be carried out en-route. Emphasise the pregnancy at the earliest opportunity during pre-alert to allow for further specialist hospital staff to be available in order to perform a peri-mortem caesarean section on arrival to resus if indicated.

11.2 Drowning

- Drowning is defined as a process resulting in primary respiratory impairment from submersion/immersion in a liquid medium and is the third leading cause of accidental death in Europe.
- Patients who have been submerged for less than 10 min have a very high chance of a good outcome, whereas those submerged for more than 25 min are associated with a low chance of good outcome. Rescue efforts of up to 90 minutes may be appropriate for children or those submerged in icy cold water (See Figure 2.12).
- Ensure personal safety and the safety of other rescuers. Establish whether the patient was alone or if there may be other patients. Ensure additional resources, including enhanced or specialist units, are requested as required.
- Hypoxia is the most common cause of arrest in drowning but hypothermia or arrhythmia should also be considered.
- Resuscitative efforts should be made where there is a possibility of an air pocket from which the patient could breathe while under water or, where the patient's airway has only been intermittently submerged (e.g. wearing a life jacket), provided there are no signs unequivocally associated with death.
- Palpation of the pulse as the sole indicator to confirm the presence or absence of cardiac arrest is unreliable. Use an ECG and waveform capnography ($EtCO_2$) monitoring to confirm cardiac arrest.
- There is no difference in the management of salt and fresh water drowning.
- Regurgitation of stomach contents and large amounts of foam can be common during resuscitation from drowning. Efforts to remove the foam may be futile; therefore, early intubation may assist airway management and ventilation. In most drowning incidents patients will aspirate small amounts of water, and this is absorbed into the central circulation. Where contaminants prevent ventilation, the patient can be turned on their side or direct suction can be used to remove the regurgitated material as best as possible.
- Administer IV fluids to correct hypovolaemia if indicated.
- If submersion occurs in cold water (< 5°C), hypothermia may develop rapidly and provides some protection against hypoxia. If hypothermia is considered to be the primary cause of the cardiac arrest, manage as per hypothermia section.

Management

- Give five initial rescue breaths while administering high flow oxygen, then follow standard ALS protocols.

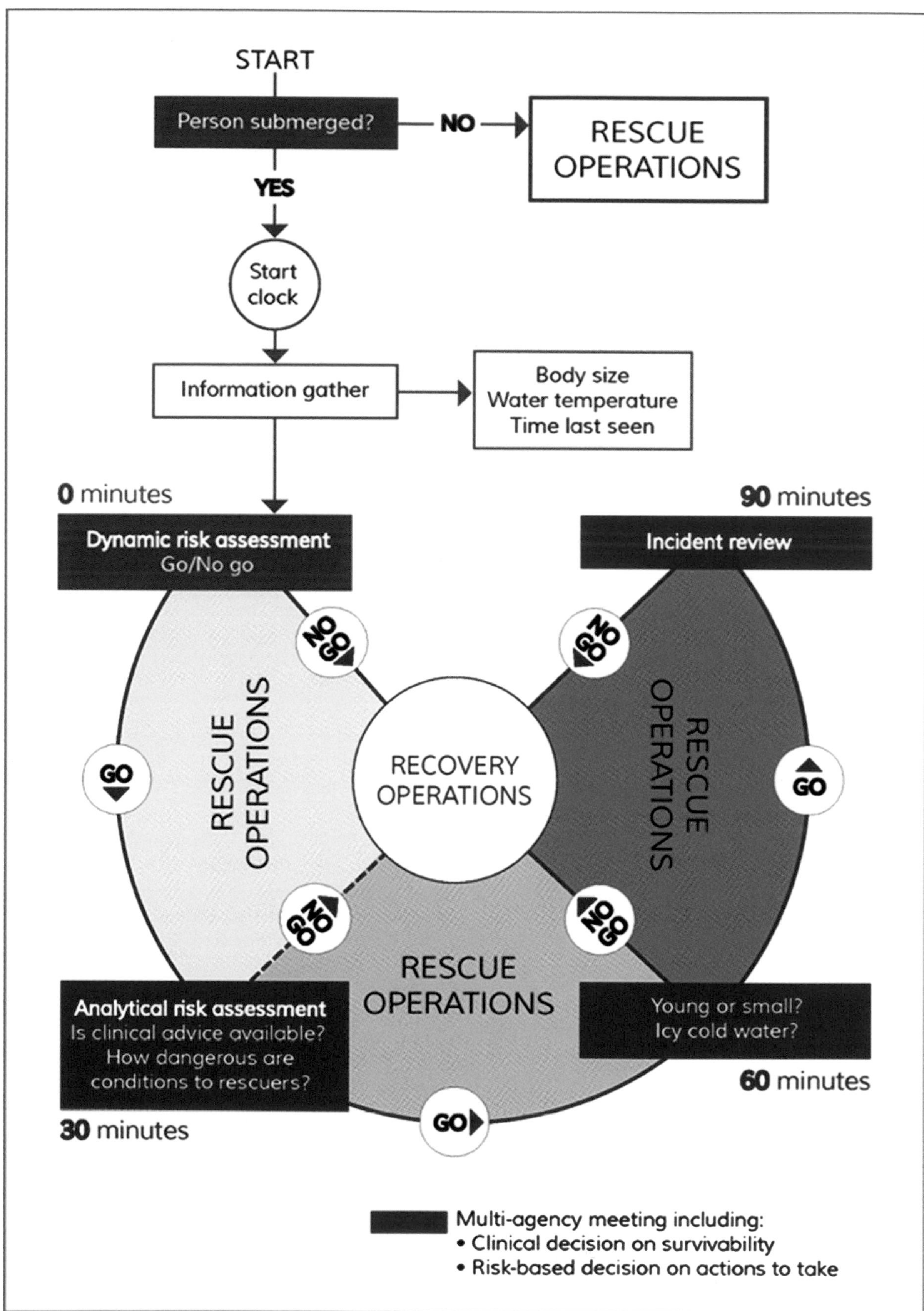

Figure 2.12 – UK risk assessment for submersion

- Consider head and neck injuries, which may be present if the patient dived into shallow water; these are present in <0.5% of all cases and rescue should take precedence over c-spine protection.
- The patient's heart may be extremely slow and external cardiac chest compressions may be required.
- Consider early tracheal intubation, as high ventilation pressure may be required because of poor compliance resulting from pulmonary oedema.

11.3 Asthma

- Cardiac arrest in the asthmatic patient is often a terminal event after a period of hypoxaemia and respiratory exhaustion, and is associated with:
  - Severe bronchospasm and mucous plugging leading to asphyxia.
  - Cardiac arrhythmias due to hypoxia, stimulant drug or electrolyte abnormalities.
  - Dynamic hyperinflation where a gradual build-up of pressure occurs which reduces venous return and blood pressure.
  - Tension pneumothorax (sometimes bilateral).
- Consideration of reversible causes (the 4Hs and 4Ts) will help identify these causes of cardiac arrest. Management of cardiac arrest in asthma patients should follow standard ALS guidelines while incorporating the following recommendations:
  - If IV or IO access cannot be established rapidly, give 1 mg IM adrenaline (1:1,000) if cardiorespiratory arrest has just occurred.
  - Ventilation may be difficult because of increased airway resistance; a two-person technique may assist.
  - If dynamic hyperinflation is suspected during CPR, manual compression of the chest wall and/or a period of planned apnoea achieved by disconnecting the BMV from the tracheal tube may reduce gas trapping.
  - There is a significant risk of gastric inflation and hypoventilation of the lungs when ventilating a severely asthmatic patient; therefore, consider early tracheal intubation where required.
  - Regularly check for evidence of reversible causes, specifically tension pneumothorax.
- Decompress suspected pneumothoraces and consider enhanced/critical care support to perform a thoracostomy. **NB** bi-lateral needle decompression will not make the situation worse and may reverse the cause of the cardiac arrest.

11.4 Opiate overdose

- Cardiac arrest following opiate overdose (OD) is usually secondary to a respiratory arrest. If cardiac arrest occurs, follow standard resuscitation guidelines while incorporating the following modifications:
  - Administering naloxone is unlikely to cause harm; it can be given where opiate OD is likely. The usual adult dose is 400 mcg IV, which should be titrated to affect every 60 seconds with the subsequent doses being 800 mcg IV (Toxbase). Administer incrementally until the patient is breathing adequately and is able to protect their airway.
  - If no response is observed after a total of 10mg IV Naloxone, consider a non-opioid related drug or other cause.
  - The administration of Naloxone should not compromise the provision of quality CPR, early defibrillation and adequate airway management and effective ventilation.
  - Prolonged resuscitation may be appropriate in this cohort of patients as good neurological outcome is possible. Cessation of resuscitation should be in consultation with a senior clinician.

11.5 Rhythm-Affecting Drugs

- Consider the effect that rhythm-affecting prescription drugs (e.g. beta blockers, tricyclic anti-depressants, cocaine, etc.) and non-opiate recreational drugs may have on cardiac output before terminating a resuscitation attempt. Follow normal ALS guidance for these patient groups.

11.6 Bariatric patients

- While normal ALS guidance and shock protocols should be followed in the resuscitation of bariatric patients, it is recognised that delivery of effective CPR may be challenging. Chest compressions will be difficult to perform in many patients, simply because of suboptimal positioning of rescuers. A step or platform may be required, or compressions can be performed from the patients' head end.
- Additional rescuers may be required to assist due to rescuer fatigue, particularly in relation to the delivery of chest compressions. It may be necessary to change the CPR provider more frequently and mechanical devices may not accommodate this patient group. Although chest compressions are most effective when performed with the patient lying on a firm surface, where it is unsafe to attempt to move the patient, they may remain on a mattress as the heavier torso compresses the surface leaving less potential for displacement during chest compressions.
- Higher inspiration pressure is needed for positive pressure ventilation due to increased intra-abdominal pressure. In all patients with extreme obesity, difficult intubation must be anticipated, with a clear failed intubation drill if necessary.
- It is important to request additional resources to assist with moving the patient with consideration

for specially adapted vehicles. Weight limits of equipment must be checked before use. Underestimation of the technical aspects of rescue operations may cause trauma or prohibit safe transfer of bariatric patients.

12. Chemical, Biological, Radiological, Nuclear (CBRN) Incidents

- The key priority of the first medical personnel on arrival at a CBRN incident is to ensure all emergency service control centres are alerted and specialist resources are summoned early.
- If there is one casualty, rescuers may approach as usual. If there are two casualties, only approach with caution, considering all options. If there are three or more casualties, one should not approach. Instead withdraw, contain the scene, report the situation, isolate oneself and await specialist resources.
- A patient in cardiac arrest as a result of a CBRN incident should only be approached and treated once the risk to rescuers is known. A chemical incident may initially present with patients in a peri or actual cardiac arrest. Proper scene management of chemical incidents is crucial for preventing further exposure and incident escalation. Early pattern recognition of chemical agent syndromes is vital, and paramedics should be aware of the constant threat of this type of incident. These can result from terrorist action, or industrial and chemical incidents, as well as isolated cases of toxic exposure.
- The signs of a CBRN incident can often be subtle or delayed, and emergency medical personnel should always be vigilant for abnormal situational or patient factors that raise suspicion of a CBRN incident. Exposure to a CBRN agent can occur through direct contact, inhalation, injection, ingestion or irradiation.

12.1 Personal Protection

- Rescuers must not approach potential casualties unless adequate personal protective equipment (PPE) is worn.
- Personal protection is paramount if a CBRN incident is suspected. If in doubt, the rescuer should withdraw to a place of safety until the CBRN threat can be accurately identified and the necessary PPE brought to the scene.
- Entering a CBRN scene without adequate PPE puts the rescuer at risk of harm and also risks spread of contamination. A CBRN patient will need decontamination before being able to receive advanced medical care.
- There are also an increasing number of individual chemical exposure incidents in the UK, this may occur as a result of suicide or agricultural accidents for example. There are a number of different agents commonly used which include:
  - hydrogen sulphide (made by mixing a combination of household chemicals)
  - aluminium phosphide (from rat poison)
  - cyanide salts
  - helium gas
  - nitrogen gas
  - carbon monoxide (e.g. from a disposable BBQ or car exhaust).

13. Trauma

- Establishing the cause of cardiac arrest may not be straightforward. A primary medical arrest can occur before a patient suffers a secondary traumatic insult. Primary medical cardiac arrests resulting in falls from height or while driving are examples that can typically result in rescuers suspecting cardiac arrest of traumatic origin.
- Pay close attention to a witness history and perform an accurate scene assessment to establish the course of events and mechanism of injury. If there is a possibility that the patient has had a primary medical cardiac arrest, follow standard BLS and ALS guidelines. Where trauma is considered to be the primary cause of the arrest, consider early enhanced care support and follow the traumatic cardiac arrest algorithm in Figure 2.13.
- Standard BLS/ALS without urgent attention to reversible pathology is unacceptable and unlikely to result in ROSC.
- Patients who are in cardiac arrest following drowning, hanging or asphyxiation should not automatically be conveyed to an MTC (unless there is significant mechanism to trigger TU bypass). However, all patients for whom ROSC has been achieved following traumatic cardiac arrest should be conveyed to an MTC unless airway and/or catastrophic haemorrhage cannot be safely managed when a pit stop at the nearest Emergency Department is indicated.
- Consider termination of the resuscitative effort if the patient presents in asystole and has not responded to 20 minutes of ALS **with likely reversible causes treated successfully (Rapid MTC conveyance is indicated where reversible causes cannot be corrected, or for patients with penetrating trauma).** The exceptions are for pregnancy, children and where hypothermia may be a contributory factor. Consider senior advice when appropriate.

13.1 Blunt Trauma

- In the pre-hospital setting, advanced life support and exclusion of reversible causes using the 4Hs and 4Ts, or the HOTT approach should take priority:

Advanced Life Support

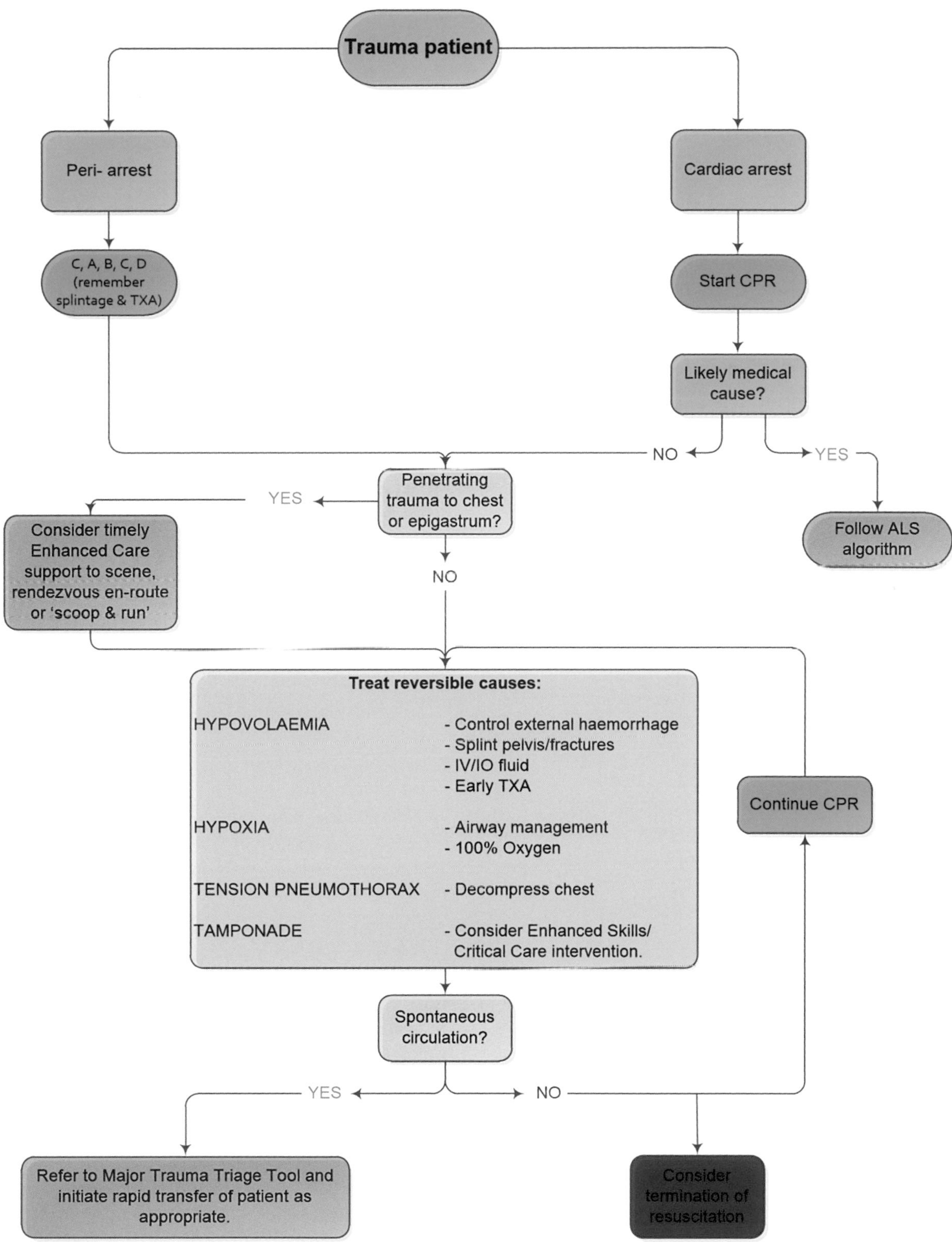

Figure 2.13 – Traumatic cardiac arrest algorithm. Source: Resuscitation Council (UK), 2015.

- Hypovolemia – control external haemorrhage, pelvic binder, long bone splinting and give fluids/blood (where carried), early administration of TXA.
- Oxygenation – including airway management.
- Tension pneumothorax – bilateral decompression, or bilateral thoracostomies (where trained) if significant chest trauma.
- Tamponade – early thoracotomy (for penetrating trauma) - consider early enhanced/critical care or rapid conveyance to closest MTC.

- Rapid treatment of reversible causes should take priority over chest compressions and ALS drug administration. However, high-quality chest compressions are important and may generate some forward flow, even in cases of severe hypovolaemia or cardiac tamponade; it is therefore important to continue chest compressions as soon as sufficient personnel are available to allocate someone to this task.
- Undertake only essential lifesaving interventions on scene. If the patient has signs of life (pulse, chest rise, breathing efforts, movements, eye opening or shockable rhythm), rapidly transfer to hospital or arrange rendezvous with enhanced/critical care support. Do not delay for spinal immobilisation.
- Effective airway management using a stepwise approach is essential to maintain oxygenation of the severely compromised trauma patient. In low cardiac output conditions, positive pressure ventilation may cause further circulatory depression or even cardiac arrest by impeding venous return to the heart. Monitor ventilation with continuous waveform capnography and adjust rate to achieve normocarbia.
- Consider performing all further interventions en-route and administer 1 g tranexamic acid IV/IO early. Refer to **Tranexamic Acid**, **Page for Age** for children.
- Hypovolaemia due to blood loss that is sufficient in volume to cause cardiac arrest is difficult to treat. Gain large bore IV access. Although IV normal saline may restore blood volume (often requiring 2-3 litres), excessive crystalloid causes coagulopathy, acidosis and hypothermia which in itself worsens outcome. Request enhanced care, particularly if it enables blood and blood products to be brought to scene without delay. Once ROSC is achieved, only give IV fluids to achieve a systolic BP no higher than 80 mmHg.
- Consider whether the patient can be conveyed for early blood or blood product intervention, or whether this can be brought to the scene or to a rendezvous point in a timely manner by enhanced care assets.
- In blunt trauma cases, where ALS (including attempts to address reversible causes) is being delivered, clinical judgement may be applied as to whether enhanced care assets may be accessed or the patient can be conveyed to a MTC (or TU if necessary) in a timely manner. If likely reversible causes of traumatic cardiac arrest have been treated and there has been no ROSC after 20 minutes of ALS, resuscitation may stop.

13.2 Penetrating Trauma

- In penetrating traumatic cardiac arrest, patients should be transferred rapidly to hospital because surgical intervention is often needed to treat the cause of the arrest. A rapid transport approach is appropriate to the nearest MTU (or TU if necessary), but crew safety should be a consideration where there are prolonged journey times in a moving vehicle.
- Enhanced care assets should be requested early for attendance at the scene (but do not delay departure from scene while waiting for these assets) and/or during conveyance.
- Rapidly address immediate issues:
  - catastrophic haemorrhage (splinting, trauma dressings, tourniquet etc.)
  - airway and breathing (consider tension pneumothorax, sucking chest wound etc.)
  - defibrillation, if indicated.
- Consider performing all further interventions en-route and administer 1 g tranexamic acid IV/IO early, over 10 minutes.
- The principles for volume resuscitation for penetrating trauma are similar to blunt trauma. However, the priority for rapid conveyance to hospital often precludes any significant pre-hospital volume being administered. Do not delay on scene to obtain IV access. Surgical intervention is the only intervention that will save the victim's life and rapid conveyance to hospital is vital to achieve this.

Bibliography

1. Resuscitation Council (UK). *Resuscitation Council Guidelines 2015: Adult Advanced Life Support.* London: Resuscitation Council, 2015. Available from: https://www.resus.org.uk/resuscitation-guidelines/adult-advanced-life-support.
2. Resuscitation Council (UK). *Resuscitation Council Guidelines 2015: Paediatric Advanced Life Support. London: Resuscitation Council, 2015.* Available from: https://www.resus.org.uk/resuscitation-guidelines/paediatric-advanced-life-support.
3. Resuscitation Council (UK). *Resuscitation Council Guidelines 2015: Peri-arrest arrhythmias.* London: Resuscitation Council UK, 2015. Available from: https://www.resus.org.uk/resuscitation-guidelines/peri-arrest-arrhythmias.
4. Resuscitation Council (UK). *Resuscitation Council Guidelines 2015: Prehospital resuscitation.* London: Resuscitation Council UK, 2015. Available from: https://www.resus.org.uk/resuscitation-guidelines/prehospital-resuscitation/.
5. Soar J, Nolan JP, Bottiger BW, et al. European Resuscitation Council Guidelines for Resuscitation 2015: Section 3. Adult advanced life support. *Resuscitation* 2015; 95: 100-147. Available from: https://www.resuscitationjournal.com/article/S0300-9572(15)00328-7/fulltext.

6. Truhlar A, Deakin CD, Soar J, et al. European Resuscitation Council Guidelines for Resuscitation 2015: Section 4. Cardiac arrest in special circumstances. *Resuscitation* 2015; 95: 148-201. Available from: https://www.resuscitationjournal.com/article/S0300-9572(15)00329-9/fulltext.

7. Maconochie I, Bingham R, Eich C, López-Herce J, Rodriguez-Nunez A, Rajka T, Van de Voorde P, Zideman D, Biarent D. European Resuscitation Council Guidelines for Resuscitation 2015 Section 6: Paediatric life support. *Resuscitation* 2015, 95: 223–248. Available from: https://www.resuscitationjournal.com/article/S0300-9572(15)00340-8/fulltext.

8. Delorenzo A, Nehme Z, Yates J, et al. Double sequential external defibrillation for refractory ventricular fibrillation out-of-hospital cardiac arrest: A systematic review and meta-analysis. *Resuscitation* 2019; 135: 124–129. Available from: http://doi.org/10.1016/j.resuscitation.2018.10.025.

9. Finn J, Jacobs I, Williams TA, et al. (2019). Adrenaline and vasopressin for cardiac arrest. *Cochrane Database of Systematic Reviews*, 327(15), 1051. Available from: http://doi.org/10.1002/14651858.CD003179.

10. Soar J, Perkin G, Maconochie I, et al. European Resuscitation Council Guidelines for Resuscitation: 2018 update - antiarrhythmic drugs for cardiac arrest. *Resuscitation* 2019; 134; 99-103. Available from: https://www.sciencedirect.com/science/article/pii/S0300957218310967/pdfft?md5=22f72cc33ecab8b1e38130bfb18dc680&pid=1-s2.0-S0300957218310967-main.pdf.

11. Perkins GD, Ji C, Deakin CD, et al, on behalf of PARAMEDIC2 collaborators. A Randomized Trial of Epinephrine in Out-of-Hospital Cardiac Arrest. *New England Journal of Medicine* 2018; 379: 711-721. Available from: https://www.nejm.org/doi/full/10.1056/NEJMoa1806842.

12. Holmberg MJ, Geri G, Wiberg S et al. Extracorporeal cardiopulmonary resuscitation for cardiac arrest: a systematic review. *Resuscitation* 2018; 131: 91–100. Available from: https://www.resuscitationjournal.com/article/S0300-9572(18)30373-3/pdf.

13. Benger J, Kirby K, Black S, et al. Effect of a Strategy of a Supraglottic Airway Device vs Tracheal Intubation During Out-of-Hospital Cardiac Arrest on Functional Outcome: The AIRWAYS-2 Randomized Clinical Trial. *JAMA*. 2018; 320: 779-791. Available from: https://www.ncbi.nlm.nih.gov/pmc/articles/PMC6142999/.

14. Poole K, Couper K, Smyth MA, et al. Mechanical CPR: Who? When? How?. *Critical Care* (2018) 22:140. Available from: https://ccforum.biomedcentral.com/track/pdf/10.1186/s13054-018-2059-0.

Return of Spontaneous Circulation

1. Introduction

- Gaining return of spontaneous circulation (ROSC) is the initial step towards recovery from out-of-hospital cardiac arrest. As such, it is important that paramedics are aware of the critical nature of the post-ROSC patient.
- Undertake an accurate and complete patient assessment and provide all interventions to ensure that the patient's condition has been optimised before transfer to hospital, except where an intervention only available in hospital is required or it is unsafe to remain on scene.
- Be prepared for re-arrest; the recurrence rate of a shockable rhythm is at its highest during this period.
- Following ROSC, patients may present with a varying degree of post-cardiac arrest syndrome. Post-cardiac arrest syndrome comprises four key elements:
  - **Brain injury** – coma, seizures, myoclonus, varying degrees of neurocognitive dysfunction and brain death; this may be exacerbated by microcirculatory failure, impaired autoregulation, hypercarbia, hyperoxia, pyrexia, hyper/hypoglycaemia and seizures.
  - **Myocardial dysfunction** – this is common after cardiac arrest, but usually improves in the following weeks.
  - **Systemic ischemia/reperfusion response** – the whole-body ischaemia/reperfusion that occurs with resuscitation from cardiac arrest activates immunological and coagulation pathways contributing to a systemic inflammatory response syndrome (SIRS).
  - **Persistence of the precipitating pathology.**
- The management of post-cardiac arrest syndrome requires ambulance paramedics to assimilate their clinical assessment and findings, with a view to targeting therapy to the patient's needs.

2. Assessment and Management

TABLE 2.9 – Return of Spontaneous Circulation: ASSESSMENT and MANAGEMENT

ASSESSMENT	MANAGEMENT
• Return of spontaneous circulation	• Early recurrence of VF is common; ensure appropriate ongoing monitoring through defibrillator pads. • Undertake a structured <C>ABCD assessment that enables appropriate treatment to be applied, as described in the immediate management below. Consider and continue to treat any reversible cause of the initial cardiac arrest. Refer to **Medical Emergencies in Adults – Overview** and **Medical Emergencies in Children – Overview**. • Measure and record a full set of observations. • Early optimisation of airway, breathing and circulatory support will assist in the heart's recovery. • Forward planning – ensure appropriate resources are on scene or requested to the scene; this may include enhanced care. • Consider the extrication plan and facilitate preparations for extrication and onward transfer. • Transfer the patient directly to the nearest appropriate hospital in accordance with local pathways for primary percutaneous coronary intervention (PPCI) or ECMO (where available). Consider discussion with nearest PPCI centre for patients following out-of-hospital cardiac arrest (of medical cause) where defined pathways do not exist. • Provide an ATMIST pre-alert call to the receiving facility.
• Airway and Breathing	• Ensure an effective airway; consider enhanced care support for advanced airway insertion or maintenance. • Maintain oxygen saturations of 94–98%; (titrating oxygen to prevent hyperoxia when necessary). Refer to **Oxygen**.

Return of Spontaneous Circulation

TABLE 2.9 – Return of Spontaneous Circulation: ASSESSMENT and MANAGEMENT *(continued)*	
	• Assist ventilations where required • Use of a mechanical ventilator (if available) is preferable to manual ventilation; ensure the settings are appropriate for age, weight and rate (Generally a tidal volume of 6–7ml/kg with a rate of 10/min). • Monitor waveform capnography. • Ventilate lungs to normocarbia (4.6–6.0 kPa); consider the reason for readings that fall outside normocarbia, i.e. is this a perfusion, ventilation or metabolic issue?
• Circulation	• Perform a 12-lead ECG. – **NB** post-ROSC ECGs frequently demonstrate a 'recovering heart'; therefore, ECGs should be obtained at regular intervals. • Ensure adequate vascular access. • Aim for a systolic blood pressure (SBP) > 80 mmHg. • Following ROSC, patients are often haemodynamically unstable, arrhythmogenic and hypotensive. In these situations, a 250 ml IV/IO bolus of 0.9% saline may be administered, repeated as necessary to a maximum of 1000 ml, aiming for a systolic blood pressure of 90 mmHg. • In the event of symptomatic bradycardia, atropine should be administered, refer to **Atropine**, **Page for Age** for children. • If bradycardia persists, external pacing should be considered. • In the event of severe haemodynamic instability unresponsive to: – atropine and/or – fluids and/or – external pacing (if available), boluses of adrenaline 0.1mg IV/IO may be titrated against blood pressure, as per local guidelines.
• Control temperature	• The evidence for the benefits of cooling post-ROSC is limited. As a minimum, patients post-ROSC should be allowed to cool passively – cover with no more clothing/blankets than is necessary to maintain patient dignity, and do not use vehicle heating. • Aim for a core temperature no higher than 36°C.
• Blood glucose level	• Measure and record blood glucose for hypo/hyperglycaemia; refer to **Glycaemic Emergencies in Adults and Children**. • Accuracy of blood glucose measurements immediately following ROSC may be impaired by capillary blood stasis. Venous blood glucose should be measured and repeated 10 minutes following ROSC.
• Combative patient	• Following ROSC, patients may be cerebrally irritated and combative. • Exclude hypoglycaemia and hypoxaemia. • Combative patients may benefit from anaesthetic management or sedation, if available. This should only be provided by defined teams or individuals in line with robust governance and scope of practice.
• Pain relief	• Consider the provision of analgesia (IV paracetamol, supplemented with small dose of opiates) for the management of patient-reported pain following resuscitation efforts/precipitating pathology of the arrest
• Seizure control	• Seizures that do not self-terminate within five minutes may be treated with a benzodiazepine, refer to **Diazepam, Page for Age** for children. • The administration of diazepam or midazolam (where available) should be carried out in line with clinical practice guidelines or PGD (in the context of midazolam).

Return of Spontaneous Circulation

Prepare for Transfer

a. Early recurrence of VF is common; ensure appropriate ongoing monitoring through defibrillator pads.
b. Transfer the patient directly to the nearest appropriate hospital in accordance with local pathways.
c. Provide an ATMIST pre-alert call to the receiving facility.

Airway & Breathing

a. Ensure an effective airway; consider enhanced support
b. Record and maintain oxygen saturations of 94–98%, refer to Oxygen.
c. Monitor waveform capnography.
d. Ventilate lungs to normocarbia (4.6–6.0 kPa)

Circulation

a. Record Blood Pressure and aim for SBP > 80 mmHg.
b. First: Fluid (crystalloid) – restore normovolaemia. Refer to Intravascular Fluid in Adults and Intravascular Fluid in Children.
c. Second: Consider vasopressor/inotrope to maintain SBP unresponsive to fluid resuscitation as per local guideline (if this exists), e.g. adrenaline.
d. In the event of symptomatic bradycardia, atropine should be administered, refer to Atropine.

ECG

Perform a 12-lead ECG

Temperature

a. Measure temperature.
b. Patients post-ROSC should be allowed to cool passively.

BM

Measure and record blood glucose for hypo/hyperglycaemia, refer to Glycaemic Emergencies in Adults and Children.

Other

a. Consider the provision of analgesia (small dose opiates or IV Paracetamol) for the management of pain
b. Seizures that do not self-terminate within five minutes may be treated with a benzodiazepine, refer to Diazepam.
c. Combative patients may benefit from anaesthetic management or sedation. Consider enhanced care.

Figure 2.14 – Assessment and management of return of spontaneous circulation (ROSC).

3. Disposition

- Acute coronary syndrome (ACS) is a frequent cause of OHCA. Patients with ROSC and presenting with ST segment elevation myocardial infarction (STEMI) or presumed new left bundle branch block (LBBB) should be conveyed to a PPCI centre where local pathways exist.
- Patients with ROSC following medical collapse should be treated in line with local pathways; wherever possible a discussion should occur with the nearest PPCI centre to understand potential suitability for direct referral.
- Patients who obtain ROSC following traumatic cardiac arrest should be conveyed in line with the local major trauma pathways, normally to a major trauma centre, assuming criteria for trauma unit bypass are met.

Bibliography

1. Nolan JP, Soar, J, Cariou, A., et al. European Resuscitation Council and European Society of Intensive Care Medicine Guidelines for Post-resuscitation Care 2015: Section 5 of the European Resuscitation Council Guidelines for Resuscitation 2015. *Resuscitation* 2019; 95: 202-222. Available from: https://cprguidelines.eu/sites/573c777f5e61585a053d7ba5/content_entry573c77e35e61585a053d7baf/573c780c5e61585a083d7bcc/ files/S0300-9572_15_00330-5_main.pdf?.
2. Nolan JP, Neumar RW, Adrie C, et al. Post-cardiac arrest syndrome: Epidemiology, pathophysiology, treatment, and prognostication: A Scientific Statement from the International Liaison Committee on Resuscitation; the American Heart Association Emergency Cardiovascular Care Committee; the Council on Cardiovascular Surgery and Anesthesia; the Council on Cardiopulmonary, Perioperative, and Critical Care; the Council on Clinical Cardiology; the Council on Stroke. *Resuscitation* 2008: 79: 350-379. Available from: https://www.ilcor.org/data/Post-cardiac_arrest_syndrome.pdf.
3. Donnino MW, Andersen LW, Berg KM, et al.Temperature Management After Cardiac Arrest An Advisory Statement by the Advanced Life Support Task Force of the International Liaison Committee on Resuscitation and the American Heart Association Emergency Cardiovascular Care Committee and the Council on Cardiopulmonary, Critical Care, Perioperative and Resuscitation. *Circulation*. 2015;132:2448-2456. Available from: https://www.ahajournals.org/doi/pdf/10.1161/CIR.0000000000000313.

Verification of Death and Termination of Resuscitation by Paramedics

1. Introduction

- The challenge for paramedics is to differentiate those patients for whom cardiac arrest is their natural end of life event and for whom resuscitation is not indicated from those where there is a chance to restore life to a quality acceptable to the patient and in accordance with their wishes through provision of optimum pre-hospital care.
- Where no explicit decision about CPR has been considered and recorded in advance, there should be an initial presumption in favour of CPR.
- However, in some circumstances where there is no recorded explicit decision (for example, for a person in the advanced stages of a terminal illness where death is imminent and unavoidable and CPR would not be successful), a carefully considered decision not to commence inappropriate CPR is appropriate.
- For patients in whom there is no chance of survival, CPR is not supported; for example:
  - where resuscitation would be both futile and distressing for the patient, relatives, friends and healthcare personnel
  - where time and resources would be ineffective undertaking such measures.
- Every effort should be made to identify patients with DNACPR form, ReSPECT forms, treatment escalation plans or advanced directives.
- The views of an attending general practitioner (GP), ambulance doctor or relevant third party should be considered.
- CPR should not be attempted, or it should be abandoned if already started by the general public or CFRs if the paramedic is as certain as they can be that a person is dying as an inevitable result of underlying disease (it is therefore their natural end of life event) and CPR would not re-start the heart and breathing for a sustained period.
- Where there is uncertainty, it is acceptable to commence BLS while further information is rapidly gathered to enable the decision to be made on whether to then stop resuscitation.

2. Conditions Unequivocally Associated with Death

- The following conditions are unequivocally associated with death in adults, and can be used by paramedics to verify death:
  - **decapitation**
  - **massive cranial and cerebral destruction**
  - **hemicorporectomy or similar massive injury**
  - **decomposition/putrefaction** – where tissue damage indicates that the patient has been dead for some hours, days or longer
  - **incineration** – the presence of full thickness burns with charring of greater than 95% of the body surface
  - **hypostasis** – the pooling of blood in congested vessels in the dependent part of the body in the position in which it lies after death
  - **rigor mortis** – the stiffness occurring after death from the post mortem breakdown of enzymes in the muscle fibres
  - **fetal maceration in a newborn** – when the child is born with such severe abnormalities that it is considered incompatible with life.
- It is appropriate not to commence CPR in these cases. However, in cases of apparent rigor mortis, hypostasis and fetal maceration, take an ECG while confirming the absence of a pulse and breathing.

Hypostasis

- Intially, hypostatic staining may appear as small round patches looking rather like bruises, but later these coalesce to merge as the familiar pattern. Above the hypostatic engorgement there is obvious pallor of the skin.
- The presence of hypostasis is diagnostic of death – the appearance is not present in a live patient. In extremely cold conditions, hypostasis may be bright red in colour, and in carbon monoxide poisoning it is characteristically 'cherry red' in appearance.

Rigor mortis

- Rigor mortis occurs first in the small muscles of the face, next in the arms, then in the legs; these changes taking 30 mins to 3 hrs. Children will show a more rapid onset of rigor. The recognition of rigor mortis can be made difficult where, rarely, death has occurred from tetanus or strychnine poisoning.
- In some, rigidity never develops (infants, cachectic individuals, and the aged), while in others it may become apparent more rapidly (in the conditions in which muscle glycogen is depleted): exertion (which includes struggling), strychnine poisoning, local heat (e.g. from a fire, hot room or direct sunlight).
- Rigor should not be confused with cadaveric spasm (sometimes referred to as instant rigor mortis), which develops immediately after death without preceding flaccidity following intense physical and/or emotional activity. Examples include death by drowning or a fall from a height. In contrast with true rigor mortis, only one group of muscles is affected and **not** the whole body. Rigor mortis will develop subsequently.
- Rigor mortis can appear quickly following a child death and resuscitation should be attempted unless there is a condition unequivocally associated with death (see **Death of a Child**).

3. Other Conditions Where Resuscitation May Be Withheld or Discontinued

- In addition to the conditions above, there are other criteria which can be used to confirm death, and which indicate that resuscitation should not be attempted, or may be discontinued:
  - The presence of a DNACPR (do not attempt cardiopulmonary resuscitation) order, an advance directive or ReSPECT form that states the wish of the patient not to undergo attempted resuscitation.
  - If a person is known to be in the final stages of an advanced and irreversible condition, in which attempted CPR would be both inappropriate and unsuccessful, CPR should not be started. Even in the absence of a recorded DNACPR decision, paramedics may be able to recognise this situation and make an appropriate decision, based on clear evidence that they should document. Where there is doubt, it may be necessary to start CPR and to review whether or not to continue in the light of any further information received during the resuscitation attempt, or to seek senior clinical advice. The relatives/carers should be informed of this decision.
  - Submersion for longer than 90 minutes (refer to **Immersion and Drowning**).

Final stages of an advanced and irreversible condition

An irreversible condition may be defined as a condition, injury or illness that meets all three of the following criteria:

1 May be treated, but can never be cured or eliminated.

2 Leaves the person unable to care or make decisions for him or herself.

3 Without life-sustaining treatment is fatal.

- There is no realistic chance that CPR would be successful if **ALL** the following exist together:
  - > 15 minutes has elapsed since the onset of cardiac arrest.
  - No evidence of bystander CPR in the 15 mins before the arrival of the ambulance.
  - Exclusion factors are absent: Drowning, hypothermia, poisoning/overdose, pregnancy, child/neonate).
  - Asystole for >30 seconds on the ECG monitor screen. CPR should only be paused for a 30-second asystole check if all other criteria are met.
- Whenever possible a confirmatory ECG demonstrating asystole should be documented as evidence of death. In this situation a 3- or 4-electrode system using limbs alone will cause minimum disturbance to the deceased. If a paper ECG trace cannot be taken, it is permissible to make a diagnosis of asystole from the screen alone (**NB** due caution must be applied in respect of electrode contact, gain and, where possible, using more than one ECG lead).
- It is important that in order to confirm death, the rhythm is unequivocally persistent and continuous asystole. If CPR is stopped when any other rhythm is present (i.e. agonal rhythm or PEA), it is important to wait until all cardiac electrical activity has ceased and the ECG shows asystole. Only at this stage should the patient be declared life extinct and any the family/relatives informed that this is the case. This is because there have been well-documented cases where spontaneous ROSC has occurred following termination of resuscitation.

4. Termination of Resuscitation

- If there is a realistic chance that CPR could be successful, then resuscitation should continue to establish the patient's response to ALS interventions (ALS is defined in the **Advanced Life Support** guideline).
- If, following ALS interventions, the patient has been **persistently and continuously** asystolic for 20 minutes and all reversible causes have been identified and corrected, resuscitation may be discontinued, except in cases listed below.
  - pregnancy
  - hypothermic patients (where hypothermia is the primary cause of the cardiac arrest)
  - suspected drugs overdose/poisoning
  - Infants, children and adolescents (i.e. all those < 18 yrs age)
- These patients should be transported to the nearest facility with on-going resuscitation, unless the circumstances would make transport futile.

4.1 Pulseless electrical activity

- Pulseless electrical activity (PEA) is a scenario that presents challenges to the decision making about the cardiac arrest management.
- Although there is ongoing myocardial electrical activity, the outcome is often poor.
- An early decision around the need for rapid removal to hospital should be considered.
- The use of cardiac ultrasound, if available, may enable more guided therapy or decision making.
- Senior clinicians may be asked to advise on situations where the patient remains in pulseless electrical activity (PEA) following 20 minutes of resuscitation, and where paramedics on scene believe continuing the resuscitation is futile. Refer to local senior clinician guidance.

Verification of Death and Termination of Resuscitation by Paramedics

- There is limited evidence to support when one should terminate a PEA cardiac arrest; however, the following factors are important to consider when making this decision:
  - the interval of time in arrest without life support
  - the absence of reversible causes
  - the presence of co-morbidities
  - the rate/width of the QRS complexes
  - the trend and absolute value of $EtCO_2$.
- Some patients undergoing prolonged CPR can survive with good outcome.
- Young age, myocardial infarction and potentially reversible causes of cardiac arrest such as hypothermia and pulmonary emboli are associated with a better outcome, especially when the arrest is witnessed and followed by prompt and effective resuscitative efforts.

4.2 Refractory VF

- A significant number of patients may present in VF which is unresponsive to repeated defibrillation shocks and amiodarone.
- Many cases of VF are secondary to myocardial ischaemia as a result of myocardial infarction, which is potentially reversible with PPCI. Resuscitation should not therefore be stopped in cases of refractory or persistent VF.
- Where practical, transport patients with persistent/refractory VF or pulseless VT to a cardiac arrest centre with ongoing CPR, because further in-hospital treatment may occasionally be successful.

4.3 Agonal rhythm

- As resuscitation progresses, organised QRS complexes often deteriorate to wide, low amplitude, irregular complexes, known as an idioventricular or agonal rhythm. This is typically at a rate < 10bpm and is not associated with effective cardiac output.
- This rhythm is usually a prelude to asystole.
- A persistent agonal rhythm can be treated as asystole and resuscitation can be terminated if it has persisted continuously for more than 20 mins.

5. Advance Decision to Refuse Treatment (ADRT) and Do Not Attempt Resuscitation (DNACPR)

5.1 Advance Decision to Refuse Treatment (ADRT)

- ADRTs are a form of advance decisions as defined within the Mental Capacity Act 2005 (MCA).
- Providing ADRTs meet all the requirements of the MCA, they will be legally binding for health and social care professionals. This makes ADRTs quite distinct from other aspects of advance care planning.
- The MCA and MCA Code of Practice clearly define that the responsibility for making an advance decision lies with the person making it.
- An advance decision enables someone aged 18 and over, while still capable, to refuse specified medical treatment for a time in the future when they may lack the capacity to consent to or refuse that treatment.
- An ADRT must be valid and applicable to current circumstances. If it is, it has the same effect as a decision that is made by a person with capacity: healthcare professionals (including paramedics) must follow the decision.
- ADRT are only valid if the patient is unconscious or lacks capacity. If the patient has capacity before arrest and states their wishes at that time, they should be followed.
- Paramedics will be protected from liability if they:
  - stop or withhold treatment because they reasonably believe that an advance decision exists, and that it is valid and applicable
  - treat a person because, having taken all practical and appropriate steps to find out if the person has made an advance decision to refuse treatment, they do not know or are not satisfied that a valid and applicable advance decision exists.
- If the advance decision refuses life-sustaining treatment, it must be:
  - in writing, which includes being written on the person's behalf or recorded in their medical notes
  - signed by the maker in the presence of a witness who must also sign the document. It can also be signed on the maker's behalf at their direction if they are unable to sign it for themselves
  - verified by a specific statement made by the maker, either included in the document or a separate statement that says that the advance decision is to apply to the specified treatment even if life is at risk. If there is a separate statement this must also be signed and witnessed.
- To establish whether an advance decision is valid and applicable, paramedics must take reasonable steps to find out if the person:
  - has done anything that clearly goes against their advance decision
  - has withdrawn their decision
  - has subsequently conferred the power to make that decision on an attorney
  - would have changed their decision if they had known more about the current circumstances.

Verification of Death and Termination of Resuscitation by Paramedics

Lasting Power of Attorney (LPA)

- There are two types of LPA: property and financial affairs and personal health and welfare.
- Only a personal health and welfare LPA allows decisions to be made on the person's behalf when they lack capacity for life-sustaining treatment if detailed within Section 5. This has to be expressly provided in the document.
- The document should be viewed before basing a decision on information provided by the named individual.
- An ADRT supersedes a LPA, unless the LPA was created later and is valid and applicable to the circumstance.

- If there is any genuine doubt about the validity of an advance decision, paramedics must act in the patient's 'best interests'.
- Paramedics must consider any evidence as an expression of previous wishes when establishing the person's best interests. This may involve the provision of clinical treatment, including resuscitation.
- It is the paramedic in charge of a patient's care and treatment who must decide what is in his/her best interests.
- Ambulance clinicians should be guided by advice from those close to a patient regarding the patient's previously expressed wishes and beliefs, even though the patient's spouse, family, friends or colleagues may not be entitled to give or withhold consent to treatment on the patient's behalf.
- Decisions must not be based on assumptions made solely on factors such as the person's age, disability or a professional's subjective view of a person's quality of life.
- When an advance decision is not followed, the reasons must be clearly documented.
- In Scotland and Northern Ireland, ADRTs are not covered by statute but it is likely that they are binding under common law. Although no cases have been taken to court in Scotland or Northern Ireland, it is likely that the principles that emerged from consideration of cases by the English courts (before the Mental Capacity Act) would also guide decision making in these jurisdictions.
- An advance refusal of CPR is likely to be legally binding in Scotland and Northern Ireland if:
  - The person was an adult at the time the decision was made (16 years old in Scotland and 18 in Northern Ireland).
  - The person had capacity when the decision was made.
  - The circumstances that have arisen are those that were envisaged by the person.
  - The person was not subjected to undue influence in making the decision.
- If an ADRT does not meet these criteria but appears to set out a clear indication of the person's wishes, it will not be legally binding but should be taken into consideration in determining the person's best interests.

5.2 Do Not Attempt Cardiopulmonary Resuscitation (DNACPR) Order

- Currently, DNACPR decisions are made, in the main, for children and adults for whom attempting CPR is inappropriate; for example, a patient who is at the end stages of a terminal illness or is suffering from a life limiting congenital abnormality.
- In these cases, a DNACPR decision can enable the person to die with dignity and appropriate support.
- A DNACPR decision applies solely to cardiopulmonary resuscitation. All other treatment and care that a patient requires is not precluded or influenced by a DNACPR decision.
- DNACPR documents should, ideally, move with patients as they are transferred from one setting to another – particularly when death is expected (i.e. end of life patient being discharged home to die).
- In the absence of the original copy, a photocopy should be considered valid.

5.3 Validation of DNACPR

- DNACPR recommendations and similar decisions are often recorded on a form approved by the organisation providing the care for the patient. The design and content of these forms can vary significantly.
- Care planning documents (particularly for children) can often contain DNACPR sections and formal letters can also be used to communicate resuscitation instructions to other professionals. These are often communicated to ambulance control and logged against the patient's address.
- It is important to note that all of the above methods are acceptable methods for recording and communicating resuscitation decisions. Ideally a DNACPR form should:
  - explicitly identify the patient
  - explicitly identify the circumstances in which the DNACPR recommendation applies
  - identify if the patient and their family are aware of the DNACPR recommendation
  - identify by whom and when the DNACPR form was produced
- If a review date is specified, expiry of that date DOES NOT invalidate the DNACPR. A decision

must be made and recorded by the paramedic (with senior clinical advice if appropriate) as to whether the document is still considered valid.

- Valid DNACPRs are applicable to patients who are in the dying phase (hours to live), peri-arrest or who have just died.
- Where a valid DNACPR exists, paramedics should support dying patients, provide appropriate comfort measures and support relatives and carers.
- Contact should be made with the patient's GP, district nursing team or equivalent, to ensure the provision of ongoing care and support and to ensure the death is managed appropriately.
- In cases where the DNACPR decision cannot be validated or is unclear, any evidence obtained should be taken into consideration in determining the person's best interests. This may require paramedics to continue to provide care and treatment (including basic life support for cardiac arrests) and seek further advice from senior clinicians.
- Paramedics will be protected from liability if they stop or withhold treatment because they reasonably believe that a DNACPR exists, and that it is valid and applicable.

5.4 Recommended Summary Plan for Emergency Care and Treatment (ReSPECT)

- A ReSPECT form summarises treatments to be considered and those that would not be wanted or would not work for the patient in an emergency. It might include recommendations of when transfer to hospital would be desirable or not.
- ReSPECT is a summary of recommendations to help the paramedic to make immediate decisions about the patient's care and treatment. It contains recommendations about whether CPR should be attempted.
- A ReSPECT form contains more than a CPR decision: it is not just a replacement for a DNACPR form; it is to promote recording an emergency care plan by many people, and may recommend active treatment, **including attempted CPR** if it should be needed.
- Like a DNACPR form, it is not legally binding; clinical judgment must still be applied and paramedics may decide not to follow the recommendations on a ReSPECT form.
- Paramedics should be prepared to justify valid reasons for overriding the recommendations on a ReSPECT form. For example a decision to treat an immediately reversible cause such as a choking person would be reasonable if it was believed that this was not the circumstance envisaged when the person decided that they did not want CPR.
- The ReSPECT form should be with the person and be readily available. (In some areas it may be accessed electronically.)

6. Deaths During a Major Incident

- In a major incident scenario, deceased patients **MUST** have a mass casualty assessment/triage card attached to them with the following details recorded:
  - the patient identified as dead.
  - the time that the patient was identified as deceased
  - the identity of the paramedic making the decision.
- Deceased patients should only be moved if they are blocking an evacuation route for other casualties, as the location is to be treated as a crime scene. Follow major incident protocols.

7. Action to Be Taken after Death Has Been Established

- Following termination of a resuscitation attempt, removal of advanced airways and/or indwelling cannulas should be in accordance with local protocol.
- Complete documentation – including all decisions regarding do not attempt resuscitation DNARCPR/advance decision to refuse treatment/ ReSPECT form.
- It is not necessary for a medical practitioner to attend to confirm the fact of death. Moreover, there is no obligation for a GP to do so when requested to attend by ambulance control.
- Services should be encouraged, in conjunction with their Coroner's service (or Procurator Fiscal in Scotland), to develop a local procedure for handling the body once death has been verified by ambulance personnel.
- A locally approved leaflet should be adopted for handing to bereaved relatives.
- Any consideration for organ donation should not influence resuscitation attempt decision making:
  - If there is no ROSC, it is unlikely organ donation will occur.
  - If there is ROSC but the patient is not suitable for critical care, they are unlikely to be admitted solely for donation purposes.
  - A long downtime usually makes organs unsuitable for donation.
  - Tissue donation occurs the next day in the mortuary not in the hospital, so transport to hospital does not change the chance of tissue donation.

8. Supporting Bystanders Witnessing Cardiac Arrest

- In many cases of OHCA a close relative or friend may have performed CPR before ambulance service help arriving.
- Relatives may find it more distressing to be separated from their family member during the resuscitation attempt, and there may be advantages to them being present.
- However, it is also important to acknowledge that these are distressing events, and so there can be disadvantages to the relative being present.
- There are a number of key principles, actions and safeguards that ambulance professionals should be aware of, and adopt, to support relatives through the witnessing of a resuscitation attempt:
  - Always acknowledge the difficulty of the situation.
  - When possible try to ensure that one member of the team is with the relative at all times. This can be challenging to achieve with limited numbers of people on scene, but will ensure the relative is supported as much as possible during the event.
  - Ensure the bystander understands they have a choice of whether or not to be present.
  - Ensure that introductions are made and names known.
  - Give clear, simple and honest explanations of what is happening.
  - Ask the relative, in a sensitive manner, not to interfere with the resuscitation process, but allow them to touch the patient when it is safe to do so should they so wish.
  - Explain the procedures in simple terms.
  - If the patient dies, explain that there will be a period where actions will need to be taken for example, that equipment will need to be removed.
- Best attempts should be made to ensure that any member of the public who has delivered CPR is supported at scene and given welfare advice.

  Bystanders should be signposted to their GP in the first instance.

8.1 Breaking Bad News

- Breaking bad news is best done with a well-prepared, honest and simple approach.
- Relatives will often not remember the details of what was said, but they will remember how they were made to feel.
- Paramedics should try to:
  - Take time to prepare personal appearance; check and tidy uniform/clothing, remove gloves and, if necessary, wash hands.
  - Confirm the name of the deceased before speaking to the relatives, establish their relationship and confirm the correct relatives where there are multiple patients.
  - Adopt a position at the same level as the relative.
  - Use simple language and avoid medical jargon.
  - Avoid long preamble such as asking about the patient's pre-morbid health.
  - Ensure the word 'dead' or 'died' is introduced early in the conversation.
  - Use periods of silence to enable the relatives to absorb and understand what they are being told.
- Remember to anticipate the types of reaction or emotional response to the bad news and be ready to support the relatives as much as possible.

8.2 Children and Young People Witnessing Cardiac Arrest

- Children and young people that witness and are present at a cardiac arrest, particularly of a close relative, may need additional support.
- Before leaving the scene, consider making a referral to their GP.
- Consider signposting parents/carers to organisations that provide specific support for bereaved children, as per local procedures.

Verification of Death and Termination of Resuscitation by Paramedics

KEY POINTS!

- **Paramedics are increasingly being called upon to diagnose death and initiate the appropriate clinical response.**
- **After cardiac arrest, resuscitation efforts including ALS must be made whenever there is a chance of survival, unless the person has made an advance directive refusing CPR in these circumstances.**
- **Some conditions are incompatible with recovery and in these cases resuscitation should not be attempted.**
- **In some situations, once the facts of the patient and situation are known, resuscitation efforts can be discontinued.**
- **Patients can and do make anticipatory decisions NOT to be resuscitated.' An advance directive must be respected and a DNACPR recommendation should be used to guide decision making on whether or not to attempt CPR.**
- **These guidelines should be read in conjunction with local policies and procedures.**
- **Rigor mortis can appear quickly following a child death and resuscitation should always be attempted unless there is a condition unequivocally associated with death.**

Bibliography

1. Soar J, Nolan JP, Bottiger BW, et al. European Resuscitation Council Guidelines for Resuscitation 2015: Section 3. Adult advanced life support. *Resuscitation* 2015; 95: 100-147. Available from: https://www.resuscitationjournal.com/article/S0300-9572(15)00328-7/fulltext.
2. Resuscitation Council (UK). Resuscitation Guidelines 2015. Prevention of cardiac arrest and decisions about CPR. Available from: https://resus.org.uk/resuscitation-guidelines/prevention-of-cardiac-arrest-and-decisions-about-cpr/
3. British Medical Association, Resuscitation Council (UK), Royal College of Nursing. Decisions relating to cardiopulmonary resuscitation, 3rd edition. 2016. Available from: https://resus.org.uk/EasySiteWeb/GatewayLink.aspx?alId=16643

Death of a Child

1. Introduction

- Being called to a death of an infant, child or adolescent is one of the most difficult experiences to encounter. Paramedics are usually the first professionals to arrive at the scene, and, at the same time as making difficult judgements about resuscitation, they have to deal with the devastating initial shock of the parents/carers.
- Despite the recent fall in incidence, sudden unexpected death in infancy (SUDI) remains the largest single cause of death in infants aged one month to one year. SUDI can also occasionally occur in children older than one year of age. The national 'Reduce the Risk' campaign of 1991 advocating infants sleep on their backs produced a dramatic reduction (70%) in sudden infant deaths.
- In 50% of SUDI, a specific cause for the death is found. The vast majority of SUDI occur from natural causes. 10% of SUDI are thought to arise from some form of maltreatment by their parents/carers and so a joint paediatrician and police investigation is required for **ALL** SUDIs. When informed of a SUDI, ambulance control should notify the police to initiate this process.
- This section draws on national experiences and is in accord with the recommendations of the Kennedy Report (2016).
- This guideline covers:
  - infants (defined as under one year old)
  - children (defined as between one year and puberty)
  - adolescents (defined as between puberty and 18 years old).
- In this guideline, the term 'child' includes infants and adolescents unless specified otherwise.

2. Objectives

- The main objectives for paramedics when called to a child death are:
  - Resuscitation (refer to **Basic Life Support in Children** and **Advanced Life Support** guidelines) should be attempted in all cases, unless there is a condition unequivocally associated with death or a valid advance decision (**Verification of Death and Termination of Resuscitation by Paramedics**).
  - Detecting a pulse in a sick infant can be extremely difficult so the absence of a peripheral pulse is not a reliable indication of death. Similarly, a sick infant may have marked peripheral cyanosis and cold extremities (refer to **Medical Emergencies in Children – Overview** and **Trauma Emergencies in Children – Overview**).
- It is better for parents/carers to know that resuscitation was attempted but failed, than to be left feeling that something that might have saved their infant was not done.
- Once resuscitation has been initiated, the infant should be transported as soon as practically possible to the nearest suitable emergency department, with resuscitation continuing en-route.

3. Care of the Family

- The initial response of professionals will affect the family profoundly.
- Having experienced this hugely distressing event, parents/carers exhibit a variety of reactions (e.g. overwhelming grief, anger, confusion, disbelief or guilt). Be prepared to deal with any of these feelings with sympathy and sensitivity, remembering some reactions may be directed towards the attending staffs as a manifestation of their distress.
- Think before you speak. Chance remarks may cause offence and may be remembered indefinitely (e.g. 'I'm sorry he looks so awful').
- Avoid any criticism of the parents/carers, either direct or implied.
- Ask the child's name and use it when referring to them (do not refer to the child as 'it').
- If possible, do not put children in body bags. It is known that relatives do not perceive very traumatic events in the way that unrelated onlookers might, and it is important they can see, touch and hold their loved one.
- Explain what you are doing at every stage.
- Allow the parents/carers to hold the child if they so wish (unless there are obvious indications of trauma or obvious suspicious circumstances that result in the police declaring a crime scene), as long as it does not interfere with clinical care.
- The parents/carers will need to accompany you when you take the child to hospital. If appropriate, offer to take one or both in the ambulance. Alternatively, ensure that they have other means of transport, and that they know where to go.
- If they have no telephone, offer to help in contacting a relative or friend who can give immediate support, such as looking after other children or making sure the premises are secure.

4. Document

- Time arrived on scene.
- The situation in which you find the child (e.g. position in cot, bedding, proximity to others, room temperature etc.).
- A brief description from the parents/carers of the events that led up to them finding the deceased child (e.g. when last seen alive, health at that time, position when found etc.). The police and

Death of a Child

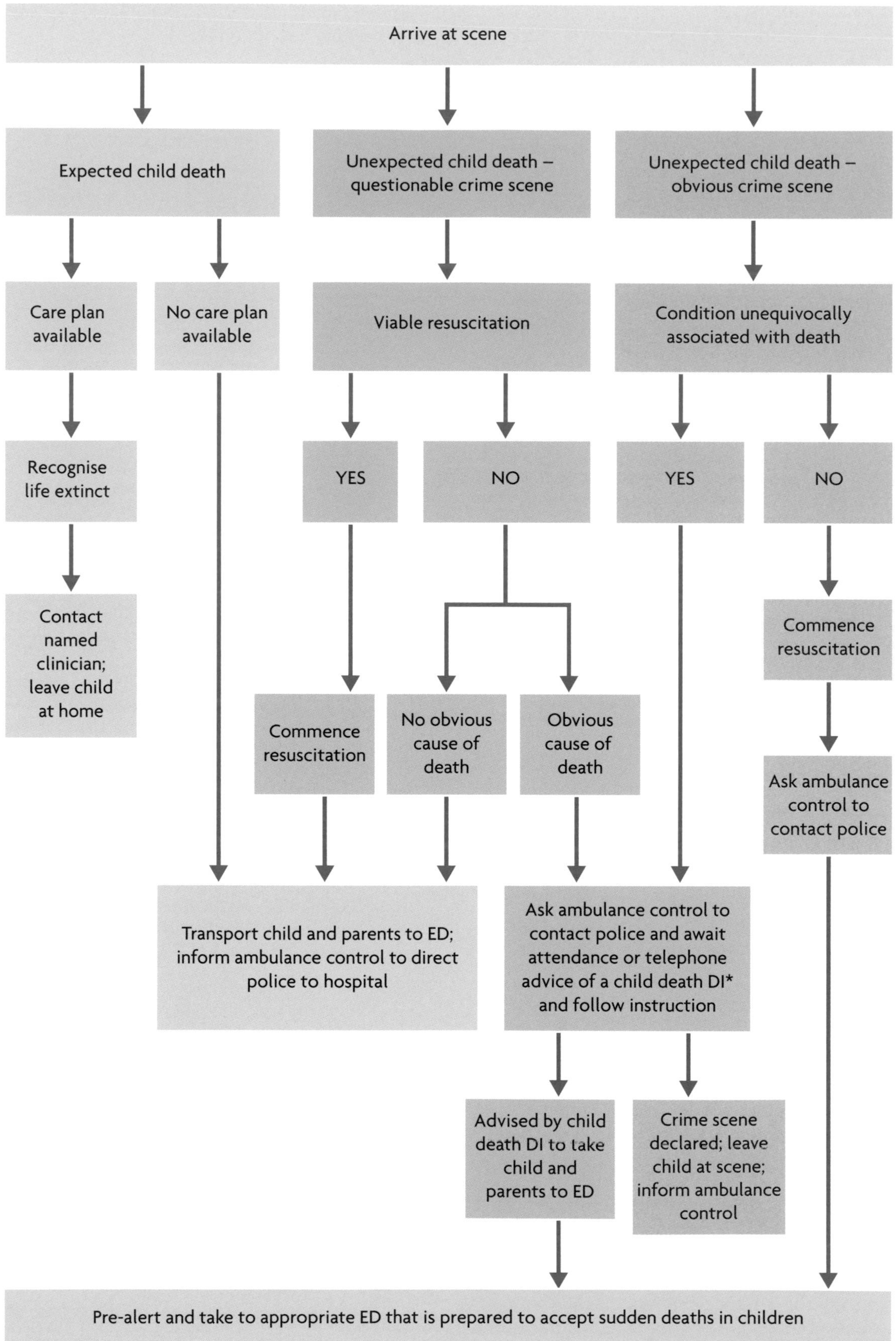

Figure 2.15 – Death of a child, including sudden unexpected death in infancy, children and adolescents (SUDICA).

*Child Death Detective Inspector – A Detective Inspector who is trained in the management of child death incidents to ensure the multi-agency investigation is commenced and evidence gathered to ascertain the full facts of the child's death.

community paediatrician will go through these events in greater detail, but the parent/carer's initial statement to you may be particularly valuable in the investigation.

- Write all this information down as soon as you have the opportunity, giving times and other details as precisely as possible.

5. Multi-Agency Approach

The Kennedy Report requires a multi-agency approach to the management of SUDI, in which all the professionals involved keep each other informed and collaborate.

5.1 Communication with other agencies

- After you have arrived at the house and confirmed that the infant is deceased, the police child abuse investigation team must be informed (refer to locally agreed procedure).
- In unexpected child deaths, advise the parents/carers that the death will be reported to the Coroner, and that they will be interviewed by the Coroner's Officer and the police in due course.
- Share the information you have collected with the police and with relevant health professionals.

Conditions unequivocally associated with death

- Decapitation.
- Massive cranial and cerebral destruction.
- Hemicorporectomy or similar massive injury.
- Decomposition/putrefaction – where tissue damage indicates that the patient has been dead for some hours, days or longer.
- Incineration – the presence of full thickness burns with charring of greater than 95% of the body surface.
- Hypostasis – the pooling of blood in congested vessels in the dependent part of the body in the position in which it lies after death.
- Fetal maceration in a newborn – when the child is born with such severe abnormalities that it is considered incompatible with life.

6. Transferring the Child

- The child should be taken to the nearest appropriate emergency department, not direct to a mortuary. This should apply even when the child has clearly been dead for some time and a doctor has certified death at home (it will on occasions be necessary to remind a doctor that taking the child to a hospital is now the preferred procedure, as recommended by Kennedy).
- The main reasons for taking the child to the hospital rather than the mortuary are that at hospital an immediate examination can be made by a paediatrician, early samples can be taken for laboratory tests, parents/carers can talk with the paediatricians and other local support services can be contacted.
- Pre-alert the emergency department of your arrival, asking them to be ready to take over resuscitation if this is ongoing.

7. Support

- The death of a child is very distressing for all those involved, and opportunities for debriefing or counselling should be available.
- Follow local procedures for post critical incident debriefing local guidelines/processes.
- Some people will feel ongoing distress. This is normal but should be recognised, and other forms of therapy, from informal support from colleagues, to formal counselling, may be required.
- As part of the ambulance service safeguarding processes, information from local paediatricians and ambulance service safeguarding leads will be available if required for further discussion.
- Unsuccessful resuscitation attempts on children weigh heavily on many people's shoulders and it is very important to remember that the vast majority of children who arrest outside hospital will die, whoever is there, or whatever is done – less than 10% of paediatric out-of-hospital cardiac arrests survive. Such outcomes are almost never the fault of those attempting resuscitation who will have done everything possible to help that child.

Death of a Child

KEY POINTS!

Death of a Child

- **A child death is one of the most emotionally traumatic and challenging events to encounter.**
- **Resuscitation should always be attempted unless there is a condition unequivocally associated with death or a valid advance decision.**
- **Communication and empathy are essential, and the family must be treated with compassion and sensitivity throughout. Findings from the Foundation for the Study of Infant Deaths have shown that parents/carers regard the actions and attitudes of those who tend to them as extremely important and speak very highly of the way both they and their child were treated.**
- **Your role is not only essential for immediate practical reasons but also has a great influence on how the family deals with the death, long after the initial crisis is over.**
- **Ensure the family is aware of where you are taking their infant/child.**
- **Collect information pertaining to the situation in which you find the child, a history of events and any significant past medical history.**
- **Follow agreed protocols with regards to inter-agency communication and informing the police.**
- **In unexpected deaths, explain to the family that the death will be reported to the Coroner and that they will be interviewed by the Coroner's Officer and the police in due course.**

Bibliography

1. Resuscitation Council (UK). *Resuscitation Guidelines 2015. Prevention of cardiac arrest and decisions about CPR.* London: Resuscitation Council, 2015. Available from: https://resus.org.uk/resuscitation-guidelines/prevention-of-cardiac-arrest-and-decisions-about-cpr/.
2. British Medical Association, Resuscitation Council (UK), Royal College of Nursing. *Decisions relating to cardiopulmonary resuscitation, 3rd edition.* London: British Medical Association, 2016. Available from: https://resus.org.uk/EasySiteWeb/GatewayLink.aspx?alId=16643.
3. Kennedy, H, Royal College of Pathologists, Royal College of Paediatrics. *Sudden unexpected death in infancy and childhood.* London: Royal College of Pathologists, 2016. Available from: https://www.rcpath.org/uploads/assets/uploaded/af879a1b-1974-4692-9e002c20f09dc14c.pdf.

Emergency Tracheostomy and Laryngectomy Pre-Hospital Management

1. Introduction

'A patient with a tracheostomy or laryngectomy is at risk of death or harm if inappropriate or inadequate care is provided. This patient group requires airway devices to be safely inserted, securely positioned and appropriately cared for, in order to continue to provide the patient with a patent airway. Failure to do so may lead to a displaced or blocked tube, which, if not dealt with immediately, may be fatal within minutes.'[1]

An increasing number of patients with long-term tracheostomies and laryngectomies are now being managed in the community. Approximately 12,000 tracheostomy procedures are performed each year in the UK.[2] Patients are discharged from hospital once the tracheostomy is stable and the patient or carer is competent with self-care along with the support from community nurses.

2. Incidence

- All trusts can expect to see more patients requiring emergency care due to the increase in head and neck cancers. These are the fifth leading cause of cancer and the sixth leading cause of cancer mortality.[3]
- Approximately 31 people receive a diagnosis every day in the UK and most are associated with risk factors such as smoking and drinking alcohol.[2] Up to 75% fall into these categories. Men over 50 are more commonly affected.
- The instances of affected younger people are also increasing due to the incidence of oral human papillomavirus (HPV). Transmission is likely to be sexually acquired; strong evidence suggests that this is an important prognostic factor associated with head and neck squamous cell carcinoma (HNSCC).[3]
- Cannabis smoke is strongly linked to the pathogenesis of HNSCC because the smoke has a far greater number of carcinogens than is found in cigarette smoke.[3] Studies are ongoing in this area and are not conclusive but are strongly linked to a younger population. Over 5,000 tracheostomy procedures per year are undertaken on patients with HNSCC.[1]
- These may be permanent or temporary tracheostomy tubes, but the higher incidence suggests the potential for a rise in patient numbers within the community with challenging airways. Clinicians must have the necessary skills and knowledge to provide the appropriate assessment and management in the pre-hospital setting.

3. Severity and Outcome

- Most patients are discharged with all the necessary equipment to manage most emergencies. The majority of patients are also discharged with a hospital passport that provides vital details in relation to the specifics of the patient, their airway management and the history of their condition.
- The most common tracheostomy airway emergencies are displacement, accidental de-cannulation and obstruction.[1]
- Obstruction of the tube is the third most common cause of death in patients with tracheostomies (Feber, 2016).[4] Maintaining a patent airway is the priority. Clinicians must be able to recognise a blocked tube in the presence of severe difficulty in breathing or apnoea. Tubes can become blocked with plugs of mucous, blood and crusts, and the clinician must be competent and trained in suction techniques. They should also be aware of the different types of tracheostomy tubes in use in order to clear the tube safely and effectively.

4. Physiology

4.1 Laryngectomy

- Laryngectomy is the total removal of the larynx and the separation of the airway from the nose, mouth and oesophagus. In a total laryngectomy the laryngectomee breathes through an opening in the neck. This becomes the patient's primary airway. The procedure is usually performed by head and neck surgeons following a diagnosis of laryngeal cancer (CA) which is unresponsive to chemotherapy and radiotherapy. Total laryngectomy results in permanent changes to the airway anatomy; the trachea is pulled forward during surgery and stitched to the anterior neck skin forming a new stoma (Figure 2.16).

4.2 Tracheostomy

- A tracheostomy is an opening in the neck performed by using a surgical incision or a percutaneous technique. A tracheostomy tube is passed into the trachea between the second and third tracheal rings, and a stoma is formed 3–5 days post-surgery. The airway is then secured. The surgical* approach is usually an elective procedure prior to planned surgery and the percutaneous** approach is generally carried out as part of a critical care emergency. All tracheostomies can be permanent or temporary (Figure 2.17).

* An open approach where inner organs or tissue are exposed (typically with the use of a scalpel).

** A percutaneous procedure is any medical procedure where access to inner organs or other tissue is done via needle-puncture of the skin.

SECTION 2 Resuscitation

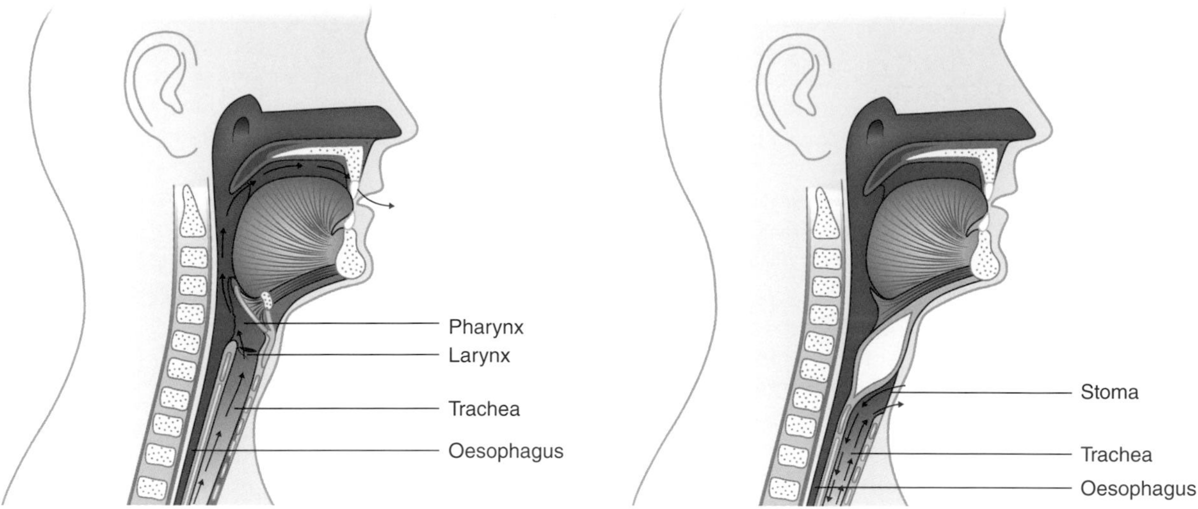

Figure 2.16 – Airway anatomy before and after laryngectomy

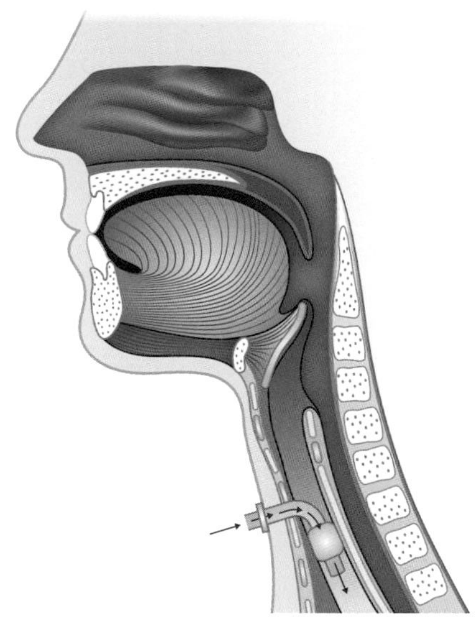

Figure 2.17 – Tracheostomy

5. Assessment and Management

For the assessment and management of tracheostomy and laryngectomy refer to Table 2.10 and Figures 2.17 to 2.19.

Emergency Tracheostomy and Laryngectomy Pre-Hospital Management

TABLE 2.10 – ASSESSMENT and MANAGEMENT of: Suction and Oxygen	
ENSURE PPE INCLUDING FACE MASK PROTECTION. REMOVE FENESTRATED TUBES BEFORE SUCTIONING. REMEMBER SUCTION IS A HYPOXIC PROCESS.	
ASSESSMENT	**MANAGEMENT**
Aims of suction and oxygenation: • Prevent respiratory distress • Maintain a patent airway • Clear excessive secretions **Indications for suction found on assessment:** • Excessive secretions not cleared by coughing • Increase in pulse, BP or respiratory rate • Decrease in O_2 saturations, prolonged capillary refill • Difficulty in mechanically ventilating the patient Assess the need for oxygen based on reliable saturation readings.	• Pre-oxygenate* the patient before the suction procedure; aim for 94–98% SpO_2 (88–92% SpO_2 for COPD patients). Explain your actions to the patient. • Remove the inner cannula and clean it if blocked. Replace and assess for improvement. • Set suction at 150–200 mmHg. • If using a hard Yankeur – do not lose sight of the tip; suction on the way out. • If using a soft catheter – go no further than 2 cm beyond the tube length; suction on the way out. • Remember to re-oxygenate* the patient after suctioning. • If you are unable to pass suction beyond the length of the tube, refer to the conscious patient algorithm.
*Hi-flow oxygen 15 l/min, tracheostomy O_2 mask at the neck, non-rebreather mask over the nose and mouth.	

TABLE 2.11 – Glossary of Commonly used Tracheostomy/Laryngectomy Terms	
Tracheotomy/tracheostomy	Technically, the suffix -otomy means 'to cut into'. The suffix -ostomy means 'opening into'. So a tracheotomy is the surgical procedure to create an opening into the trachea to enable a tracheostomy.
Inner and outer cannula	The inner part of the tracheostomy tube can be removed, cleaned or replaced. The outer part of the tube stays in place.
Cuff 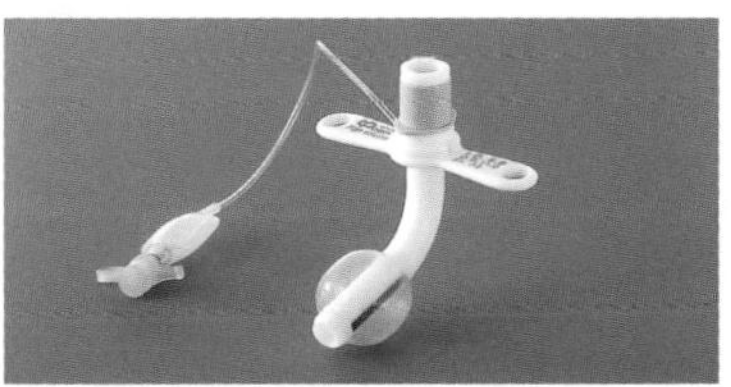 Republished with permission of Fuji Systems	The balloon at the end of the tracheostomy tube that can be inflated, similar to that of inflatable cuffs on ET tubes.
De-cannulation	Removal or accidental removal of the whole tracheostomy tube.
Fenestrated tracheostomy tube 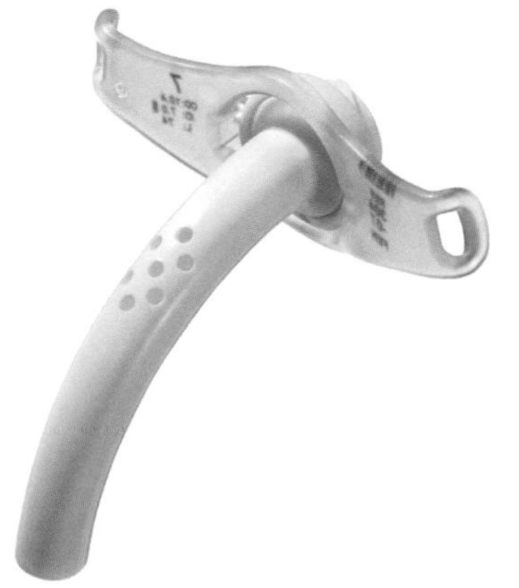 Republished with permission of Kapitex.	The word fenestration comes from the French word fenêtre, meaning window. A fenestration is an opening in the shaft of the tube allowing air to pass through. This allows people to speak when it is correctly fitted. **NB**: must be removed when applying suction.

SECTION 2 Resuscitation

TABLE 2.11 – Glossary of Commonly used Tracheostomy/Laryngectomy Terms *(continued)*

Flange Republished with permission of Kapitex	The part of the tracheostomy tube that fits against the anterior neck and around the stoma. It also carries written information about the tube. The flange provides anchoring for securing straps and stops the tube from slipping into the stoma.
Laryngectomee	A person who has had a laryngectomy.
Laryngectomy	The surgical removal of the larynx.
Mucus plug	An accumulation of mucus that can obstruct the lumen of the tracheostomy tube.
Speaking valve Republished with permission of Kapitex	Usually a one-way valve that fits on the tracheostomy tube. It allows air to pass into the tracheostomy, but closes with exhalation, forcing air into the mouth and nose which allows speech. Used only on cuffless tubes or in 'cuff down' mode.
Stoma	Literally translates as 'mouth' in seventeenth-century Latin. It refers to the skin around the opening.
Suctioning	Removal of tracheal secretions or blood in the airway.
Heat moisture exchanger (HME) Republished with permission of Intersurgical	A device that fits on the tracheostomy tube. It collects exhaled water vapour, allowing it to be inhaled, which aids humidification.
Buchanan bibs Republished with permission of Kapitex	Buchanan DeltaNex® is a three-layer system with a hydrolox foam core and a breathable soft cotton outer mesh. It is designed specifically for airway protection, to filter fine particles and allow moisture transfer. It is a bib of plastic foam covered with knitted fabric of honeycomb pattern. The neck band includes Velcro strips for fastening onto the strip on the bib and fastening around the neck.
Phonation	Using the voice.

Emergency Tracheostomy and Laryngectomy Pre-Hospital Management

TABLE 2.12 – Stepwise Approach to Airway Management

A tracheostomy tube in situ with a dressing, neck tie, cuffed tube and a heat moisture exchanger (HME). 1. Any attachment that covers the tube must be removed if the patient is experiencing difficulty in breathing. Ensure that the tube is in neutral alignment.	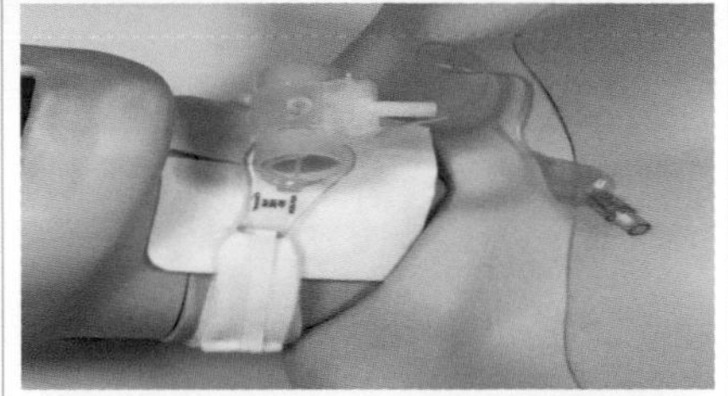
2. The inner part of the tracheostomy tube can be removed by twisting and gently extracting. It can then be cleaned or replaced. The outer part of the tube stays in place. The 15 mm connection is compatible with the BVM attachment and the catheter mount.	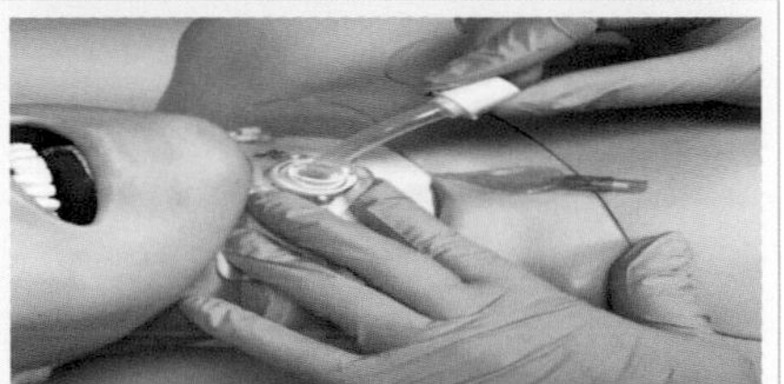
3. If there are **no airway problems** and the **airway is patent** you can use a **CUFFED** tube with the inner tube in place as an advanced airway. The cuff must be inflated to achieve positive pressure ventilations. $EtCO_2$ must be recorded to confirm advance airway. **Look for equal bilateral chest rise.**	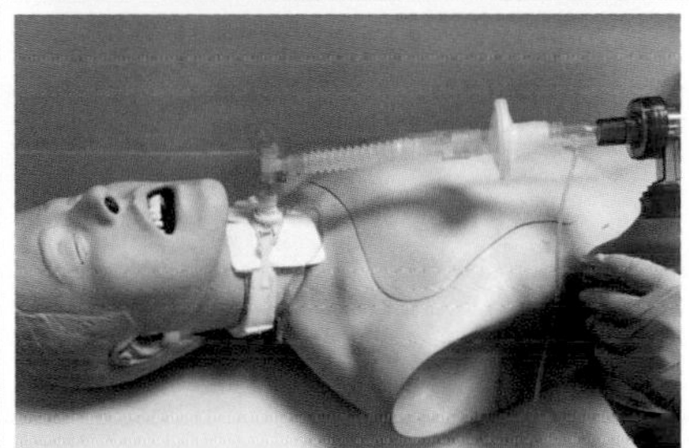
4. If the tube is blocked it must be removed. Open the stoma with a finger if it has closed, gently insert a bougie and carefully railroad a size 6 ET tube up to the first black line. Inflate the cuff. This is a two-person procedure; be gentle in your technique and remember the delicate nature of tracheal tissue.	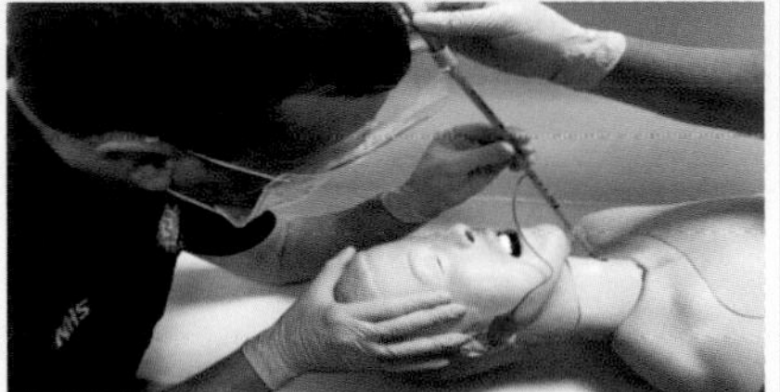
5. Once the cuff is inflated, attach the catheter mount, filter, $EtCO_2$ line and the BVM. **Do not let go of the tube, do not use a Thomas™ tube holder.** Best practice is to appoint someone to hold the tube and monitor the airway constantly. This is a two-person technique**. Look for equal bilateral chest rise.**	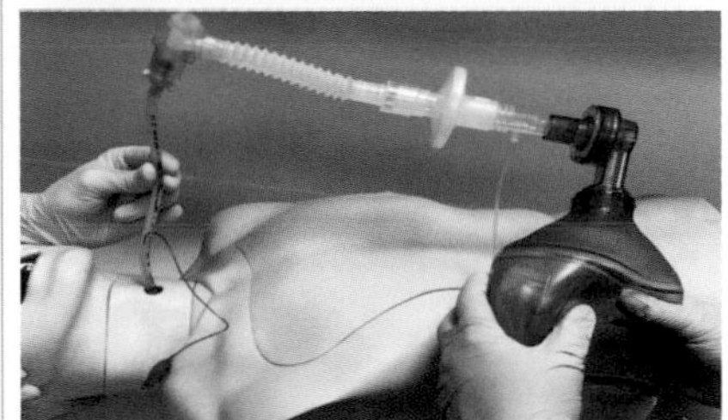
6. If the tube is blocked it must be removed. The nose and mouth must be occluded to prevent any air escape. Use a small paediatric mask attached to an adult bag and valve, seal over the stoma and ventilate the patient. This is best carried out as a two-person technique. **Look for equal bilateral chest rise.**	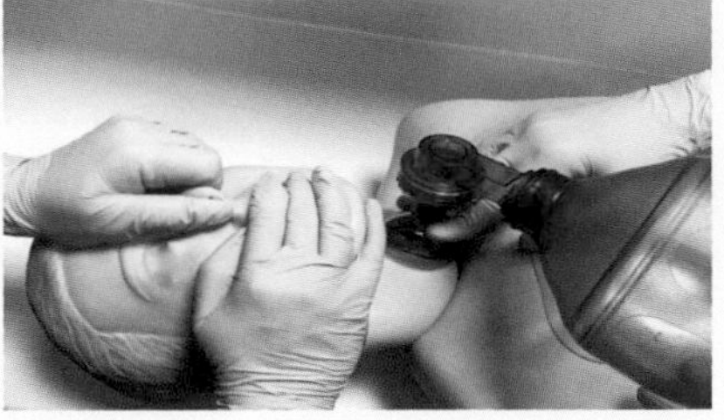
Images republished with kind permission of Dorothy Antrim, London Ambulance Service.	

Emergency Tracheostomy and Laryngectomy Pre-Hospital Management

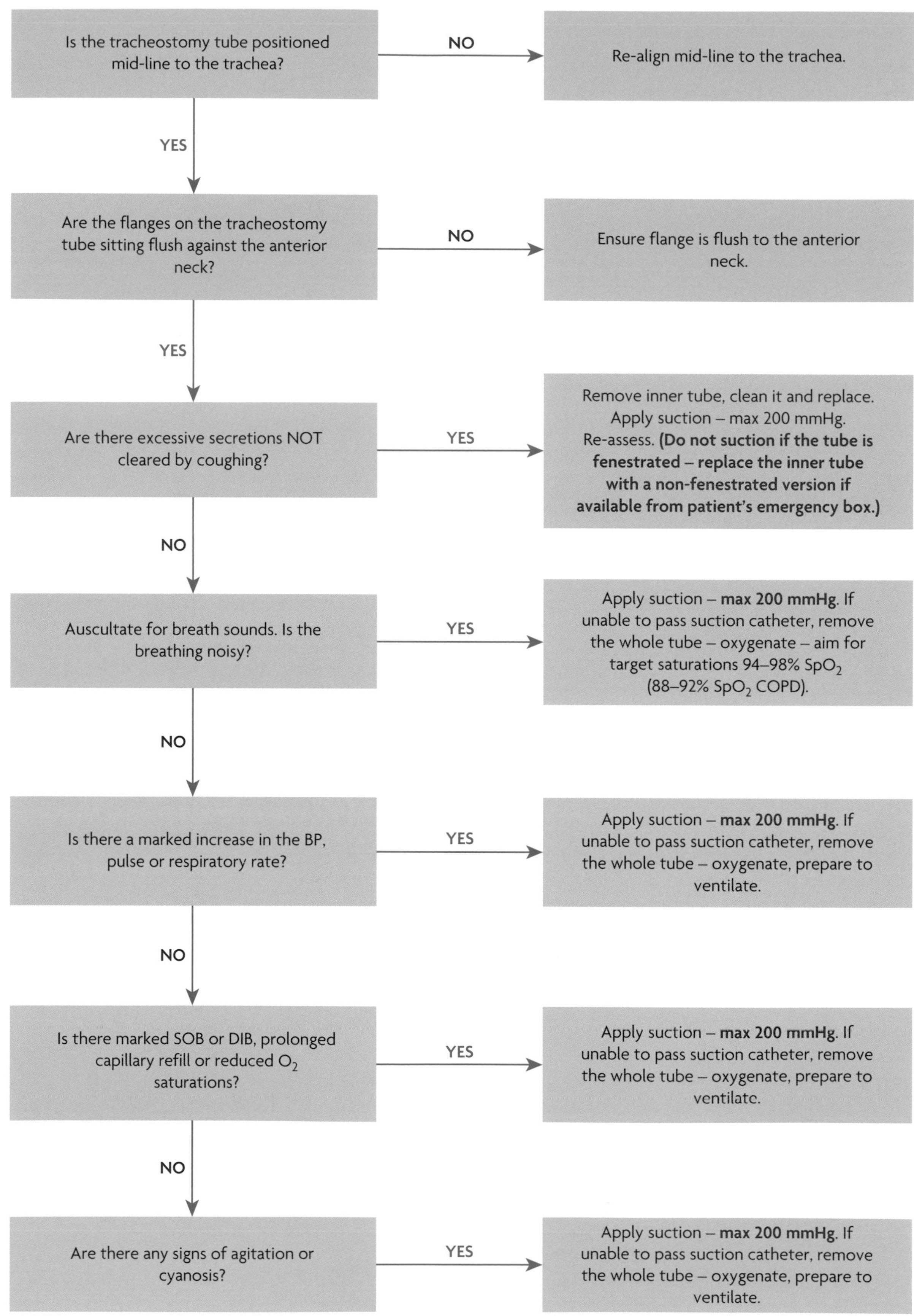

Figure 2.18 – Steps for confirming tracheostomy patency on the conscious patient.

Emergency Tracheostomy and Laryngectomy Pre-Hospital Management

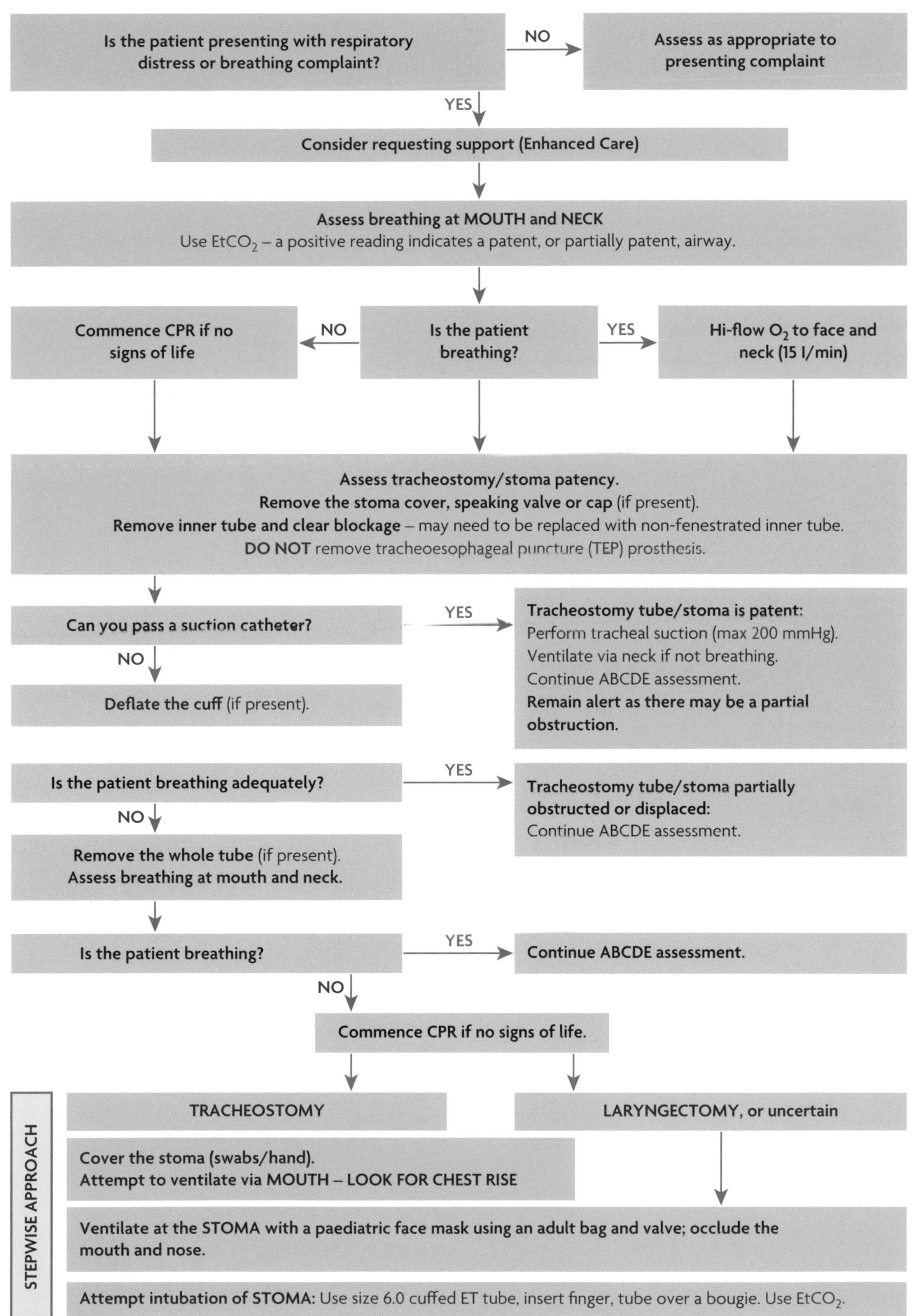

Figure 2.19 – Emergency tracheostomy and laryngectomy management.

SECTION 2 Resuscitation

Emergency Tracheostomy and Laryngectomy Pre-Hospital Management

KEY POINTS!

- **A third of deaths associated with tracheostomy and laryngectomy patients are due to hypoxia caused by a blocked tube.**
- **Early recognition of a blocked tube is vital.**
- **Inability to pass suction catheters beyond the tube indicates a blockage.**
- **Accidental removal of the whole tracheostomy tube (de-cannulation) is a TIME-CRITICAL emergency.**
- **Try to remember to take the patient's emergency box to hospital; it contains their appropriately sized tubes.**
- **NEVER reintroduce a tracheostomy tube.**
- **Emphasis must be on oxygenation to reverse the hypoxia together with reassurance.**
- **Always be prepared to ventilate airway-compromised patients.**

Acknowledgement

Acknowledgements to Jacqueline Mitchell, CNS Tracheostomy Specialist at Guy's and St Thomas' NHS Foundation Trust.

Bibliography

1. McGrath BA. Executive summary key recommendations. In BA McGrath, *Comprehensive Tracheostomy Care*. Chichester: John Wiley & Sons Ltd, 2014: xix.
2. Wilkinson KA, Freeth H, Kelly K. On the right trach. A review of care received by patients who underwent a tracheostomy. *British Journal of Hospital Medicine* 2014, 76(3): 163–165.
3. Goon PKC, Stanley MA, Ebmeyer J, Steinsträsser L, Upile T et al. HPV and head and neck cancer: A descriptive update. *Head and Neck Oncology* 2009, 1: 36.
4. Feber T. Tracheostomy care for community nurses: Basic principles. *British Journal of Community Nursing* 2016, 11(5): 186–193.

3

Medical Emergencies

Medical Emergencies in Adults – Overview

1. Introduction

Although the care of a wide range of medical conditions will be quite specific to the presenting condition, there are general principles of care that apply to most medical cases, regardless of underlying condition(s).

2. Patient Assessment

In order to gather as much relevant information as possible, without delaying care, the accepted format of history taking is as follows:

- Presenting complaint – why the patient or carer called for help at this time.
- The history of presenting complaint – details of when the problem started, exacerbating factors and previous similar episodes. **NB** The patient history can provide valuable insight into the cause of the current condition.
- Direct questioning about associated symptoms, by system. Ask about all appropriate systems. Refer to **Table 3.1**.
- Past medical history, including current medication.
- Family history.
- Social history.

Combined with a good physical examination (primary and secondary survey), this format of history taking should ensure that you correctly identify those patients who are time critical, urgent or routine. The history taken must be fully documented. In many cases, a well-taken history will point to the diagnosis.

The presence of MedicAlert® type jewellery (bracelets or necklets) can provide information on the patient's pre-existing health risk (e.g. diabetes, anaphylaxis, Addison's disease etc.) that may be relevant to the current medical emergency.

2.1 Primary Survey

- The primary survey should take 60–90 seconds for assessment and follow the approach set out in **Table 3.1**. This rapid assessment should quickly identify patients with actual or potential life-threatening conditions or symptoms.
- Assessment and management should proceed in a 'stepwise' manner and abnormalities should be managed as they are encountered; that is, do not move onto breathing and circulation until the airway is managed. Every time an intervention has been carried out, re-assess the patient.
- If haemorrhage cannot be controlled or airway and breathing cannot be corrected, evacuate immediately, continuing resuscitation as appropriate en-route.

<table>
<tr><th colspan="3">TABLE 3.1 – ASSESSMENT and MANAGEMENT of: Medical Emergencies</th></tr>
<tr><td colspan="2">• All stages should be considered but some more detailed elements may be omitted if not considered appropriate.</td><td>At each stage consider the need for:
• Early senior clinical support.</td></tr>
<tr><td colspan="3">• Start correcting any <C>ABCD problems as below.
• Undertake a TIME CRITICAL transfer to nearest appropriate receiving hospital.
• Continue patient management en-route
• Provide an ATMIST information call.</td></tr>
<tr><td>STAGE</td><td>ASSESSMENT</td><td>MANAGEMENT</td></tr>
<tr><td>C</td><td>Catastrophic haemorrhage
Look for evidence of external catastrophic haemorrhage.
Consider whether occult catastrophic haemorrhage could be occurring. For example, following trauma or as a result of an aneurysm rupture.</td><td>Stem external bleeding
Apply a tourniquet and/or apply direct pressure to the site.
Dress the site with appropriate haemorrhage/trauma dressing.
Elevate the site if possible.</td></tr>
<tr><td>A</td><td>AIRWAY – assess the airway (refer to Airway and Breathing Management).
Look for obvious obstructions, e.g. teeth/dentures, foreign bodies, vomit, blood. Refer to Foreign Body Airway Obstruction.</td><td>Correct any airway problems immediately by:
• Positioning – head tilt, chin lift, jaw thrust.
• Suction (if available and appropriate).</td></tr>
</table>

Medical Emergencies in Adults – Overview

TABLE 3.1 – ASSESSMENT and MANAGEMENT of: Medical Emergencies *(continued)*		
	Listen for noisy airflow, e.g. snoring, gurgling or no airflow. Refer to **Dyspnoea**. **Feel for** air movement. Airway constriction is a life-threatening condition and can result from an immune response to an allergen – refer to **Allergic Reactions including Anaphylaxis**.	• Oropharyngeal airway. • Nasopharyngeal airway. • Supraglottic airway (SGA) (if appropriate). • Endotracheal intubation (if appropriate, appropriately trained and only if waveform capnography is available). • Needle cricothyroidotomy.
B	**BREATHING** – expose the chest and assess (refer to **Airway and Breathing Management**). **Inspect:** • Respiratory rate (<10 or >30). • Adequacy and depth of chest movements. • Symmetry of chest movement. • Effectiveness of ventilation. • Cyanosis or pallor peripherally and centrally. • Position of trachea in suprasternal notch. **Palpate:** • Any instability of chest wall and note any areas of tenderness • Note depth and equality of chest movement. **Percuss for:** • Dullness or hyperresonance. **Auscultate:** • Altered breathing patterns with a stethoscope – ask the patient to take deep breaths in and out briskly through their mouth if possible – listen on both sides of the chest: – above the nipples in the mid-clavicular line – laterally in the mid-axillary line – below the shoulder blade (front and back). • Auscultate to assess air entry and compare sides. Equality of air entry. • Crepitations at the rear of the chest (crackles, heard low down in the lung fields at the rear – may indicate fluid in the lung in heart failure). • Wheezing, noisy respiration on inspiration or expiration.	• Correct any breathing problems immediately. • Consider patient positioning (e.g. sitting upright for respiratory problems). • If breathing is absent, refer to appropriate **Resuscitation** guidelines. • If the breathing is inadequate, refer to **Airway and Breathing Management**. • Treat underlying cause of unilateral chest movement if tension pneumothorax. • Monitor the patient's SpO_2, administer oxygen to achieve saturations of >94% if the patient presents as hypoxaemic on air, refer to **Oxygen**. • **NB** this is except for patients with COPD or other risk factors for hypercapnia (refer to **Oxygen**). • In patients with a decreased level of consciousness (Glasgow Coma Scale (GCS) <15) administer the initial supplemental oxygen dose until the vital signs are normal, then reduce the oxygen dose and aim for a target saturation (SpO_2) >94%. Refer to **Altered Level of Consciousness**. • In patients with sickle cell crisis administer supplemental oxygen via an appropriate mask/nasal cannula until a reliable SpO_2 measurement is available; then adjust the oxygen flow to aim for target saturation within the range of 94–98%. Refer to **Sickle Cell Crisis**. Consider assisted ventilation at a rate of 12–20 respirations per minute if any of the following are present: • Oxygen saturation (SpO_2) <90% on levels of supplemental oxygen. • Respiratory rate <10 or >30 bpm. • Inadequate chest expansion.

(continued)

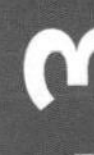

Medical Emergencies in Adults – Overview

TABLE 3.1 – ASSESSMENT and MANAGEMENT of: Medical Emergencies *(continued)*

	• Stridor (higher pitched noise on inspiration), suggestive of upper respiratory obstruction. • Additional crackles and wheeze on inspiration may be associated with inhalation of blood or vomit.	**NB Restraint (positional) asphyxia** – If the patient is required to be physically restrained (e.g. by police officers) in order to prevent them injuring themselves or others, or for the purpose of being detained under the Mental Health Act, then it is paramount that the method of restraint allows both for a patent airway and adequate respiratory volume. **Under these circumstances it is essential to ensure that the patient's airway and breathing are adequate at all times.**
STAGE **C**	**ASSESSMENT** • Assess for evidence of external haemorrhage (e.g. epistaxis, haemoptysis, haematemesis, melaena). For suspected gastrointestinal bleeding, refer to **Gastrointestinal Bleeding**. • Assess skin colour and temperature. • Palpate for a radial pulses – if absent feel for a carotid pulse. **NB** The estimation of blood pressure by pulse is inaccurate and unreliable; however, the presence of a radial pulse suggests adequate perfusion of major organs. The presence of a femoral pulse suggests perfusion of the kidneys, while a carotid pulse and coherent mental state suggests adequate perfusion of the brain. • Assess pulse rate, volume and rhythm. • Check capillary refill time centrally (forehead or sternum – normal <2 seconds). Consider hypovolaemic shock and be aware of its early signs: • Pallor. • Cool peripheries. • Anxiety, abnormal behaviour. • Increased respiratory rate. • Tachycardia. **Recognition of shock** Shock is difficult to diagnose. In certain groups of patients the signs of shock may appear late (e.g. patients with acute adrenal insufficiency (adrenal crisis), pregnant women, patients on medication such as beta-blockers, and the physically fit). Blood loss of 750–1000 ml will produce little evidence of shock; blood loss of 1000–1500 ml is required before more classical signs of shock appear. **NB** This loss is from the circulation **NOT** necessarily visible externally.	**MANAGEMENT** • Arrest external haemorrhage. • In cases of internal or uncontrolled haemorrhage undertake a **TIME CRITICAL** transfer to further care; provide an alert/information call. • Patients with sepsis will usually benefit from early fluid therapy and an appropriate hospital alert/information call. Refer to **Sepsis**. **Fluid therapy** • If fluid replacement is indicated refer to **Intravascular Fluid Therapy in Adults**. • Rapid fluid replacement into the vascular compartment can overload the cardiovascular system particularly where there is pre-existing cardiovascular disease and in older people. Gradual rehydration over many hours rather than minutes may be indicated for rehydration. **NB** Monitor fluid replacement closely in these cases.

Medical Emergencies in Adults – Overview

TABLE 3.1 – ASSESSMENT and MANAGEMENT of: Medical Emergencies *(continued)*		
D	**DISABILITY** ● Note the initial level of responsiveness on AVPU scale, and time of assessment. **A** – Alert. **V** – Responds to voice. **P** – Responds to painful stimulus. **U** – Unresponsive. ● Detail how to check pain. ● Assess and note pupil size, equality and response to light. **NB** In patients with fixed pinpoint pupils, suspect opiate use. ● Check for purposeful movement in all four limbs. ● Check sensory function. ● Assess blood glucose levels in all patients with diabetes, impaired consciousness, convulsions, collapse or alcohol consumption, a history of Addison's disease or other forms of adrenal insufficiency.	● Check blood glucose level to rule out hypo – or hyperglycaemia as the cause; refer to **Glycaemic Emergencies in Adults and Children**. ● Also check blood glucose levels in all patients with history of diabetes, impaired consciousness, seizures, collapse or alcohol/drug consumption ● Consider adrenal crisis as a cause and provide drug therapy as required; refer to appropriate drug guidelines. In adrenal crisis refer to **Hydrocortisone**. ● If the level of consciousness deteriorates or respiratory depression develops in cases where an overdose with opiate type drugs may be a possibility, consider administering naloxone, refer to **Naloxone Hydrochloride**. ● For patients with decreased consciousness and active seizure, refer to **Convulsions in Adults**.
Vital Signs and NEWS2 **NB** complete a full set of observations for all patients, repeat after intervention or when any value is outside normal parameters.	Respiratory rate	Measure and record respiratory rate.
	Pulse	Measure and record pulse.
	Oxygen saturation	Monitor the patient's SpO_2, administer oxygen to achieve saturations of >94%. If the patient presents as hypoxaemic on air, refer to **Oxygen**.
	Blood pressure and fluids	Measure and record blood pressure. If required, administer fluids; refer to **Intravascular Fluid Therapy in Adults** and **Intravascular Fluid Therapy in Children**.
	Blood glucose	If appropriate, measure and record blood glucose for hypo/hyperglycaemia; refer to **Glycaemic Emergencies in Adults and Children**.
	Temperature	Measure and record temperature.
	NEWS2	These observations will enable you to calculate a NEWS2 score; refer to **Sepsis**.
ECG		If required, monitor and record 12-Lead ECG. Assess for abnormality; refer to **Cardiac Rhythm Disturbance**.
Assess the patient's pain		Where present, assess the **SOCRATES** of pain and record initial and subsequent pain scores. Consider analgesia if appropriate; refer to **Pain Management in Adults** and **Pain Management in Children**.
Documentation		Complete documentation to include all clinical findings, advice from other clinicians, onward referral and worsening advice given.

Medical Emergencies in Adults – Overview

2.2 Secondary Survey

- A secondary survey should only commence after the primary survey has been completed and an assessment of the patient's critical status has been made.
- The secondary survey is a more thorough 'head-to-toe' assessment of the patient including their past medical history (refer to **Table 3.2**). It is important to monitor the patient's vital signs during the survey.
- A complete and thorough secondary survey may not be possible in some patients with **TIME CRITICAL** conditions.
- Follow additional medical guidelines as indicated by the patient's condition (e.g. cardiac rhythm disturbance).

TABLE 3.2 – Clinical Assessment

- Continually re-assess <C>ABCD throughout clinical assessment.
- Assess all patients holistically considering the implications of any of the following:
  - Congenital defects/malformations – kyphosis/scoliosis – causing compression.
  - Dentition – this may indicate level of nutrition.
  - Jugular vein distension – cardiac history.
  - Oedema (ankles/orbital) – failure or kidney disease.
  - Central cyanosis.
  - Finger clubbing/splinter haemorrhage – respiratory or cardiac history.
  - Bruising – injury (consider non-accidental injury in vulnerable patient groups).
  - Surgical scars – previous procedures.

Respiratory

- Inspect, palpate, percuss and auscultate the chest, examining for signs which could indicate a respiratory cause for the presenting condition:
  - Accessory muscles/recession/nasal flaring.
  - Chest shape and symmetry.
  - Palpate for tactile fremitus which may indicate mucus plug or pneumonia.
  - Central trachea.
- Assess for pneumothorax – in small pneumothorax no clinical signs may be detected. A pneumothorax causes breathlessness, reduced air entry and chest movement on the affected side. If this is a tension pneumothorax, then the patient will have increasing respiratory distress; distended neck veins and tracheal deviation (late sign) away from affected side may also be present.

Cardiac

- Auscultate and palpate, examining for signs which could indicate a cardiac cause for the presenting condition.
- Assess skin colour and temperature.
- Record pulse oximeter reading including heart rate.
- Assess heart sounds and bruits.
- Palpate bilateral pulses for equality.
- Obtain a blood pressure reading using a sphygmomanometer; consider bilateral and standing and sitting blood pressures – consider postural drop.

Neurological

- Establish Glasgow Coma Scale (refer to **Altered Level of Consciousness**).
- Assess cranial nerves.
- Consider gait.

Medical Emergencies in Adults – Overview

TABLE 3.2 – Clinical Assessment *(continued)*

- Assess tone, strength and sensation to separate limbs and dermatomes.
- Consider assessing reflexes.
- **NB** Patients on long-term steroids or who have adrenal insufficiency may deteriorate rapidly because of steroid insufficiency. If significantly unwell, the patient should be given hydrocortisone and fluids if required, refer to **Hydrocortisone**, **Intravascular Fluid Therapy in Adults** and **Intravascular Fluid Therapy in Children**.
- Some patients, especially those with spinal cord injury above T6, are particularly susceptible to the potentially life-threatening condition autonomic dysreflexia, which is characterised by a rapid rise in blood pressure, bradycardia, tachycardia, arrhythmia, headache or sweating due to unregulated sympathetic hyperactivity. This can cause cerebral haemorrhage and death.
- A small number of patients who have had a severe stroke or who have severe forms of Parkinson's disease, multiple sclerosis, cerebral palsy or spina bifida may also be susceptible to autonomic dysreflexia.
  - Patients with spinal cord injury or neurological conditions may have neurogenic bowel dysfunction. They may depend on routine interventional bowel care, including manual removal of faeces. Autonomic dysreflexia can be caused by non-adherence to a patient's usual bowel routine or during or following interventional bowel care.
- Patients that present to ambulance services may have difficulty when their normal bowel routine does not occur, for example due to illness or injury. The condition autonomic dysreflexia should always be considered.

Gastrointestinal

- Auscultate, percuss and palpate, examining for signs which could indicate a gastrointestinal cause for the presenting condition.
- Auscultate for bowel sounds and bruits.

Percuss for hypo/hyper resonance (e.g. dull = solid, high pitch = gas, shifting dullness = fluid)

- Feel for tenderness and guarding in all four quadrants.

Musculoskeletal/Skin

- Check for MSC in four limbs:
  - Test for movement and power.
  - Apply light touch to evaluate sensation.
  - Assess pulse and skin temperature.
- Assess for rashes, localised inflammation, bruising, swelling, erythema or other abnormalities.
- Assess for jaundice.

ADDITIONAL INFORMATION

The following may assist in determining the diagnosis:

- Relatives, carers or friends with knowledge of the patient's history.
- Packets or containers of medication (including domiciliary oxygen) or evidence of administration devices (e.g. nebuliser machines).
- Warning stickers, often placed by the front door or the telephone, directing the health professional to a source of detailed information (one current scheme involves storing the patient details in a container in the fridge, as this is relatively easy to find in the house).
- Patient-held warning cards denoting previous thrombolysis, at-risk COPD patients, or those taking monoamine oxidase inhibitor (MAOI) medication.
- Patients' individualised treatment plans.

Medical Emergencies in Adults – Overview

Appendix

TABLE 3.3 – Glasgow Coma Scale	
Item / **Element**	**Score**
Eyes Opening:	
Spontaneously	4
To speech	3
To pain	2
None	1
Motor Response:	
Obeys commands	6
Localises pain	5
Withdraws from pain	4
Abnormal flexion	3
Extensor response	2
No response to pain	1
Verbal Response:	
Orientated	5
Confused	4
Inappropriate words	3
Incomprehensible sounds	2
No verbal response	1

KEY POINTS!

Medical Emergencies in Adults (Overview)

- **Detect TIME CRITICAL problems early.**
- **Minimise time on scene.**
- **Continuously re-assess <C>ABCD.**
- **Initiate treatments en-route if the patient is deteriorating.**
- **Provide an ATMIST information call for TIME CRITICAL patients.**

Medical Emergencies in Children – Overview

1. Introduction

- A problem-based approach to paediatric emergencies is to be encouraged. Identifying the features of possible serious illnesses (and addressing them) is more important than identifying the child's underlying diagnosis.
- Assessment priorities include the detection of respiratory distress, circulatory impairment or decreased consciousness.
- Good patient assessment will allow potentially life-threatening illnesses or injuries to be recognised sooner. This should allow treatments and interventions to be given at the earliest opportunity, including rapid hospital transfer for urgent assessment and further treatments when needed.

2. History

- In most cases, a well-taken history will point to the diagnosis. When combined with the findings of your physical examination, this format of history taking should allow **TIME CRITICAL** patients, urgent patients and routine patients to be correctly identified.
- History taking should adhere to the following format and be fully documented:
  - **Presenting complaint** — why did the patient or carer call for help?
  - The **history** of the presenting complaint – details of when the problem started, exacerbating factors and previous similar episodes.
  - Direct questioning about associated **symptoms**, by system. Ask about all appropriate systems.
  - **Past medical history**, including current medication.
  - **Family history**.
  - **Social history**.
- The following should also be considered:
  - **Previous** treatment/contact with healthcare services or episodes of a similar nature.
  - **Feeding and appetite** –

    note how the child is typically fed: bottle/breast/solids.

    Button battery ingestion may need to be considered (refer to **Overdose and Poisoning in Adults and Children**).
  - **Activity/Apathy** — does the child act and respond appropriately?
  - **Urine and faeces** — is this more or less than usual? Wet/dry nappies can be used as a measure of hydration/dehydration.
  - **Growth** — is the child's growth following expected and previously measured centiles?
  - **Sleeping** — is this normal for the child?
  - **Pregnancy** — maternal illness or drug ingestion during pregnancy may have affected the child.
  - **Birth** — antenatal complications, premature labour and birth complications may impact a child's weight and development.
  - **Immunisation and Health Screening**.
  - **Development** — is the child meeting their expected developmental milestones, e.g. hearing, speech or motor ability? Have there been any backward steps/developmental regression? The child's Red Book or other documentation may provide useful supporting information.
- Remember that the history of the child and parent provides invaluable insights into the cause of the current condition.
- In making an assessment, make use of the following sources of additional information:
  - Relatives, carers or friends.
  - Packets or containers of medication.
  - Administration devices, e.g. inhalers, spacers etc.
  - MedicAlert® type jewellery, e.g. bracelets, detailing underlying health issues (diabetes, anaphylaxis, drug allergy etc.), as well as a 24-hour telephone number to obtain a more detailed patient history.
  - Child protection concerns may become apparent during the initial medical assessment and should be appropriately dealt with (refer to **Safeguarding Children**).
- Having called the emergency services, it is also important to address parental ideas, concerns and expectations, regarding their child's current health.

Medical Emergencies in Children – Overview

3. Assessment and Management

TABLE 3.4 – ASSESSMENT and MANAGEMENT of: Medical Emergencies in Children	
• All stages should be considered but some more detailed elements may be omitted when not clinically appropriate.	• At each stage, consider the need for early senior clinical support. • Start correcting any <C>**ABCDE** problems. • Undertake a **TIME CRITICAL** transfer to nearest appropriate receiving hospital. • Continue patient management en-route. • Provide an ATMIST information call.
Catastrophic haemorrhage • Look for evidence of significant external haemorrhage. • Consider occult sources of internal bleeding, especially following trauma.	**Arrest external bleeding** • Apply a tourniquet and/or apply direct pressure to the site. • Dress the site with an appropriate haemorrhage or trauma dressing. • Elevate the site if possible.
AIRWAY — assess the airway (refer to **Airway and Breathing Management**). • Manage the child's airway in a stepwise manner. • Exercise extreme caution when managing epiglottitis (refer to **Respiratory Illness in Children**). **Position the head to open the airway.** **Abnormal upper airway sounds** • **Look for** physical obstructions, e.g. teeth, foreign bodies, vomit or blood (refer to **Foreign Body Airway Obstruction (Child)**). • **Listen for** noisy airflow, e.g. snoring, gurgling or no airflow (refer to **Dyspnoea**): – Inspiratory noises (stridor) suggest an airway obstruction near the larynx. – A snoring noise (stertorous breathing) may be present when there is obstruction in the pharynx, e.g. enlarged tonsils. • **Feel for** air movement: – Airway constriction is a life-threatening condition and can result from an immune response to an allergen (refer to **Allergic Reactions including Anaphylaxis**).	**AIRWAY MANAGEMENT** **Manual extension manoeuvres, head tilt, chin lift or jaw thrust** • The younger the child, the less neck extension will be required. A newborn's head should be placed in the neutral position, while an older child should be extended into a 'sniffing the morning air' position. • Do not place pressure on the soft tissues under the chin or in front of the neck - this can obstruct the airway. **Aspiration, foreign body removal** • Blind finger sweeps must be avoided as they may push material further down the airway or damage the soft palate. • Refer to **Foreign Body Airway Obstruction (Child)**. **Oropharyngeal airway (OPA)** • Ensure the OPA is of the appropriate size (refer to **Page for Age**) and inserted using the correct technique. Discontinue insertion or remove if the child gags (refer to **Paediatric Resuscitation**). **Nasopharyngeal airway** • Correct sizing is essential (refer to **Page for Age**). • In small children, a size smaller than estimated may be required. • Care should be taken not to damage tonsillar or adenoidal tissues. **Endotracheal intubation** • The hazards associated with intubation in children are considerable and usually outweigh the advantages. It should only be attempted where other more basic methods of ventilation have failed and only when capnography is available (ETT sizes are listed on **Page for Age**). • Only attempt paediatric intubation if authorised to do so and follow local protocols.

Medical Emergencies in Children – Overview

<table>
<tr><th colspan="2">TABLE 3.4 – ASSESSMENT and MANAGEMENT of: Medical Emergencies in Children (continued)</th></tr>
<tr><td></td><td>Needle cricothyroidotomy
● Needle cricothyroidotomy is considered a method of last resort.
● Surgical airways should not be performed on children under the age of 12 years.
● The initial oxygen (O_2) flow rate in litres per minute should be set to equal the child's age in years and gradually increased (in 1 litre min^{-1} increments) until adequate chest wall movements are seen.
● Allow ~4 sec for exhalation.</td></tr>
<tr><td>BREATHING — assessment and recognition of potential respiratory impairment
Measure the respiratory rate (see Page for Age).
● Tachypnoea, a rapid respiratory rate, in a child at rest indicates a need for increased ventilation and suggests:
– an airway problem
– a lung problem
– a circulatory problem, or
– a metabolic problem.
Recession (indrawing, retraction)
● Intercostal recession (indrawing of the space between the ribs) and subcostal recession (along the costal margins at the point of diaphragmatic attachment) is seen when respiratory effort is high, due to the pliable nature of children's rib cages. In infants, the sternum itself may even be drawn in (sternal recession), but as children get older, the rib cage becomes less pliable and other signs of accessory muscle use (other than recession) are seen (see below). If recession is seen in older children, it suggests severe respiratory difficulty.
Accessory muscle use
● As in adult life, when the work of breathing is increased, the sternocleidomastoid muscle may be used as an accessory respiratory muscle. This can cause head bobbing (the head bobs up and down with each breath) in infants.
Flaring of the nostrils
● This is a subtle sign that is easily missed. It indicates significant respiratory distress.
Inspiratory or expiratory noises
● Wheezing indicates lower airway narrowing and is most commonly heard on expiration. The volume of the wheeze is NOT an indicator of severity - it may diminish with increasing respiratory distress because less air is being moved.</td><td>BREATHING MANAGEMENT
● All sick children require adequate oxygenation.
● Administer high levels of supplemental oxygen (O_2) via a non-rebreathing mask.
● If the child finds the face mask distressing, ask the parent to help by holding the mask as close to the child's face as possible. If this still produces distress, wafting O_2 across the face directly from the tubing, with the face mask detached from the tubing, is better than nothing.
● In children with sickle cell disease or cardiac disease, high levels of O_2 should be administered routinely, whatever their oxygen saturation.
● Consider assisted ventilation at a rate equivalent to the normal respiratory rate for the age of the child (refer to paediatric resuscitation charts for normal values) if:
– The child is hypoxic (SpO_2 <90%) and remains so after being placed on high flows and concentration O_2.
– Respiratory rate is slower (3 times normal), than normal.
– Expansion is inadequate.
● Use an appropriately sized mask to ensure a good seal.
● Try to avoid hyperventilation to minimise the risks of gastric insufflation or barotrauma. The bag-valve-mask should have a pressure release valve as an added safety measure. If this is not available, extreme care must be taken not to over expand the lungs. No bag smaller than 500 ml volume should be used for bag-valve-mask ventilation unless the child is <2.5 kg, i.e. pre-term baby size.
Wheezing
● The management of asthma is discussed elsewhere (refer to Asthma).
● See paediatric respiratory illness for further guidance on childhood respiratory illnesses.</td></tr>
</table>

(continued)

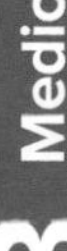

Medical Emergencies in Children – Overview

<table>
<tr><th colspan="2">TABLE 3.4 – ASSESSMENT and MANAGEMENT of: Medical Emergencies in Children (continued)</th></tr>
<tr><td>
Inspiratory noises (stridor)
● This suggests an imminent danger to the airway due to reduction in airway circumference to approximately 10% of normal. Again, the volume of stridor does NOT reflect severity and may also diminish with increasing respiratory distress as less air is moved.
Grunting
● This is produced by exhalation against a partially closed laryngeal opening (glottis). This is more likely to be seen in infants and is a sign of severe respiratory distress.
Effectiveness of breathing — chest expansion and breath sounds
● Note the degree of expansion on both sides of the chest and whether it is equal.
Auscultate the chest with a stethoscope
● A silent chest is a pre-terminal sign, as it indicates that very little air is moving in or out of the chest.
Pulse oximetry
● This can be used at all ages to measure oxygen saturation (readings are less reliable in the presence of shock, hypothermia and other conditions such as carbon monoxide poisoning and severe anaemia).
● For additional signs of breathing compromise, refer to Table 3.5.
</td><td></td></tr>
<tr><td>
CIRCULATION — assessment and recognition of potential circulatory failure (Shock)
● Circulatory assessments in children are difficult as each physical sign may have a number of confounding variables.
● When assessing whether a child is shocked, it is important to assess and evaluate each of the signs below:
Heart Rate: (see Page for Age)
● Tachycardia results from loss of circulatory volume. Heart rates, particularly in infants, can be very high (up to 220 beats per minute). (Heart rates greater than 220bpm are seen in Supraventricular Tachycardia).
● An abnormally slow pulse, or bradycardia, is defined as less than 60 bpm or a rapidly falling heart rate associated with poor systemic circulation. Bradycardia is a pre-terminal sign and becomes apparent before cardiac arrest (see above).
</td><td>
● CIRCULATORY MANAGEMENT
Arrest external haemorrhage
● Do not attempt to gain intravenous (IV) or intraosseous (IO) access at the scene. Obtain access en-route unless delay is unavoidable.
Cannulation
● Attempt cannulation with the widest bore cannula that can be confidently placed. The vehicle can be stopped briefly to allow for venepuncture and disposal of the sharp with transport being recommenced before applying the IV dressing.
● The IO route may be required where venous access has failed on two occasions or no suitable vein is apparent within a reasonable timeframe. The IO route is the preferred route for vascular access in all cases of cardiac arrest in young children.
● Blood glucose level should be measured in (i) all children in whom vascular access is being obtained and (ii) any child with decreased conscious level (refer to Altered Level of Consciousness).
</td></tr>
</table>

Medical Emergencies in Children – Overview

TABLE 3.4 – ASSESSMENT and MANAGEMENT of: Medical Emergencies in Children *(continued)*

<table>
<tr>
<td>

Pulse volume

- Peripheral pulses become weak and then absent as shock advances.
- Children peripherally vasoconstrict their extremities as shock progresses, initially cooling skin distally and then more proximally as shock advances.
- There is no validated relationship between the presence of certain peripheral pulses and the systemic blood pressure in children.

Capillary refill

- This should be measured on the forehead or sternum.
- A capillary refill time of >2 seconds indicates poor perfusion, although this is influenced by a number of factors, including cold and poor lighting conditions.

Blood pressure

- Varies with age.
- Is difficult to reliably measure, increasing on-scene times, and therefore is not routinely measured in pre-hospital practice.
- Hypotension is a very late (and pre-terminal sign) in shocked children and so other signs of circulatory inadequacy will manifest (and should have been recognised) long before hypotension occurs.
- For other signs of circulatory compromise, refer to **Table 3.6**.

</td>
<td>

Fluid administration

- Use sodium chloride 0.9% to treat shock.
- Fluids should be measured in millilitres and documented as volume administered — not as the volume of fluid chosen.
- Fluids should be administered as boluses rather than 'run in'.
- Hand-over at the receiving unit must include details of volume and type of fluid administered.

Fluid volumes

- 20 ml/kg boluses of 0.9% Sodium Chloride are used to resuscitate medically ill children with shock from circulatory failure, to restore vital signs to normal.
- No more than two boluses should be given except on medical advice (refer to **Intravascular Fluid Therapy in Children** and **0.9% Sodium Chloride**).

Exceptions

- In diabetic ketoacidosis, fluids are administered more cautiously to reduce the risk of cerebral oedema (refer to **Glycaemic Emergencies in Adults and Children**).
- In diabetic ketoacidosis, fluid should be withheld unless severe shock is present, in which case 10 ml/kg should be administered over 10–15 minutes (refer to **Glycaemic Emergencies in Adults and Children**).
- If a child has heart failure or renal failure give a 10 ml/kg bolus but stop if the patient deteriorates. Transfer to hospital as a priority.
- Seek medical advice when exceptional circumstances are present, such as a long transfer time.

</td>
</tr>
<tr>
<td>

DISABILITY – Recognition of potential neurological failure

- Note the initial level of responsiveness on the AVPU scale, and time of assessment:

  A — Alert.

  V — Responds to voice.

  P — Responds to painful stimulus.

  U — Unresponsive.

Response to a painful stimulus

- Pinch a digit or pull frontal hair. A child who is unconscious or who only responds to pain has a significant degree of coma (refer to Glasgow Coma Scale — Appendix 1. **NB** The 'adult' GCS should be used in children over 4 years of age).

</td>
<td>

DISABILITY MANAGEMENT

The aim of management of any child with a cerebral insult is to minimise further insult by optimising their circumstances. This usually concerns management strategies designed to:

- prevent hypoxia (see above)
- normalise circulation without causing fluid overload
- identify and treat hypoglycaemia (refer to **Glycaemic Emergencies in Adults and Children**).

Other conditions that can be treated out of hospital and are discussed elsewhere include:

- convulsions (refer to **Convulsions in Children**)
- opiate poisoning (refer to **Overdose and Poisoning in Adults and Children**)
- meningococcal septicaemia (refer to **Meningococcal Meningitis and Septicaemia**).

</td>
</tr>
</table>

(continued)

Medical Emergencies in Children – Overview

Summary

- The primary assessment of the child should establish whether the child is seriously ill.
- Immediate correction of any problems must be undertaken without delay at the scene.
- Continually monitor and re-assess the child en-route to hospital.
- Children who are found to be seriously ill must be considered to have a **TIME CRITICAL** condition and be taken to the nearest suitable receiving hospital without delay.
- A hospital **ATMIST** call should be made whenever a seriously ill child is transported.
- Paediatric drug dosages are calculated as 'mg per kilogram' (refer to **Page for Age** and specific medicine guidelines for dosages and information).
- Drug doses **MUST** be checked before **ANY** drug administration, no matter how confident the practitioner may be.

Appendix

TABLE 3.8 — Modified Glasgow Coma Scale For Children Under 4-Years of Age

Item	Element	Score
Eyes opening:		
	Spontaneously	4
	To speech	3
	To pain	2
	None	1
Motor response:		
	Obeys commands	6
	Localises pain	5
	Withdraws from pain	4
	Abnormal flexion	3
	Extensor response	2
	No response to pain	1
Verbal response:		
	Orientated (appropriate words or social smiles, and fixes on and follows objects)	5
	Confused (cries, but is consolable)	4
	Inappropriate words (persistently irritable)	3
	Incomprehensible sounds (restless, agitated)	2
	No verbal response (silent)	1

KEY POINTS!

Medical Emergencies in Children

- **The child and parent's history will provide a valuable insight into the cause of the child's current condition.**
- **Hypoxia and hypovolaemia need urgent correction.**
- **Emergency airway management rarely requires intubation.**
- **Check the blood glucose in all seriously ill children and those with a decreased level of consciousness.**
- **<C>ABCDE problems should be corrected and managed en route to further care. Do not delay on scene.**
- **It is important to address ideas, concerns and expectations, especially of the parents, who are often concerned, hence the call to emergency services.**

Acute Coronary Syndrome

1. Introduction

The National Institute for Health and Care Excellence (NICE) outlines that:

'The term "acute coronary syndromes" encompasses a range of conditions including unstable angina, non-ST-segment-elevation myocardial infarction (NSTEMI) and ST-segment-elevation myocardial infarction (STEMI). All are due to a sudden reduction of blood flow to the heart, usually caused by the rupture of an atherosclerotic plaque within the wall of a coronary artery, and may cause the formation of a blood clot.

The most common symptom of acute coronary syndromes is severe pain in the chest and/or in other areas (for example, the arms, back or jaw), which can last for several hours. Other symptoms include sweating, nausea and vomiting, breathlessness and feeling faint.

People with acute coronary syndromes may have a poor prognosis without prompt and accurate diagnosis. Treatments are available to help ease the pain, improve the blood flow and to prevent any future complications.

The highest priority in managing STEMI is to restore an adequate coronary blood flow as quickly as possible using drug treatment and/or revascularisation. This applies to all people with STEMI, including those who have been resuscitated after cardiac arrest. The time taken to restore coronary blood flow is very important because heart muscle starts to be lost as soon as the coronary artery is blocked.

In people with NSTEMI and unstable angina, the aim of treatment is to alleviate pain and anxiety and prevent recurrence of ischaemia. For people with unstable angina, treatment also aims to prevent or limit progression to acute myocardial infarction. The type of treatment is determined by the person's individual risk of future adverse cardiovascular events (heart attack and stroke, repeat treatment or death).'[1]

2. Incidence

- In 2016/17 the Myocardial Ischaemia National Audit Project (MINAP), which covers England, Wales and Northern Ireland, recorded more than 95,000 'heart attack' (ACS) patients on the database. This is likely to be an underestimate. Of those with a confirmed diagnosis of myocardial infarction on the MINAP database, 40% have ST segment elevation myocardial infarction (STEMI) and 60% non-STEMI.
- Over 80% of patients with STEMI present via ambulance services.
- In England, 99% of STEMI patients who receive reperfusion treatment have primary percutaneous coronary intervention (PPCI).
- According to the British Heart Foundation (BHF) an estimated 7 million people in the UK are living with heart and circulatory diseases. With an ageing and growing population, and improved survival rates from heart and circulatory events, these numbers are expected to rise still further. The most recent BHF statistics, published in November 2018, estimate that:
- Heart and circulatory diseases cause a quarter (25 per cent) of all deaths in the UK; over 150,000 deaths each year – an average of 420 people each day or one death every three minutes.
- Around 42,000 people under the age of 75 in the UK die from CVD each year.
- Around 80 per cent of people with heart and circulatory diseases have at least one other health condition.
- Coronary heart disease (CHD) is the single biggest cause of death in the UK and is a major cause of premature mortality (i.e. death in people aged under 75).

3. Severity and Outcome

- Case fatality rates at 30 days following hospital admission declined between 2002 and 2010 from 18.5% to 12.2% in men and from 20.0% to 12.5% in women, but are determined by factors such as age, co-morbidity, type of AMI and use of treatments (e.g. PPCI, secondary prevention medicines) recommended in NICE and other guidelines. For non-STEMI, unadjusted all-cause mortality at 180 days decreased from 10.8% to 7.6% from 2003–2013.
- The risk of cardiac arrest from ventricular fibrillation (VF) or other arrhythmia is highest in the first few hours from symptom onset. VF can occur without warning. For some patients, cardiac arrest is the first presentation of ACS.

4. Assessment and Management

- The diagnosis and management of a patient with suspected ACS requires a detailed clinical assessment and the recording of a 12-lead electrocardiogram. Reperfusion treatments for STEMI are critically time dependent and immediate clinical assessment of all patients with a suspected ACS is essential.
- Clinical risk factors should be considered together when assessing the likelihood of myocardial ischaemia relating to ACS. Such factors include increasing age, sex, family history of coronary heart disease, prior history of ischaemic heart disease and peripheral vascular disease, diabetes mellitus and renal impairment. High-risk features include:
  - worsening angina
  - prolonged pain (>20 minutes)
  - pulmonary oedema
  - hypotension
  - arrhythmias.

Acute Coronary Syndrome

TABLE 3.9 – ASSESSMENT and MANAGEMENT of: Acute Coronary Syndrome *(continued)*	
• Assess patient's pain	• Where present, assess the **SOCRATES** of pain and record initial and subsequent pain scores. • Consider analgesia if appropriate (refer to **Pain Management in Adults** and **Pain Management in Children**).
• Documentation	• Complete documentation to include all clinical findings, advice from other clinicians and onward referral.
	Additional Information: • National and international standards and guidelines for ACS care consistently emphasise the importance of rapid access to defibrillation and reperfusion, and specialist cardiological care. • Pre-alerting the hospital can speed up appropriate treatment of STEMI patients. • **MINAP national data suggest 'call to balloon' times are increasing in patients receiving PPCI. Make every effort to reduce delay to hospital.** • Pre-hospital thrombolysis may be an option where PPCI is not available, but is rarely given in England where 99% of reperfusion patients receive PPCI. Patients who receive thrombolytic treatment should subsequently be transferred urgently to a PPCI-capable hospital. • Patients post ROSC with ST elevation should be taken to a PPCI-capable hospital. • The role of emergency angiography (and PCI if indicated) in patients resuscitated from cardiac arrest but without ST-segment elevation on the pre-hospital 12-lead ECG is uncertain. Research is ongoing in London (the ARREST trial) to evaluate this strategy. Such patients should be treated according to locally agreed pathways of care. It is important to establish a history of the events prior to the cardiac arrest. • The diagnosis of non-STEMI cannot be made pre-hospital as it requires use of biomarkers. Point of care POC troponin assays are insufficiently sensitive to 'rule out' ACS in the pre-hospital environment and are not recommended at this time. The Pre-hospital Evaluation of Sensitive Troponin (PRESTO) Study led by the University of Manchester is currently evaluating this approach with NHS ambulance services.

TABLE 3.10 – Features of Different Types of Pain
Features that suggest a diagnosis of myocardial ischaemia include: • Central chest pain. • Crushing or constricting in nature. • Persists for >15 minutes. • Pain may also present: – in the shoulders – in upper abdomen – referred to the neck, jaws and arm.
Features that suggest a diagnosis of stable angina include: • Pain typically related to exertion and tending to last minutes, but should it persist for >15 minutes, or despite usual treatment, ACS is more likely.

Acute Coronary Syndrome

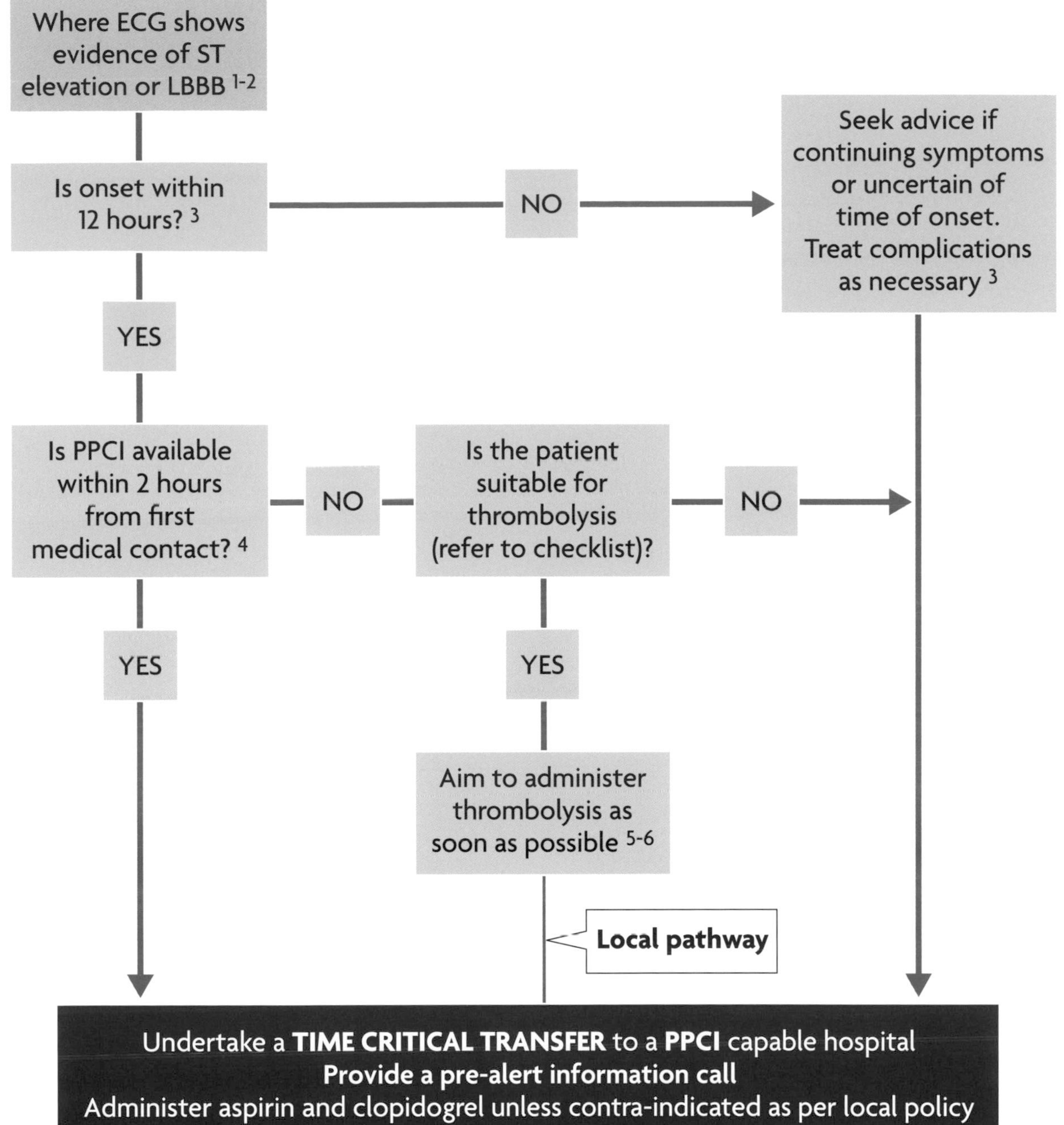

Where ECG shows evidence of ST elevation or LBBB 1-2
Is onset within 12 hours? 3
NO
Seek advice if continuing symptoms or uncertain of time of onset. Treat complications as necessary 3
YES
Is PPCI available within 2 hours from first medical contact? 4
NO
Is the patient suitable for thrombolysis (refer to checklist)?
NO
YES
YES
Aim to administer thrombolysis as soon as possible 5-6
Local pathway
Undertake a TIME CRITICAL TRANSFER to a PPCI capable hospital
Provide a pre-alert information call
Administer aspirin and clopidogrel unless contra-indicated as per local policy

1. Up to a third of patients with MI will have atypical presentations such as shortness of breath or collapse, without chest pain. This is particularly so in women, patients with diabetes or the elderly. **Have a low threshold for performing a 12-lead ECG in any patient presenting as 'unwell'** Seek advice in 'atypical' patients who have ST elevation or LBBB (see below) as urgent reperfusion may still be indicated.

2. ST-segment elevation (measured at the J-point): at least two contiguous leads with ST-segment elevation 2.5 mm in men aged under 40, 2 mm in men over 40 years, or 1.5 mm in women and/or 1 mm in the other leads [in the absence of left ventricular (LV) hypertrophy or left bundle branch block LBBB)]

3. If there is uncertainty about the time of symptom onset, or any ongoing chest pain/discomfort or haemodynamic upset beyond 12 hours, seek advice as urgent reperfusion may still be indicated.

4. Refer to local policies for target 'call to balloon' time.

5. Thrombolytic treatment should not be regarded as the end of the emergency care of a STEMI patient. Rapid transfer to an appropriate hospital for timely therapy to prevent re-infarction, and assessment of the need for rescue PPCI, is essential.

6. Refer to tenecteplase guidelines for the checklist to identify eligibility for pre-hospital thrombolysis.

Figure 3.1 – The management of patients presenting with STEMI or LBBB.

Acute Coronary Syndrome

KEY POINTS!

Acute Coronary Syndrome

- **Acute coronary syndrome refers to a spectrum of conditions.**
- **Risk of VF is high in the early stages of ACS. Always take a defibrillator to the patient.**
- **Patients with ECG evidence of STEMI should be assessed for suitability for reperfusion with PPCI or thrombolysis according to local care pathways. The vast majority of STEMI patients now receive PPCI as their reperfusion treatment.**
- **Patients with non-STEMI remain at high risk and should be treated as a MEDICAL EMERGENCY.**

Bibliography

1. National Institute for Health and Care Excellence. *Acute coronary syndromes in adults.* London: NICE, 2014. Available from: https://www.nice.org.uk/guidance/qs68/chapter/Introduction.
2. National Institute for Health and Care Excellence. *Unstable Angina and NSTEMI: The early management of unstable angina and non-ST-segmentelevation myocardial infarction* (CG94). London: NICE, 2013. Available from: https://www.nice.org.uk/guidance/cg94.
3. Scottish Intercollegiate Guidelines Network (SIGN). *Acute coronary syndrome.* Edinburgh: SIGN, 2016. Available from: https://www.sign.ac.uk/assets/sign148.pdf.
4. Ibanez B, James S, Agewall S, et al. 2017 ESC Guidelines for the management of acute myocardial infarction in patients presenting with ST-segment elevation: The Task Force for the management of acute myocardial infarction in patients presenting with ST-segment elevation of the European Society of Cardiology (ESC). *Eur Heart J* 2018, 29(2): 119–177.
5. British Heart Foundation. *Heart statistics publications.* Birmingham: British Heart Foundation, 2018. Available from: https://www.bhf.org.uk/what-we-do/our-research/heart-statistics/heart-statistics-publications.
6. Sepehrvand N, James S, Stub D, et al. Effects of supplemental oxygen therapy in patients with suspected acute myocardial infarction: a meta-analysis of randomised clinical trials. Heart 2018, 104(20): 1691–1698.
7. Sparv D, Hofmann R, Gunnarsson A, et al. DETO2X-SWEDEHEART Investigators. The analgesic effect of oxygen in suspected acute myocardial infarction: A substudy of the DETO2X-AMI trial. *JACC Cardiovasc Interv* 2018, 11(16): 1590–1597.
8. Quinn T, Johnsen S, Gale CP, et al. Myocardial Ischaemia National Audit Project (MINAP) Steering Group. Effects of prehospital 12-lead ECG on processes of care and mortality in acute coronary syndrome: A linked cohort study from the Myocardial Ischaemia National Audit Project. *Heart* 2014, 100(12): 944–950.
9. Manchester University NHS Foundation Trust. *The Pre-hospital Evaluation of Sensitive Troponin (PRESTO) Study.* Washington, D.C.: U.S. National Library of Medicine, 2019. Available from: https://clinicaltrials.gov/ct2/show/NCT03561051.

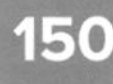

Abdominal Pain

1. Introduction

- Abdominal pain is a common presenting symptom to ambulance services. The specific cause can be difficult to identify in pre-hospital care and a definitive diagnosis may require in-hospital investigations.
- The nature, location and pattern of the pain together with associated symptoms, may indicate a possible cause (refer to Table 3.11). Many of the causes for abdominal pain can be self-limiting. However, it is important to recognise the risk associated with those conditions that need further input, as well as those that need more urgent life-saving interventions.
- The elderly, those with alcohol dependence and immunosuppressed patients may have atypical presentations.
- This guideline covers adults, infants and children. In this guideline, the term 'child' includes infants, unless specified otherwise.
- Abdominal pain can arise from both acute and chronic abdominal conditions:
  - **Acute conditions:** e.g. appendicitis, cholecystitis, intestinal obstruction, ureteric colic, gastritis, perforated peptic ulcer, gastroenteritis, pancreatitis, diverticular disease, leaking or ruptured abdominal aortic aneurysms and gynaecological disorders.
  - **Chronic conditions:** e.g. irritable bowel syndrome (IBS), inflammatory bowel syndromes (ulcerative colitis and Crohn's disease), gastric and duodenal ulcers and intra-abdominal malignancy.

TABLE 3.11 – Causes of Abdominal Pain in Adults and Children

Condition	Characteristics of Pain	Associated Symptoms
Abdominal migraine	• Presents typically as recurrent bouts of generalised abdominal pain.	• Nausea and vomiting. • No headache, followed by sleep and recovery.
Acute cholecystitis Accounts for approximately 30% of patients attending ED for acute abdominal pain.	• A sharp pain in the right upper quadrant of the abdomen. • May experience right shoulder-tip pain. • The pain is worse when breathing deeply and on palpation of the right upper quadrant.	• Nausea and vomiting. • Increased temperature >38°C. • History of fat intolerance.
Acute pancreatitis Inflammation of the pancreas.	• Constant pain in the upper left quadrant or middle of the abdomen. • The pain may radiate to the patient's back.	• Abdominal tenderness. • Hypotension. • Nausea and vomiting. • Dehydration. • Shock. • History of alcohol abuse or gallstones.
Appendicitis Frequently misdiagnosed. Approximately one-third of women of childbearing age with appendicitis are considered as having pelvic inflammatory disease or UTI. Appendicitis accounts for more than 40,000 hospital admissions in England each year (more common in children aged 12–16).	• A constant pain, increasing in intensity often starting in the peri-umbilical area. • The pain may settle in the right lower quadrant; but the location may vary in the early stages. • Tenderness on percussion, guarding (muscular rigidity). The site of maximal tenderness is often said to be over McBurney's point, which is two-thirds of the way along a line drawn from the umbilicus to the anterior superior iliac spine.	• Nausea. • Vomiting (profuse vomiting may indicate development of peritonitis). • Loss of appetite. • Constipation. • Increased low grade temperature >37.5°C. • Diarrhoea. • Facial flushing, dry tongue, halitosis. • Tachycardia.

(continued)

SECTION 3 Medical Emergencies

Abdominal Pain

TABLE 3.11 – Causes of Abdominal Pain in Adults and Children *(continued)*

Condition	Characteristics of Pain	Associated Symptoms
	• There is rebound tenderness in the right iliac fossa and coughing and walking may exacerbate the pain. • Older patients may present with generalised pain, distension and decreased bowel sounds. • In children, if asked to hop the child will refuse as this causes pain. • Rovsing's sign – palpation of the left lower quadrant increases the pain felt in the right lower quadrant. • Psoas sign – extending the right thigh with the person in the left lateral position elicits pain in the right lower quadrant. • Obturator sign – internal rotation of the flexed right thigh elicits pain in the right lower quadrant.	**NB** Assess the for potential complications: • Tachycardia and sudden relief of pain may be signs of a perforated appendix. • Palpable abdominal mass and swinging pyrexia may be signs of an appendix abscess. • High fever (more than 40°C), severe abdominal tenderness, and absent bowel sounds may be signs of peritonitis.
Constipation	• Abdominal tenderness.	• Infrequent bowel activity. • Foul smelling wind and stools. • Excessive flatulence. • Irregular stool texture. • Passing occasional enormous stools or frequent small pellets. • Withholding or straining to stop passage of stools. • Soiling or overflow. • Abdominal distension. • Poor appetite. • Lack of energy. • Unhappy, angry or irritable mood and general malaise.
Diverticular disease Inflammation of diverticula in the large intestine.	• Abdominal pain in the lower left quadrant.	• Nausea and vomiting. • Altered bowel habit. • Bloating. • Increased temperature >38°C.
Ectopic pregnancy Pregnancy not implanted in the uterus. It affects 1 pregnancy in 80 and accounts for 13% of all pregnancy-related deaths.	• Pain in the lower abdomen, pelvic area or back. • **NB** Patients may present atypically but pain is almost always present.	• Nausea. • Missed last menstrual period (though can occur before this). • History of pelvic inflammatory disease. • Previous ectopic pregnancy. If the pregnancy ruptures, patients may report: • Severe lower abdominal pain. • Shoulder tip pain. • Feeling faint/collapse.

Abdominal Pain

TABLE 3.11 – Causes of Abdominal Pain in Adults and Children *(continued)*		
Condition	**Characteristics of Pain**	**Associated Symptoms**
Gastritis An inflammation of the gastric lining can be caused by medication (aspirin, non-steroidal anti-inflammatory drugs), alcohol, *Helicobacter pylori* or stress.	• Upper abdominal pain. • Lower/central chest pain/epigastric pain.	• Nausea and vomiting. • Loss of appetite. • Haematemesis.
Hepatitis	• Abdominal pain.	• This is due to liver swelling.
Infective diarrhoea	• Intermittent generalised abdominal pain.	• Blood mixed with stools – ask about travel history and recent antibiotic therapy.
Inflammatory bowel disease, midgut volvulus		• Blood in stools.
Intestinal obstruction A partial or complete obstruction of the small or large intestine. Intussusception (bowel obstruction caused by a segment of intestine sliding inside another part of the intestines). Most commonly found in infants; another peak in incidence occurs at 6 years of age. Volvulus (a loop of intestine twisting around itself resulting in obstruction).	• Abdominal pain that is cramping in nature. • Intermittent colicky pain associated with bouts of screaming and drawing up legs.	• Abdominal distension. • Nausea and vomiting. • Absolute constipation (late stage). • 'Currant jelly stool' – blood and mucus. • Faecal vomiting. • Bile stained vomiting. • Absence of normal flatus. • Abdominal distension. • Increased bowel sounds. • Visible distended loops of bowel. • Visible peristalsis. • Scars. • Swellings at the site of hernial orifices and of the external genitalia.
Ischaemic bowel Ischaemic bowel is a group of conditions that are associated with reduced blood flow and potential infarction of the intestines. This can occur within both the small intestine and the large intestine. This is a medical emergency with mortality rates up to 90% in missed recognition or delayed diagnosis and treatment.	• Moderate to severe colic type or constant and poorly localised pain. • Severe left iliac fossa pain.	• Physical findings and observations that are out of proportion to the degree of pain reported. • Gastrointestinal symptoms such as nausea and vomiting, PR bleeds and bowel problems may also be present. • In early presentation the abdominal examination may not show any significant findings, but later stages may include signs of peritonitis.

(continued)

Abdominal Pain

TABLE 3.11 – Causes of Abdominal Pain in Adults and Children *(continued)*		
Condition	**Characteristics of Pain**	**Associated Symptoms**
The main contributing cause is a thrombus and specific risk factors include AF, particularly where patient is not medicated, mitral stenosis, vasopressors and strangulated hernias.		
Leaking or ruptured abdominal aortic aneurysms (AAA) Consider AAA in patients >50 years who present with the symptoms listed. Most deaths occur in older people.	• Sudden severe abdominal pain or backache. • Renal colic type pain – a new diagnosis of renal colic in a patient over 50 years of age raises the concern of abdominal aortic aneurysm even in the absence of a palpable mass. • **NB** Given that <25% of all AAA patients present with classic signs and symptoms, there is a risk of misdiagnosis.	• Collapse. • Hypotension with bilateral lower limb ischaemia or mottling (a late sign). • History of smoking. • Hypertension and hypercholesterolaemia.
Lower lobe pneumonia (children)	• Abdominal pain.	• Fever. • Cough. • Tachypnoea. • Desaturation.
Pelvic inflammatory disease A common cause of abdominal pain in females but rarely presents as an acute collapse.	• Pain in the lower abdomen, pelvic area or back. • Abdominal tenderness.	• Vaginal discharge. • Nausea. • Fever
Peritonitis	• Refusal or inability to walk. • Slow walk or stooped forward. • Pain on coughing or moving.	• Lying motionless. • Decreased/absent abdominal wall movements with respiration. • Abdominal distention. • Abdominal tenderness – localised/ generalised. • Abdominal guarding/rigidity. • Percussion tenderness. • Palpable abdominal mass. • Bowel sounds – absent/decreased (peritonitis). • Associated non-specific signs – tachycardia, fever.
Peptic ulcer An erosion of the lining of the stomach or small intestine forming an ulcer.	• Central burning abdominal pain. • Back pain. • Perforation may lead to abrupt onset epigastric pain.	• Nausea and vomiting – haematemesis. • Fatigue. • Weight loss.

Abdominal Pain

TABLE 3.11 – Causes of Abdominal Pain in Adults and Children *(continued)*

Condition	Characteristics of Pain	Associated Symptoms
Torsion of the testis **NB** This is a surgical emergency and if suspected the patient should be admitted to the nearest appropriate ED immediately.	• Sudden onset of severe pain in lower abdominal region or in the scrotum.	• Acute swelling of the scrotum (swelling is not *always* present). • Nausea and vomiting often occur. **NB** These symptoms indicate torsion of the testis until proven otherwise.
Urinary tract pathology Infection arising from the kidneys, ureters, bladder and/or urethra. Urinary tract obstruction.	• Pain in the lower abdomen and/or back. • Cramping.	• Pain/burning sensation when urinating. • Needing to urinate frequently. • Urinary frequency and nocturia. • Offensive urine. • Nausea and vomiting. • Cloudy/bloody urine with a malodour. • Lethargy. • Irritability. • Poor feeding. • Jaundice fever. • If the infection involves the kidneys the patient may have increased temperature >38°C, and fatigue. • Rigors may be present.

TABLE 3.12 – Common Causes of Abdominal Pain in Children

< 2 Years	2 to 12 Years	12 to 16 Years
• Gastroenteritis. • Constipation. • Intussusception. • Infantile colic. • UTI. • Incarcerated inguinal hernia. • Trauma. • Pneumonia. • Diabetes.	• Gastroenteritis. • Mesenteric adenitis. • Constipation. • UTI. • Onset of menstruation. • Psychogenic. • Trauma. • Pneumonia. • Diabetes.	• Mesenteric adenitis. • Acute appendicitis. • Menstruation. • Mittelschmerz. • Ovarian cyst torsion. • UTI. • Pregnancy. • Ectopic Pregnancy. • Testicular torsion. • Psychogenic. • Trauma. • Pneumonia. • Diabetes.

Abdominal Pain

2. Severity and Outcome

- The most common diagnosis of patients presenting to emergency departments (ED) with abdominal pain is non-specific abdominal pain, followed by renal colic.
- Many cases are relatively minor in nature (e.g. constipation, urinary tract infection (UTI)); however, 25% of patients contacting the ambulance service with abdominal pain have serious underlying conditions.
- In patients >65 years there is a 6–8 times higher mortality rate due to atypical clinical presentations and the presence of co-morbidities.

3. Pathophysiology

Abdominal pain can be localised and referred, due to overlapping innervations of the organs contained in the abdomen (e.g. small and large intestines).

4. Assessment and Management

For the assessment and management of abdominal pain refer to Table 3.13.

TABLE 3.13 – ASSESSMENT and MANAGEMENT of: Abdominal Pain

ASSESSMENT	MANAGEMENT
• Assess <C>ABCD	• If any of the following **TIME CRITICAL** features present: – major **<C>ABCD** problems (refer to **Medical Emergencies in Adults – Overview** and **Medical Emergencies in Children – Overview**). – suspected leaking or ruptured aortic aneurysm – ectopic pregnancy – sepsis resulting from perforation – torsion of the testis – traumatic disruption of abdominal organs, e.g. liver, spleen, then: • Start correcting any **<C>ABCD** problems. • Undertake a **TIME CRITICAL** transfer to nearest appropriate receiving hospital – for patients with suspected leaking or ruptured aortic aneurysm follow local care pathway. • Continue patient management en-route. • Provide an ATMIST information call.
• Differential diagnoses	• If no immediately life-threatening signs are identified during the primary survey, then continue to a secondary survey to understand causes of pain and form differential diagnoses. Refer to Table 3.11. **NB** For indigestion type pain have a high index of suspicion that it may be cardiac in origin.
• Examination	• Assess the patient's abdomen, where possible in a supine position. Flexing the knees to 90 degrees relaxes the abdominal wall. The physical abdominal examination should include: – auscultating the abdomen for bowel sounds and their frequency – palpating for tenderness, rebound tenderness and guarding. **NB** Hyperactive bowel sounds in children commonly stem from gastroenteritis; however, consider bowel obstructions or gastro-intestinal (GI) haemorrhage/infection as a risk when completing the assessment.
• History	• During history taking, be aware of bowel obstructions caused by surgical emergencies, such as intussusception (bowel obstruction caused by a segment of intestine sliding inside another part of the intestines) or volvulus (a loop of intestine twisting around itself resulting in obstruction). These presentations are a surgical emergency and need to be conveyed to an ED within an hour of presentation. **NB** Bites, stings and poisons: ask about the possibility of bites, stings or ingestion of poisons. Adder envenomation can result in abdominal pain and vomiting.

TABLE 3.13 – ASSESSMENT and MANAGEMENT of: Abdominal Pain *(continued)*	
• If patient is female and of child bearing age, consider additional causes	• Suggest pregnancy test. • Consider ectopic pregnancy, pelvic inflammatory disease or other STD. • Other gynaecological problems. • Mittelschmerz (one-sided lower abdominal pain associated with ovulation). • Torsion of the ovary. • Pelvic inflammatory disease.
• Known congenital or pre-existing condition	• Previous abdominal surgery (adhesions). • Nephrotic syndrome (primary peritonitis). • Mediterranean background (familial mediterranean fever). • Hereditary spherocytosis (cholethiasis). • Cystic fibrosis (meconium ileus equivalent). • Cystinuria. • Porphyria. • Current drug treatment if any. • Recent travel. • Presence of similar symptoms in others.
• Associated symptoms/ conditions	• Altered bowel habit. • Nausea and vomiting – haematemesis/malaena may indicate gastrointestinal pathology – refer to **Gastrointestinal Bleeding**. • Vaginal bleeding/pregnancy/previous ectopic pregnancy – refer to **relevant Maternity Care guidelines.** • Burning on urination. • Menstrual and sexual history in females of childbearing age (is there any possibility of pregnancy?). **NB** For details of signs and symptoms of specific conditions, refer to Table 3.11.
• Respiratory rate	• Measure and record respiratory rate.
• Pulse	• Measure and record pulse.
• Oxygen saturation	• Monitor the patient's SpO_2, administer oxygen to achieve saturations of >94% if the patient presents as hypoxemic on air (refer to **Oxygen**).
• Blood pressure and fluids	• Measure and record blood pressure. If required, administer fluids (refer to **Intravascular Fluid Therapy in Adults** and **Intravascular Fluid Therapy in Children**).
• Blood glucose	• If appropriate, measure and record blood glucose for hypo/hyperglycaemia (refer to **Glycaemic Emergencies in Adults and Children**).
• Temperature	• Measure and record temperature.
• NEWS2	• These observations will enable you to calculate a NEWS2 Score (refer to **Sepsis**).
• ECG	• If required, monitor and record 12-lead ECG. Assess for abnormality (refer to **Cardiac Rhythm Disturbance**).
• Assess the patient's pain	• Where present, assess the SOCRATES of pain and record initial and subsequent pain scores. • Consider analgesia if appropriate (refer to **Pain Management in Adults** and **Pain Management in Children**).

(continued)

TABLE 3.13 – ASSESSMENT and MANAGEMENT of: Abdominal Pain *(continued)*	
• Documentation	• Complete documentation to include all clinical findings, advice from other clinicians, onward referral and worsening advice given.
• Transfer to further care	• Transfer to further care (consider most appropriate centre). • Transfer all children with bile stained (green) vomit. • A new diagnosis of renal colic in a patient over 50 years of age raises the concern of abdominal aortic aneurysm even in the absence of a palpable mass.

Community Management

All patients with abdominal pain being left in the community MUST be discussed with another healthcare professional, such as the general practitioner (GP) or out-of-hours GP, due to the complex nature of the presentation and potential implication for missed diagnosis.

Should the patient be discharged on scene, provide the following advice to the patient/parent/carer:

- Reassure the patient and encourage them to rest.
- If they are not vomiting, advise regular paracetamol for pain relief.
- Advise the patient to avoid aspirin.
- Encourage the patient to drink plenty of clear fluids (e.g. cooled boiled water).
- Do not push the patient to eat if they feel unwell.
- If the patient is hungry, encourage them to eat bland food (e.g. crackers, rice, bananas or toast).
- Many patients with abdominal pain get better without intervention over a few hours or days. However, if problems persist, encourage them to seek further medical advice.

SECTION 3 Medical Emergencies

KEY POINTS!

Abdominal Pain

- **The most important diagnoses to consider are those that are life-threatening, either as the result of internal haemorrhage or perforation of a viscus and sepsis.**
- **For indigestion type pain have a high index of suspicion that it may be cardiac in origin. Obtain a 12-lead ECG for older patients and patients with cardiac risks presenting with upper abdominal pain.**
- **If a patient is in pain, adequate analgesia should be given.**
- **A precise diagnosis of the cause of abdominal pain is often not possible without access to tests and investigations in hospital or via primary care.**

Acknowledgements

We would like to gratefully acknowledge the contribution of South Western Ambulance Service to this JRCALC guideline.

Bibliography

1. Kavanagh S. The acute abdomen: Assessment, diagnosis and pitfalls. *UK MPS Casebook* 2004, 12(1): 11–18.
2. Manterola C, Vial M, Moraga J, Astudillo P. Analgesia in patients with acute abdominal pain. *Cochrane Database of Systematic Reviews* 2011, 1. Available from: http://www.mrw.interscience.wiley.com/cochrane/clsysrev/articles/CD005660/frame.html: doi 10.1002/14651858.CD005660.pub3.
3. Agarwal T, Butt MA. Small bowel obstruction. *Emergency Medicine Journal* 2007, 24(5): 368.
4. Amoli HA, Golozar A, Keshavarzi S, Tavakoli H, Yaghoobi A. Morphine analgesia in patients with acute appendicitis: A randomised double-blind clinical trial. *Emergency Medicine Journal* 2008, 25(9): 586–589.
5. Beck J, Jang TB. Short answer question case series: Controversies in the diagnosis and management of diverticulitis. *Emergency Medicine Journal* 2012, 29(6): 517–518.
6. Beck J, Jang TB. Short answer question case series: Diagnosis of acute cholecystitis. *Emergency Medicine Journal* 2012, 29(5): 430–431.
7. Beckingham IJ, Bornman PC. Acute pancreatitis. *British Medical Journal* 2001, 322(7286): 595–598.
8. Car J. Urinary tract infections in women: Diagnosis and management in primary care. *British Medical Journal* 2006, 332(7533): 94–97.
9. Cartwright SL, Knudson MP. Evaluation of acute abdominal pain in adults. *American Family Physician* 2008, 77(7): 971–978.

10. Chan SSW, Ng KC, Lyon DJ, Cheung WL, Cheng AFB, Rainer TH. Acute bacterial gastroenteritis: A study of adult patients with positive stool cultures treated in the emergency department. *Emergency Medicine Journal* 2003, 20(4): 335–338.

11. Chong CF, Wang TL, Chen CC, Ma HP, Chang H. Preconsultation use of analgesics on adults presenting to the emergency department with acute appendicitis. *Emergency Medicine Journal* 2004, 21(1): 41–43.

12. Gray J, Wardrope J, Fothergill DJ. The ABC of community emergency care: 7 Abdominal pain: Abdominal pain in women, complications of pregnancy and labour. *Emergency Medicine Journal* 2004, 21(5): 606–613.

13. Hall J, Driscoll P. The ABC of community emergency care: 10 Nausea, vomiting and fever. *Emergency Medicine Journal* 2005, 22(3): 200–204.

14. Humes DJ, Simpson J. Acute appendicitis. *British Medical Journal* 2006, 333(7567): 530–534.

15. Kingsnorth A, O'Reilly D. Acute pancreatitis. *British Medical Journal* 2006, 332(7549): 1072–1076.

16. Lehnert T, Sorge I, Till H, Rolle U. Intussusception in children: Clinical presentation, diagnosis and management. *International Journal of Colorectal Disease* 2009, 24(10): 1187–1192.

17. Lewis SRR, Mahony PJ, Simpson J. Appendicitis. *British Medical Journal* 2011, 343: d5976.

18. Little P, Merriman R, Turner S, Rumsby K, Warner G, Lowes JA, et al. Presentation, pattern, and natural course of severe symptoms, and role of antibiotics and antibiotic resistance among patients presenting with suspected uncomplicated urinary tract infection in primary care: Observational study. *British Medical Journal* 2010, 340: b5633.

19. Lynch RM. Accuracy of abdominal examination in the diagnosis of non-ruptured abdominal aortic aneurysm. *Accident and Emergency Nursing* 2004, 12(2): 99–107.

20. Metcalfe D, Holt PIE, Thompson MM. The management of abdominal aortic aneurysms. *British Medical Journal* 2011, 342: d1384.

21. Ranji SR, Goldman L, Simel DL, Shojania KG. Do opiates affect the clinical evaluation of patients with acute abdominal pain? *Journal of the American Medical Association* 2006, 296(14): 764–774.

22. Royal College of Obstetricians and Gynaecologists. *Management of Acute Pelvic Inflammatory Disease* (Green-top Guideline 32). London: RCOG, 2008. Available from: https://www.rcog.org.uk/en/guidelines-research-services/guidelines/gtg32/.

23. Sakalihasan N, Limet R, Defawe OD. Abdominal aortic aneurysm. *The Lancet* 2005, 365(9470): 1577–1589.

24. Touzios JG, Dozois EJ. Diverticulosis and acute diverticulitis. *Gastroenterology Clinics of North America* 2009, 38(3): 513–525.

25. Trowbridge RL, Rutkowski NK, Shojania KG. Does this patient have acute cholecystitis? *Journal of the American Medical Association* 2003, 289(1): 80–86.

26. National Collaborating Centre for Women's and Children's Health. *Urinary Tract Infection in Children: Diagnosis, treatment and long-term management* (CG54). London: Royal College of Obstetricians and Gynaecologists, 2007. Available from: http://www.nice.org.uk/nicemedia/pdf/CG54fullguideline.pdf.

27. National Institute for Health and Care Excellence. *Diarrhoea and Vomiting in Children: Diarrhoea and vomiting caused by gastroenteritis: diagnosis, assessment and management in children younger than 5 years* (CG84). Available from: https://www.nice.org.uk/guidance/cg84, 2009.

28. Scottish Intercollegiate Guidelines Network. *Management of Acute Upper and Lower Gastrointestinal Bleeding* (Guideline 105). Edinburgh: SIGN, 2008.

29. Gloucestershire Clinical Commissioning Group. 2015. *The Big 6*.

30. Clinical Knowledge Summaries. Appendicitis. Available from: https://cks.nice.org.uk/appendicitis, 2016.

31. Bickley LS. *Bates' Guide to Physical Examination and History Taking*. Philadelphia, PA: Lippincott Williams & Wilkins, 2013.

Allergic Reactions including Anaphylaxis

1. Introduction

- The incidence of allergic reactions continues to rise. It is estimated that allergic reactions affect 30% of adults and 40% of children, while anaphylaxis affects up to 2% of the population.
- The most common triggers are food, drugs and venom but in 30% of cases the trigger is unknown.
- Injected allergens commonly result in cardiovascular compromise, with hypotension and shock predominating. While inhaled and ingested allergens typically cause rashes, vomiting, facial swelling, upper airway swelling and wheeze. Slow release drugs prolong absorption and exposure to the allergen.
- Anaphylaxis is defined as a severe, life-threatening, generalised or systemic hypersensitivity reaction. This is characterised by rapidly developing life-threatening airway and/or breathing and/or circulation problems, usually associated with skin and mucosal changes.

2. Severity and Outcome

- The severity of symptoms varies from a localised urticaria to life-threatening respiratory and/or cardiovascular compromise – anaphylaxis.
- Some patients relapse after an apparent recovery (biphasic response); therefore, patients who have experienced an anaphylactic reaction should be transferred to hospital for further evaluation. The risk of an individual suffering a recurrent anaphylactic reaction is estimated to be approximately 1:12 per year.
- Patients with other allergic conditions, such as asthma or atopic eczema, are most at risk of developing anaphylaxis and risk of death is increased in those with pre-existing asthma, particularly if the asthma is poorly controlled.
- Patients who have experienced previous episodes of anaphylaxis may wear a 'Medic Alert' bracelet or necklace and carry an adrenaline auto-injector (e.g. Anapen®, EpiPen®). It is now advised that all patients who have previously experienced an anaphylactic reaction are prescribed two auto-injectors that should be carried at all times.
- The mortality associated with anaphylaxis is estimated to be <1%. Death occurs after contact with the trigger usually as a result of respiratory arrest from airway obstruction.

3. Triggers

- Allergic reaction and anaphylaxis can be caused by a broad range of triggers including food, drugs and insect stings. Food is a common trigger in children, while drugs are a more common trigger in older people. Virtually any food or class of drug can be implicated, although the classes of foods and drugs responsible for the majority of reactions are well described. For common triggers refer to Table 3.14.
- The time it takes for the symptoms of anaphylaxis to develop depends on how the trigger enters the body. Death occurs quickly after contact with the trigger or allergen, with approximately 50% of fatalities due to circulatory collapse (shock) and the rest due to respiratory failure (asphyxia).
- Fatal food reactions cause respiratory arrest after 30-35 minutes, insect stings cause collapse from shock after 10-15 minutes and deaths caused by intravenous medication often occur within just 5 minutes.

4. Assessment and Management

Anaphylaxis is likely when all of the following criteria are met (exposure to a known allergen for the patient also supports the diagnosis and the reaction is usually unexpected):

- Sudden onset and rapid progression of symptoms.
- Life-threatening airway and/or breathing and/or circulation problems.

TABLE 3.14 – Common Triggers of Allergic Reactions
1 – Foods
Nuts (e.g. peanuts, walnut, almond, brazil, and hazel), pulses, sesame seeds, milk, eggs, fish/shellfish.
2 – Venom – insect sting/bites
Insect stings and bites (e.g. wasps and bees). **NB** Bees may leave a venom sac which should be scraped off (not squeezed).
3 – Drugs
Antibiotics (e.g. penicillin, cephalosporin, ciprofloxacin, and vancomycin), non-steroidal anti-inflammatory drugs, angiotensin converting enzyme inhibitor, gelatins, protamine, vitamin K, amphotericin, etoposide, acetazolamide, pethidine, local anaesthetic, diamorphine, streptokinase.
4 – Other causes
Latex, hair dye, semen and hydatid.

Allergic Reactions including Anaphylaxis

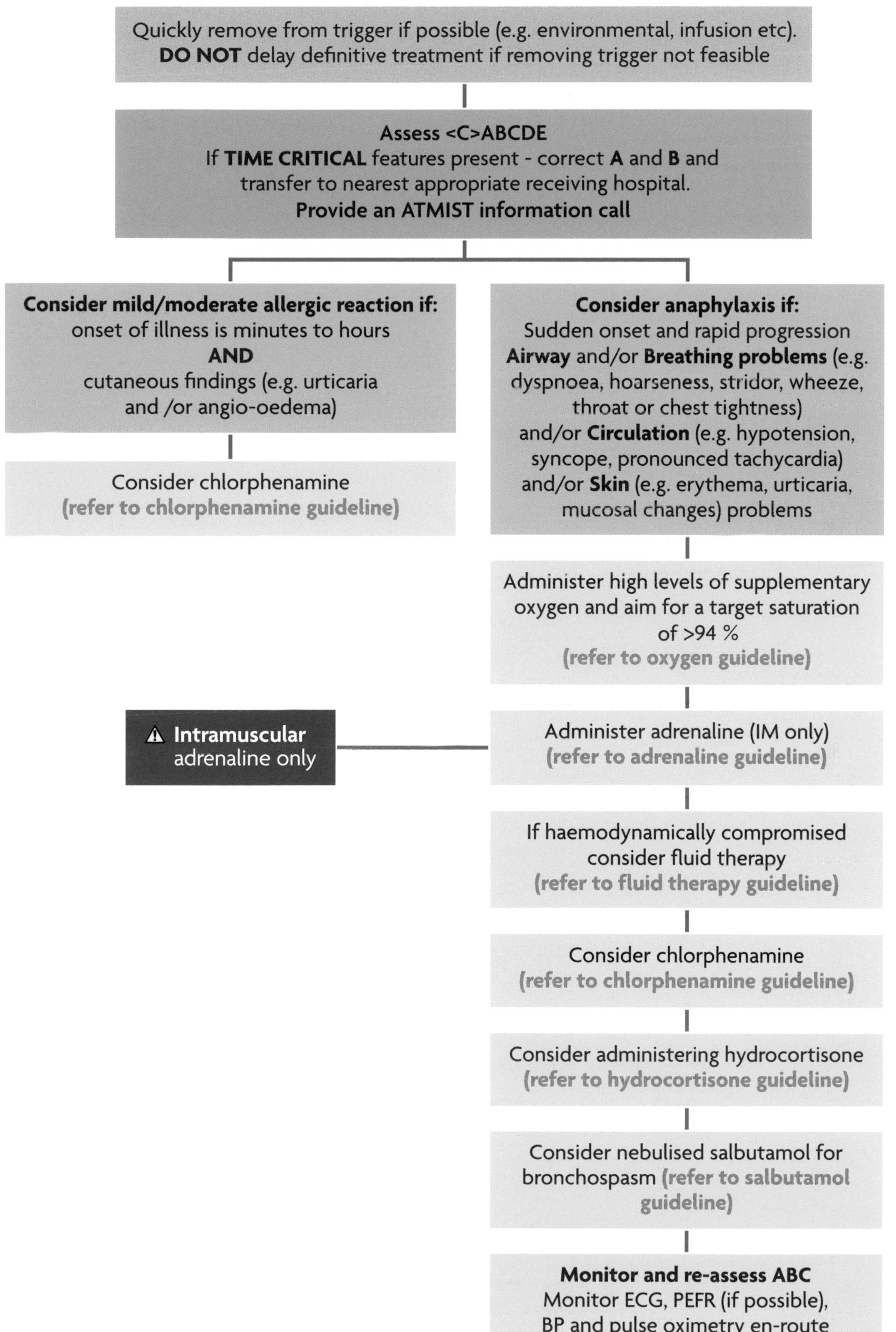

Quickly remove from trigger if possible (e.g. environmental, infusion etc).
DO NOT delay definitive treatment if removing trigger not feasible
Assess <C>ABCDE
If TIME CRITICAL features present - correct A and B and transfer to nearest appropriate receiving hospital.
Provide an ATMIST information call
Consider mild/moderate allergic reaction if:
onset of illness is minutes to hours
AND
cutaneous findings (e.g. urticaria and /or angio-oedema)
Consider chlorphenamine
(refer to chlorphenamine guideline)
Consider anaphylaxis if:
Sudden onset and rapid progression
Airway and/or Breathing problems (e.g. dyspnoea, hoarseness, stridor, wheeze, throat or chest tightness)
and/or Circulation (e.g. hypotension, syncope, pronounced tachycardia)
and/or Skin (e.g. erythema, urticaria, mucosal changes) problems
Administer high levels of supplementary oxygen and aim for a target saturation of >94 %
(refer to oxygen guideline)
Intramuscular adrenaline only
Administer adrenaline (IM only)
(refer to adrenaline guideline)
If haemodynamically compromised consider fluid therapy
(refer to fluid therapy guideline)
Consider chlorphenamine
(refer to chlorphenamine guideline)
Consider administering hydrocortisone
(refer to hydrocortisone guideline)
Consider nebulised salbutamol for bronchospasm (refer to salbutamol guideline)
Monitor and re-assess ABC
Monitor ECG, PEFR (if possible), BP and pulse oximetry en-route

Figure 3.2 – Allergic reactions including anaphylaxis algorithm.

Allergic Reactions including Anaphylaxis

- Skin and/or mucosal changes (flushing, urticaria, angioedema).

The skin and/or mucosal changes that occur in allergic reactions and anaphylaxis include:

- Erythema (superficial reddening of the skin, caused by dilatation of the capillaries).
- Urticaria (a raised itchy rash, also known as hives, nettle rash, weals or welts).
- Angioedema (swelling in the dermis, subcutaneous and submucosal tissues).

Isolated skin or mucosal changes without life-threatening airway, breathing or circulatory problems do not signify an anaphylactic reaction. Skin and mucosal changes can be subtle or absent in up to 20% of reactions.

Angioedema most commonly occurs with urticaria, but may occur in isolation. It can occur anywhere on the body, but most often involves the eye, lips, hands and feet. Less commonly, submucosal swelling affects the airway. Angioedema may be considered part of the continuum of anaphylaxis, but in isolation, without respiratory difficulty or circulatory collapse, is not anaphylaxis.

The mechanism for angioedema and anaphylaxis is the same, in that both histamine and bradykinin are involved. However, in anaphylaxis the reaction is more marked, resulting in an increase in vascular permeability and circulatory collapse.

Anaphylaxis can occur despite a long history of previously safe exposure to a potential trigger. Reactions can be rapid, slow or biphasic.

For a list of signs and symptoms which may occur during an allergic reaction or anaphylaxis refer to Table 3.15.

For the assessment and management of anaphylaxis and allergic reactions refer to Table 3.16.

SECTION 3 Medical Emergencies

TABLE 3.15 – Signs and symptoms of an allergic reaction or anaphylaxis

Airway problems	• Throat and tongue swelling (laryngeal/pharyngeal oedema). • Difficulty in breathing and swallowing. • Hoarse voice. • Stridor (high-pitched inspiratory noise caused by upper airway obstruction).
Breathing problems	• Bronchospasm. • Tachypnoea/Dyspnoea. • Wheeze/Stridor. • Fatigue. • Confusion caused by hypoxia. • Cyanosis (usually a late feature). • SpO_2 <92%. • Respiratory arrest.
Circulatory problems	• Hypotension. • Tachycardia. • Pale and clammy skin. • Dizziness. • Decreased conscious level. • Myocardial ischaemia. • Bradycardia (usually a late feature). • Cardiac arrest.
Other	• Skin/Mucosal changes (urticarial/hives). • Diarrhoea and/or vomiting. • Abdominal pain. • Anxiety.

Allergic Reactions including Anaphylaxis

TABLE 3.16 – Assessment and Management of: Allergic Reactions and Anaphylaxis

ASSESSMENT	MANAGEMENT
● Trigger	● Quickly remove the patient from the trigger. Do not delay definitive treatment if this is not possible or where the trigger is unknown. ● Where an insect sting is the trigger, early removal is more important than the method of removal. If the trigger has been ingested, attempts to make the patient vomit are not recommended.
● Assess <C>ABCD	● If any of the following **TIME CRITICAL** features are present: – Major **<C>ABCD** problems refer to **Medical Emergencies in Adults – Overview** and **Medical Emergencies in Children – Overview**. – Administer high levels of supplementary oxygen to achieve saturations of >94% if the patient presents as hypoxemic on air, refer to **Oxygen**. ● Start correcting any **<C>ABCD** problems. ● Undertake a **TIME CRITICAL** transfer to nearest appropriate receiving hospital. ● Continue patient management en-route. ● Provide an ATMIST information call.
● For anaphylaxis	1. Administer Adrenaline **SAFETY NOTE 1:1,000 IM ONLY**. Intra-muscular adrenaline is the most important drug for the treatment of anaphylactic reactions, refer to **Adrenaline**, refer to **Page for Age** for children's doses. **NB** Drug Check MUST be completed before administration including clarification of route to be used (**IM ONLY**). 2. Histamine release during an anaphylactic reaction leads to increased vascular permeability, causing large volumes of fluid to leak from the patient's circulation. If haemodynamically compromised, refer to **Intravascular Fluid Therapy in Adults** and **Intravascular Fluid Therapy in Children**. 3. Antihistamines are the second line of treatment for anaphylactic reactions to help counteract histamine induced vasodilation and bronchoconstriction, refer to **Chlorphenamine**, refer to **Page for Age** for children's doses. 4. Consider hydrocortisone, refer to **Hydrocortisone**, refer to **Page for Age** for children's doses. 5. Consider nebulised Salbutamol for bronchospasm, refer to **Salbutamol**, refer to **Page for Age** for children's doses.
● Mild or moderate allergic reaction	● Consider a mild/moderate allergic reaction if the onset of the presentation has progressed over minutes to hours, and there are skin and/or mucosal changes in the absence of life-threatening features. In this scenario, adrenaline is not appropriate. – For mild and moderate allergic reactions oral antihistamine is the treatment of choice; in moderate reactions consider IM administration. – For a mild reaction not requiring IM chlorphenamine, consider the appropriateness of advising the patient to purchase their own over-the-counter anti-histamine. If this is not possible, consider referral for oral chlorphenamine supply.
● Respiratory rate	● Measure and record respiratory rate.
● Pulse	● Measure and record pulse.
● Oxygen saturation	● Monitor the patient's SpO_2, administer oxygen to achieve saturations of >94% if the patient presents as hypoxemic on air, refer to **Oxygen**.

(continued)

Allergic Reactions including Anaphylaxis

TABLE 3.16 – Assessment and Management of Allergic Reactions and Anaphylaxis *(continued)*	
ASSESSMENT	**MANAGEMENT**
• Blood pressure and fluids	• Measure and record blood pressure, if required administer fluids, refer to **Intravascular Fluid Therapy in Adults** and **Intravascular Fluid Therapy in Children**.
• Blood glucose	• If appropriate, measure and record blood glucose for hypo/ hyperglycaemia, refer to **Glycaemic Emergencies in Adults and Children**.
• Temperature	• Measure and record temperature.
• NEWS2	• These observations will enable you to calculate a NEWS2 Score, refer to **Sepsis**.
• ECG	• If required, monitor and record 12-Lead ECG. Assess for abnormality, refer to **Cardiac Rhythm Disturbance**.
• Assess the patient's pain	• Where present, assess the **SOCRATES** of pain and record initial and subsequent pain scores. • Consider analgesia if appropriate, refer to **Pain Management in Adults** and **Pain Management in Children**.
• Transfer to further care	• All patients who have experienced an anaphylactic reaction as some patients may relapse hours after an apparent recovery from anaphylaxis (biphasic response) • Patients who have experienced an allergic reaction and do not require attendance at the Emergency Department should be advised to see their GP for consideration of oral steroids (where not already prescribed), as a useful adjunct to chlorphenamine. For first presentations of an allergic reaction consider informing the patient's GP.
• Documentation	• Complete documentation to include all clinical findings, advice from other clinicians, onward referral and worsening advice given.

KEY POINTS!

Allergic Reactions including Anaphylaxis

- **Remove from trigger if possible.**
- **Anaphylaxis can occur despite a long history of previously safe exposure to a potential trigger.**
- **Consider anaphylaxis in the presence of acute cutaneous symptoms and airway or cardiovascular compromise.**
- **Anaphylaxis may be rapid, slow or biphasic.**
- **Adrenaline is key in managing anaphylaxis.**
- **The benefit of using appropriate doses of adrenaline far exceeds any risk.**
- **Half doses of adrenaline are no longer recommended for anaphylaxis in patients who are prescribe beta-blockers or tricyclic anti-depressants and a standard adult dose should be administered.**

Acknowledgements

We would like to gratefully acknowledge the contribution of South Western Ambulance Service to this JRCALC guideline.

Allergic Reactions including Anaphylaxis

Bibliography

1. Deakin CD, Morrison LJ, Morley PT, Callaway CW, Kerber RE, Kronick SL, et al. Part 8: Advanced life support: 2010 International Consensus on Cardiopulmonary Resuscitation and Emergency Cardiovascular Care Science with Treatment Recommendations. *Resuscitation* 2010, 81(1): e93–174.
2. National Institute for Health and Clinical Excellence. *Anaphylaxis: Assessment to confirm an anaphylactic episode and the decision to refer after emergency treatment for a suspected anaphylactic episode* (CG134). London: NICE, 2011. Available from: https://www.nice.org.uk/guidance/cg134.
3. Brown SGA. Clinical features and severity grading of anaphylaxis. *Journal of Allergy and Clinical Immunology* 2004, 114(2): 371–6.
4. Kane KE, Cone DC. Anaphylaxis in the pre-hospital setting. *Journal of Emergency Medicine* 2004, 27(4): 371–7.
5. McLean-Tooke APC, Bethune CA, Fay AC, Spickett GP. Adrenaline in the treatment of anaphylaxis: what is the evidence? *British Medical Journal* 2003, 327(7427): 1332–5.
6. Langran M, Laird C. Management of allergy, rashes, and itching. *Emergency Medicine Journal* 2004, 21(6): 728–41.
7. Lieberman P, Nicklas RA, Oppenheimer J, Kemp SF, Lang DM, Bernstein DI, et al. The diagnosis and management of anaphylaxis practice parameter: 2010 update. *Journal of Allergy and Clinical Immunology* 2010, 126(3): 477–80.e1–42.
8. Pumphrey RSH. Lessons for management of anaphylaxis from a study of fatal reactions. *Clinical & Experimental Allergy* 2000, 30(8): 1144–50.
9. Sampson HA, Muñoz-Furlong A, Campbell RL, Adkinson NF Jr, Allan Bock S, Branum A, et al. Second symposium on the definition and management of anaphylaxis: summary report – second National Institute of Allergy and Infectious Disease/Food Allergy and Anaphylaxis Network symposium. *Annals of Emergency Medicine* 2006, 47(4): 373–80.
10. Brown AFT, McKinnon D, Chu K. Emergency department anaphylaxis: a review of 142 patients in a single year. *Journal of Allergy and Clinical Immunology* 2001, 108(5): 861–6.
11. Sheikh A, Shehata YA, Brown SGA, Simons FER. Adrenaline for the treatment of anaphylaxis: Cochrane Systematic Review. *Allergy* 2009, 64(2): 204–12.
12. Pumphrey RSH, Gowland MH. Further fatal allergic reactions to food in the United Kingdom, 1999–2006. *Journal of Allergy and Clinical Immunology* 2007, 119(4): 1018–19.
13. Visscher PK, Vetter RS, Camazine S. Removing bee stings. *The Lancet* 1996, 348(9023): 301–2.
14. Brown SGA, Blackman KE, Stenlake V, Heddle RJ. Insect sting anaphylaxis: prospective evaluation of treatment with intravenous adrenaline and volume resuscitation. *Emergency Medicine Journal* 2004, 21(2): 149–54.

Altered Level of Consciousness

1. Introduction

- Pre-hospital presentation of altered level of consciousness (ALoC) can be a major challenge.
- In patients with ALoC it is important to undertake a rapid assessment for **TIME CRITICAL** conditions.
- It is important to understand, where possible, the cause of altered consciousness which can range from diabetic collapse, to factitious illness (refer to Table 3.17 and Table 3.18).
- The patient history may provide valuable insight into the cause of the current condition. Consider the following in formulating your diagnosis; ask relatives or bystanders:
  - is there any history of recent illness or pre-existing chronic illness (e.g. diabetes, steroid-dependent adrenal insufficiency or epilepsy)?
  - any past history of mental health problems?
  - any preceding symptoms such as headache, fits, confusion?
  - any history of trauma?

NB Remember, an acute condition may be an exacerbation of a chronic condition or a 'new' illness superimposed on top of a pre-existing problem, such as adrenal crisis triggered by infective gastroenteritis.

However, often there is little available information – in these circumstances the scene may provide clues to assist in formulating a diagnosis:

- Environmental factors (e.g. extreme cold, possible carbon monoxide sources)?
- Evidence of tablets, ampoules, pill boxes, syringes, including domiciliary oxygen (O_2), or administration devices (e.g. nebuliser machines)?
- Evidence of alcohol, or medication abuse?

This guideline contains guidance for managing patients with transient loss of consciousness (section 1) and coma (section 2).

TABLE 3.17 – Red Flag Conditions

Condition
Adrenal insufficiency (risk of adrenal crisis with hypoglycaemia) (refer to **Hydrocortisone**).
Epilepsy (refer to **Stroke/Transient Ischaemic Attack (TIA)**).
Head injury (refer to **Head Injury**).
Hyperglycaemia (refer to **Glycaemic Emergencies in Adults and Children**).
Hypoglycaemia (refer to **Glycaemic Emergencies in Adults and Children**).
Overdose (refer to **Overdose and Poisoning in Adults and Children**).
Stroke/TIA (refer to **Stroke**).
Subarachnoid haemorrhage (refer to **Headache**).

TABLE 3.18 – Some Conditions That May Result In DLoC (Decreased level of consciousness)

Alterations in pO_2 (hypoxia) and/or pCO_2 (hyper/hypocapnia)
Inadequate airway.
Inadequate ventilation or depressed respiratory drive.
Persistent hyperventilation.
Inadequate perfusion
Cardiac arrhythmias.
Distributive shock.
Hypovolaemia.
Neurogenic shock.
Raised intracranial pressure.
Altered metabolic states
Hypoglycaemia and hyperglycaemia.
Intoxication or poisoning
Alcohol intoxication.
Carbon monoxide poisoning.
Drug overdose.
Medical conditions
Adrenal crisis.
Epilepsy.
Hypo/hyperthermia.
Meningitis.
Stroke.
Subarachnoid haemorrhage.
Head injury

2. SECTION 1 – Transient Loss of Consciousness (TLoC)

- Transient loss of consciousness (TLoC) may be defined as spontaneous loss of consciousness with complete recovery i.e. full recovery of consciousness without any residual neurological deficit.
- An episode of TLoC is often described as a 'blackout' or a 'collapse'. There are various causes of TLoC, including:
  - cardiovascular disorders (which are the most common)
  - neurological conditions such as epilepsy, and psychogenic attacks.
- The diagnosis of the underlying cause of TLoC is often inaccurate and delayed.

2.1 Assessment and Management

For the assessment and management of transient loss of consciousness refer to Table 3.19.

Altered Level of Consciousness

TABLE 3.19 – Assessment and Management of: Transient Loss of Consciousness

ASSESSMENT (ADULTS)	MANAGEMENT (ADULTS)
• Assess <C>ABCD	• If any of the following **TIME CRITICAL** features are present: – major **<C>ABCD** problems – unexpected OR persistent loss of consciousness, ECG Abnormalities, TLoC during exertion, new unexplained breathlessness. then: • Start correcting any **<C>ABCD** problems. • Undertake a **TIME CRITICAL** transfer to nearest appropriate receiving hospital. • Continue patient management en-route. • Provide an ATMIST information call.
• Ascertain from the patient or witnesses what happened before, during and after the event	**Record details about:** • Circumstances of the event. • The patient's posture immediately before loss of consciousness. • Prodromal symptoms (such as sweating or feeling warm/hot). • Appearance (whether eyes were open or shut) and colour of the patient during the event. • Presence or absence of movement during the event (limb-jerking and its duration). • Any tongue-biting (record whether the side or the tip of the tongue was bitten). • Injury occurring during the event (record site and severity). • Duration of the event (onset to regaining consciousness). • Presence or absence of confusion during the recovery period. • Weakness down one side during the recovery period. • Details of any previous TLoC, including number and frequency. • The patient medical history and any family history of cardiac disease (personal history of heart disease or family history of sudden cardiac death). • Current medication that may have contributed to TLoC (diuretics). • Routine observations (pulse rate, respiratory rate and temperature) – repeat if clinically indicated. • Lying and standing blood pressure if clinically appropriate. • Other cardiovascular and neurological signs.
• ECG	• Monitor and record 12-Lead ECG. Assess for abnormality, refer to **Cardiac Rhythm Disturbance**.
• If an underlying cause is suspected	• Undertake relevant examinations and investigations, for example, check blood glucose levels if hypoglycaemia is suspected – refer to relevant guideline.
• Assess for uncomplicated faint and situational syncope	Diagnose uncomplicated faint (uncomplicated vasovagal syncope) on the basis of the initial assessment when: • There are no features that suggest an alternative diagnosis (**NB** brief seizure activity can occur during uncomplicated faints and is not necessarily diagnostic of epilepsy). **AND** • There are features suggestive of uncomplicated faint (the 3 'P's) such as: – **posture** – prolonged standing, or similar episodes – **provoking** factors (such as pain or a medical procedure) – **prodromal** symptoms (such as sweating or feeling warm/hot before TLoC). Diagnose situational syncope on the basis of the initial assessment when: • There are no features from the initial assessment that suggest an alternative diagnosis. **AND** • Syncope is clearly and consistently provoked by straining during micturition (usually while standing) or by coughing or swallowing.

(continued)

TABLE 3.19 – Assessment and Management of: Transient Loss of Consciousness *(continued)*	
• Care pathway	• Only patients with a GCS 15, with normal blood glucose and responsible adult supervision present may be left at scene. For example, if a diagnosis of uncomplicated faint or situational syncope is made, there is nothing in the initial assessment to raise clinical or social concern and there are no red flags present, the patient may be left at home. • **Advise the patient to take a copy of the clinical record and the ECG record to their GP and follow local protocols to safely hand over clinical responsibility.** • Take the opportunity, if appropriate, to discuss and record any lifestyle factors which may influence the cause of any TLoC episode.
Red Flags	The presence of any of the following during physical examination should be considered a red flag, resulting in conveyance to the Emergency Department: • New ECG abnormalities (listed below). • Physical signs of heart failure. • Transient loss of consciousness during exertion. • Family history of sudden cardiac death in people aged younger than 40 years and/or an inherited cardiac condition. • New or unexplained breathlessness. • A heart murmur. Conveyance should be considered for anyone aged older than 65 years of age who has experienced a TLoC without prodromal symptoms. Where not conveyed these patients must be discussed directly with a doctor. The following ECG abnormalities are considered red flags and the patient must be conveyed to the Emergency Department for assessment: • New conduction abnormalities (complete right or left bundle branch block or any degree of heart block). • Evidence or prolonged (> 440ms for males or >460ms for females) or shortened QTc intervals (<350ms for both). • Any ST segment or T wave abnormalities (e.g. brugada syndrome, abnormal T wave inversion). • Pathological Q waves. • Paced rhythm. • Inappropriate persistent bradycardia. • Ventricular arrhythmia. • Ventricular pre-excitation. • Sustained atrial arrhythmias.

3. SECTION 2 – Coma

3.1 Introduction

- Coma is defined as U on the AVPU scale or a Glasgow Coma Score (GCS) (refer to Appendix) of 8 or less; however, any patient presenting with a decreased level of consciousness (GCS<15) mandates further assessment and, possibly, treatment.
- There are a number of causes of coma; refer to Tables 3.17 and 3.18.

3.2 Assessment and management

For the assessment and management of coma refer to Table 3.20.

TABLE 3.20 – Assessment and Management of: Coma (GCS <8)	
ASSESSMENT (ADULTS)	**MANAGEMENT (ADULTS)** **NB** TAKE A DEFRIBILLATOR TO THE INCIDENT – many calls to unconscious patients are cardiac arrests.
• Assess **<C>ABCD**	• Start correcting any **<C>ABCD** problems. • Undertake a **TIME CRITICAL** transfer to the nearest appropriate receiving hospital. • Continue patient management en-route. • Provide an ATMIST information call.

TABLE 3.20 – Assessment and Management of: Coma (GCS <8) *(continued)*	
• Oxygen	• Administer high levels of supplementary oxygen and aim for a target saturation within the range of 94–98% (refer to **Oxygen**).
• Assess for hypoxia	• Apply pulse oximetry. • Obtain IV access if appropriate.
• Assess heart rhythm for arrhythmias	• Undertake a 12-lead ECG.
• Assess level of consciousness	• Assess using the AVPU scale or Glasgow Coma Scale (GCS) (refer to Appendix): A – Alert V – Response to voice P – Responds to painful stimulus U – Unresponsive. • Assess and note pupil size, equality and response to light. • Check for purposeful movement in all four limbs and note sensory function.
• Assess blood glucose level	• If hypoglycaemic (<4.0 mmol/l) or suspected, refer to **Glycaemic Emergencies in Adults and Children**.
• Blood pressure	• Measure blood pressure. • Correct blood pressure with fluid administration if required, refer to **0.9% Sodium Chloride**.
• Assess for significant injury especially to the head	• If trauma detected or suspected, immobilise spine and refer to Spinal Injury and Spinal Cord Injury.
• Assess for other causes	• Breath for ketones, alcohol and solvents. • Evidence of needle tracks/marks. • MedicAlert® type jewellery (bracelets or necklets) which detail the patient's primary health risk (e.g. diabetes, anaphylaxis, Addison's disease etc) – also list a 24-hour telephone number to obtain a more detailed patient history. • Warning stickers, often placed by the front door or the telephone, directing the health professional to a source of detailed information (one current scheme involves storing the patient details in a container in the fridge, as this is relatively easy to find in the house). • Patient-held warning cards, for example, those taking monoamine oxidase inhibitor (MAOI) medication. • **For management refer to relevant guideline(s).**
• Assess for respiratory depression	• In cases of severe respiratory depressions, refer to **Airway and Breathing Management**. • If the level of consciousness deteriorates or respiratory depression develops in cases where an overdose with opiate-type drugs may be a possibility, consider naloxone (refer to **Naloxone Hydrochloride**). • In a patient with fixed pinpoint pupils suspect opiate use/overdose. **NB** any patient with a decreased level of consciousness may have a compromised airway.
• Re-assess <C>ABCD	• Document any changes/note trends in: – GCS – altered neurological function – base line observations.

Appendix

Glasgow Coma Scale		
Item	**Element**	**Score**
Eyes opening:		
	Spontaneously	4
	To speech	3
	To pain	2
	None	1
Motor response:		
	Obeys commands	6
	Localises pain	5
	Withdraws from pain	4
	Abnormal flexion	3
	Extensor response	2
	No response to pain	1
Verbal response:		
	Orientated	5
	Confused	4
	Inappropriate words	3
	Incomprehensible sounds	2
	No verbal response	1

KEY POINTS!

Decreased Level of Consciousness

- **Maintain patent airway.**
- **Support ventilation if required.**
- **Address treatable causes.**
- **History – obtain as much information as possible.**
- **Consider an alert/information call.**

Bibliography

1. National Collaborating Centre for Acute Care. *Head Injury: Triage, assessment, investigation and early management of head injury in infants, children and adults* (CG56). London: National Collaborating Centre for Acute Care at The Royal College of Surgeons of England, 2007. Available from: https://www.nice.org.uk/guidance/cg176.
2. National Institute for Health and Clinical Excellence. *Stroke: The diagnosis and initial management of acute stroke and transient ischaemic attack* (CG68). London: NICE, 2008.
3. National Institute for Health and Clinical Excellence. *The Epilepsies: The diagnosis and management of the epilepsies in adults and children in primary and secondary care* (CG137). London: NICE, 2012. Available from: https://nice.org.uk/guidance/CG137.
4. National Institute for Health and Clinical Excellence. *Transient Loss of Consciousness in Adults and Young People* (CG109). London: NICE, 2012. Available from: https://www.nice.org.uk/guidance/qs71.
5. Task Force for the Diagnosis and Management of Syncope, European Society of Cardiology, European Heart Rhythm Association, Heart Failure Association, Heart Rhythm Society, Moya A, Sutton R, Ammirati F, Blanc JJ, Brignole M, Dahm JB, et al. Guidelines for the diagnosis and management of syncope (version 2009). *European Heart Journal* 2009, 30(21): 2631–71.

Asthma in Adults and Children

1. Introduction

- Asthma is the most common of all medical conditions. Asthma has varying levels of severity and patients usually present to pre-hospital care with one of four presentations: mild/moderate, severe, life-threatening, and near fatal (refer to Table 3.21).
- This guideline covers asthma in adults and children. A child is defined as between one year and puberty.
- Typically in patients requiring hospital admission the symptoms will have developed gradually over a number of hours (>6 hours).
- There may be a history of increasing wheeze or breathlessness which is often worse at night or early in the morning. Respiratory infections, allergy and physical exertion are common triggers.
- Known asthmatics will be on regular medication, taking inhalers ('preventers' and/or 'relievers') and sometimes oral medications such as Montelukast (Singulair®) and theophyllines.
- Some patients with asthma will have an individualised treatment plan with detailed information regarding their daily symptom control as well as what to do in an acute exacerbation.
- **Inhaled foreign body**: Consider an inhaled foreign body in a child experiencing their first wheezy episode, especially if there is a history of playing with small toys and the wheeze was of sudden onset and is unilateral. These children must be transferred for medical assessment. If they are unwell during transport, bronchodilators may provide some clinical benefit.
- Patients over 50 years of age who are long-term smokers with a history of exertional breathlessness and no other known cause of breathlessness should be treated as having COPD, refer to **Chronic Obstructive Pulmonary Disease**.

2. Incidence

- Asthma is rare in the older population and practitioners should be aware that many people will describe a range of other respiratory conditions as 'asthma', and therefore other causes of breathlessness need to be considered.
- In adults, asthma may often be complicated and mixed in with a degree of bronchitis, especially in smokers. This can make the condition much more difficult to treat, both routinely and in emergencies. The majority of asthmatic patients take regular 'preventer' and 'reliever' inhalers.

3. Severity and Outcome

- The obstruction in its most severe form can be **TIME CRITICAL** and in the UK some 2,000 people a year die as a result of asthma. Patients with severe asthma and one or more risk factor(s) (refer to Table 3.21) are at risk of death.
- In patients ≤40 years, deaths from asthma peak in July/August in contrast to patients aged >40 years where deaths peak in December/January.

TABLE 3.21 – Risk Factors for Developing Near-Fatal Asthma

Medical

- Anaphylaxis.
- Previous near-fatal asthma (e.g. previous ventilation or respiratory acidosis).
- Previous hospital admission for asthma especially if in the last year requiring three or more classes of asthma medication.
- Previous admission requiring intensive care.
- Heavy use of ß2 agonist, especially with poor or no response.
- Repeated emergency department attendance for asthma care especially if in the last year.
- Brittle asthma.

Psychological/behavioural

- Non-compliance with treatment or monitoring.
- Failure to attend appointments.
- Fewer GP contacts.
- Frequent home visits.
- Self-discharge from hospital.
- Psychosis, depression, other psychiatric illness or deliberate self-harm.
- Current or recent major tranquilliser use.
- Denial.
- Alcohol or drug abuse.
- Obesity.
- Learning difficulties.
- Employment problems.
- Income problems.
- Social isolation.
- Childhood abuse.
- Severe domestic, marital or legal stress.

Asthma in Adults and Children

TABLE 3.22 – Features of Severity

Near-fatal asthma

- Raised $PaCO_2$ and/or requiring mechanical ventilation with raised inflation pressures.

Life-threatening asthma

Any one of the following in a patient with severe asthma:

- Altered conscious level.
- Exhaustion.
- Arrhythmia.
- Hypotension.
- Cyanosis.
- Silent chest.
- Poor respiratory effort.
- PEF <33% best or predicted.
- SpO_2 <92%.
- PaO_2 <8 kPa.
- 'Abnormal' $PaCO_2$ (Normal range: 4.6–6.0 kPa).

Acute severe asthma

Any one of:

- PEF 33–50% best or predicted.
- Inability to complete sentences in one breath.
- Pulse:
  - >110/minute in adults
  - >125/minute in children >5 years
  - > 140/minute in children 2-5 years
- Respiration:
  - >25/minute in adults
  - >30/minute in children >5 years
  - >40/minute in children 2-5 years

Mild/moderate asthma exacerbation

- Able to speak in sentences.
- Increasing symptoms.
- PEF >50–75% best or predicted.
- No features of acute severe asthma.
- Heart rate:
  - ≤140/min in children aged 2–5 years.
  - ≤125/min in children >5 years.
- Respiratory rate:
  - ≤40/min in children aged 2–5 years.
  - ≤30/min in children >5 years.

4. Pathophysiology

- Asthma is caused by inflammation of the bronchi, making them narrower. The muscles around the bronchi become irritated and contract, causing sudden worsening of the symptoms. The inflammation can also cause the mucus glands to produce excessive sputum which further blocks the air passages.
- The obstruction and subsequent wheezing are caused by three factors within the bronchial tree:

  a swelling of the bronchial tube mucosal lining cells

  b spasm and constriction of bronchial muscles

  c increased production of bronchial mucus.
- These three factors combine to cause blockage and narrowing of the small airways in the lung. Because inspiration is an active process involving the muscles of respiration, the obstruction of the airways is overcome on breathing in. Expiration occurs with muscle relaxation, and is severely delayed by the narrowing of the airways in asthma. This generates the wheezing on expiration that is characteristic of this condition.
- Asthma is managed with a variety of inhaled and tablet medications. Inhalers are divided into two broad categories: preventer and reliever.

  1 The preventer inhalers are normally anti-inflammatory drugs and these include steroids and other milder anti-inflammatories such as Tilade. The common steroid inhalers are beclomethasone (Becotide), budesonide (Pulmicort), fluticasone (Flixotide) and tiotropium (Spiriva). These drugs act on the lung over a period of time to reduce the inflammatory reaction that causes the asthma. Regular use of these inhalers often eradicates all symptoms of asthma and allows for a normal lifestyle.

  2 The reliever inhalers include salbutamol (Ventolin), terbutaline (Bricanyl) and ipratropium bromide (Atrovent). These inhalers work rapidly on the lung to relax the smooth muscle spasm when the patient feels wheezy or tight chested. They are used in conjunction with preventer inhalers. Inhalers are often used through large plastic spacer devices, such as the Volumatic® or Aerochamber®. This allows the drug to spread into a larger volume and allows the patient to inhale it more effectively. In mild and moderate asthma attacks some

patients may be treated with high doses of 'relievers' through a spacer device. This has been shown to be as effective as giving a salbutamol nebuliser.

5. Assessment

- Assess **<C>ABCD** (refer to **Medical Emergencies in Adults – Overview** and **Medical Emergencies in Children – Overview**), but specifically assess for the severity of the asthma attack (refer to asthma algorithm – Figure 3.4 and Table 3.21).

6. Management

- Refer to the asthma algorithm (Figure 3.4 and Table 3.24) for the management of mild/moderate, severe, life-threatening, and near-fatal.
- Always ask if the patient has an individualised asthma treatment plan and follow it, unless clinical circumstances dictate otherwise.

For less severe attacks

- Where possible the patient's own ß2 agonist should be given (ideally using a spacer) as first line treatment. Increase the dose by two puffs every 2 minutes according to response up to ten puffs.
- If symptoms are not controlled by ten puffs, then start nebulised salbutamol whilst transferring to the emergency department. **NB** In children under 2 years old who have a poor initial response to Salbutamol (administered with adequate technique), consider an alternative diagnosis and other treatment options, refer to **Respiratory Illness in Children**.
- Patients (or friends/bystanders) who have previously experienced a severe asthma attack may be more likely to call for help early in the development of an attack, and the symptoms may appear mild on arrival of the ambulance.
- Some patients may be appropriate for alternative care pathways, for example, early referral to a general practitioner. However, apparently minor symptoms should not preclude onward referral especially where an alternative pathway is not readily accessible. Local care pathways should be followed where patients are considered for non-conveyance. However, caution should be exercised in known severe asthmatics and robust safety netting of patients must be in place.

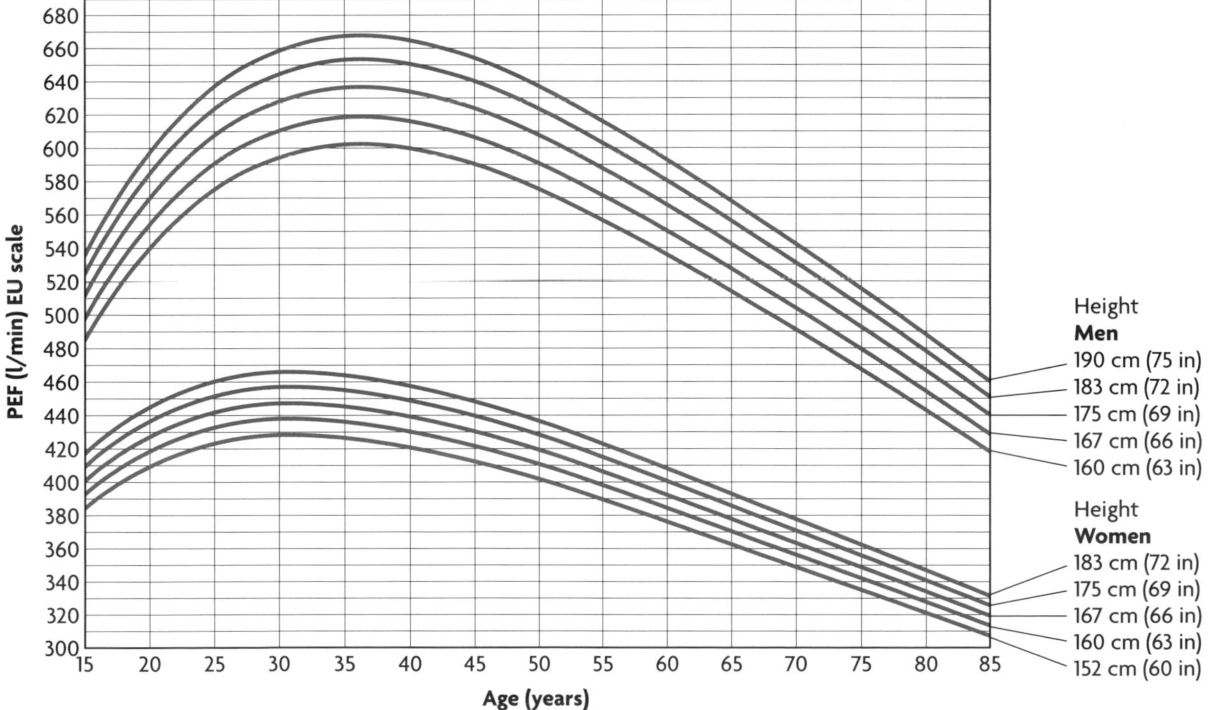

Figure 3.3 – Peak flow charts – Peak expiratory flow rate – normal values. For use with EU/EN13826 scale PEF meters only.

Adapted by Clement Clarke for use with EN13826 / EU scale peak flow meters from Nunn AJ Gregg I, Br Med J 1989:298;1068–70.

Asthma in Adults and Children

TABLE 3.23 – Peak Expiratory Flow Rates		
Height (m)	**Height (ft)**	**Predicted EU PEFR (L/min)**
0.85	2′9″	87
0.90	2′11″	95
0.95	3′1″	104
1.00	3′3″	115
1.05	3′5″	127
1.10	3′7″	141
1.15	3′9″	157
1.20	3′11″	174
1.25	4′1″	192
1.30	4′3″	212
1.35	4′5″	233
1.40	4′7″	254
1.45	4′9″	276
1.50	4′11″	299
1.55	5′1″	323
1.60	5′3″	346
1.65	5′5″	370
1.70	5′7″	393

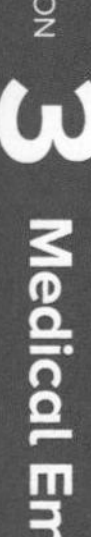

TABLE 3.24 – ASSESSMENT and MANAGEMENT of: Asthma	
ASSESSMENT	**MANAGEMENT**
• Assess **<C>ABCD**	• If any of the following **TIME CRITICAL** features present: – major <C>ABCD problems, refer to **Medical Emergencies in Adults – Overview** and **Medical Emergencies in Children – Overview**. – extreme difficulty in breathing or requirement for assisted ventilations. **NB** asthma is predominantly a disease of exhalation, therefore care should be taken not to over-ventilate. Adequate expiration must be achieved. – exhaustion – cyanosis – silent chest – SpO_2 <92% – PEF <33% best or predicted. • Start correcting any <C>ABCD problems. • Undertake a TIME CRITICAL transfer to nearest appropriate receiving hospital. • Continue patient management en-route. • Provide an ATMIST information call.

Asthma in Adults and Children

TABLE 3.24 – ASSESSMENT and MANAGEMENT of: Asthma *(continued)*	
• Respiratory rate	• Measure and record respiratory rate.
• Pulse	• Measure and record pulse.
• Oxygen saturation	• Monitor the patient's SpO_2, administer oxygen to achieve saturations of >94% if the patient presents as hypoxemic on air, refer to **Oxygen**.
• Specifically assess for the severity of the asthma attack (refer to Figure 3.4 and Table 3.21)	• Move to a calm quiet environment. • Encourage use of own inhaler, using a spacer if available. Ensure correct technique is used (refer to Figure 3.4). **NB** In children under 2 who have a poor response to salbutamol, consider an alternative cause, refer to **Respiratory Illness in Children**. • If unresponsive: – Administer high levels of supplementary oxygen. – Administer nebulised salbutamol, refer to **Salbutamol**, refer to **Page for Age** for children's doses.
• Mild/moderate asthma	• For cases of mild asthma that respond to treatment consider alternative care pathway where appropriate. **NB** exercise caution in known severe asthmatics. • Where available, refer to local guidance for Prednisolone administration and supply.
• Severe asthma	• Administer high levels of supplementary oxygen. • Administer nebulised salbutamol, refer to **Salbutamol**, refer to **Page for Age** for children's doses. • If no improvement, administer ipratropium bromide, refer to **Ipratropium Bromide**, refer to **Page for Age** for children's doses. • Administer steroids, refer to **Hydrocortisone**, refer to **Page for Age** for children's doses. • Continuous salbutamol nebulisation may be administered unless clinically significant side effects occur, refer to **Salbutamol**, refer to **Page for Age** for children's doses.
• Life-threatening asthma	• Give early consideration and low threshold to activate enhanced care support. • Continuous salbutamol nebulisation may be administered unless clinically significant side effects occur, refer to **Salbutamol**, refer to **Page for Age** for children's doses. • If there is no improvement, administer ipratropium bromide, refer to **Ipratropium Bromide**, refer to **Page for Age** for children's doses. • Administer adrenaline **SAFETY NOTE 1:1000 IM ONLY**, refer to **Adrenaline**, refer to **Page for Age** for children's doses. **NB:** Drug Check MUST be completed before administration including clarification of route to be used (IM ONLY). • Administer steroids, refer to **Hydrocortisone**, refer to **Page for Age** for children's doses.

(continued)

Asthma in Adults and Children

TABLE 3.24 – ASSESSMENT and MANAGEMENT of: Asthma *(continued)*	
• Life-threatening asthma	• Require bag-valve-mask ventilation with raised inflation pressures. **NB** Asthma is predominantly a disease of exhalation, care should be taken not to over ventilate. Adequate expiration must be achieved. • Assess for bilateral tension pneumothorax. • Transfer rapidly to nearest receiving hospital. • Provide an ATMIST information call. • Continue patient management en-route.
• Blood pressure and fluids	• Measure and record blood pressure, if required administer fluids, refer to **Intravascular Fluid Therapy in Adults** and **Intravascular Fluid Therapy in Children**.
• Blood glucose	• If appropriate, measure and record blood glucose for hypo/hyperglycaemia, refer to **Glycaemic Emergencies in Adults and Children**.
• Temperature	• Measure and record temperature.
• NEWS2	• These observations will enable you to calculate a NEWS2 Score, refer to **Sepsis**.
• ECG	• If required, monitor and record 12-Lead ECG. Assess for abnormality, refer to **Cardiac Rhythm Disturbance**.
• Assess the patient's pain	• Where present, assess the SOCRATES of pain and record initial and subsequent pain scores. • Consider analgesia if appropriate, refer to **Pain Management in Adults** and **Pain Management in Children**.
• Documentation	• Complete documentation to include all clinical findings, advice from other clinicians, onward referral and worsening advice given.

Peak expiratory flow rate (PEFR)

- Peak flow is a rapid measurement of the degree of obstruction in the patient's lungs. It measures the maximum flow on breathing out, or expiring and therefore can reflect the amount of airway obstruction. Whenever possible, peak flow should be performed before and after nebulised treatment. Many patients now have their own meter at home and know what their normal peak flow is. Clearly, when control is good, their peak flow will be equivalent to a normal patient's measurement, but during an attack it may drop markedly (refer to Figure 3.3).
- There is no place for PEFR measurements in preschool children as developmentally they do not have the technical ability to reliably perform this task.
- PEFR should be attempted where possible before and after nebulised therapy in mild to moderate asthma. However, care should be taken in severe life-threatening attacks as it could exacerbate the attack and the patient may deteriorate. Predicted PEFR is shown in Figure 3.3.

Asthma in Adults and Children

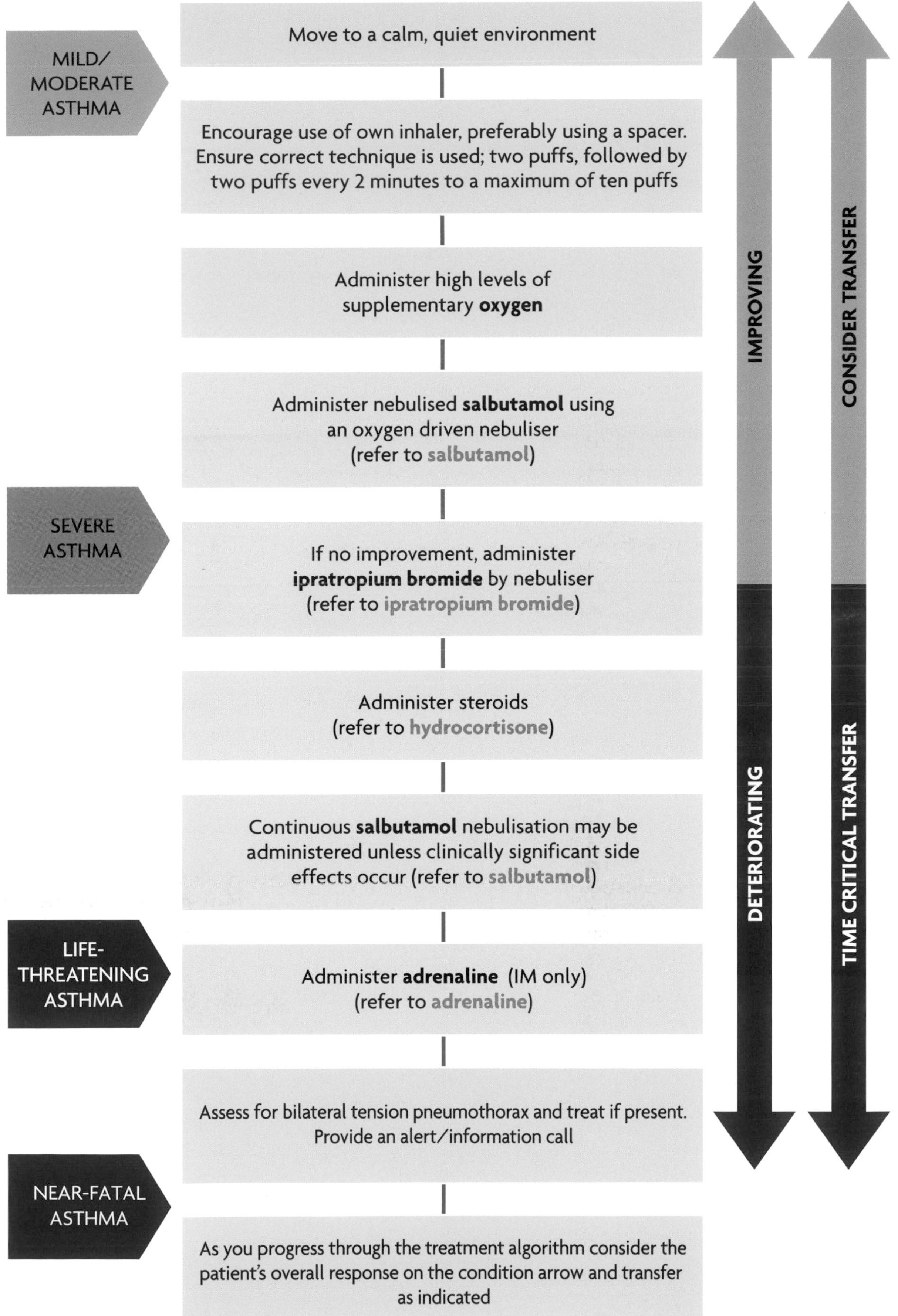

Figure 3.4 – Asthma assessment and management algorithm.

Asthma in Adults and Children

KEY POINTS!

Asthma in Adults and Children

- **Asthma is a common life-threatening condition.**
- **Its severity is often not recognised.**
- **Accurate documentation is essential.**
- **A silent chest is a pre-terminal sign.**
- **Bronchodilators are the mainstay of treatment.**
- **Ipatropium bromide should be considered in severe cases.**
- **Clinical assessment should determine the severity of the asthma attack.**
- **Consider adrenaline for life-threatening asthma.**

Bibliography

1. Soar J, Perkins GD, Abbas G, Alfonzo A, Barelli A, Bierens JJLM, et al. European Resuscitation Council Guidelines for Resuscitation 2010 Section 8: Cardiac arrest in special circumstances: electrolyte abnormalities, poisoning, drowning, accidental hypothermia, hyperthermia, asthma, anaphylaxis, cardiac surgery, trauma, pregnancy, electrocution. *Resuscitation* 2010, 81(10): 1400–1433.
2. The British Thoracic Society, Scottish Intercollegiate Guidelines Network. *British Guideline on the Management of Asthma* (Guideline 101). London/ Edinburgh: BTS and SIGN, 2008 (revised May 2012). Available from: https://www.brit-thoracic.org.uk/document-library/clinical-information/asthma/btssign-asthma-guideline-2014/.
3. Rubin BK, Dhand R, Ruppel GL, Branson RD, Hess DR. Respiratory care year in review 2010. Part 1: Asthma, COPD, pulmonary function testing, ventilator-associated pneumonia. *Respiratory Care* 2011, 56(4): 488–502.
4. Nunn AJ, Gregg I. New regression equations for predicting peak expiratory flow in adults. *British Medical Journal* 1989, 298(6680): 1068–70.

SECTION 3 Medical Emergencies

Cardiac Rhythm Disturbance

1. Introduction

- Cardiac arrhythmia is a common complication of acute myocardial ischaemia or infarction and may precede cardiac arrest or complicate the early post-resuscitation period.
- Rhythm disturbance may also present in many other ways and be unrelated to coronary heart disease.
- The management of disorders of cardiac rhythm is a specialised subject, often requiring detailed investigation and management strategies that are not available outside hospital.
- Diagnosis of the precise rhythm disturbance may be complicated and the selection of optimal treatment difficult. Very often, expert advice will be required, yet this expertise is rarely immediately available in the emergency situation.

2. Principles of Treatment

- Management is determined by the condition of the patient as well as the nature of the rhythm. Manage the patient using the standard <C>ABCDE approach.
- In all cases follow the oxygen guideline and aim for a target saturation within the range of 94–98%.
- Gain venous access.
- Always take a defibrillator to any patient with suspected cardiac rhythm disturbance.
- Establish cardiac rhythm monitoring as soon as possible.

Document the arrhythmia. This should be done with a 12-lead ECG whenever possible. If only a 3-lead ECG is available, lead II provides the best waveform for arrhythmia analysis.

- Provide a printout for the hospital, and, if possible, archive the record electronically so that further copies can be available at a later time if needed. Repeat the recording if the rhythm should change at any time. Record the ECG rhythm during any intervention (vagotonic procedures or the administration of drugs).
- If patients are not acutely ill there may be time to seek appropriate advice.
- The presence of adverse signs or symptoms will dictate the need for urgent treatment. The following adverse factors indicate a patient who is unstable because of the arrhythmia:
  - evidence of low cardiac output: pallor, sweating, cold clammy extremities, impaired consciousness or hypotension (SBP <90 mmHg)
  - excessive tachycardia, defined as a heart rate of >150 bpm
  - excessive bradycardia, defined as a heart rate of <40 bpm
  - heart failure implies the arrhythmia is compromising left ventricular function. This may cause breathlessness, confusion and hypotension or other features of reduced cardiac output
  - ischaemic chest pain implies that the arrhythmia (particularly tachyarrhythmia) is producing myocardial ischaemia. It is particularly important if there is underlying coronary disease or structural heart disease in which ischaemia is likely to lead to life-threatening complications including cardiac arrest.

3. Bradycardia

Introduction

- A bradycardia is defined as a ventricular rate <60 bpm, but it is important to recognise patients with a relative bradycardia in whom the rate is inappropriately slow for their haemodynamic state.

4. Risk of Asystole

Assessment and management

For the assessment and management of bradycardia and risk of asystole refer to Table 3.25.

5. Tachycardia

Introduction

- These guidelines are intended for the treatment of patients who maintain a cardiac output in the presence of the tachycardia.
- Pulseless ventricular tachycardia is treated according to the cardiac arrest algorithm for the treatment of pulseless VT/VF.
- Broad complex tachycardia.
- Narrow complex tachycardia.

Assessment and management

For the assessment and management of tachycardia, broad complex tachycardia, and narrow complex tachycardia refer to Table 3.26.

Cardiac Rhythm Disturbance

TABLE 3.25 – ASSESSMENT and MANAGEMENT of: Bradycardia and Risk of Asystole	
Bradycardia: A ventricular rate <60 bpm, but it is important to recognise patients with a relative bradycardia in whom the rate is inappropriately slow for their haemodynamic state.	
ASSESSMENT	**MANAGEMENT**
Assess to determine if one or more adverse signs are present: – Systolic blood pressure <90 mmHg. – Ventricular rate <40 bpm. – Ventricular arrhythmias compromising BP requiring treatment. – Heart failure.	**If one or more signs are present:** ● Follow oxygen guidelines – aim for target saturation within the range 94–98%. ● Gain IV access. ● Administer atropine[a] (refer to **Atropine**) and repeat after 3–5 minutes if necessary, or transcutaneous pacing. ● Undertake a 12-lead ECG. ● Transfer to further care.
Risk of asystole: If the patient is initially stable (i.e. no adverse signs are present) or a satisfactory response is achieved with atropine, next determine the risk of asystole.	
Assess for risk of asystole – this is indicated by: – Previous episode of asystole. – Möbitz II AV block. – Complete (third degree) AV block, especially with a broad QRS complex or an initial ventricular rate <40 bpm. – Ventricular standstill >3 seconds.	**If there is a risk of asytole (i.e. one or more signs are present)** or the patient shows adverse signs and has not responded satisfactorily to atropine, transvenous pacing is likely to be required. One or more of the following interventions may improve the patient's condition during transport: ● Transcutaneous pacing should be undertaken if available. **If transcutaneous pacing is not available:** ● Fist pacing may produce ventricular contraction – give serial rhythmic blows with the closed fist over the lower left sternal edge to pace the heart at a rate of 50–70 bpm. NOTES: a **Do not** give atropine to patients with cardiac transplants; their hearts will not respond to vagal blocking by atropine and paradoxical high degree AV block or sinus arrest may result. b Complete heart block with a narrow QRS complex escape rhythm may not require pacing. The ectopic pacemaker (which is situated in the atrioventricular junction) may provide a stable rhythm at an adequate rate. c Initiate transcutaneous pacing (if equipment is available): – if there is no response to atropine – if patient is severely symptomatic, particularly when high degree block (Möbitz type II or third degree AV block) is present. **NB** Transcutaneous pacing may be painful; use analgesia. Verify mechanical capture. Monitor the patient carefully; try to identify the cause of the bradycardia.

a Caution – Doses of atropine lower than 500 mcg may paradoxically cause further slowing of ventricular rate. Use atropine cautiously in acute myocardial ischaemia or infarction; an increased rate may worsen ischaemia.

Cardiac Rhythm Disturbance

<table>
<tr><th colspan="2">TABLE 3.26 – ASSESSMENT and MANAGEMENT of: Tachycardia, Broad Complex Tachycardia and Narrow Complex Tachycardia</th></tr>
<tr><th>ASSESSMENT</th><th>MANAGEMENT</th></tr>
<tr><td>Tachycardia
● These guidelines are intended for the treatment of patients who maintain a cardiac output in the presence of the tachycardia.
● Pulseless ventricular tachycardia is treated with immediate attempts at defibrillation following the algorithm for the treatment of pulseless VT/VF.</td><td>1 Support the ABCs.
2 Administer high levels of supplemental oxygen – aim for a target saturation 94–98%.
3 Gain IV access.
4 Establish cardiac rhythm monitoring.
5 Record and monitor BP and SpO_2.
6 Record a 12-lead ECG if possible, if not, record a rhythm strip.
7 If the rhythm changes at any time, make a further recording.
8 Make a continuous record of the rhythm during any therapeutic intervention (whether a drug or physical manoeuvre like carotid sinus massage).
9 The response to treatment can provide important additional information about the arrhythmia.
10 Identify and treat reversible causes; give analgesia if indicated.
11 Try to define the cardiac rhythm from the ECG. Determine the QRS duration and determine whether the rhythm is regular or irregular. If the QRS duration is 120 msec or more, the rhythm is a broad complex tachycardia. If less than 120 msec, the rhythm is a narrow complex tachycardia.</td></tr>
<tr><td>Broad complex tachycardia</td><td>● The rhythm is likely to be ventricular tachycardia, particularly in the context of ischaemic heart disease, patients showing adverse signs (reduced consciousness, SBP <90 mmHg, chest pain or heart failure), or in the peri-arrest situation.
● In all cases, maintain the supportive measures above and monitor the patient during transport.
● Provide an alert/information call according to local guidelines.
● Atrial fibrillation with aberrant conduction may produce an irregular broad complex tachycardia, but the diagnosis is difficult to make with certainty and often requires expert examination of the ECG. This emphasises the importance of recording the ECG when the arrhythmia is present. Ambulance personnel may greatly assist the subsequent diagnosis and management of patients by obtaining good quality ECG recordings. It is advantageous if these can also be archived electronically so that additional copies are available in the future.</td></tr>
<tr><td>Narrow complex tachycardia</td><td>If the rhythm is narrow complex (QRS <120 msec) AND REGULAR, it is likely to be either:
– sinus tachycardia. This is a physiological response, for example to pain, fever, blood loss or heart failure. Treatment is directed towards the cause. Trying to slow the rate is likely to make the situation worse
– supraventricular tachycardia (SVT). This is often seen in patients without other forms of heart disease. There may be a history of previous attacks
– atrial flutter with regular AV conduction (often 2:1 and a rate of 150 bpm).
● In cases of SVT, start with vagal manoeuvres. In some cases the patient may be aware of techniques that have terminated previous episodes. The Valsalva manoeuvre (forced expiration against a closed glottis) may be effective and is conveniently achieved (especially in supine patients) by asking the patient to blow into a 20 ml syringe with sufficient force to push back the plunger. If this fails, perform carotid sinus massage provided no carotid bruit is heard on auscultation. A bruit may indicate the presence of atheromatous plaque, rupture of which may cause cerebral embolism and stroke.</td></tr>
</table>

(continued)

Cardiac Rhythm Disturbance

TABLE 3.26 – ASSESSMENT and MANAGEMENT of: Tachycardia, Broad Complex Tachycardia and Narrow Complex Tachycardia *(continued)*	
	• Record the ECG (preferably multi-lead) during each manoeuvre. If the arrhythmia is successfully terminated by vagal procedures, it is very likely to have been SVT. If the rhythm is atrial flutter, slowing of ventricular rate may occur and allow the identification of flutter waves on the ECG. • Maintain the supportive measures above and monitor the patient during transport. • **AN IRREGULAR** narrow complex rhythm is most commonly atrial fibrillation, less commonly atrial flutter with variable block. Maintain the supportive measures above and monitor the patient during transport. • In all cases, ensure the patient is received into a suitable emergency department maintaining cardiac monitoring throughout. Ensure detailed hand-over to appropriate staff and that ECGs are safely handed over.

KEY POINTS!

Cardiac Rhythm Disturbance

- **Gain venous access.**
- **Always take a defibrillator to any patient with suspected cardiac rhythm disturbance.**
- **Establish cardiac rhythm monitoring as soon as possible, preferably with a 12-lead ECG.**
- **Record the ECG rhythm during any intervention and archive. Ensure all ECGs are safely handed over to receiving staff and archive so further copies can be retrieved if necessary.**

Bibliography

1. Deakin CD, Nolan JP, Soar J, Sunde K, Koster RW, Smith GB, et al. European Resuscitation Council Guidelines for Resuscitation 2010 Section 4: Adult advanced life support. *Resuscitation* 2010, 81(10): 1305–1352.
2. Soar J, Perkins GD, Abbas G, Alfonzo A, Barelli A, Bierens JJLM, et al. European Resuscitation Council Guidelines for Resuscitation 2010 Section 8: Cardiac arrest in special circumstances: electrolyte abnormalities, poisoning, drowning, accidental hypothermia, hyperthermia, asthma, anaphylaxis, cardiac surgery, trauma, pregnancy, electrocution. *Resuscitation* 2010, 81(10): 1400–1433.
3. Deakin CD, Nolan JP, Sunde K, Koster RW. European Resuscitation Council Guidelines for Resuscitation 2010 Section 3: Electrical therapies: automated external defibrillators, defibrillation, cardioversion and pacing. *Resuscitation* 2010, 81(10): 1293–1304.
4. Arntz H-R, Bossaert LL, Danchin N, Nikolaou NI. European Resuscitation Council Guidelines for Resuscitation 2010 Section 5: Initial management of acute coronary syndromes. *Resuscitation* 2010, 81(10): 1353–63.
5. de Caen AR, Kleinman ME, Chameides L, Atkins DL, Berg RA, Berg MD, et al. Part 10: Paediatric basic and advanced life support: 2010 International Consensus on Cardiopulmonary Resuscitation and Emergency Cardiovascular Care Science with Treatment Recommendations. *Resuscitation* 2010, 81(1): e213–59.
6. Deakin CD, Morrison LJ, Morley PT, Callaway CW, Kerber RE, Kronick SL, et al. Part 8: Advanced life support: 2010 International Consensus on Cardiopulmonary Resuscitation and Emergency Cardiovascular Care Science with Treatment Recommendations. *Resuscitation* 2010, 81(1): e93–174.
7. Wyllie J, Perlman JM, Kattwinkel J, Atkins DL, Chameides L, Goldsmith JP, et al. Part 11: Neonatal resuscitation: 2010 International Consensus on Cardiopulmonary Resuscitation and Emergency Cardiovascular Care Science with Treatment Recommendations. *Resuscitation* 2010, 81(1): e260–287.
8. Sunde K, Jacobs I, Deakin CD, Hazinski MF, Kerber RE, Koster RW, et al. Part 6: Defibrillation: 2010 International Consensus on Cardiopulmonary Resuscitation and Emergency Cardiovascular Care Science with Treatment Recommendations. *Resuscitation* 2010, 81(1): e71–85.
9. Bossaert L, O'Connor RE, Arntz H-R, Brooks SC, Diercks D, Feitosa-Filho G, et al. Part 9: Acute coronary syndromes: 2010 International Consensus on Cardiopulmonary Resuscitation and Emergency Cardiovascular Care Science with Treatment Recommendations. *Resuscitation* 2010, 81(1): e175–212.

Chronic Obstructive Pulmonary Disease

1. Introduction

- Chronic obstructive pulmonary disease (COPD) is a chronic progressive disorder characterised by airflow obstruction.
- A diagnosis of COPD is usually made in the presence of airflow obstruction in people >35 years of age, who are or were previously smokers and may have one or more risk factors (refer to Table 3.27).
- Patients over 50 years of age who are long-term smokers with a history of exertional breathlessness and no other known cause of breathlessness should be treated as having COPD.
- Patients with COPD usually present to the ambulance service with an acute exacerbation of the underlying illness. COPD is a concomitant/secondary illness in many incidents with other chief complaints.
- Patients with COPD are at increased risk of hypercapnic respiratory failure (Type 2) and respiratory acidosis due to carbon dioxide retention. It is vital for any patient who has a history of this to be issued an "alert card" by their specialist, so that respiratory failure is not worsened by high levels of oxygen administration. Ambulance clinicians should be aware of the British Thoracic Society and Oxygen guidelines; however these patients may require a tailored approach.
- Excessive oxygen administration in these patients can lead to:
  - Worsened ventilation-perfusion matching due to attenuation of hypoxic pulmonary vasoconstriction
  - Decreased binding affinity of haemoglobin for carbon dioxide
  - Decreased minute ventilation.

2. Incidence

- It is estimated that approximately 3 million people have COPD affecting 2–4% of the population over 45 years of age. However, only 1.5% of the population are diagnosed with the condition.
- In the UK, COPD is the fifth leading cause of death and it is estimated that by 2020 it will be the third leading cause of death worldwide.

3. Severity and Outcome

- COPD results in disability and impaired quality of life leading to 30,000 deaths per annum in the UK.
- COPD is the second leading cause of emergency admission, with 130,000 cases per annum, in the UK and direct costs estimated at £800 million and indirect costs of £24 million.

4. Pathophysiology

- Airflow obstruction is the result of airway and parenchymal damage due to chronic inflammation.
- COPD increases the risk of co-morbidities such as lung cancer and cardiovascular disease.
- An acute exacerbation refers to a worsening of the patient's symptoms (refer to Table 3.28). There is no single feature that defines an exacerbation, although there are a number of known causes (refer to Table 3.30), however, in 30% of cases the cause is unknown.

TABLE 3.27 – Signs/Symptoms of COPD

Signs/symptoms
• Exertional breathlessness.
• Chronic cough.
• Regular sputum production.
• Frequent winter 'bronchitis'.
• Wheeze.
• No clinical features of asthma.

TABLE 3.28 – Features of an Acute Exacerbation of COPD

Features
• Increased dyspnoea – particularly on exertion.
• Increased sputum volume/purulence.
• Increased cough.
• Upper airway symptoms (e.g. colds and sore throats).
• Increased wheeze.
• Chest tightness.
• Reduced exercise tolerance.
• Fluid retention.
• Increased fatigue.
• Acute confusion.
• Worsening of a previously stable condition.
Severe features
• Marked dyspnoea.
• Tachypnoea.
• Purse lip breathing.
• Use of accessory respiratory muscles (sternomastoid and abdominal) at rest.
• Acute confusion.
• New-onset cyanosis.
• New-onset peripheral oedema.
• Marked reduction in activities of daily living.

Chronic Obstructive Pulmonary Disease

- COPD patients generally have lower than normal SpO_2 levels and British Thoracic Society oxygen guidelines should be followed to maintain a target saturation of 88–92% SpO_2.
- Some exacerbations are mild and self-limiting whilst others are more severe, potentially life-threatening, and require intervention – not all features will be present (refer to Table 3.28).
- Some conditions may present with symptoms similar to an exacerbation of COPD – consider these when diagnosing an exacerbation of COPD (refer to Table 3.29).

TABLE 3.29 – Conditions with Similar Features to an Acute Exacerbation of COPD
Features
• Asthma.
• Pneumonia.
• Pneumothorax.
• Left ventricular failure/pulmonary oedema.
• Pulmonary embolus.
• Lung cancer.
• Upper airway obstruction.
• Pleural effusion.
• Recurrent aspiration.

5. Assessment and Management

For assessment and management of chronic obstructive pulmonary disease refer to Table 3.31 and Figure 3.5.

TABLE 3.30 – Causes of Exacerbation of COPD
Infections
• Rhinoviruses (common cold).
• Influenza.
• Parainfluenza.
• Coronavirus.
• Adenovirus.
• Respiratory syncytial virus.
• *C. pneumoniae.*
• *H. influenzae.*
• *S. pneumoniae.*
• *M. catarrhalis.*
• *S. aureus.*
• *P. aeruginosa.*
Pollutants
• Nitrogen dioxide.
• Particulates.
• Sulphur dioxide.
• Ozone.

TABLE 3.31 – ASSESSMENT and MANAGEMENT of: Chronic Obstructive Pulmonary Disease

ASSESSMENT	MANAGEMENT
• Assess <C>ABCDE	• If any of the following **TIME CRITICAL** features present: – major **<C>ABCDE** problems – extreme breathing difficulty (by reference to patient's usual condition) – cyanosis (although peripheral cyanosis may be 'normal' in some patients) – exhaustion – hypoxia (oxygen saturation <88%) unresponsive to oxygen (O_2) – COPD patients normally have a lower than normal oxygen saturation (SpO_2). • Start correcting any **<C>ABCDE** problems. • Undertake a **TIME CRITICAL** transfer to nearest appropriate receiving hospital. • Continue patient management en-route. • Provide an ATMIST information call.
• Position	• Position the patient for comfort and ease of respiration, often sitting forwards, but be aware of potential hypotension.
• Ventilation	• Consider non-invasive ventilation if not responding to treatment.

Chronic Obstructive Pulmonary Disease

TABLE 3.31 – ASSESSMENT and MANAGEMENT of: Chronic Obstructive Pulmonary Disease *(continued)*

• Ask the patient if they have an individualised treatment plan	• Follow the individualised treatment plan or alert card if available. • The patient will often be able to guide their care. • Alert cards outline emergency treatment, with specific target oxygen saturation as decided by the specialist, according to most recent investigations. As part of general history taking and scene survey, ambulance clinicians should be mindful of the need to find out if such a card exists. Many patients may also have a special message passed from the GP surgery to the Ambulance Clinical Hub. • A typical card will be similar to the one shown below, as recommended by the British Thoracic Society (BTS 2017). **OXYGEN ALERT CARD** **Name:** ______ **I have a chronic respiratory condition and I am at risk of having a raised carbon dioxide level in my blood during flare-ups of my condition (exacerbations)** **Please use my ______% Venturi mask to achieve an oxygen saturation of** **_____% to _____% during exacerbations of my condition** Use compressed air to drive nebulisers (with nasal oxygen a 2 l/min) If compressed air is not available, limit oxygen-driven nebulisers to 6 minutes Republished with kind permission of the British Thoracic Society. BTS Guideline for oxygen use in adults in healthcare and emergency settings 2017. Thorax Vol 72, Suppl 1 • Patients with COPD can easily become anxious, making it feel harder to breathe. They may have received advice about using specific breathing control techniques to help reduce breathlessness; one example is pursed-lips breathing. Encourage the patient to use these techniques if appropriate and if the patient has found them helpful previously.
Specifically assess: **Diagnosis**	• Assess whether this is an acute exacerbation of COPD – refer to Table 3.28 for the features of COPD. • Or another condition – refer to Table 3.29 and **Dyspnoea** for conditions with similar features to an acute exacerbation of COPD. **NB** Chest pain and fever are uncommon symptoms of COPD – therefore consider other possible causes.
Airway	• Maintain airway patency. NB Noises (e.g. 'bubbling' or wheeze) associated with breathing indicating respiratory distress.
• Bronchodilators	• Administer nebulised salbutamol (refer to **Salbutamol**). • In severe cases, administer ipratropium bromide (refer to **Ipratropium Bromide**). • If inadequate response after 5 minutes, a further dose of nebulised salbutamol may be administered. • Ipratropium can only be administered ONCE; salbutamol may be repeated at regular intervals unless the side effects of the drug become significant. **NB** Limit oxygen-driven nebulisation to 6 minutes. If journey time is significant, consider a further 6 minutes of nebulisation therapy ONLY if clinically indicated, but aim for a target saturation within the range of 88–92%.
• Respiratory rate	• Measure and record respiratory rate.

(continued)

SECTION 3 Medical Emergencies

Chronic Obstructive Pulmonary Disease

TABLE 3.31 – ASSESSMENT and MANAGEMENT of: Chronic Obstructive Pulmonary Disease *(continued)*	
• Oxygen. If the primary illness in a patient with COPD requires high concentration oxygen (refer to **Oxygen**) then this should **NOT BE WITHHELD**. The patient should be continually monitored closely for changes in respiratory rate and depth and the inspired concentration adjusted accordingly. In the short time that a patient is in ambulance care, hypoxia presents a much greater risk than hypercapnia in most cases.	• Measure oxygen saturation. Pulse oximetry, whilst important in COPD patients, will not indicate carbon dioxide (CO_2) levels which are assessed by capnography or more commonly, blood gas analysis in hospital. • Administer supplemental oxygen; aim for a target saturation within the range of 88–92% or the prespecified range – refer to the patient's individualised treatment plan or alert card if available. **NB** The aim of oxygen therapy is to prevent life-threatening hypoxia – administer cautiously as a proportion of COPD sufferers are chronically hypoxic and when given oxygen may develop increasing drowsiness and loss of respiratory drive. If this occurs, reduce oxygen concentration and support ventilation if required.
• Pulse	• Measure and record pulse.
• Blood pressure and fluids	• Measure and record blood pressure, if required administer fluids, refer to **Intravascular Fluid Therapy in Adults** and **Intravascular Fluid Therapy in Children**.
• Blood glucose	• If appropriate, measure and record blood glucose for hypo/hyperglycaemia, refer to **Glycaemic Emergencies in Adults and Children.**
• Temperature	• Measure and record temperature.
• NEWS2	• These observations will enable you to calculate a NEWS2 Score, refer to **Sepsis.**
• ECG	• If required, monitor and record 12-Lead ECG. Assess for abnormality, refer to **Cardiac Rhythm Disturbance.**
• Assess the patient's pain	• Where present, assess the **SOCRATES** of pain and record initial and subsequent pain scores. • Consider analgesia if appropriate, refer to **Pain Management in Adults** and **Pain Management in Children**.
• Documentation	• Complete documentation to include all clinical findings, advice from other clinicians, onward referral and worsening advice given.
• Transfer	• Consider alternative care pathway where appropriate, refer to table 3.32. • Arrange a follow up, such as visiting a nurse, a GP review or referral to other support before discharge.

Chronic Obstructive Pulmonary Disease

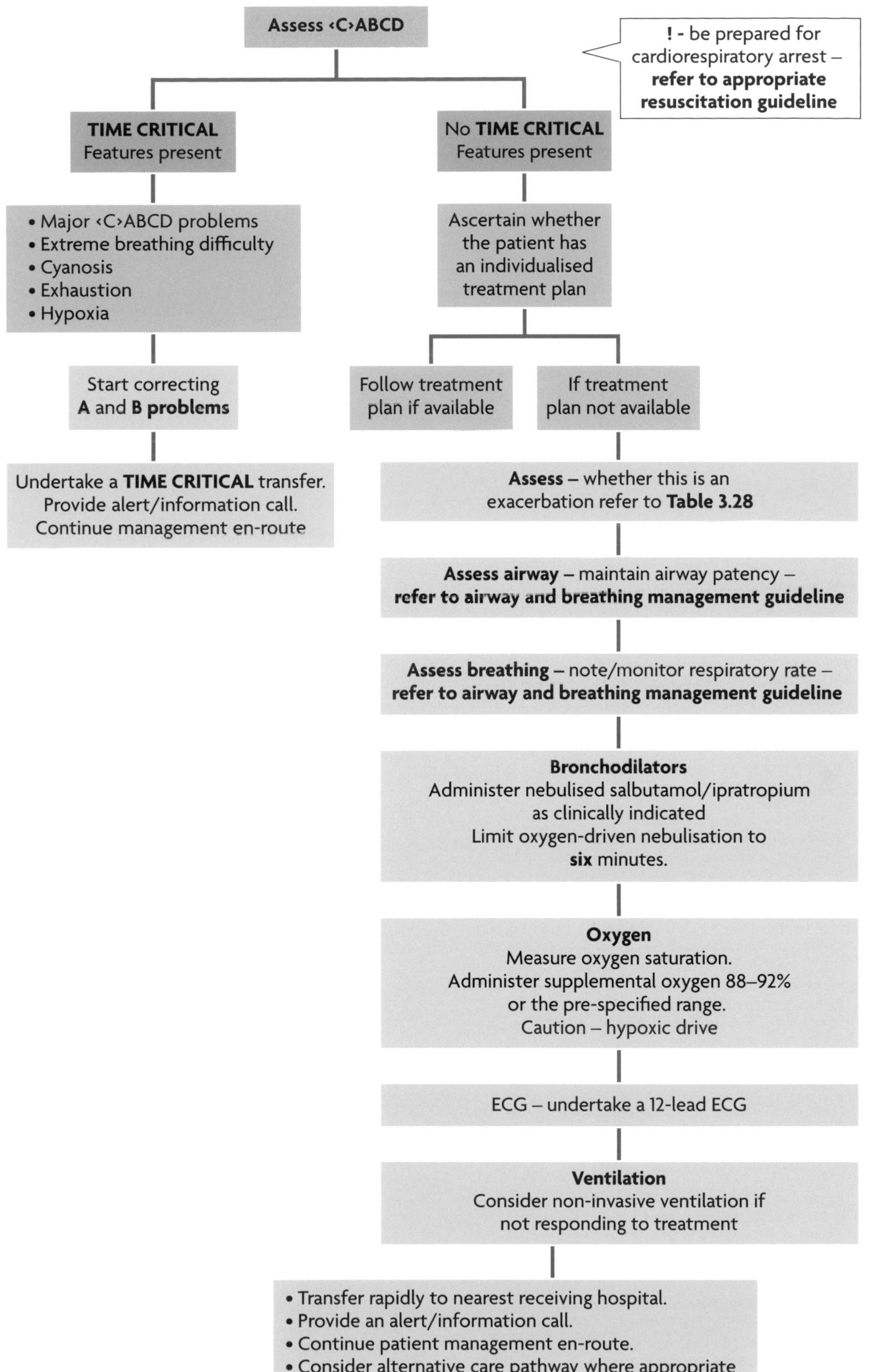

Assess <C>ABCD
! - be prepared for cardiorespiratory arrest – refer to appropriate resuscitation guideline
TIME CRITICAL Features present
No TIME CRITICAL Features present
• Major <C>ABCD problems
• Extreme breathing difficulty
• Cyanosis
• Exhaustion
• Hypoxia
Ascertain whether the patient has an individualised treatment plan
Start correcting A and B problems
Follow treatment plan if available
If treatment plan not available
Undertake a TIME CRITICAL transfer. Provide alert/information call. Continue management en-route
Assess – whether this is an exacerbation refer to Table 3.28
Assess airway – maintain airway patency – refer to airway and breathing management guideline
Assess breathing – note/monitor respiratory rate – refer to airway and breathing management guideline
Bronchodilators
Administer nebulised salbutamol/ipratropium as clinically indicated
Limit oxygen-driven nebulisation to six minutes.
Oxygen
Measure oxygen saturation.
Administer supplemental oxygen 88–92% or the pre-specified range.
Caution – hypoxic drive
ECG – undertake a 12-lead ECG
Ventilation
Consider non-invasive ventilation if not responding to treatment
• Transfer rapidly to nearest receiving hospital.
• Provide an alert/information call.
• Continue patient management en-route.
• Consider alternative care pathway where appropriate

Figure 3.5 – Assessment and management of chronic obstructive pulmonary disease algorithm.

Chronic Obstructive Pulmonary Disease

TABLE 3.32 – Factors to consider when deciding where to treat a person with COPD

Factor	Treat at home	Treat in hospital
Able to cope at home	Yes	No
Breathlessness	Mild	Severe
General condition	Good	Poor/deteriorating
Level of activity	Good	Poor/confined to bed
Cyanosis	No	Yes
Worsening peripheral oedema	No	Yes
Level of consciousness	Normal	Impaired
Already receiving long-term oxygen therapy	No	Yes
Social circumstances	Good	Living alone/not coping
Acute confusion	No	Yes
Rapid rate of onset	No	Yes
Significant co-morbidity (particularly cardiac disease and insulin-dependent diabetes)	No	Yes
SpO_2 <90%	No	Yes

KEY POINTS!

Chronic Obstructive Pulmonary Disease

- **Early respiratory assessment (including oxygen saturation) is vital.**
- **If in doubt, provide oxygen therapy, titrating en-route, aiming for oxygen saturation of 88–92%.**
- **Provide nebulisation with salbutamol and assess response.**

Bibliography

1. National Institute for Health and Clinical Excellence. Chronic obstructive pulmonary disease in over 16s: diagnosis and management. London: NICE, 2018. Available from: https://www.nice.org.uk/guidance/ng115/chapter/Recommendations#managing-exacerbations-of-copd.
2. British Thoracic Society Emergency Oxygen Guideline Development Group. BTS Guideline for Oxygen Use in Adults in Healthcare and Emergency Settings. Thorax: An International Journal of Respiratory Medicine. 2017, 72:1. Available from: https://www.brit-thoracic.org.uk/document-library/clinical-information/oxygen/2017-emergency-oxygen-guideline/bts-guideline-for-oxygen-use-in-adults-in-healthcare-and-emergency-settings/.
3. Rubin BK, Dhand R, Ruppel GL, Branson RD, Hess DR. Respiratory care year in review 2010. Part 1: Asthma, COPD, pulmonary function testing, ventilator-associated pneumonia. Respiratory Care 2011, 56(4): 488–502.
4. Austin MA, Wills KE, Blizzard L, Walters EH, Wood-Baker R. Effect of high flow oxygen on mortality in chronic obstructive pulmonary disease patients in pre-hospital setting: randomised controlled trial. British Medical Journal 2010, 341: c5462.
5. Austin MA, Wood-Baker R. Oxygen therapy in the pre-hospital setting for acute exacerbations of chronic obstructive pulmonary disease. Cochrane Database of Systematic Reviews 2006, 3: doi 10.1002/14651858.CD005534.pub2. Available from: http://www.mrw.interscience.wiley.com/cochrane/clsysrev/articles/CD005534/frame.html.
6. National Institute for Health and Clinical Excellence. Chronic Obstructive Pulmonary Disease: Management of chronic obstructive pulmonary disease in adults in primary and secondary care (partial update) (CG101). London: NICE, 2010. Available from: http://www.nice.org.uk/nicemedia/live/13029/49397/49397.pdf.
7. NHS Evidence. COPD. Available from: http://www.evidence.nhs.uk/topic/chronic-obstructive-pulmonarydisease?q=copd, 2012.
8. Ram FSF, Picot J, Lightowler J, Wedzicha JA. Non-invasive positive pressure ventilation for treatment of respiratory failure due to exacerbations of chronic obstructive pulmonary disease. Cochrane Database of Systematic Reviews 2004, 3: doi 10.1002/14651858.CD004104.pub3.
9. Schmidbauer W, Ahlers O, Spies C, Dreyer A, Mager G, Kerner T. Early pre-hospital use of non-invasive ventilation improves acute respiratory failure in acute exacerbation of chronic obstructive pulmonary disease. Emergency Medicine Journal 2011, 28(7): 626–7.
10. The Global Initiative for Chronic Obstructive Lung Disease. Global Strategy for Diagnosis, Management, and Prevention of COPD. Available from: http://goldcopd.org/gold-2017-global-strategy-diagnosis-management-prevention-copd/, 2011.
11. Uronis H, McCrory DC, Samsa G, Currow D, Abernethy A. Symptomatic oxygen for non-hypoxaemic chronic obstructive pulmonary disease. Cochrane Database of Systematic Reviews 2011, 6: doi 10.1002/14651858.

CD006429.pub2. Available from: http://www.mrw.interscience.wiley.com/cochrane/clsysrev/articles/CD006429/frame.html.

12. O'Driscoll BR, Howard LS, Davison AG, on behalf of the British Thoracic Society. BTS guideline for emergency oxygen use in adult patients. Thorax 2008, 63(suppl. 6): vi1–vi68.

13. Healthcare Commission. Clearing the Air: A national study of chronic obstructive pulmonary disease. London: Healthcare Commission, 2006.

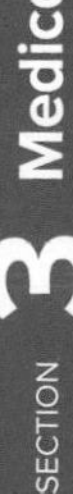

Convulsions in Adults

1. Introduction

- A convulsion is an involuntary contraction and relaxation of the muscles producing rigidity and violent shaking of the body and limbs. Convulsions are often associated with altered/ reduced consciousness; refer to **Altered Level of Consciousness**.
- The most common causes of convulsions are seizures in the context of epilepsy, provoked (acute symptomatic) seizures, psychogenic non-epileptic seizures (PNES), vasovagal syncope and cardiogenic events. The full list of causes is long and beyond the scope of this guideline. Other JRCALC guidelines are potentially relevant to the assessment of these patients and are cited here where appropriate.
- Eclampsia is a complication of pregnancy which may occur in women who are ≥20 weeks pregnant (including post-partum) and can give rise to seizures. Eclamptic seizures are beyond the scope of this guideline. Refer to **Pregnancy-induced Hypertension (including Eclampsia)** for the assessment and management of convulsions in patients who are ≥20 weeks pregnant.

2. Epileptic Seizures

- Epileptic seizures are caused by abnormal electrical activity in the brain. There are many types of epileptic seizures. The manifestations of seizures depend on which part of the brain is affected. This guideline focuses on bilateral tonic-clonic seizures (BTCS), which are the most common type of seizure, and present as stiffening of the whole body (tonic phase), gradually merging into vigorous shaking (clonic phase). During a BTCS patients typically have their eyes open and are unresponsive to commands or sensory stimuli. Most BTCS terminate within 90 seconds of their onset, afterwards patients are often confused and/or drowsy.
- A BTCS that has not stopped after 5 minutes, or a series of such seizures without recovery in-between which lasts for 5 minutes or more, is defined as convulsive status epilepticus (CSE). This is a medical emergency and requires rapid treatment. However, many patients with prolonged convulsions are having a psychogenic seizure, which can resemble a BTCS, see section 3. It may be difficult to distinguish between BTCS and PNES but some features are important in making this distinction (refer to Table 3.33).
- Seizures often start in only one part of the brain (a focal seizure) and then spread through the brain to cause a BTCS. Consciousness may be retained in focal seizures (also called an aura). The manifestations of all types of epileptic seizures are very diverse and their description is beyond the scope of this guideline which focuses on BTCS.
- Epilepsy is a chronic disorder in which patients are at increased risk of unprovoked seizures. Epileptic seizures also occur as 'provoked' (acute symptomatic) seizures caused by irritation of the brain, for instance by head injury, stroke, alcohol, hypoglycaemia, drug overdose or infection. The provoking factor may itself require emergency treatment.
- Many patients with epilepsy have an emergency care plan. They may also have a supply of emergency medication (usually midazolam), which can be administered by carers or healthcare professionals according to the care plan.

3. Psychogenic Non-Epileptic Seizures (PNES)

- PNES are a common cause of prolonged convulsions. PNES are the most important differential diagnosis of epileptic convulsions in the emergency setting. PNES are usually an involuntary psychological response to distress and are commonly associated with a history of emotional trauma (abuse or neglect, potentially in childhood). Patients with PNES have commonly received an erroneous diagnosis of epilepsy and many are treated with antiepileptic drugs which are ineffective in this condition. Those who have received a diagnosis of PNES may know their condition by another name e.g. non-epileptic attack disorder (NEAD), dissociative seizures, functional seizures, conversion disorder or pseudo-seizures.
- In contrast to convulsions caused by epilepsy, convulsive activity in PNES often continues for more than 5 minutes and PNES are commonly mistaken for status epilepticus. See Table 3.33 for a guide on distinguishing PNES from status epilepticus. Even prolonged PNES do not put the patient at risk of physiological derangement or brain damage. Emergency drug treatment is not effective and is potentially dangerous because it puts patients at risk of the side effects including respiratory depression, aspiration and death. Many patients with PNES have an emergency care plan which should be taken into account in decisions about treatment.
- Because of the similarity of PNES and convulsive status epilepticus it is important to note and to record the characteristics of the convulsions as accurately as possible. This aids assessment and treatment during the convulsion but it also assists specialists in making the diagnosis in retrospect. For the same reason, families and carers may have been asked to video record the events by specialists, and they should be encouraged to do so.

Convulsions in Adults

TABLE 3.33 – Features which help to distinguish between BTCS and PNES	
Signs that favour Bilateral Tonic Clonic Seizures	**Signs that favour Psychogenic Non-Epileptic Seizures**
BTCS: during convulsion	**PNES: during convulsion**
● Consistent, repeated, rhythmic myoclonic jerking	● Fluctuating intensity/location
● 'Shock like' movement	● Brief pauses, tremor or slow flexion/extension movements
● Arms & legs mostly synchronised/symmetrical	● Arms & legs often not synchronised/symmetrical
● Convulsion may spread from focal to generalised and tonic merging to clonic	● Convulsion may move from one body area to another
● Unresponsive (GCS 3 [4 if grunting])	● May respond in some way (e.g. to speech, blink reflex, or on NPA or IV insertion)
● Lateral tongue biting common	● Tongue biting rare/minor/involves tip
● Eyes often open	● Eyes mostly shut (opening may be resisted)
● Mouth often open	● Mouth often shut
● Pupils not reacting	● Pupils reacting
● No purposeful movements	● May carry out purposeful movements
● Low SpO_2 or cyanosis	● Normal SpO_2, no cyanosis, hyperventilation
● Typically short (<90 secs) or repeated without recovery between (constant prolonged are rare)	● May be prolonged (>3 mins)
● Pelvic thrusting rare	● Pelvic thrusting common
● Arching of the head, neck, and spine rare	● Arching of the head, neck, and spine common
● Clonic head movements to one side may occur	● Side-to-side movements of the head/body
● Initial scream, then grunting	● Crying during/after convulsion
● Plantar response may be abnormal (big toe up)	● Plantar response normal (big toe flexed down)
BTCS: post-ictal (after the convulsion)	**PNES: post-ictal (after the convulsion)**
● Gradual slowing down of convulsion	● Rapid end to convulsion
● Gradual post-ictal recovery	● Rapid post-ictal recovery
● Noisy laboured post-ictal breathing	● Normal post-ictal breathing (or slow after hyperventilation)
BTCS: history	**PNES: history**
● Onset under 10 years old	● Onset over 15 years old
● Alcohol misuse	● Recurrent 'status epilepticus' (a misdiagnosis)
● Provoked seizure (e.g. brain injury)	● PTSD or psychological distress

4. Syncope

- Vasovagal syncope (fainting) is the most common cause of transient loss of consciousness. It is caused by a temporary disruption to the supply of oxygen and glucose to the brain due to a fall in cerebral blood pressure. Vasovagal syncope usually happens when the person is upright, especially just after standing up, but it can occur whilst sitting especially when provoked by intercurrent illness, medical procedures, drugs, dehydration, alcohol and loss of bodily fluids, such as might occur with vomiting, bleeding or diarrhoea. In men, syncope is sometimes provoked by passing of urine while standing. People who faint usually feel dizzy and sweaty, get blurred vision and may experience distortion of hearing before they collapse. Brief but vigorous jerking may occur. This can mimic an epileptic seizure, although the jerking usually stops within less than twenty seconds, once normal cerebral circulation is restored. When the patient is supine, recovery is rapid, and the patient may be able to hear what is going on around them before they can respond verbally. Patients may faint again if they sit up before their blood pressure and heart rate have stabilised.

- Syncope can also be caused by cardiac dysrhythmia (tachycardia or bradycardia) when it is known as cardiac syncope, refer to **Cardiac Rhythm Disturbance**, but this is much less common than vasovagal syncope. Cardiac syncope can occur whilst resting but it is more likely to occur during exercise. Pre-existing heart disease is a risk factor for cardiac syncope. Cardiac syncope can cause impairment of consciousness lasting for over one minute and decerebrate posturing (tonic extension of the limbs and neck), but is not likely to cause convulsive movements lasting longer than 20 seconds.

5. Alcohol

- Alcohol is an important cause of convulsions and collapse. Acute intoxication is a cause of reduced/lost consciousness. Alcohol withdrawal and delirium tremens is a cause of seizures and requires urgent medical treatment. Chronic alcohol overuse predisposes to seizures. Consider referring the patient to an alcohol misuse service as per locally agreed pathways.

6. Driving

- The DVLA has specific and legal regulations regarding convulsions and other causes of lost/altered consciousness. Epileptic seizures and the other conditions mentioned in this guideline are a common medical cause of collapse at the wheel. It is a legal requirement for drivers to inform the DVLA themselves if they have a medical condition that could affect driving.
- When it is appropriate, particularly when discharging a patient who is a driver and not conveying them to a health care facility ambulance clinicians should:
  - advise the patient on the possible impact of their medical condition for safe driving ability.
  - advise the patient on their legal requirement to notify the DVLA about seizures.
  - document any of the above if it is discussed with the patient.

Note that the patient could be fined up to £1,000 if they do not tell the DVLA about a medical condition that affects their driving, and that they could be prosecuted if they are involved in an accident as a result.

If an ambulance clinician is concerned that the patient cannot or will not notify the DVLA themselves it would be appropriate to liaise with the patient's GP and to document these actions.

7. Assessment and Management

Assessment and management of convulsions varies according to whether the convulsion is ongoing/recurrent or has stopped, see Figure 3.6. If the convulsion is ongoing or recurrent, refer to Table 3.34. If the convulsion has stopped, refer to Table 3.35.

8. Emergency Medical Treatment

First dose benzodiazepines

Refer to **Midazolam** and **Diazepam**.

Other doses of benzodiazepines previously administered during this episode of care, for example by carers, should be considered and subtracted from the maximum cumulative dose unless there was clear evidence it was not absorbed.

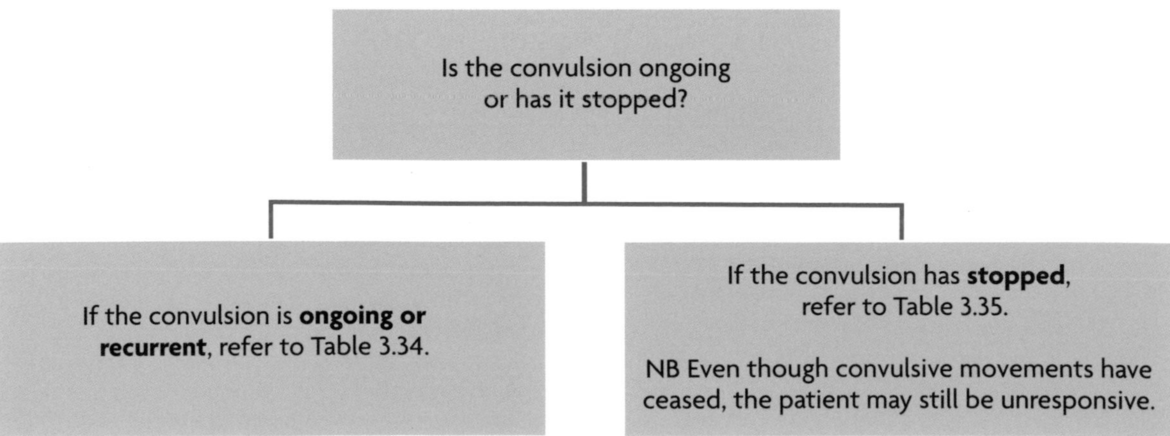
Is the convulsion ongoing or has it stopped?
If the convulsion is ongoing or recurrent, refer to Table 3.34.
If the convulsion has stopped, refer to Table 3.35.
NB Even though convulsive movements have ceased, the patient may still be unresponsive.

Figure 3.6 – Initial assessment and management of convulsions in adults.

Convulsions in Adults

TABLE 3.34 – Assessment and Management of: ONGOING/RECURRENT Adult Convulsions

General	
ASSESSMENT Assess **<C>ABCDE**	**MANAGEMENT** ● Assess for, and simultaneously manage, immediately life-threatening conditions using the **<C>ABCDE** approach.
Correct position	● Position the patient for safety and comfort. Protect from dangers especially aspiration and head injuries during the convulsion.
History	● Take a focussed history while simultaneously managing **<C>ABCDE**. Establish key information from carers/witnesses (if there are any available). The history should be taken from the most appropriate person(s) and at the most appropriate time throughout the assessment/ management of the patient. Consider all causes of convulsions especially potential provoking factors for epileptic seizures. Try to establish: – an estimate of the duration of the convulsion. – whether the patient already has a diagnosis of epilepsy or PNES (and if there is a history of previous convulsions regardless of formal diagnoses made by doctors). – if this is an isolated seizure or if there has been a cluster of seizures. – whether any medication has already been administered to terminate the seizure. – if there were any symptoms preceding the seizure providing hints to its underlying cause and the need for additional emergency interventions (eg. treatment of hypoglycaemia, thiamine deficiency, meningitis). – if the patient is pregnant and the gestational age ≥20 weeks suspect eclampsia and refer to **Pregnancy-induced Hypertension (including Eclampsia)**. – relevant past medical history (including diabetes, hypertension, heart disease) and medication use. – alcohol intake. – potential provoking factors.
Observe/inspect	● Observe and record types of movements (see Table 3.33).
Airway	
Assess and manage as appropriate	● Consider an oropharyngeal airway but do not attempt to force an oropharyngeal airway into a convulsing patient if there is trismus or if it is not tolerated. Inability to tolerate an airway adjunct is suggestive of a GCS>3, which is not consistent with a BTCS. A nasopharyngeal airway can be a useful adjunct.
Breathing	
Assess breathing rate and quality	● BTCS cause cessation of effective respiration. PNES may involve breath holding interspersed with periods of hyperventilation. Refer to **Hyperventilation Syndrome** guideline if relevant. ● For BTCS administer high concentration oxygen using a reservoir mask at 15 L/min, until a reliable oximetry measurement can be obtained; clinicians should then aim for an oxygen saturation of 94–98% (or 88–92% if the patient is at risk of hypercapnic respiratory failure e.g. COPD). Refer to **Oxygen** guideline. ● If assessment indicates this convulsion is PNES, then oxygen should **not** normally be administered; measure oxygen saturation and only administer oxygen if it is actually required (SpO_2 of 93% or less).

(continued)

TABLE 3.34 – Assessment and Management of: ONGOING/RECURRENT Adult Convulsions *(continued)*	
	● In CSE, if pulse oximetry is low and/or end tidal CO_2 is high, and respirations are ineffective, then assist ventilations with a bag-valve-mask device (with suitable airway adjuncts, and supplemental oxygen); this may be difficult during a convulsion (but will be possible if there are pauses between convulsions, or in the post-ictal period). ● Administration of medicines for the convulsion should not be delayed, as treating the convulsion can improve ventilation (indeed there is a higher rate of respiratory compromise in status epilepticus where patients are not treated with benzodiazepines, than in those who are). Refer to Figure 3.7 and the **Midazolam** and **Diazepam** guidelines.
Circulation	
Blood pressure	● Measure BP as soon as possible. Consider eclampsia as a cause of hypertension if the patient is pregnant (gestational age ≥20 weeks). Refer to **Pregnancy-induced Hypertension (including Eclampsia)** guideline.
Heart rate and rhythm IV access	● Monitor heart rate and rhythm. Cardiac dysrhythmia can cause transient loss of consciousness and convulsions (hypoxic seizures). However, sinus tachycardia is normal during epileptic seizures or PNES. Refer to **Cardiac Rhythm Disturbance** guideline if relevant. Record a 12-lead ECG when possible where the diagnosis is unclear. Document your interpretation of the ECG. ● Rarely epileptic seizures or status epilepticus can trigger abnormal heart rhythms requiring ECG monitoring or even defibrillation. ● Assess the need for IV access taking into account individual circumstances. Consider the possible need for IV administration of emergency drugs taking into account the choice of drug and the alternative routes of administration.
Disability	
Consciousness	● Assess consciousness using AVPU and GCS. Take special care to record how the patient responds to voice and provide an opportunity for the patient to respond by grunting or moving part of a limb (e.g. squeezing the hand of the examiner). Ongoing convulsions in patients who are responsive are likely to be PNES. Refer to Table 3.33.
Blood glucose level	● Measure capillary blood glucose and document the result. If glucose is <4mmol/L, treat according to **Glycaemic Emergencies in Adults and Children** guideline.
Exposure	
Temperature	● Measure temperature. A raised temperature may indicate that the patient has an infection. Consider cerebral infections especially meningococcal meningitis. Refer to **Meningococcal Meningitis and Septicaemia** if this is suspected. Epileptic epileptic seizures can cause a rise in body temperature in the absence of infection.
Injuries	● A head injury may be the cause of a convulsion, i.e. a provoked seizure. This may have occurred in the context of a major trauma or RTC. Treat the **Head Injury** and the convulsion in parallel. ● Convulsions may cause injuries. Treat injuries as appropriate. Common minor injuries are facial contusions, dental injuries, joint dislocation and trauma to the tongue and lips. These should be noted even if they do not require immediate treatment because they are important factors for specialists to consider when trying to make a diagnosis in retrospect.
Incontinence	● Urinary incontinence regularly occurs in epileptic seizures and PNES. It is also reported by patients with vasovagal episodes (rarely). It is not a good discriminator between epileptic seizures and PNES, but it is an important feature and it should be noted.

Convulsions in Adults

TABLE 3.34 – Assessment and Management of: ONGOING/RECURRENT Adult Convulsions *(continued)*	
Rash	• Look for a non-blanching rash. A purpuric rash and fever is highly predictive of meningococcal infection / meningitis, which can cause seizures. Refer to **Meningococcal Meningitis and Septicaemia** guideline.
Pregnancy	• Examine the abdomen of female patients. Is there a palpable uterus that indicates a second/third trimester pregnancy and the possibility of eclampsia? If so, refer to **Pregnancy-induced Hypertension (including Eclampsia)**.
Description of the seizure	• Because of the similarity of PNES to convulsive status epilepticus it is important to note and to record the characteristics of the convulsions as accurately as possible. This aids assessment and treatment during the convulsion but it also assists specialists in making the diagnosis in retrospect. For the same reason, families and carers may have been asked to video record the events by specialists and they should be encouraged to do so.
Conveyance and referral	
	Most seizures will stop spontaneously. A small proportion will require emergency medical treatment for CSE; many will respond to this treatment and the seizure will terminate. A priority is therefore timely and effective delivery of a dose(s) of a benzodiazepine drug via the optimal route of administration and then appropriate supportive care. A small proportion of patients will not respond to benzodiazepine treatment and will require a time critical transport to hospital. Preparing and transferring the patient for conveyance is therefore a competing priority, decisions about how long to treat at the scene, when to transport and to what extent these treatment and conveyance can happen simultaneously need to be made on a case-by-case basis. The following factors should be taken into account: • Time since onset of seizure(s) • Diagnosis (status epilepticus, PNES, uncertainty) • Relative ease or difficulty of extricating the patient to the ambulance • Distance from hospital and transport time • Availability of an effective drug and route of administration • Co-existing acute or chronic medical conditions

TABLE 3.35 – Assessment and Management of: STOPPED Adult Convulsions	
General	
ASSESSMENT	**MANAGEMENT**
Assess **<C>ABCDE**	• Assess for, and simultaneously manage, immediately life-threatening conditions using the **<C>ABCDE** approach. • Most patients will spontaneously make a full recovery after a convulsion. The aim for these patients is to support them as they recover. However, all patients should undergo a careful assessment once their convulsion has stopped to identify the small number with a serious underlying illness as well as those patients who have sustained serious injuries during the seizure.
Correct position	• Position the patient for comfort and protect from dangers, especially aspiration if the patient remains obtunded. Consider placing in the recovery position.

(continued)

Convulsions in Adults

TABLE 3.35 – Assessment and Management of: STOPPED Adult Convulsions *(continued)*	
History	• Take a focussed history, including previous episodes, while simultaneously managing **<C>ABCDE**. After an epileptic seizure patients are often confused, drowsy and agitated. It can take minutes or hours to return to normal consciousness and they are unlikely to be able to give a reliable history immediately after a seizure. After a PNES and syncope the recovery is usually more rapid. Establish key information from carers/witnesses (if there are any available). The history should be taken from the most appropriate person(s) and at the most appropriate time throughout the assessment/management of the patient. Consider all causes of convulsions especially potential provoking factors for epileptic seizures. Try to establish: – an estimate of the duration of the seizure. – whether the patient already has a diagnosis of epilepsy or PNES (and if there is a history of previous convulsions regardless of formal diagnosis). – if this an isolated seizure or if there has been a cluster of seizures. – whether any medication has already been administered to terminate the seizure. – if there were any symptoms preceding the seizure providing hints to its underlying cause / need for additional emergency interventions (eg. treatment of hypoglycaemia, thiamine deficiency, meningitis). – if the patient is pregnant and the gestational age ≥20 weeks suspect eclampsia and refer to **Pregnancy-induced Hypertension (including Eclampsia)**. – relevant past medical history (including diabetes, hypertension, heart disease) and medication use. – alcohol intake. – potential provoking factors.
Airway	
Assess and manage as appropriate	• Consider an oropharyngeal or nasopharyngeal airway.
Breathing	
Assess breathing rate and quality	• Respiration usually rapidly returns to normal after cessation of a convulsion. • Measure oxygen saturations and only administer oxygen if it is actually required (SpO_2 of 93% or less). Refer to **Oxygen** guideline. • If assessment indicates this convulsion is PNES, then oxygen should **not** normally be administered.
Circulation	
Blood pressure	• Measure BP. Consider eclampsia as a cause of hypertension if the patient is pregnant (gestational age ≥20 weeks).
Heart rate and rhythm	• Monitor heart rate and rhythm. Perform a 12-lead ECG if the diagnosis is unclear. Document your interpretation of the ECG. Cardiac arrhythmias are an important cause of transient loss of consciousness and suspected seizures, so an ECG is an important part of the assessment of a patient after a convulsion.
IV access	• Assess the risk of another convulsion and the potential need for IV access taking into account individual circumstances. Consider the possible need for IV administration of emergency drugs taking into account the choice of drug and the alternative routes of administration.

Convulsions in Adults

TABLE 3.35 – Assessment and Management of: STOPPED Adult Convulsions *(continued)*	
Disability	
Consciousness	• Assess consciousness using AVPU and GCS. If improving, wait 10 minutes and repeat. Take special care to record how the patient responds to voice and provide an opportunity for the patient to respond by grunting or moving part of a limb (e.g. squeezing the hand of the examiner). Refer to Table 3.33. • After an epileptic seizure, patients are often left confused, tired and aching (this is the postictal state). The confusion usually resolves relatively rapidly leaving the patient alert with a GCS of 15/15. Tiredness, aching and amnesia may persist longer than this, but it is not a cause for concern.
Blood glucose level	• Measure capillary blood glucose and document the result. If glucose is <4mmol/L, treat according to **Glycaemic Emergencies in Adults and Children** guideline.
Exposure	
Temperature	• Measure temperature. A raised temperature may indicate that the patient has an infection. Consider cerebral infections especially meningococcal meningitis. Refer to **Meningococcal Meningitis and Septicaemia** if this is suspected. Epileptic seizures can also lead to a temporary rise in body temperature in the absence of infection.
Injuries	• Treat injuries as appropriate. • A head injury may be the cause of a convulsion, i.e. a provoked seizure. This may have occurred in the context of a major trauma or RTC. Treat the head injury and the convulsion in parallel. • Convulsions may cause injuries. Common minor injuries are facial contusions, dental injuries, joint dislocation and trauma to the tongue from biting. These should be noted even if they do not require immediate treatment because they are important factors for specialists to consider when trying to make a diagnosis in retrospect.
Incontinence	• Urinary incontinence regularly occurs in epileptic seizures and PNES. It is also reported by patients with vasovagal episodes (rarely). It is not a good discriminator between epileptic seizures and PNES, but it is an important feature and it should be noted.
Rash	• Look for a non-blanching rash. A purpuric rash and fever is highly predictive of meningococcal infection / meningitis, which can cause seizures. Refer to **Meningococcal Meningitis and Septicaemia** guideline.
Pregnancy	• Examine the abdomen of female patients. Is there a palpable uterus that indicates a second/third trimester pregnancy and the possibility of eclampsia? If so, refer to **Pregnancy-induced Hypertension (including Eclampsia)**.
Description of the seizure	• An accurate assessment, including a detailed description of events, is very important during and after a convulsion. Based on witness accounts and the events that you witnessed write a detailed account of the events.
Conveyance and referral	
	• All patients with a first seizure must be conveyed to hospital. • The decision whether to convey a patient to hospital after a convulsion is difficult. The overall risk of adverse events is low and most patients do not require the facilities of a hospital emergency department. But it is important to accurately identify those patients who do need transport to hospital. The following factors should be considered when making this decision: – Single or serial convulsions. – Known seizure disorder.

(continued)

SECTION 3 Medical Emergencies

Convulsions in Adults

TABLE 3.35 – Assessment and Management of: STOPPED Adult Convulsions *(continued)*	
	– Extent of neurological recovery. – Level of support / supervision. Availability of suitable care pathways. – Care plan. – Injuries. – Treatment with benzodiazepines (these patients should always be transported to hospital unless their care plan states otherwise). – Co-morbidities including frailty. – The patient's wishes, assuming that they have mental capacity. Refer to **Mental Capacity Act** guideline. – Refer to **Pregnancy-induced Hypertension (including Eclampsia)**. ● For patients who are not conveyed: – Document the justification for the decision not to convey. – Advise them to make an appointment with their epilepsy specialist or GP to discuss the events and provide them with a copy of the PRF if possible. – Use an alternative care pathway if one is available, for example referral to an epilepsy specialist nurse team. – Advise patients/carers to dial 999 if there are further convulsions. – Provide written advice if possible or leave a relevant patient information leaflet. – Advise the patient about driving and DVLA regulations.

Midazolam

- If buccal midazolam is immediately available use this (do not use PR diazepam or delay administration by attempting IV access).
- Ambulance clinicians can administer the patient's own buccal midazolam provided they are competent to administer buccal medications and are familiar with midazolam's indications, actions and side effects, which are very similar to diazepam although midazolam is shorter acting.
- Midazolam is probably more effective than diazepam.

Diazepam

- If no midazolam is available, and IV access is unlikely to be obtained quickly, administer PR diazepam.
- If IV access has previously been achieved, IV diazepam can be given instead.

After the 1st dose

- Convulsive status epilepticus is an emergency, and can cause permanent brain damage or even death. If IV access is difficult then IO access (where available) should be used.
- The aim should be to have IV access within 10 minutes of the first dose.

Second dose benzodiazepines

- If the convulsion is continuing **10 minutes** after the first benzodiazepine has been given, a dose of IV diazepam should be administered.
- Only if IV or IO access has proved impossible should the second dose be given buccally (midazolam) or PR (diazepam).
- Do not delay the second dose.
- If the convulsion continues 10 minutes after the second dose, then seek senior clinical advice to consider:
  - alternative diagnoses, including PNES.
  - reasons for lack of effect, such as poor administration/absorption, patient size or inadequate dose.
  - any access to alternative second line anti-convulsant.
  - the risks/benefits of a third dose of benzodiazepine. The risk of side effects increases with the number of doses and the effectiveness of the drug decreases over the duration of the convulsion.
- Consider asking for senior clinical advice from a prescriber to consider a third dose of IV/IO benzodiazepine, if no alternative anticonvulsant available and the patient is still another 15 minutes or more from hospital i.e. a total of 25 minutes from the end of last dose.
- After prolonged convulsions or drug treatment prepare for airway obstruction, respiratory depression, hypotension and cardiac arrhythmia, particularly if they have also received opiates, additional benzodiazepines or alternative central nervous system depressants.

Convulsions in Adults

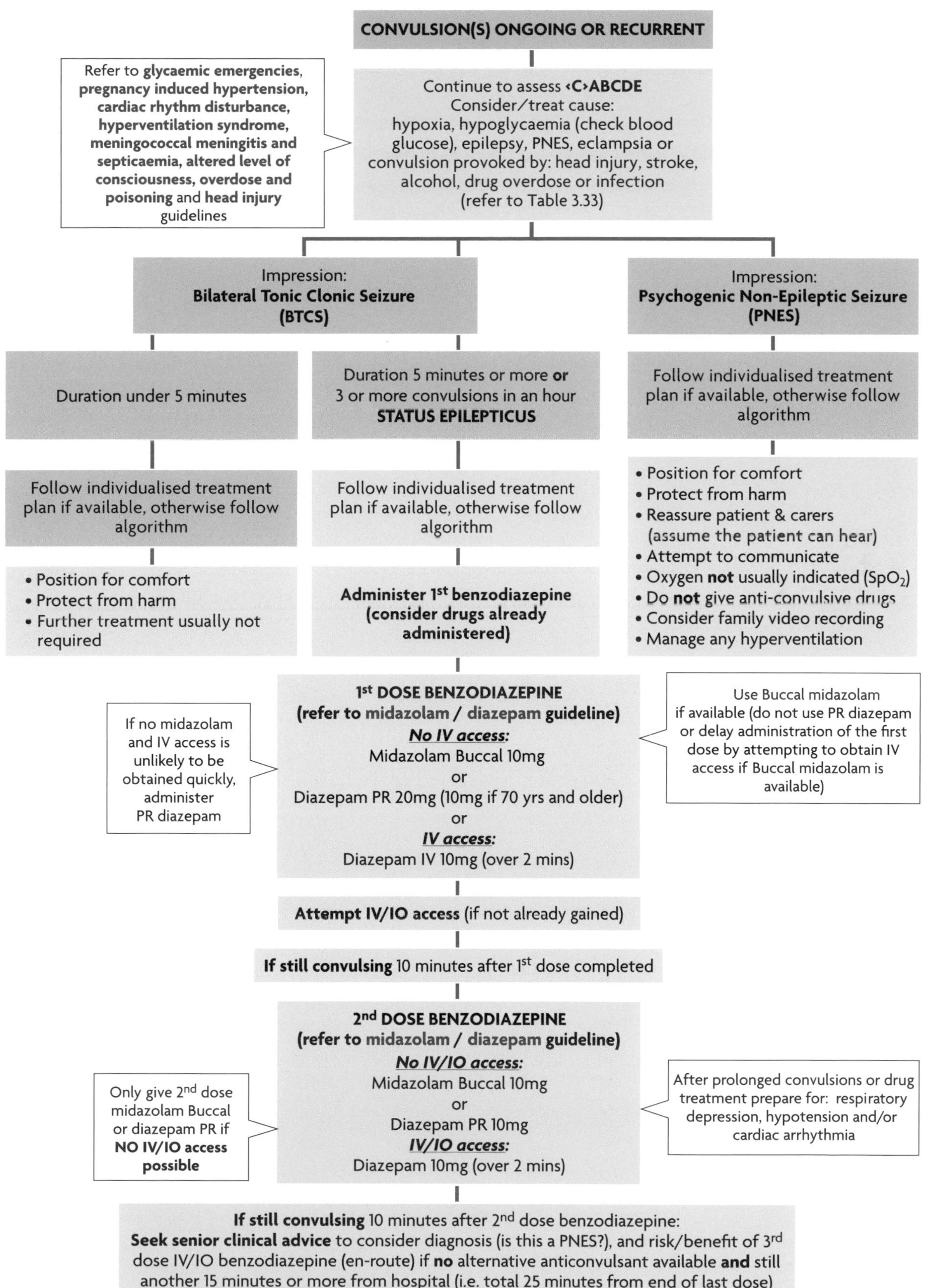

CONVULSION(S) ONGOING OR RECURRENT
Refer to glycaemic emergencies, pregnancy induced hypertension, cardiac rhythm disturbance, hyperventilation syndrome, meningococcal meningitis and septicaemia, altered level of consciousness, overdose and poisoning and head injury guidelines
Continue to assess ‹C›ABCDE
Consider/treat cause:
hypoxia, hypoglycaemia (check blood glucose), epilepsy, PNES, eclampsia or convulsion provoked by: head injury, stroke, alcohol, drug overdose or infection
(refer to Table 3.33)
Impression:
Bilateral Tonic Clonic Seizure (BTCS)
Impression:
Psychogenic Non-Epileptic Seizure (PNES)
Duration under 5 minutes
Duration 5 minutes or more or 3 or more convulsions in an hour
STATUS EPILEPTICUS
Follow individualised treatment plan if available, otherwise follow algorithm
Follow individualised treatment plan if available, otherwise follow algorithm
Follow individualised treatment plan if available, otherwise follow algorithm
• Position for comfort
• Protect from harm
• Further treatment usually not required
Administer 1st benzodiazepine (consider drugs already administered)
• Position for comfort
• Protect from harm
• Reassure patient & carers (assume the patient can hear)
• Attempt to communicate
• Oxygen not usually indicated (SpO2)
• Do not give anti-convulsive drugs
• Consider family video recording
• Manage any hyperventilation
If no midazolam and IV access is unlikely to be obtained quickly, administer PR diazepam
1st DOSE BENZODIAZEPINE
(refer to midazolam / diazepam guideline)
No IV access:
Midazolam Buccal 10mg
or
Diazepam PR 20mg (10mg if 70 yrs and older)
or
IV access:
Diazepam IV 10mg (over 2 mins)
Use Buccal midazolam if available (do not use PR diazepam or delay administration of the first dose by attempting to obtain IV access if Buccal midazolam is available)
Attempt IV/IO access (if not already gained)
If still convulsing 10 minutes after 1st dose completed
Only give 2nd dose midazolam Buccal or diazepam PR if NO IV/IO access possible
2nd DOSE BENZODIAZEPINE
(refer to midazolam / diazepam guideline)
No IV/IO access:
Midazolam Buccal 10mg
or
Diazepam PR 10mg
IV/IO access:
Diazepam 10mg (over 2 mins)
After prolonged convulsions or drug treatment prepare for: respiratory depression, hypotension and/or cardiac arrhythmia
If still convulsing 10 minutes after 2nd dose benzodiazepine:
Seek senior clinical advice to consider diagnosis (is this a PNES?), and risk/benefit of 3rd dose IV/IO benzodiazepine (en-route) if no alternative anticonvulsant available and still another 15 minutes or more from hospital (i.e. total 25 minutes from end of last dose)

Figure 3.7 – Emergency medical treatment algorithm for adult convulsions: ongoing or recurrent

Convulsions in Adults

KEY POINTS!

- **Psychogenic non-epileptic seizures (PNES) are the most important differential diagnosis of epileptic convulsions.**
- **Most bilateral tonic-clonic seizures (BTCS) are self-limiting and do not require drug treatment.**
- **All patients with a first seizure should be conveyed to hospital.**
- **Administer medicines if a convulsion lasts longer than 5 minutes or the patient has 3 or more convulsions in an hour.**
- **Consider referral to an epilepsy specialist nurse team or an alternative care pathway for patients who are not conveyed.**
- **If the patient is pregnant and gestational age ≥22 weeks, suspect eclampsia.**

Convulsions in Children

1. Introduction

- Convulsions (also called 'tonic-clonic seizure' or 'fit') arise from abnormal electrical activity in the brain. They are usually **generalised** (affecting both sides of the body), but may also be **focal**, affecting just one side of the body. Fever is the commonest cause for convulsions (febrile convulsions) but they can also be caused by epilepsy, CNS infections (meningitis or encephalitis), hypoglycaemia, hypoxia, electrolyte imbalances, head injuries or (rarely) hypertension. Occasionally, cardiac arrest can be the presenting feature of an initial convulsion.
- Most convulsions stop within 4 minutes (>90%). After 5 minutes, a convulsion is unlikely to stop spontaneously. Prolonged fits become harder to stop with anticonvulsants. As a consequence, if a convulsion has not stopped within 5 minutes of its start, emergency (rescue) medication should be given.
- During febrile illnesses, small children (aged 6 months to 5 years) may develop febrile convulsions. These are not epilepsy. They can be seen in up to 1 in 20 children.
- A child having convulsions that are not triggered by fever requires further investigation.

2. Incidence

- 1 in 200 people have active epilepsy.
- It is twice as common in children as in adults.
- It can be related to another underlying condition such as cerebral palsy or a genetic disorder.
- Both meningitis and encephalitis cause fever and may cause convulsions (although these would not normally be classed as febrile convulsions).

3. Severity and Outcome

Febrile convulsions

- 66% of children only ever have the one febrile convulsion; the remainder may have further episodes during subsequent infections.
- 5% of children with febrile convulsions go on to develop epilepsy.

Convulsive Status Epilepticus (CSE)

- Convulsive status epilepticus is the most common neurological emergency in children.
- 1 in 20 febrile convulsions presents with CSE.
- 1 in 20 epileptic children have CSE (more common in children with Dravet syndrome and Lennox-Gastaut syndrome).
- CSE is defined as a convulsive seizure lasting 30 minutes or longer, or repeated tonic-clonic convulsions occurring over a 30 minute period without recovery of consciousness between each seizure.
- Prolonged convulsions (45–60 minutes or more) can result in death (observed mortality rate: 4%). They can also cause serious and irreversible consequences such as stroke, learning difficulties, visual impairment, behavioural problems and epilepsy. Adverse outcomes are more common in young children (<5 years of age).

4. Assessment

(Refer to Table 3.36)

- Correct hypoxia and seek an underlying cause for the seizure. Ensure the child is not hypoglycaemic.
- Document if the child was unwell or feverish before the convulsion, any serious past medical history and any important events immediately preceding the convulsion (e.g. head injury).
- When managing a febrile convulsion, it is not sufficient to simply manage the convulsion. It is vitally important to seek and identify the underlying infection producing the child's fever, especially if managing in the community (although this should not delay immediate treatment priorities or hospital transport).
- Seizures are a feature of meningitis – if the seizure has stopped and the child's condition permits, look for clinical signs (e.g. the typical rash of meningococcal septicaemia (and treat when present)).
- Establishing that a convulsion has fully stopped can be difficult. Following a tonic-clonic convulsion, the repeated, regular, rhythmic jerks of the limbs (the clonic phase of the seizure) become less frequent and eventually stop. In the following minutes, the child may show some or all of the following post-ictal ('post-convulsion') features:
  - brief and irregular jerks of one or more limbs
  - eye deviation
  - nystagmus (jerky eye movements to one side and then back to the midline)
  - noisy breathing.
- Since these features do not **necessarily** mean the child is still convulsing, additional emergency (rescue) medication (benzodiazepines) should not be given.
- Even when the above features are found to be part of an ongoing seizure, they are not thought to be harmful.
- Conversely, further doses of benzodiazepines can cause significant respiratory depression and respiratory arrest. When uncertain, do not give further benzodiazepines but transfer the child rapidly to hospital, for further assessment and ongoing treatment.

Convulsions in Children

5. Management

(Refer to Table 3.36 and Figures 3.8–3.9)

- This follows <C>ABCDE priorities, treating the convulsion once ABC issues have been addressed.
- Manage airway, breathing and circulation as usual (also remember to measure the blood glucose as hypoglycaemia can cause seizures). An oropharyngeal airway may be helpful to maintain airway patency (alternatively, if the jaw is clenched a nasopharyngeal airway may prove useful). Administer oxygen and treat shock in the usual way. Oxygen saturation monitoring and capnography (if available) should be applied.
- Epileptic children in the UK now carry individualised "Epilepsy Passports," containing essential information about their epilepsy, their emergency care plan and key professional

TABLE 3.36 – ASSESSMENT and MANAGEMENT of: Convulsions in Children	
ASSESSMENT	**MANAGEMENT**
Assess <C>ABCD	Treat problems as they are found. ● The airway must be cleared. – Oropharyngeal or nasopharyngeal airways may be helpful. ● Administer high levels of supplemental oxygen – refer to **Oxygen**. ● Assist ventilations with a BVM if necessary. ● Check blood glucose level and manage if low – refer to **Glycaemic Emergencies in Adults and Children**. ● Monitor vital signs. ● Manage the convulsion (see below).
Medication	● Administer an anticonvulsant. The first choice anticonvulsant is usually given buccally (midazolam) or rectally (diazepam): i. if the first convulsion lasts ≥5 minutes or ii. if the child has another convulsion that lasts ≥5 minutes within 10 minutes of the end of the first convulsion or iii. if the child continues to have brief (<5 minute) convulsions and has had three of these in a hour or has not regained consciousness between each convulsion. Ask whether the child has their own supply of medication. ● If the child **has** their own supply of medication: – if the child has their own buccal midazolam this should be used. – ask whether they have already received a dose, if not then administer the patient's own buccal midazolam*. ● If the child does **not** have their own buccal midazolam medication: – (and they have not yet received an anticonvulsant) give **buccal midazolam** (if carried) or (if midazolam is not available) **rectal diazepam** (refer to **Midazolam / Diazepam**)*. ● If the child **has already received an anticonvulsant** (e.g. rectal **diazepam** or **buccal midazolam**): – If the convulsion is continuing **10 minutes** after this first anticonvulsant, one dose of an intravenous or intra-osseous anticonvulsant should be given e.g. **diazepam** IV/IO (refer to **Diazepam**). ● If it is not possible to gain intravenous or intra-osseous access for the second dose of medication, the child **should** be given another full dose of buccal or rectal medication; as continuing convulsive activity is more dangerous than the risk of side effects e.g. respiratory depression. ● In very rare cases a child may continue in convulsive status epilepticus 10 minutes after a second full dose of benzodiazepine. If at that point in time the hospital is still over 15 minutes away (total 25 minutes after the second dose) then a third dose of anticonvulsant may be considered. This must **only** be intravenous or intra-osseous.* * **Be ready to support ventilation as respiratory depression may occur.**

TABLE 3.36 – ASSESSMENT and MANAGEMENT of: Convulsions in Children *(continued)*	
Other care	• Record the child's temperature. • If transporting to hospital, ongoing assessments of ABCDEs and continuous ECG and oxygen saturation monitoring (and $EtCO_2$ if available) should be undertaken, continuing **oxygen** therapy as needed. • If meningococcal septicaemia is diagnosed, treat with **benzylpenicillin** en-route to hospital (refer to **Benzylpenicillin**). • A child who has suffered a seizure and has a fever is likely to be distressed, therefore Paracetamol should be considered (refer to **Paracetamol**). • A febrile child should wear light clothing only. If the child begins to shiver (e.g. after stripping off all layers down to a nappy) this will potentially raise core temperature and will be counter productive.
Transfer to further care	The following should all be transported to hospital: • Any child who is still convulsing or in status epilepticus must be transferred to further care as soon as possible, preferably after the first dose of anticonvulsant – undertake a **TIME CRITICAL** transfer, provide an alert/information call. • Any child with suspected meningococcal septicaemia or meningitis – undertake a **TIME CRITICAL** transfer, provide an alert/information call. • All first febrile convulsions even if the child has recovered. • All children with seizures who have required more than one dose of anticonvulsant. • Any child ≤ 2 years old who has had a seizure (even if totally recovered). • Any child who has not fully recovered from their seizure. The following children may not require transport to hospital: • Children following a febrile convulsion: – that is **not their first** and – **who have completely recovered** and – **where the carer is happy for the child not to be transported** • may be left at home, providing that urgent review by the general practitioner (GP) or out of hours (OOH) GP is arranged to establish the cause of the fever. If this cannot be arranged by the attending crew, the child must be transported to hospital. • Children who have recovered from a convulsion and **who are known to have epilepsy (and have followed their normal pattern) and have not required more than one dose of medication need not be transported** if they are otherwise well.

contacts. These should be located, where possible, without delaying treatment.

- Most convulsions stop spontaneously (within 4 minutes).
- Anticonvulsant treatment should be given if the convulsion **has lasted 5 minutes or more or if the child has had three or more focal or generalised convulsions in an hour**. Pre-hospital treatments include **buccal midazolam** and **diazepam** (both rectal and intravenous preparations). Buccal midazolam is more effective than rectal diazepam but often diazepam is the only drug available. Both drugs may cause respiratory depression although this is uncommon.
- Do not delay the first dose of anticonvulsant medication whilst attempting venous access, for example use buccal or rectal routes.
- Before administration, ensure that the appropriate anticonvulsant dose for the child's weight and age is chosen, giving the **full** dose at the appropriate times. It is **not** appropriate to either i) gradually 'titrate the dose upwards' or ii) to only give a partial dose if the convulsion stops (even if the seizure has stopped, that full dose must be given). If this approach is followed, seizure recurrence is much less likely.
- A focal convulsion lasting longer than 5 minutes should be managed and treated in the same way as a generalised convulsion.
- If the convulsion is continuing 10 minutes after the first dose of medication has been given, a second dose of anticonvulsant can be given. Ideally, this should be given intravenously or intra-osseously e.g. **diazepam** IV/IO (refer to **Diazepam**) but if this is not possible a second dose can be given buccally or rectally. (This also applies if a carer has given the first dose of medication before the clinician arrives on scene.)

Convulsions in Children

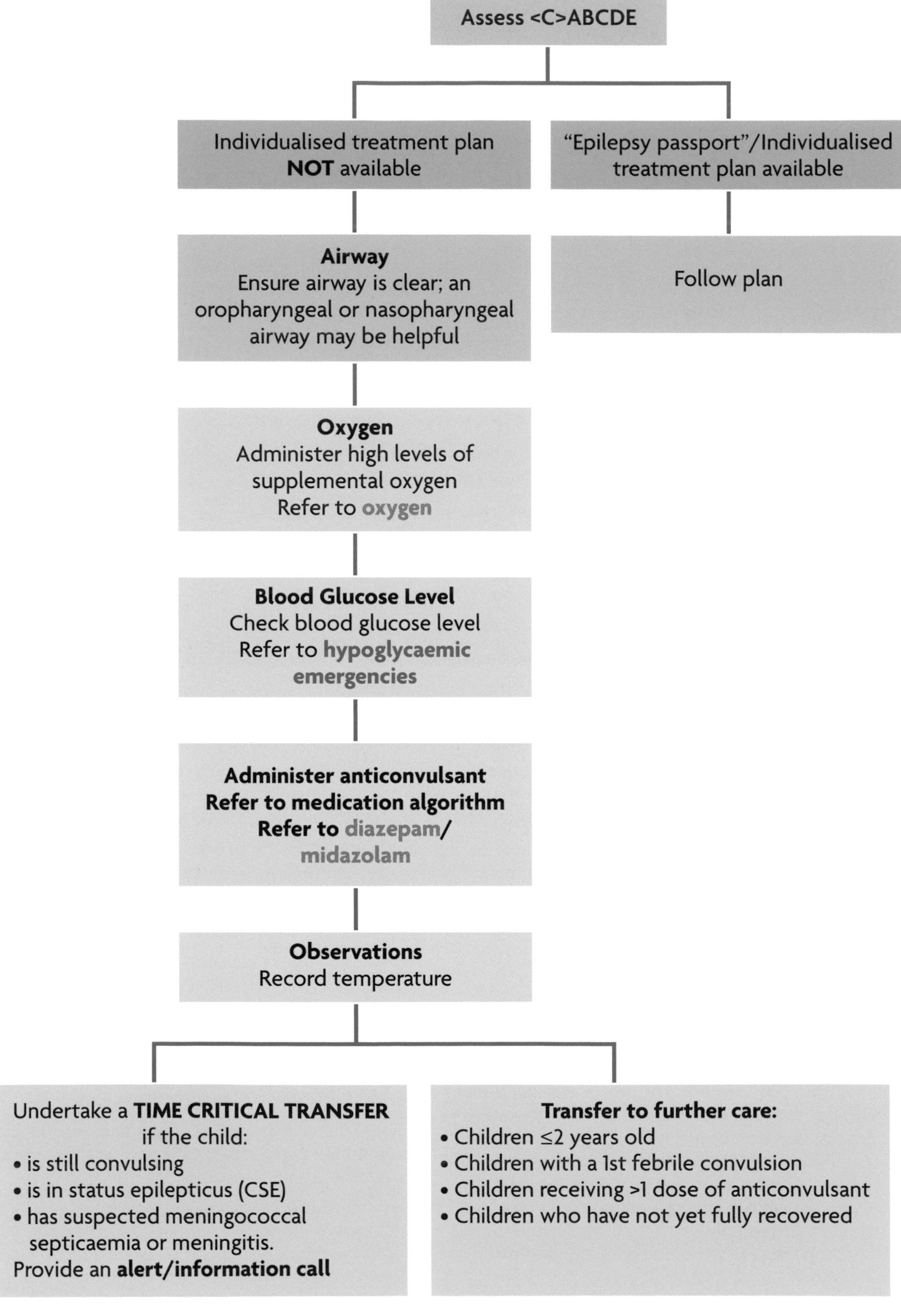

Figure 3.8 – Assessment and management algorithm of convulsions in children.

SECTION 3 Medical Emergencies

Convulsions in Children

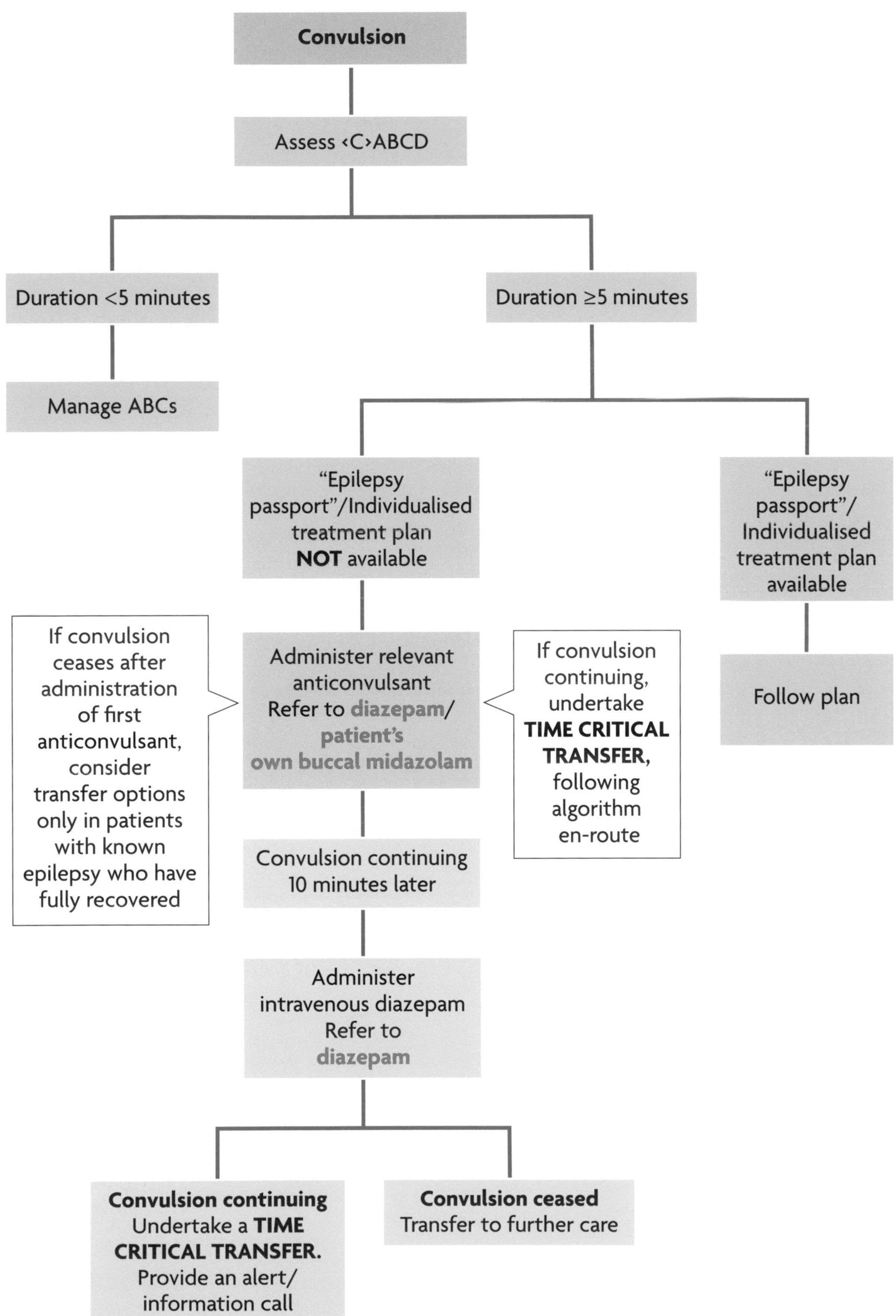

Figure 3.9 – Medication algorithm for convulsions in children.

- Further doses of benzodiazepine should not be given even when there is uncertainty about whether the convulsion has stopped or not (see 'Assessment' above).
- Children may sometimes experience brief (i.e. <5 minute) repeated or 'serial' convulsions. Such children should be given an anticonvulsant if they have experienced three convulsions in an hour.

Hospital transfer

- Often it is safest to treat the convulsion before moving the child, although if the seizure has not stopped after one dose of anticonvulsant the child will have to be transferred while still convulsing.
- Pre-alert the hospital if the child continues to fit during the journey or appears to be otherwise very unwell.
- All children having their first convulsion should be transported to hospital for investigation.
- If the child has fully recovered and is a known epileptic it may not be necessary to take them to hospital.

KEY POINTS!

Convulsions (Children)

- **Prolonged convulsions, called convulsive status epilepticus (CSE), is a medical emergency and may result in death or serious neurological impairments.**
- **Febrile convulsions are a very common cause for a childhood convulsion and occur between the ages of 6 months and 5 years.**
- **Most convulsions stop spontaneously within 4 minutes.**
- **A convulsion lasting 5 minutes (or more) should be treated with anticonvulsants.**
- **Buccal midazolam is the most widely available rescue medication used in childhood epilepsy.**
- **First choice anticonvulsants are usually given buccally or rectally, with buccal midazolam being the preferred treatment option.**
- **Wherever possible, the second dose of anticonvulsant should always be given intravenously (e.g. diazepam).**
- **The full dose for the child's age must be given when treating a convulsion.**
- **A child should not usually receive more than two doses of pre-hospital anticonvulsant.**
- **Always consider (and actively seek) the underlying cause for the convulsion.**
- **All first convulsions must be transported to hospital.**

Bibliography

1. National Institute for Health and Clinical Excellence. *The Epilepsies: The diagnosis and management of the epilepsies in adults and children in primary and secondary care* (CG137). London: NICE, 2012. Available from: https://nice.org.uk/guidance/CG137.
2. Woollard M, Pitt K. Antipyretic pre-hospital therapy for febrile convulsions: does the treatment fit? A literature review. *Health Education* 2003, 62(1): 23–8.
3. Yoong M, Chin RFM, Scott RC. Management of convulsive status epilepticus in children. *Archives of Disease in Childhood Education and Practice Edition* 2009, 94(1): 1–9.
4. The Status Epilepticus Working Party, Appleton R, Choonara I, Martland T, Phillips B, Scott R, et al. The treatment of convulsive status epilepticus in children. *Archives of Disease in Childhood* 2000, 83(5): 415–19.
5. Sadleir LG, Scheffer IE. Febrile seizures. *British Medical Journal* 2007, 334(7588): 307–11.
6. Baysun S, Aydin ÖF, Atmaca E, Gürer YKY. A comparison of buccal midazolam and rectal diazepam for the acute treatment of seizures. *Clinical Pediatrics* 2005, 44(9): 771–6.
7. Sadleir LG, Scheffer IE. Febrile seizures. *British Medical Journal* 2007, 334(7588): 307–11.

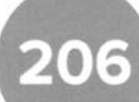

Dyspnoea

1. Introduction

- Dyspnoea is defined as '*a subjective experience of breathing discomfort that consists of qualitatively distinct sensations that vary in intensity*'.
- Dyspnoea is an important clinical symptom that may indicate underlying pathology for a large range of conditions (refer to Table 3.37), particularly those affecting the respiratory and cardiac systems.
- Acute episodes of dyspnoea often have a pulmonary or cardiac cause. Asthma, cardiogenic pulmonary oedema, chronic obstructive pulmonary disease (COPD), pneumonia, cardiac ischaemia, and interstitial lung disease are common causes and account for approximately 85% of all ED cases of dyspnoea. In 15% of cases dyspnoea is unexplained.

2. Severity and Outcome

- Dyspnoea is an important clinical symptom which in some circumstances can be severe or life-threatening. Dyspnoea varies in intensity and can be a distressing symptom, especially for patients at the end of life. **For details of the severity and outcome for specific conditions refer to individual guidelines.**

3. Pathophysiology

- Dyspnoea is a multi-dimensional process involving physiological and psychological systems. Table 3.38 details symptoms, signs and history associated with the potential causes of dyspnoea.

TABLE 3.37 – Causes of Dyspnoea

Pulmonary causes	**Cardiac causes**	**Other causes**
Acute exacerbation of asthma.	Acute heart failure.	Anaphylaxis.
Bronchiectasis.	Cardiac arrhythmia.	Chemicals/poisons.
Acute exacerbation of COPD.	Cardiac tamponade.	Diabetic ketoacidosis.
Flail chest.	Ischaemic heart disease.	Diaphragmatic splinting.
Interstitial lung disease.	Myocardial infarction.	Hyperventilation.
Lung/lobar collapse.	Valvular dysfunction.	Panic attack/anxiety.
Massive haemothorax.	Pericarditis.	Severe hypovolaemia.
Pleural effusion.		Metabolic causes.
Pneumonia.		Obesity.
Pneumothorax.		Pain.
Pulmonary embolism.		Severe anaemia.
Upper airway obstruction.		End of life.
		Carbon monoxide exposure

TABLE 3.38 – Differential Diagnosis for Common Conditions

Condition	**Symptoms**	**Signs**	**Auscultation or audible sounds**	**History**
Acute exacerbation of asthma Refer to **Asthma**	Dyspnoea Cough Unable to complete sentences	Wheeze Tachypnoea Tachycardia Pulsus paradoxus Hyperresonant chest Accessory muscle use	Decreased or absent breath sounds if severe Wheeze	Previous asthma Recent increase in inhaler use Allergen exposure

(continued)

Dyspnoea

TABLE 3.38 – Differential Diagnosis for Common Conditions *(continued)*

Condition	Symptoms	Signs	Auscultation or audible sounds	History
Acute Coronary Syndrome, for example, STEMI or NSTEMI Refer to **Acute Coronary Syndrome**	Central chest pain for >15 minutes, constricting or crushing that radiates to arm/ neck	Tachycardia Arrhythmia	Wheeze Crackles	Symptoms suggestive of ischaemic heart disease (IHD) or previous investigations for chest pain
Acute Heart Failure Refer to **Heart Failure**	Dyspnoea especially on exertion Orthopnoea/ paroxysmal nocturnal dyspnoea Cough producing frothy, white or pink phlegm	Peripheral oedema Tachycardia	Rales Heart murmur Crepitations	Angina Hypertension History of heart failure, for example, left ventricular failure, right ventricular failure or cor pulmonale Valvular dysfunction or congenital heart problems
Anaphylaxis Refer to **Allergic Reactions including Anaphylaxis**	Dyspnoea Dysphagia Chest tightness	Tachycardia Tachypnoea Erythema Urticaria Angioedema Pharyngeal or laryngeal oedema[1]	Decreased breath sounds Wheeze Stridor	Allergen exposure
Chronic Obstructive Pulmonary Disease (COPD) Refer to **Chronic Obstructive Pulmonary Disease**	Progressive dyspnoea Chest tightness Cough – purulent sputum	New-onset cyanosis Peripheral oedema Accessory muscle use Pursed lip breathing[2]	Rales Wheeze	Smoking >35 years of age
End of life dyspnoea Refer to **End of Life Care**	Dyspnoea	Tachypnoea	Decreased breath sounds	Long term respiratory conditions such as COPD
Foreign Body Airway Obstruction (FBAO) Refer to **Foreign Body Airway Obstruction**	Dyspnoea Inability to speak Cough	Clutching at neck	Stridor Wheeze	Eating – especially fish, meat, or poultry Illicit drug ingestion or substance misuse
Hyperventilation Refer to **Hyperventilation Syndrome**	Dyspnoea Acute agitation and anxiety Chest pain which may resemble angina pectoris Palpitations	Sudden dyspnoea Hyperpnoea Tachypnoea Numbness and tingling in the limbs and around the mouth		**NB** ensure other more serious conditions are excluded before considering this diagnosis

Dyspnoea

TABLE 3.38 – Differential Diagnosis for Common Conditions *(continued)*				
Condition	**Symptoms**	**Signs**	**Auscultation or audible sounds**	**History**
Pneumonia Refer to **Medical Emergencies in Adults – Overview** and **Medical Emergencies in Children – Overview.**	Dyspnoea Fever Cough	Tachycardia	Rhonchi	Smoking IHD
Pneumothorax Rrefer to **Thoracic Trauma**	Dyspnoea Sudden onset pleuritic chest pain	Dyspnoea	Decreased breath sounds	Trauma Previous pneumothorax COPD Asthma Smoking Tall, thin stature
Pulmonary Embolism Refer to **Pulmonary Embolism**	Dyspnoea Pleuritic chest pain Cough or haemoptysis Possible DVT Leg oedema Syncope Hypotension Fever	Tachycardia Tachypnoea Fever ECG: Non-specific ST wave changes Hypotension	Focal rales Crepitations Decreased breath sounds	Prolonged immobilisation Recent surgery Thrombotic disease Active cancer

- The respiratory system is designed to match alveolar ventilation with metabolic demand. Disruption of this process may lead to the conscious awareness of breathing and dyspnoea. Dyspnoea is an uncomfortable sensation and may include chest tightness, air hunger, effortful breathing, the urge to cough and a sense of suffocation.

4. Assessment and Management

- Diagnosis of the underlying cause of the patient's presenting illness can be difficult, and may require in-hospital investigations. Assessment must include a detailed history and a thorough physical examination. For the assessment and management of patients with dyspnoea refer to Table 3.39.

TABLE 3.39 – Assessment and Management of: Dyspnoea	
NB Take a defibrillator at the earliest opportunity and keep this with the patient until handover.	
ASSESSMENT	**MANAGEMENT**
• Assess **<C>ABCD**	• If any of the following **TIME CRITICAL** features present: – major **<C>ABCD** problems refer to **Medical Emergencies in Adults – Overview** and **Medical Emergencies in Children – Overview** – extreme airway/breathing difficulty or cyanosis, refer to **Airway and Breathing Management** – features of life-threatening asthma, refer to **Asthma** – features of tension pneumothorax or major chest trauma, refer to **Thoracic Trauma** – acute myocardial infarction, refer to **Acute Coronary Syndrome** – anaphylaxis, refer to **Allergic Reactions including Anaphylaxis**

(continued)

Dyspnoea

TABLE 3.39 – Assessment and Management of: Dyspnoea *(continued)*	
	– Foreign Body Airway Obstruction, refer to **Foreign Body Airway Obstruction** – loss of consciousness, refer to **Altered Level of Consciousness**, then: • Start correcting any **<C>ABCD** problems. • Undertake a **TIME CRITICAL** transfer to nearest appropriate receiving hospital. • Continue patient management en-route • Provide an ATMIST information call.
• Position	• Position the patient for comfort, usually sitting upright.
• Ask the patient if they have an individualised treatment plan	• Be aware that the patient may have a treatment plan or care plan. • Patients with long term conditions will often be able to guide their care and have a care plan, ReSPECT form or DNACPR form in place.
• If the patient is not TIME CRITICAL, obtain a thorough history to help identify the cause of dyspnoea	**Specifically assess:** • Effort and effectiveness of ventilation – rate and depth. • Medical Research Council (MRC) Dyspnoea Scale. • Duration of difficulty breathing – sudden or gradual onset? • Pain associated with breathing – any pattern of breathing/depth of respiration? • Do certain positions exacerbate breathing (e.g. unable to lie down, must sit upright)? • Does the patient have a cough? • If yes, is the cough productive: – **sputum or bubbling**: consider infection or heart failure – **frothy white/pink sputum**: consider acute heart failure – **yellow/green sputum**: consider chest infection – **haemoptysis**: consider PE, chest infection or carcinoma of the lung. • Has the patient increased their medication recently? • Signs of anaphylaxis: – Urticarial rash – facial swelling – circulatory collapse.
Percuss the chest	To determine if there are collections of fluid in the lungs.
Auscultate the chest	To determine adequacy of air entry on both sides of the chest. To determine chest sounds: – audible wheeze on expiration – consider asthma, ACS, anaphylaxis, COPD or heart failure (especially in older patients with no history of asthma) – audible stridor (upper airway narrowing) consider anaphylaxis, or FBAO – crepitations (fine crackling in lung bases) – ACS, heart failure – rhonchi (harsher, rattling sound) indicating collections of fluid in larger airways – pneumonia. – rales (clicking, rattling or crackling noises) - heart failure, COPD, pulmonary embolism
Consider possible causes, refer to Table 3.37 and Table 3.38	
• Known cause	• If the cause of dyspnoea is known follow relevant guideline, as per Table 3.38.
• Unknown cause	• If cause of dyspnoea unknown refer to **Medical Emergencies in Adults – Overview** and **Medical Emergencies in Children – Overview** and follow management below.

Dyspnoea

TABLE 3.39 – Assessment and Management of: Dyspnoea *(continued)*	
• Ventilation	Consider assisted ventilation at a rate of 12–20 breaths per minute if: • SpO_2 is <90% on high concentration O_2. • Respiratory rate is <10 or >30. • Expansion is inadequate, refer to **Airway and Breathing Management**.
• Fluid	• Administer fluid as required, refer to **Intravascular Fluid Therapy (Adults)** and **Intravascular Fluid Therapy (Children)**.
• Pain management	• Administer pain relief if indicated, refer to **Pain Management in Adults** and **Pain Management in Children**.
• Transfer to further care	• All patients with an unexplained cause of dyspnoea. • Where the cause is known refer to the relevant guideline for care pathway.

TABLE 3.40 – MRC Dyspnoea Scale	
Grade 1	Breathless only with strenuous exercise
Grade 2	Short of breath when hurrying on the level or up a slight hill
Grade 3	Slower than most people of the same age on a level surface OR Have to stop when walking at my own pace on the level
Grade 4	Stop for breath walking 100 meters OR After a walking few minutes at my own pace on the level
Grade 5	Too breathless to leave the house
Used with the permission of the Medical Research Council	

KEY POINTS!

Dyspnoea

- **Is dyspnoea a result of respiratory, cardiac, both or other causes?**
- **Consider time critical causes.**
- **Assess degree of dyspnoea and response to treatment.**
- **Consider possible causes and refer to relevant guidelines for assessment and management.**

Further Reading

Further important information and evidence in support of this guideline can be found in the Bibliography.[4,5,6,7,8,9,10,11]

Bibliography

1. Lansing RW, Gracely RH, Banzett RB. The multiple dimensions of dyspnea: review and hypotheses. *Respiratory Physiology and Neurobiology* 2009, 167(1): 53–60.
2. Nardi AE, Freire RC, Zin WA. Panic disorder and control of breathing. *Respiratory Physiology and Neurobiology* 2009, 167(1): 133–43.
3. Peiffer C. Dyspnea relief: more than just the perception of a decrease in dyspnea. *Respiratory Physiology and Neurobiology* 2009, 167(1): 61–71.
4. Parshall MB, Schwartzstein RM, Adams L, Banzett RB, Manning HL, Bourbeau J, et al. An official American Thoracic Society statement: update on the mechanisms, assessment, and management of dyspnea. *American Journal of Respiratory and Critical Care Medicine* 2012, 185(4): 435–52.
5. Michelson E, Hollrah S. Evaluation of the patient with shortness of breath: an evidence based approach. *Emergency Medicine Clinics of North America* 1999, 17(1): 221–37.

6. Karras DJ, Sammon ME, Terregino CA, Lopez BL, Griswold SK, Arnold GK. Clinically meaningful changes in quantitative measures of asthma severity. *Academic Emergency Medicine* 2000, 7(4): 327–34.

7. National Institute for Health and Clinical Excellence. *Chest Pain of Recent Onset: Assessment and diagnosis of recent onset chest pain or discomfort of suspected cardiac origin* (CG95). London: NICE, 2010. Available from: https://www.nice.org.uk/guidance/cg95.

8. NHS Evidence. *Dyspnoea.* 2010.

9. National Institute for Health and Care Excellence. *Angio-oedema and anaphylaxis* Clinical Knowledge Summaries. Available from: https://cks.nice.org.uk/angio-oedema-and-anaphylaxis#!diagnosissub:2, 2018.

10. National Institute for Health and Care Excellence. *Chronic obstructive pulmonary disease* Clinical Knowledge Summaries. Available from: https://cks.nice.org.uk/chronic-obstructive-pulmonary-disease, 2018.

11. National Institute for Health and Care Excellence. *Pulmonary embolism* Clinical Knowledge Summaries. Available from: https://cks.nice.org.uk/pulmonary-embolism#!diagnosissub, 2015.

Febrile Illness in Children

1. Introduction

- There are many important differences between children and adults in their anatomy, their physiology and their immunity, as well as differences in the types of illnesses they encounter and the ways these conditions present, develop and progress.
- The assessment and management of children poses many potential pitfalls for the unwary and inexperienced, and present healthcare providers with significant challenges, wherever the setting.
- Children may struggle to verbalise and communicate their condition to you, adding to the challenges faced when assessing and caring for them.

'Major' and 'minor' childhood illnesses

- Sick children are notoriously difficult to assess, except when they are obviously very ill or injured, with grossly deranged vital signs. The younger the child, the more difficult the assessment.
- Before considering 'minor' illnesses in children, it is crucial to both appreciate and understand that 'major' childhood illnesses (including life-threatening conditions such as meningococcal disease and sepsis) do not commonly present in extremis, but typically present with relatively innocent features that can easily be mistaken for minor illnesses.
- Children's vital signs may well be deranged when their illness (or injury) is advanced (significant), and these abnormalities should be readily detected. However, earlier in the same illness, these same children may appear relatively well and exhibit 'normal' physiology. There is a risk that the significance of these children's illnesses may not be appreciated, if assessed early in the course of their illness.
- In critically ill children, temperature is not routinely recorded as part of the 'ABC' assessment as it delays treatment without altering management.
- Temperature should however be measured in the less ill child, where it forms part of the picture of their illness and is an essential sign that informs clinical decision making.
- Staff should be familiar with NICE's Feverish Illness in Children guidance (on which this guideline is based).

Fever

- Normal body temperature is 37°C. A temperature of 38°C and above is likely to be significant.
- Fever is part of the immune system's response to infection and is not thought to be harmful (although lay people often assume that it is).
- It can herald a significant underlying infection hence the importance of identifying its cause.
- Throughout most of childhood, the height of the fever bears little relationship to the gravity of the illness, although in babies aged under 6 months, a high temperature is much more likely to be significant.
- When facing serious infections, small babies often have unstable body temperatures and may paradoxically present with a low body temperature.
- Febrile illnesses in children aged between 6 months and 5 years can produce a seizure – a febrile convulsion – following a rapid rise in body temperature (refer to **Convulsions in Children**).
- A child with a fever is a very common presentation. Such children may have a self-limiting viral condition or else another obvious cause, such as an ear infection or upper respiratory tract infection. However, for some febrile children no obvious cause will be found and a small number of these will have a serious illness.
- Ambulance clinicians have an important role to play in the reduction of the mortality rate for children with feverish illness, which remains higher in the UK than in many other European countries. The main priorities are to:
  - Identify any immediately life-threatening features.
  - Assess whether the child has (i) a serious illness requiring intervention or (ii) a self-limiting illness, without necessarily diagnosing a specific condition.
  - Determine a likely source of the illness to direct specific treatment.
  - Make appropriate management decisions based upon the results of the assessment.
- NICE defines a fever as 'an elevation of body temperature above the normal daily variation'. It recognises that this is often hard to define, as normal temperature varies depending on the individual, the body site where temperature is measured, and the time of day.

2. Incidence

- Febrile illness is the commonest medical problem in childhood. Younger children are the most vulnerable due to the immaturity of their immune systems. By the age of 18 months, an otherwise healthy child would be expected to have had around eight acute febrile illnesses.

3. Severity and Outcome

- Infectious diseases are a major cause of childhood mortality and morbidity.
- Most febrile illnesses are due to self-limiting viral infections requiring little or no intervention.

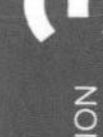

However, fever is a common presenting feature of serious bacterial infections (SBI) such as meningitis, septicaemia, urinary tract infections and pneumonia, and distinguishing between a simple viral infection and a more serious bacterial infection is a real diagnostic challenge. 1% of the UK's under-5 population will have an SBI each year.

4. Assessment

(a) FEBRILE CHILD ASSESSMENT

Carry out a primary survey immediately on any ill child to exclude any evidence of life-threatening illness. For the assessment and management of a febrile child, refer to Table 3.41.

- Use the traffic light system shown in Table 3.42 to support the assessment and management of the child.
- When assessing children with learning disabilities, take the individual child's learning disability into account when interpreting the traffic light table.

(b) TEMPERATURE MEASUREMENT

- Any reported parental perception of a fever should be considered valid and taken seriously.
- Do not take temperatures orally in the under 5s. Even in older children, it may be easier to avoid using the oral method.
- In order to obtain an accurate temperature, an appropriate thermometer must be used:
  - In children **under** 4 weeks of age, use an electronic thermometer placed in the child's axilla. **NB**: The thermometer must be left in place for at least the minimum recommended time, otherwise it may under-record.

TABLE 3.41 – ASSESSMENT and MANAGEMENT of: a Febrile Child

Assess <**C**>**ABCD**	If any of the following **TIME CRITICAL** features are present: • Major <**C**>**ABCD** problems, refer to **Medical Emergencies in Children – Overview**. • Active seizure, refer to **convulsions**. Start correcting any <**C**>**ABCD** problems. Undertake a **TIME CRITICAL** transfer to nearest appropriate receiving hospital. Continue patient management en-route. Provide an ATMIST information call.
Respiratory rate	Measure and record respiratory rate. For specific ranges, refer to Table 3.44.
Pulse	Measure and record pulse. For specific ranges, refer to Table 3.44.
Oxygen saturation	Monitor the patient's SpO_2, administer oxygen to achieve saturations of >92% if the patient presents as hypoxemic on air (refer to **Oxygen**).
Blood pressure and fluids	Measure and record blood pressure; if required administer fluids (refer to **Intravascular Fluid Therapy (Children)**).
Blood glucose	If appropriate, measure and record blood glucose for hypo/hyperglycaemia (refer to **Glycaemic Emergencies in Adults and Children**).
Overall assessment	AVPU Consider the overall impression of the child (e.g. playful, lively, disinterested, miserable, floppy etc.) Capillary refill
Temperature	Measure and record temperature.
Take and record a full history	• Length of illness. Other symptoms besides fever, specifically asking about: • urinary symptoms • abdominal pain • abnormal skin colour, cold hands and feet, muscle pains • headache, photophobia, neck stiffness • other complaints, such as a painful joints, sore throat, ear pain etc.

TABLE 3.41 – ASSESSMENT and MANAGEMENT of: a Febrile Child *(continued)*	
	Is fluid intake adequate? A febrile child needs extra fluids to prevent dehydration. If they are vomiting, they may become dehydrated and be unable to absorb medication. Diarrhoea also increases fluid losses, increasing the risk of dehydration. Underlying (chronic) medical problems, including advice that the parent may have been given by specialists regarding actions to be taken if their child develops a fever. (This should include whether the child is under current investigation or management by a doctor.) Medications, antibiotics or steroids (or other drugs reducing immunity). To assess a child properly, you will need to be aware of the action of any drug that they are taking as this may be relevant. If in doubt, this must be checked. Any other illness in the family, the nursery or school etc? Recent foreign travel – consider malaria or other tropical illness.
ECG	If required, monitor and record 12-lead ECG. Assess for abnormality (refer to **Cardiac Rhythm Disturbance**).
Assess the patient's pain	Where present, assess the SOCRATES of pain and record initial and subsequent pain scores. Consider analgesia if appropriate (refer to **Pain Management**).
Documentation	Complete documentation to include all clinical findings, advice from other clinicians, onward referral and worsening advice given.

TABLE 3.42 – Traffic Light System for Assessing Paediatric Fever			
	Green – Low Risk	**Amber – Intermediate Risk**	**Red – High Risk**
Colour (of skin, lips or tongue)	• Normal colour	• Pallor reported by parent/carer	• Pale/mottled/ashen/blue
Activity	• Responds normally to social cues • Content /smiles • Stays awake or awakens quickly • Strong normal cry/ not crying	• Not responding normally to social cues • No smile • Wakes only with prolonged stimulation • Decreased activity	• No response to social cues • Appears ill to a healthcare professional • Does not wake or if roused does not stay awake • Weak, high-pitched or continuous cry
Respiratory		• Nasal flaring • Tachypnoea: respiratory rate – >50 breaths/minute, age 6–12 months – >40 breaths/minute, age >12 months • Oxygen saturation ≤95% in air • Crackles in the chest	• Grunting • Tachypnoea: respiratory rate >60 breaths/minute • Moderate or severe chest indrawing

(continued)

Febrile Illness in Children

TABLE 3.42 – Traffic Light System for Assessing Paediatric Fever *(continued)*

	Green – Low Risk	Amber – Intermediate Risk	Red – High Risk
Circulation and hydration	• Normal skin and eyes • Moist mucous membranes	• Tachycardia: – >160 beats/minute, age <12 months – >150 beats/minute, age 12–24 months – >140 beats/minute, age 2–5 years • Capillary refill time ≥3 seconds • Dry mucous membranes • Poor feeding in infants • Reduced urine output	• Reduced skin turgor
Other	• None of the amber or red symptoms or signs	• Age 3–6 months, temperature ≥39°C • Fever for ≥5 days • Rigors • Swelling of a limb or joint • Non-weight bearing limb/not using an extremity	• Age <3 months, temperature ≥38°C* • Non-blanching rash • Bulging fontanelle • Neck stiffness • Status epilepticus • Focal neurological signs • Focal seizures

*Some vaccinations have been found to induce fever in children aged under 3 months.

Note: The traffic light system does not seek to make a specific diagnosis but simply identifies which symptoms and signs should receive the highest priority, guiding subsequent management.

  - In children **over** 4 weeks of age, use either an electronic thermometer or a tympanic thermometer.
- Earlier treatment with antipyretics (e.g. paracetamol, ibuprofen) must be considered, as it may mask the child's fever.
- Chemically sensitive strips placed on the forehead are inaccurate and should not be used.
- Mercury-containing, glass thermometers are no longer used for safety reasons.

Important clinical points

Tachycardia frequently accompanies a fever and is suggestive of an underlying infection, while **tachypnoea** suggests an underlying respiratory illness.

A child's resting heart rate increases 10 bpm for every 1°C rise in body temperature.

A **disproportionate tachycardia** – i.e. above the accepted normal range (refer to Table 3.44) having taken account of the fever – is seen in early sepsis and meningococcal disease. Such children must receive further medical assessment.

Other features suggesting sepsis include cold hands and feet, abnormal skin colour and muscle pains in the legs.

Infants and small children with meningococcal disease rarely exhibit 'classical' textbook signs (**neck stiffness, photophobia** and **non-blanching rash**), but more commonly present with features that might suggest a non-specific viral illness such as an upper respiratory tract infection (URTI) or gastroenteritis.

In such circumstances, seek (and document) evidence to rule out the possibility of meningococcal disease.

- Conduct an assessment of dehydration (refer to **Gastroenteritis in Children** guideline).
- Examine all other systems (including skin) to determine the source of the fever and estimate the disease severity.
- A positive sign must be 'seen' rather than assumed – (e.g. otitis media cannot be

diagnosed on a history of 'earache' alone). Direct visualisation of the tympanic membrane using an auroscope is required to diagnose otitis media.

- **NB It is possible for a child to have a common infection as well as a more serious underlying one; a child with coryza and runny nose could still have meningitis.**

c) SPECIFIC FEBRILE ILLNESSES

The following potential diagnoses must each be specifically considered; some typical signs and symptoms are shown in Table 3.43:

- **Meningococcal septicaemia** – often the child does not present as acutely as tradition would have it.
- **Meningitis** (preschool children rarely have neck stiffness).
- **Urinary tract infection (UTI)** – UTIs can progress to life-threatening septicaemia. They are particularly common in babies and young children and can cause permanent kidney damage. Symptoms can again be very non-specific and include: poor feeding, lethargy and abdominal pains. In hospital practice, clean catch urine samples are collected on every febrile child to exclude UTIs.
- **Pneumonia** – typical chest signs may be absent.
- **Herpes simplex encephalitis** – classical pointers include focal neurological signs and focal seizures.
- **Septic arthritis/osteomyelitis** – fever plus very tender swollen joint(s)/bone(s), with a refusal to weight-bear.
- **Kawasaki's disease** – a collection of signs including: fever for >5 days; cervical lymphadenopathy; mucosal changes in the upper respiratory tract (e.g. redness and cracked lips); peripheral limb changes (e.g. oedema, peeling skin); a non-specific, blanching 'measles-like' rash; bilateral conjunctival redness.

5. Management

Using the **Traffic Light System for Assessing Paediatric Fever** as shown in Table 3.42.

Red Traffic Light Features

Children with any of the NICE Red Traffic Light features or additional Red Flags must be conveyed to an ED with appropriate paediatric services for further specialist assessment.

Provide an ATMIST pre-alert and convey under emergency driving conditions where required. Consider sepsis or meningitis as possible causes and provide care en-route according to Trust/ JRCALC guidelines.

TABLE 3.43 – Symptoms and Signs Suggestive of Specific Diseases

Diagnosis to be considered	Symptoms and signs in conjunction with fever
Meningococcal disease	Non-blanching rash, particularly with 1 or more of the following: • an ill-looking child • lesions larger than 2 mm in diameter (purpura) • capillary refill time of ≥3 seconds • neck stiffness
Bacterial meningitis	Neck stiffness Bulging fontanelle Decreased level of consciousness Convulsive status epilepticus
Herpes simplex encephalitis	Focal neurological signs Focal seizures Decreased level of consciousness
Pneumonia	Tachypnoea (respiratory rate >60 breaths/min, age 0–5 months; >50 breaths/min, age 6–12 months; >40 breaths/min, age >12 months) Crackles in the chest Nasal flaring Chest indrawing Cyanosis Oxygen saturation ≤95%

(continued)

Febrile Illness in Children

TABLE 3.43 – Symptoms and Signs Suggestive of Specific Diseases *(continued)*	
Diagnosis to be considered	**Symptoms and signs in conjunction with fever**
Urinary tract infection	Vomiting Poor feeding Lethargy Irritability Abdominal pain or tenderness Urinary frequency or dysuria
Septic arthritis	Swelling of a limb or joint Not using an extremity Non-weight bearing
Kawasaki disease	Fever for more than 5 days and at least 4 of the following: ● bilateral conjunctival injection ● change in mucous membranes ● change in the extremities ● polymorphous rash ● cervical lymphadenopathy

Amber Traffic Light Features

Children with amber traffic light features may be considered for an alternative treatment pathway. Children presenting with multiple amber features must be considered for hospital assessment.

Note: if a child has amber traffic light features and a decision is made **not** to transport the child OR a child has green traffic light features but a cause for the fever has not been found, the following 'safety nets' **MUST** be put in place:

- The patient MUST be discussed with a GP or paediatric healthcare professional, following local protocols, for urgent follow-up arrangements giving a specified time and place (e.g. for the child to be seen within the next 2–6 hours, exact timing to be decided by the attending staff).
- Direct verbal hand-over to the doctor is important but may not always be possible.
- The arrangements must be made by the attending ambulance staff.
- **It is not adequate to tell the parents to make their own arrangements to see the GP.**

Green Traffic Light Features

Children who have only green traffic light features may be managed at home. Record that the child has been assessed as having only green features on the patient clinical record and ensure that negative findings are noted to demonstrate the absence of amber or red features, e.g. no nasal flaring.

Ensure that parents/carers are provided with a patient information leaflet if one is available. They should receive specific, written worsening advice, including expectations on length of illness. Ensure that they are aware of the following:

- Suitable antipyretic interventions available.
- The importance of offering the child regular fluids (if breastfeeding then continue as normal).
- How to identify a non-blanching rash.
- Checking the child during the night.
- Keeping the child away from nursery/school while the fever persists and to notify the nursery/school of the illness.
- The common signs of dehydration:
  - sunken fontanelle
  - dry mouth
  - sunken eyes
  - absence of tears
  - poor overall appearance.

Advise parents/carers to seek further advice if:

- The child has a fit.
- The child develops a non-blanching rash.

Febrile Illness in Children

TABLE 3.44 – 'Normal' Paediatric Physiological Values		
Age	**Respiratorty rate (bpm)**	**Heart rate (bpm)**
<1 year	30–40	110–160
1–2 yrs	25–35	110–150
2–5 yrs	25–30	95–140
5–12 yrs	20–25	80–120
Over 12 yrs	15–20	60–100

TABLE 3.45 – Red Flags

Febrile children fulfilling the following red flag criteria **must** be transported to hospital:

- Any febrile baby <1 month old (irrespective of the absolute temperature).
- Any febrile child <3 months old without an obvious cause (as a minimum, an urgent urine sample will be required).
- Any febrile child <3 years without an obvious cause, if a urine sample cannot be arranged at the time through the GP.
- Those with any signs of serious illness (refer to **Medical Emergencies in Children** guideline).
- Any child with a significant fever but no localising symptoms or signs, who has received antibiotics within the last 48 hours (signs of meningitis can be masked by antibiotic use; so called 'partially treated' meningitis).
- Any child on steroids or other medication known to suppress the immune system.
- Any child, regardless of age, where there is any concern that they could be seriously ill.
- Any child where the social or psychological environment suggests that they may not receive adequate supervision or care if left at home.
- Those with a medical protocol saying that transport is necessary.

- They are worried that the child is becoming dehydrated.
- Nappies are becoming drier or changed much less frequently.
- They feel that the child's health is getting worse.
- They are more worried than when they last received advice.
- The fever lasts longer than 5 days.
- They are distressed or concerned that they are unable to look after their child.

Use local referral pathways to inform the child's GP as required. Arrange for infants and children presenting with unexplained fever of 38°C or higher to have a urine sample tested after 24 hours at the latest.

Important clinical points – antipyretics and antibiotics

- Tepid sponging is not recommended. Do not over or under dress a child with fever.
- Giving an **antipyretic** such as paracetamol or ibuprofen purely to treat the fever is not necessary, but parental sensitivities should be observed.
- An analgesic/antipyretic may help relieve misery and other unpleasant symptoms that often accompany febrile illnesses (e.g. aches, pains and other symptoms which the child is often unable to fully describe).
- Antipyretics do not protect against febrile convulsions. Giving antipyretics to a child who has either just had a seizure or who is thought to be at risk of having a seizure has not been shown to be beneficial.
- Note: Antipyretics are effective, even in children with serious bacterial infections. It would therefore be wrong to assume that a clinical improvement seen following an antipyretic excludes a serious underlying infection.
- Combinations of paracetamol and ibuprofen should not be given. Only consider alternating these agents if the distress persists or recurs before the next dose is due.
- Paracetamol is normally given every 6 hours and ibuprofen every 8 hours, so care needs to be taken not to exceed the maximum dose of each drug in a 24-hour period. A treatment diary may be useful if the parents or carers find it difficult to remember which was the last drug given and at what time.
- **Antibiotics** should not be given to a febrile child where the diagnosis is not known. This can delay the subsequent diagnosis of a serious infection such as meningitis.

Febrile convulsions

Febrile convulsions commonly occur in children who are aged between 6 months and 3 years and have a temperature greater than 38°C. Most febrile convulsions occur in those aged approximately 18 months, although children up to 5 years of age can be affected.

Ambulance clinicians must not apply the diagnosis of febrile convulsion to patients aged over 5 years; older children require a paediatrician to rule out other causes of the convulsion first.

For the management of active febrile convulsions refer to **Convulsions In Children**.

Febrile Illness in Children

KEY POINTS!

Febrile Illness in Children

- **Febrile illness is the commonest paediatric presentation and suggests underlying infection.**
- **Always seek the underlying cause of the fever.**
- **All febrile children must be assessed with a full history and examination.**
- **Physiological parameters must be measured, documented and compared against age-specific, 'normal' values.**
- **Significant tachycardia suggests sepsis.**
- **Use the NICE 'traffic light' system.**
- **The early features of serious infections are often non-specific (e.g. meningococcal disease often mimics URTIs and gastroenteritis).**
- **Small children rarely exhibit the 'classical' meningococcal signs – neck stiffness, photophobia or non-blanching rash; these features are more likely in older children and teenagers. In all age groups important early features include fever, cold hands and feet, abnormal skin colour and muscle pains or confusion.**
- **Improvement following antipyretics does not rule out a serious underlying infection.**
- **Antibiotics should not be blindly given to a febrile child where the diagnosis is not known.**
- **Where a justifiable clinical reason not to transport a child to hospital has been found and a decision made to stay at home, these decisions must be carefully documented.**
- **Provide a 'safety net,' with written information, to any febrile child not transferred to hospital.**
- **If uncertain, seek advice from either their GP or out-of-hours doctor.**
- **The GP should be routinely informed of any consultation.**

Bibliography

1. National Collaborating Centre for Women's and Children's Health. *Urinary Tract Infection in Children: Diagnosis, treatment and long-term management* (CG54). London: Royal College of Obstetricians and Gynaecologists, 2007. Available from: http://www.nice.org.uk/nicemedia/pdf/CG54fullguideline.pdf.
2. Hanna CM, Greenes DS. How much tachycardia in infants can be attributed to fever? *Annals of Emergency Medicine* 2004, 43(6): 699–705.
3. Hay AD, Costelloe C, Redmond NM, Montgomery AA, Fletcher M, Hollinghurst S, et al. Paracetamol plus ibuprofen for the treatment of fever in children (PITCH): Randomised controlled trial. *British Medical Journal* 2008, 337: a1302.
4. National Collaborating Centre for Women's and Children's Health. *Feverish Illness in Children: Assessment and initial management in children younger than 5 years* (CG47). London: National Institute for Health and Clinical Excellence, 2007.
5. National Collaborating Centre for Women's and Children's Health. *Patient's Information Sheet.* London: National Institute for Health and Clinical Excellence, 2007.
6. National Collaborating Centre for Women's and Children's Health. *Bacterial Meningitis and Meningococcal Septicaemia: Management of bacterial meningitis and meningococcal septicaemia in children and young people younger than 16 years in primary and secondary care* (CG102). London: National Institute for Health and Clinical Excellence, 2010. Available from: https://www.nice.org.uk/guidance/cg102.
7. Woollard M, Pitt K. Antipyretic pre-hospital therapy for febrile convulsions: Does the treatment fit? A literature review. *Health Education* 2003, 62(1): 23–28.
8. Sharp A. Management of febrile convulsions within the pre-hospital environment. *Journal of Paramedic Practice* 2016. 8(9): 447–451.
9. National Institute for Health and Clinical Excellence. *Febrile Convulsions.* NICE Clinical Knowledge Summaries: NICE, 2013. Available from: https://cks.nice.org.uk.
10. National Institute for Health and Clinical Excellence. *Feverish Illness in Children: Assessment and Initial Management in children younger than five years.* NICE, 2013. Available from: https://www.nice.org.uk/guidance/cg160/resources/fever-in-children-younger-than-5-years-pdf-246224941765.
11. National Institute for Health and Care Excellence. *Fever in Under 5s: Assessment and initial management* [CG160]. London: NICE 2017. Available at: https://www.nice.org.uk/guidance/cg160.

Gastrointestinal Bleeding

1. Introduction

Gastrointestinal (GI) bleeding is a common medical emergency accounting for 7,000 admissions per year in Scotland alone.

Gastrointestinal haemorrhage is commonly divided into:

- Upper gastrointestinal haemorrhage.
- Lower gastrointestinal haemorrhage.

2. Incidence

- Upper GI bleeding is more common than lower GI bleeding and is more prevalent in socioeconomically deprived areas.
- Upper GI bleeding accounts for up to 85% of gastrointestinal bleeding events.

3. Severity and Outcome

- The severity of gastrointestinal bleeding can range from clinically insignificant blood loss to significant life-threatening haemorrhage.
- Death is uncommon in patients less than 40 years of age, it is estimated that the overall mortality rate in the UK for patients admitted with acute GI bleeding is approximately 7%. The majority of deaths occur in older people, particularly those with co-morbidities. There are many factors that are associated with a poor outcome including liver disease, acute haemodynamic disturbance, clotting abnormalities, continued bleeding, haematemesis, haematochezia, and elevated blood urea.
- Upper GI bleeding tends to be more severe and in extreme circumstances can rapidly lead to hypovolaemic shock.

4. Pathophysiology

- The upper gastrointestinal tract comprises the oesophagus, stomach and duodenum. For common causes of bleeding refer to Table 3.46.

TABLE 3.46 – Common Causes of Upper Gastrointestinal Bleeding

Common causes
● Peptic ulcers: – Duodenal ulcers – Gastric ulcers ● Oesophageal varices ● Gastritis ● Oesophagitis ● Mallory–Weiss tears ● Caustic poison ● Tumour

- The lower gastrointestinal tract comprises the lower part of the small intestine, the colon, rectum and anus. Common causes of bleeding include diverticular disease, inflammatory bowel disease, haemorrhoids, and tumour.

ACUTE UPPER GI BLEEDING

- More than 50% of cases are due to peptic ulcers which, together with oesophagitis and gastritis, account for up to 90% of all upper GI bleeding in older people. 85% of deaths associated with upper GI bleeding occur in persons older than 65 years.
- Patients presenting with upper GI bleeding may have a history of aspirin or non-steroidal anti-inflammatory drug (NSAID) use.
  - Only 50% of patients present with haematemesis alone, 30% with melaena and 20% with haematemesis and melaena
  - Patients with haematemesis tend to have greater blood loss than those with melaena alone. Patients older than 60 years account for up to 45% of all cases (60% of these are women).

Peptic ulcers

- Peptic ulcers are commonly associated with the use of aspirin, non-steroidal anti-inflammatory drugs, corticosteroids, anticoagulants, alcohol and cigarettes.

Oesophageal varices

- It is estimated that variceal bleeding is the cause of 10% of cases. These patients can bleed severely, with up to 8% dying within 48 hours from uncontrolled haemorrhage. It is commonly associated with alcoholic cirrhosis and increased portal pressure (causing progressive dilation of the veins and protrusion of the formed varices into the lumen of the oesophagus). Spontaneous rupture of the varices will cause the patient to become haemodynamically unstable within a very short period of time due to large volumes of blood loss.

Mallory–Weiss tears

- Approximately 10% are caused by oesophageal tears, which are more common in the young. Predisposing factors include hiatal hernia and alcoholism. Initiating factors are persistent coughing or severe retching and vomiting, often after an alcoholic binge; haematemesis presents after several episodes of non-bloody emesis. Bleeding can be mild to moderate.

Gastritis

- Drugs, infections, illnesses, and injuries can cause inflammation of the lining of the stomach and lead to bleeding.

Gastrointestinal Bleeding

Oesophagitis

- Gastroesophageal reflux disease or alcohol can lead to inflammation and ulcers in the lining of the oesophagus which may lead to bleeding.

Tumour

- In the oesophagus, stomach or duodenum can cause bleeding.

ACUTE LOWER GI BLEEDING

Patients with a lower GI bleed commonly present with bright red blood/dark blood with clots per rectum (PR); bright red blood PR in isolation excludes upper GI bleeding in over 98% of cases (unless the patient appears hypovolaemic). Lower GI bleeding is less likely to present with signs of haemodynamic compromise, is more prevalent in men and also has a common history of aspirin or NSAID use. The mean age for lower GI bleeding is 63–77 years, with mortality around 4% (even serious cases have rarely resulted in death). Common causes include:

Diverticular disease

- Diverticular bleeding accounts for up to 55% of cases. Patients commonly present with an abrupt but painless PR bleed. The incidence of diverticular bleeding increases with age.

Inflammatory bowel disease

- Major bleeding from ulcerative colitis and Crohn's disease is rare. Inflammatory bowel disease accounts for less than 10% of cases.

Haemorrhoids

- Haemorrhoids account for less than 10% of cases. Bleeding is bright red and usually noticed on wiping or in the toilet bowl. The incidence is high in pregnancy, a result of straining associated with constipation and hormonal changes. Further evaluation may be needed if the patient complains of an alteration of bowel habit and blood mixed with the stool.

Tumour

- Tumour in the large bowel can cause bleeding.

Differential diagnosis

- Post rectal bleeding can cause significant embarrassment for the patient and care must be taken when assessing female patients that PV bleeding is excluded.

5. Assessment and Management

For the assessment and management of gastrointestinal bleeding refer to Table 3.47.

TABLE 3.47 – ASSESSMENT and MANAGEMENT of: Gastrointestinal Bleeding

ASSESSMENT	MANAGEMENT
• Assess <C>ABCD	• If any of the following **TIME CRITICAL** features present: – major **<C>ABCD** problems, refer to **Medical Emergencies in Adults – Overview** and **Medical Emergencies in Children – Overview**. – haematemesis – large volume of bright red blood – haemodynamic compromise – decreased level of consciousness. • Start correcting any **<C>ABCD** problems. • Undertake a **TIME CRITICAL** transfer to nearest appropriate receiving hospital. • Continue patient management en-route. • Provide an ATMIST information call.
• Assess blood loss	Where does the bleeding originate – upper or lower GI tract? • **Haematemesis** – vomited fresh/dark red/brown/black or 'coffee ground' blood (depending on how long it has been in the stomach). Did this occur after an increase in intra-abdominal pressure (e.g. retching or coughing). • Ascertain how many episodes of non-bloody emesis. • **Melaena** – malodorous, liquid, black stool or bright red/dark blood with clots per rectum (PR). It can be difficult to estimate blood loss when mixed with faeces. • Estimate blood loss – if not visible ask the patient or relatives/carers to estimate colour/volume – PR blood loss is difficult to estimate. (**NB** The blood acts as a laxative, but repeated blood-liquid stool, or just blood, is associated with more severe blood loss than maroon/black solid stool.) • Has the patient suffered unexplained syncope – this may indicate concealed GI bleeding. Ensure PV bleeding is excluded in females.

Gastrointestinal Bleeding

TABLE 3.47 – ASSESSMENT and MANAGEMENT of: Gastrointestinal Bleeding *(continued)*	
• History	• **When did the bleeding begin?** • Is/has the patient: – currently taking or recently taken aspirin or NSAID? – currently taking iron tablets? – consumed food or drink containing red dye(s)? – currently taking beta-blockers or calcium-channel blockers – may mask tachycardia in the shocked patient? – currently taking or recently taken anticoagulatory or antiplatelet therapy? • **Is there a history of:** – bleeding disorders? – liver disease? – abdominal surgery in particular abdominal aortic surgery? – alcohol abuse? – syncope?
• Oxygen saturation	• Monitor the patient's SpO_2, administer oxygen to achieve saturations of >94% if the patient presents as hypoxaemic on air, refer to **Oxygen**.
• Respiratory rate	• Measure and record respiratory rate.
• Pulse	• Measure and record pulse.
• ECG	• If required, monitor and record 12-Lead ECG. Assess for abnormality, refer to **Cardiac Rhythm Disturbance**.
• Assess the patient's pain	• GI bleeding is not generally associated with pain. • Where present, assess the SOCRATES of pain and record initial and subsequent pain scores. • Consider analgesia if appropriate, refer to **Pain Management in Adults** and **Pain Management in Children**.
• Fluid	• Measure and record blood pressure, if required administer fluids, refer to **Intravascular Fluid Therapy in Adults** and **Intravascular Fluid Therapy in Children**. • Tranexamic acid is not indicated in GI haemorrhage due to a lack of current evidence for benefit.
• Blood glucose	• If appropriate, measure and record blood glucose for hypo/hyperglycaemia, refer to **Glycaemic Emergencies in Adults and Children**.
• Temperature	• Measure and record temperature.
• NEWS2	• These observations will enable you to calculate a NEWS2 Score, refer to **Sepsis**.
• Transfer to further care	• Continue patient management en-route. • Provide an alert/information call.
• Documentation	• Complete documentation to include all clinical findings, advice from other clinicians, onward referral and worsening advice given.

KEY POINTS!

Gastrointestinal Bleeding

- **Haematemesis or melaena indicates an upper GI source.**
- **Bright red or dark blood with clots per rectum indicates a lower GI source.**
- **Almost all deaths from GI bleeds occur in older people.**
- **Approximately 80% of all GI bleeds stop spontaneously or respond to conservative management.**
- **Tranexamic acid is not indicated in GI haemorrhage due to a lack of current evidence for benefit.**

Gastrointestinal Bleeding

Bibliography

1. Bennett C, Klingenberg SL, Langholz E, Gluud LL. *Tranexamic acid for upper gastrointestinal bleeding (Review).* London: Cochrane Library and Wiley, 2014. Available from: https://www.cochranelibrary.com/cdsr/doi/10.1002/14651858.CD006640.pub3/epdf/standard.
2. Scottish Intercollegiate Guidelines Network. *Management of Acute Upper and Lower Gastrointestinal Bleeding* (Guideline 105). Edinburgh: SIGN, 2008.
3. Cappell MS, Friedel D. Initial management of acute upper gastrointestinal bleeding: from initial evaluation up to gastrointestinal endoscopy. *Medical Clinics of North America* 2008, 92: 491–509.
4. Edwards AJ, Maskell GF. Acute lower gastrointestinal haemorrhage. *British Medical Journal* 2009, 339: b4156.
5. Michels SL, Collins J, Reynolds MW, Abramsky S, Paredes-Diaz A, McCarberg B. Over-the-counter ibuprofen and risk of gastrointestinal bleeding complications: a systematic literature review. *Current Medical Research and Opinion* 2012, 28(1): 89–99.
6. Palmer K. Acute upper gastrointestinal haemorrhage. *British Medical Bulletin* 2007, 83(1): 307–24.
7. Szajerka T, Jablecki J. Upper gastrointestinal bleeding in a young female with AIDS: a case report. *International Journal of STD & AIDS* 2012, 23(3): e33–4.
8. van Leerdam ME. Epidemiology of acute upper gastrointestinal bleeding. *Best Practice & Research in Clinical Gastroenterology* 2008, 22(2): 209–24.
9. Alkhatib AA, Elkhatib FA, Maldonado A, Abubakr SM, Adler DG. Acute upper gastrointestinal bleeding in elderly people: presentations, endoscopic findings, and outcomes. *Journal of the American Geriatrics Society* 2010, 58(1): 182–5.
10. Kent AJ, O'Beirne J, Negus R. The patient with haematemesis and melaena. *Acute Medicine* 2011, 10(1): 45–9.

Glycaemic Emergencies in Adults and Children

1. Introduction

- A person without diabetes maintains their blood glucose level within a narrow range.
- This is achieved by a balance between glucose entering the blood stream (from the gastrointestinal tract or from the breakdown of stored energy sources) and glucose leaving the circulation through the action of insulin.
- Increasingly, prevalence of both Type 1 and Type 2 diabetes is on the rise, in both adults and children. Type 1 diabetes, previously known as juvenile diabetes, is increasingly diagnosed in the adult population and there are known incidences of diagnosis of Type 2 diabetes in children. It is important to note that Type 2 diabetes is not always associated with severe obesity.

2. Considerations for Patients with Diabetes

2.1 Blood Glucose Monitors

- Prior to testing blood glucose, the patient's fingers must be cleaned using sterile water and a gauze swab. This prevents contamination of blood glucose results from residual deposits on the skin. Alco-wipes are not a suitable alternative as research suggests their use may adversely affect blood glucose readings. Rinsing hands thoroughly in tap water is an acceptable alternative.[1,2]
- Blood glucose monitors should be routinely checked for accuracy using control solutions as provided by manufacturers. Patients with Type 1 diabetes should have their own blood glucose monitors and ambulance clinicians may encounter a wide variety of different devices, which may not be regularly checked. Therefore, it is recommended that clinicians use service-issue blood glucose monitors only.
- Patients with Type 2 diabetes may not have their own blood glucose monitor, and blood glucose levels may only be tested sporadically at their GP's surgery.

2.2 Blood Ketone Meters

Most Type 1 diabetes patients will have a blood ketone meter issued to them. These are operated in the same way as a blood glucose meter. If available, blood ketone meters may assist the ambulance clinician in determining diabetic ketoacidosis (DKA) in the hyperglycaemic patient.

- A blood ketone level of <0.6 mmol/l is normal.
- A blood ketone level >0.6 mmol/l usually requires the patient to administer additional rapid-acting insulin as per 'sick day rules' (see below).
- Ketone levels of >0.6 and <3.0 mmol/l may require hospital assessment in the presence of illness and/or vomiting. However, if the patient is able to reliably eat and drink and administer additional doses of rapid acting insulin (as per 'sick day rules') it may be possible to avoid hospital attendance. In children, specialist diabetes teams should always be contacted for advice.
- A blood ketone level of >=3.0mmol/l is predictive of diabetic ketoacidosis and will require hospital assessment.
- Pregnant women with Type 1 diabetes are more prone to ketosis and thus ketoacidosis, even when glucose levels may be relatively normal.
- Ketoacidosis occasionally occurs in those with Type 2 diabetes during acute illness.[3,4] DKA has also been observed in those Type 2 patients who take a 'flozin tablet to control their diabetes (dapagliflozin, canagliflozin, empagliflozin). It is not uncommon for blood glucose levels to be relatively normal in this situation ('euglycaemic ketoacidosis'). While this is a rare complication of 'flozin treatment, consider ketoacidosis if the patient appears unwell or has symptoms suggestive of DKA.

2.3 Sick Day Rules

- Illness generally raises blood glucose levels and increases the risk of ketone body production. This can result in diabetic ketoacidosis (DKA) if adequate insulin and hydration is not maintained.[5]
- Increased levels of stress hormones during illness may also contribute to high blood glucose levels. Diarrhoea and vomiting may reduce blood glucose levels with a possibility of hypoglycaemia rather than hyperglycaemia. However, ketones (known as starvation ketones) may still be produced in significant quantities.
- NICE guidelines recommend that people with Type 1 diabetes mellitus (T1DM) should be provided with clear guidance for the management of diabetes during periods of illness. Thus many patients with T1DM will be able to competently manage transient episodes of hyperglycaemia at home. Timely and appropriate sick day management may prevent progression to DKA and consequent admission to hospital.

General Sick Day Rule Principles

- Never stop the insulin.
- Insulin dosages may need to be increased or decreased depending on blood glucose or ketone levels. Most patients (or parents of paediatric patients) will be aware of the relevant correction dosages. Paediatric patients will be able to contact their specialist team for further advice and support if needed.
- Encourage fluids to prevent dehydration.
- Increase the frequency of monitoring of blood glucose levels. A minimum of one test every two hours is generally suggested.

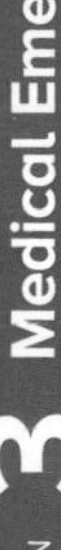

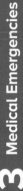

- If available, blood ketone levels should also be closely monitored. Urinalysis for ketones is less reliable, taking longer to be detected and normalised, but in the absence of a blood ketone meter, urine ketones may still be used to guide patients on additional insulin doses.

2.4 Insulin Pumps

- Increasing numbers of Type 1 diabetes patients, especially children, now wear insulin pumps. These deliver a continuous flow of rapid-acting insulin via a subcutaneous cannula, combined with a bolus delivery at mealtimes to cover the carbohydrate content of the meal.
- At no time should these devices be removed or altered by ambulance clinicians.
- Due to the use of rapid-acting insulin, patients using insulin pump therapy will generally not need to consume a slow release carbohydrate, such as a biscuit or toast, once blood glucose levels have returned to normal. If in doubt consult the patient or the child's caregivers.
- Patients using insulin pumps are at a high risk of DKA in cases of cannula blockage or pump failure. If needing to transfer a patient with Type 1 diabetes on insulin pump therapy, encourage the patient to bring a supply of pump consumables with them. Hospitals do not routinely stock insulin pump consumables, potentially risking an interruption in insulin delivery for the patient, which may lead to ketosis and DKA.

2.5 Continuous Glucose Monitors (CGMs) and Flash Glucose Monitoring

- These devices are also becoming more common. These are subcutaneous devices that read interstitial fluid glucose levels at approximately 5-minute intervals.
- These monitors can not be relied on by ambulance clinicians in lieu of blood glucose testing, as interstitial glucose lags behind that of blood glucose and does not always give accurate readings.

2.6 Driving

- It is a legal requirement for drivers to inform the DVLA of their insulin-treated diabetes. Patients with Type 2 diabetes on tablet or non-insulin injectable therapy are not required to inform the DVLA of their condition. However, patients with Type 2 diabetes taking medication that may predispose them to hypoglycaemia (e.g. gliclazide, glipizide, glimepiride, glibenclamide, tolbutamide and metiglinide or repaglinide) are required to inform the DVLA if they have recurrent episodes of hypoglycaemia.[6]
- When it is appropriate – particularly when discharging a patient who is a driver after a hypoglycaemic episode and not conveying them to a health care facility – ambulance clinicians should:
  - advise the patient on the impact of their medical condition for safe driving ability
  - advise the patient on their legal requirement to notify the DVLA if they have insulin-treated diabetes
  - document any of the above if it is discussed with the patient.

Note that the patient could be fined up to £1,000 if they do not tell the DVLA about a medical condition that affects their driving, and they could be prosecuted if they are involved in an accident as a result.

There are differences in requirements to report to the DVLA between Group 1 (cars and motorbikes) and Group 2 (bus or lorry) drivers and differences between Type 1 and Type 2 patients. Current legislation (January 2018)[7] states that:

- Nocturnal hypoglycaemic events do not require reporting to the DVLA.
- Those on insulin or who take tablets for diabetes that may predispose them to hypoglycaemia (as above) should, when assistance has been required to treat **DAYTIME** hypoglycaemia, report it to the DVLA **IF** episodes have occurred **within the past 12 months, and the last event has occurred within the last 3 months**, when this has been the:
  - second episode (Group 1, car and motorbike) or
  - first episode (Group 2, bus and lorry).

If an ambulance clinician is concerned that the patient cannot or will not notify the DVLA themselves after recurrent episodes of hypoglycaemia requiring assistance, it would be appropriate to liaise with the patient's GP and again, document these actions.

3. Hypoglycaemia

- Hypoglycaemia is the term used to describe low blood glucose levels.[8]
- In the patient with diabetes, the definition of hypoglycaemia is a blood glucose of <4.0 mmol/l.[9] This should not be confused with the lower level of <3.0 mmol/l used for patients without diabetes. There are three types of hypoglycaemia: mild, moderate and severe. In mild cases, the person can treat themselves, whereas in severe cases, third party assistance will be required.
- Correction of hypoglycaemia is a medical emergency. If left untreated hypoglycaemia may lead to the patient suffering permanent brain damage and may even prove fatal.
- Hypoglycaemia occurs when glucose metabolism is disturbed (refer to Table 3.48).

Glycaemic Emergencies in Adults and Children

TABLE 3.48 – Risk Factors for Hypoglycaemia

Medical risk factors[10]	Lifestyle risk factors
• Insulin or other hypoglycaemic drug treatments. • Tight glycaemic control. • Previous history of severe hypoglycaemia. • Undetected nocturnal hypoglycaemia. • Long duration of Type 1 diabetes. • Duration of insulin therapy in Type 2 diabetes. • Lipohypertrophy at injection sites. • Impaired awareness of hypoglycaemia. • Preceding hypoglycaemia (<3.5 mmol/l). • Severe hepatic dysfunction. • Renal dialysis therapy. • Impaired renal function. • Inadequate treatment of previous hypoglycaemia. • Terminal illness. • Sepsis. • Endocrine illness (including Addisonian crisis). • Sudden cessation of peritoneal dialysis. • Hypothermia (especially in very young babies). • Sudden cessation of tube or IV feeding. • Very sick or traumatised children. • Very young babies (especially pre-term). • Ketotic hypoglycaemia of infancy.	• Drug ingestion, e.g. oral hypoglycaemic drugs, beta-blockers, alcohol. • Inadequate carbohydrate intake. • Increased exercise (relative to usual)/excessive physical activity. • Irregular lifestyle (or supervision if the patient is a child). • Increasing age. • Excessive or chronic alcohol intake. • Early pregnancy. • Breast feeding. • No or inadequate blood glucose monitoring.

- Any person whose level of consciousness is decreased, who is having a convulsion, is seriously ill or traumatised should have hypoglycaemia excluded.
- Some patients can detect the early symptoms for themselves, but others may be too young or deteriorate rapidly and without apparent warning.
- Abnormal neurological features may occur, for example, one-sided weakness, identical to a stroke.
- Signs and symptoms can vary from person to person. Symptoms may be masked due to medication or other injuries, for example, with beta-blocking agents (refer to Table 3.49).
- The classical symptoms of hypoglycaemia may **NOT** be present, and children may have a variety of unusual symptoms with low blood glucose (refer to Table 3.49).
- In diabetes mellitus (DM) hypoglycaemia is due to a relative excess of exogenously administered insulin over available glucose.

TABLE 3.49 – Signs and Symptoms of Hypoglycaemia

• **Autonomic**[11,12]	• Sweating • Trembling/shaking • Palpitations/pounding heart • Hunger
• **General malaise**	• Headache • Nausea
• **Neuroglycopenic**[13]	• Incoordination • Confusion • Speech difficulty • Drowsiness • Odd behaviour • Aggression/combative behaviour • Fitting • Unconsciousness

SECTION 3 Medical Emergencies

Glycaemic Emergencies in Adults and Children

3.1 Hypoglycaemia in the Absence of Diabetes

This is a rare occurrence with many different causes. It can generally be divided into two types:[14,15]

- **Reactive hypoglycaemia** – may be the result of gastrointestinal surgery or enzyme deficiency and may occasionally be found in patients with pre-diabetes as the body struggles to regulate insulin production.
- **Fasting hypoglycaemia** – may occur as a result of medication such as salicylates, certain antibiotics, pentamidine and quinine; with excessive alcohol intake – especially binge drinking; serious illnesses, especially those affecting the liver, heart or kidneys; hormonal abnormalities; or the presence of certain types of tumours, particularly those in the pancreas.

Note that hypoglycaemia in the absence of diabetes is diagnosed by the lower blood glucose of <3.0 mmol/l.

3.2 Impaired Awareness of Hypoglycaemia

- Impaired awareness (IA) arises in those whose perception of hypoglycaemia is reduced or absent and as such the possibility of severe hypoglycaemic events is increased. IA is more commonly associated with insulin therapy[16] and may be induced by recurrent hypoglycaemic episodes and/or strict glycaemic control, which cause a dampening of the sympathetic response.[17] It is the dampening or absence, of any sympathetic response that leads to an under-recognition of the onset of hypoglycaemia, progression to neuroglycopenia and subsequently an inability to self-treat. The condition can be objectively identified using a number of validated tools[18] and is reversible for many through strict avoidance of hypoglycaemia for a period of weeks or months.[19,20,21]
- In the general population of those diagnosed with diabetes treated with insulin, the prevalence of IA varies between 8% to 25%[22] and increases with the duration of insulin therapy.[23] However, more recent evidence suggests the prevalence may be significantly higher (53% to 57%) in the ambulance service hypoglycaemia population.[24]

3.3 Assessment and Management of Hypoglycaemia

For the assessment and management of hypoglycaemia, refer to Tables 3.50 and 3.51 and Figure 3.10. The principles of assessment and management are essentially the same in adults and children both with and without diabetes.
NB Note that the lower blood glucose level for hypoglycaemia in the patient without diabetes is 3.0 mmol/l.

TABLE 3.50 – ASSESSMENT and MANAGEMENT of: Hypoglycaemia

ASSESSMENT	MANAGEMENT
• Undertake <C>ABCD assessment • Consider and look for medical alert/information signs (alert bracelets, chains and cards) • Assess blood glucose level	• Start correcting <C>ABCD problems (refer to **Medical Emergencies in Adults – Overview** and **Medical Emergencies in Children – Overview**). • Measure and record blood glucose level (pre-treatment measure). • Clean the patient's fingers prior to testing blood glucose levels as they may have been in contact with sugary substances (e.g. sweets). It is vital that fingers are cleaned with sterile water prior to obtaining a blood glucose reading and NOT alcohol wipes as these may give a false high reading. • Glucagon may take 10 minutes to take effect and requires the patient to have adequate glycogen stores – thus, it may be ineffective if glycogen stores have been exhausted through, for example, frequent episodes of hypoglycaemia, alcohol use or poor carbohydrate content of diet. This is likely in any patients who have any NON-diabetic causes of hypoglycaemia, although it is worth trying.
SEVERE: patient unconscious (GCS ≤8)/convulsing or very aggressive	• Check <C>ABCD and correct as necessary. • Administer IV glucose 10% over 15 minutes (refer to **Glucose 10%** for dosages). • Only administer glucagon IM if IV access is not possible (onset of action is 10 minutes, but can take up to 15 minutes). Glucagon is less effective in those who take a sulphonylurea (e.g. gliclazide, glipizide, tolbutamide, glimepiride), are chronically malnourished or take excess alcohol, so IV glucose is preferred in these groups. **NB** IM glucagon to be given ONCE ONLY.

TABLE 3.50 – ASSESSMENT and MANAGEMENT of: Hypoglycaemia *(continued)*	
	• Keep nil by mouth as there is an increased risk of aspiration/choking. • Titrate to effect – an improvement in clinical state and glucose level should be observed rapidly. • Re-assess blood glucose level after 10 minutes. • If <4.0 mmol/l administer a further dose of IV 10% glucose. • Re-assess blood glucose level after a further 15 minutes. • Consider rapid transfer to the nearest suitable receiving hospital if no improvement. • Monitor vital signs and conscious level en-route. Check glucose again if patient deteriorates, or half hourly. • Provide a pre-alert/information call if necessary.
MILD to **MODERATE:** patient conscious, orientated, able to swallow	• If capable, cooperative and deemed to have a safe swallow, administer 15–20 grams of quick-acting carbohydrate, such as one of the following: – 5–7 Dextrosol® tablets (or 4–5 Glucotabs®) or – 1 bottle (60 ml) Glucojuice® or – 150–200 ml pure fruit juice, e.g. orange (avoid pure fruit juice if a renal dialysis patient because of potassium content) or – 1–2 tubes of 40% glucose gel or – 3–4 heaped teaspoons of sugar dissolved in water (**NB** this is not an effective treatment for patients taking acarbose as it prevents the breakdown of sucrose to glucose). • Do not give chocolate as it is slower acting. • If **NOT** capable and cooperative, but able to swallow, administer 1–2 tubes of 40% glucose gel to the buccal mucosa or give IV glucose 10% or IM glucagon (refer to **Glucagon**) if IV access is not possible. • Reassess blood glucose level after 10–15 minutes and ensure blood glucose level has improved to at least 4.0 mmol/l in addition to an improvement in level of consciousness. • If no improvement, repeat oral treatment up to three times in total. **NB** IM glucagon to be given **ONCE ONLY**. • If no improvement after three treatments or 30–45 minutes, give IV glucose 10% (refer to **Glucose 10%**). • Refer to Table 3.51. • Once blood glucose is >4 mmol/l, give a starchy snack, e.g. two biscuits; one slice of bread/toast; 200–300 ml glass of milk (not soya); a normal meal if due (must contain carbohydrate). • **NB** Patients given glucagon require a larger portion of long-acting carbohydrate to replenish glycogen stores (double the suggested amount above). • **NB** Patients who self-manage their insulin pumps (CSII) may not need a long-acting carbohydrate. • Transfer to the nearest suitable receiving hospital if the patient requires further treatment, otherwise the patient can usually be safely left at home. If the patient is a child, ensure they are left with a responsible adult.

Glycaemic Emergencies in Adults and Children

TABLE 3.51 – Care Pathway

Patients who do not need conveyance to hospital

- The following patients may not need conveyance to hospital:
  - patients whose episode was mild or moderate and who are now fully recovered after treatment
  - patients with a sustained blood glucose level of >5.0 mmol/l
  - patients who have been able to eat/drink a glucose and carbohydrate-containing food where relevant.
- If the patient is a child, they must be in the care of a responsible adult.
- Advise patients/carers to call for help if any symptoms of hypoglycaemia recur.
- Ambulance services must arrange for a message to be forwarded to a primary healthcare team or diabetes nurse as per local pathways. All patients with hypoglycaemia who are requiring third party assistance should be referred to a specialist diabetes team. Where these pathways do not exist, the patient's GP must be informed.
- Patient consent is not required in order to make a referral, although the patient should be informed that a referral is being made.
- Consider giving the patient and carers a patient information leaflet.
- Consider advising the patient about their responsibilities in relation to driving.

Patients who require further care

Consider conveying to hospital patients that are older, frail, have a low BMI, live alone, are on multiple medications.

- The following patients should be transferred to further care, with continuing patient management en-route:
  - those who have had recurrent treatment within the previous 48 hours
  - patients whose episode was severe and had a very slow response and recovery after treatment
  - patients taking **sulphonylureas (glibenclamide, glipizide, gliclazide, tolbutamide, glimepiride). These can be longer acting and result in a prolonged or recurrent hypoglycaemic event. Be aware that you may need to monitor these patients for a longer time period and use clinical judgement**
  - patients with no previous history of diabetes who have suffered their first hypoglycaemic episode
  - patients with a blood glucose level ≤4.0 mmol/l after treatment
  - patients who have not returned to normal mental status within 10 minutes of treatment
  - patients with any additional disorders or other complicating factors (e.g. renal dialysis, chest pain, cardiac arrhythmias, Addison's disease, alcohol consumption, dyspnoea, seizures or focal neurological signs/symptoms)
  - patients with signs of infection (urinary tract infection, upper respiratory tract infections) and/or are unwell ('flu-like symptoms).

4. Hyperglycaemia

- Hyperglycaemia is the term used to describe high blood glucose levels. Symptoms include unusual thirst (polydipsia), urinary frequency (polyuria) and tiredness. They are usually of slower onset in comparison to those of hypoglycaemia but can develop relatively quickly (days to weeks) in those with newly presenting Type 1 diabetes.
- Patients with diabetes mellitus are very likely to develop a raised blood glucose in response to infection and will have instructions as to how to deal with this – so called 'sick day rules' (see above).
- Hyperglycaemia may also occur transiently in patients who are severely physically stressed (e.g. during a convulsion).
- It is important to distinguish a simple raised blood glucose from the condition of diabetic ketoacidosis, which is much more serious. A raised blood glucose is not a pre-hospital emergency unless diabetic ketoacidosis is present. However, the underlying reason for the raised blood glucose may well be an emergency in its own right.
- In adults, if capillary blood glucose is more than 7.8 mmol/l but less than 11.1 mmol/l this may indicate that the patient is at risk of Type 2 diabetes, or has non-diabetic hyperglycaemia (raised blood glucose levels but not in the diabetic range, also known as 'impaired glucose regulation'), or 'stress hyperglycaemia' (transient rise in blood glucose levels due to acute illness in a patient without diabetes, which settles to

Glycaemic Emergencies in Adults and Children

MILD

The patient is conscious, orientated and able to swallow.

- Give 15–20 g quick acting carbohydrate, such as:
  - 4–5 Glucotabs or
  - 1 bottle (60 ml) Glucojuice® or
  - 1–2 tubes 40% glucose gel or
  - 3–4 heaped teaspoons of sugar dissolved in water or
  - 150–200 ml pure fruit juice.
- Re-test blood glucose after 15 mins.
- If blood glucose remains <4 mmol/l, repeat above treatment up to twice more at 15-minute intervals until a blood glucose of >4 mmol/l is obtained.
- If blood glucose fails to rise >4 mmol/l AFTER 3 cycles of oral treatment (i.e. 45 mins), consider IV 10% glucose or IM glucagon.

MODERATE

The patient is conscious and able to swallow, but may be confused, disoriented and/or combative.

If capable and cooperative:

- Give 15–20 g quick acting carbohydrate, such as:
  - 4–5 Glucotabs or
  - 1 bottle (60 ml) Glucojuice® or
  - 1–2 tubes 40% glucose gel or
  - 3–4 heaped teaspoons of sugar dissolved in water or
  - 150–200 ml pure fruit juice.

If **NOT** capable and cooperative, but able to swallow:

- Administer 1–2 tubes of glucose gel 40% to the buccal mucosa or give 1 mg glucagon IM (refer to **Glucagon**).
- Re-test blood glucose after 15 mins. If <4 mmol/l, repeat administration of 40% glucose gel. **NB** IM glucagon cannot be repeated.
- If 40% glucose gel cannot be administered due to patient disposition, consider IV 10% glucose (refer to **Glucose 10%**).
- If blood glucose remains <4 mmol/l, repeat above treatment up to twice more at 15-minute intervals until a blood glucose of >4 mmol/l is obtained.

SEVERE

The patient is unconscious/fitting or combative or where there is increased risk of aspiration/choking.

- Check ABC and correct as necessary.
- Administer IV glucose 10% over 15 minutes (refer to **Glucose 10%** for dosages).
- If IV not possible administer IM glucagon (may take up to 15 minutes to work and IM glucagon ONCE ONLY).
- Re-assess blood glucose level after 10 minutes.
- If blood glucose remains <4.0 mmol/l, administer a further dose of IV 10% glucose.
- Repeat treatment until a blood glucose of >4 mmol/l is obtained.
- If no improvement, convey to nearest suitable receiving hospital.
- Check glucose again if patient deteriorates.
- Provide a pre-alert/information call if necessary.

Blood glucose level should now be 4 mmol/l or above.

- Once a blood glucose of >4 mmol/l is achieved, give a starchy snack, e.g. two biscuits; one slice of bread/toast; 200–300 ml glass of milk (not soya); a normal meal if due (must contain carbohydrate).
- **NB** Patients given glucagon require a larger portion of long-acting carbohydrate to replenish glycogen stores (double the suggested amount above).
- **NB** Patients who self-manage their insulin pumps (CSII) may not need a long-acting carbohydrate.
- In most cases patients who have fully recovered and maintain glucose levels >4 mmol/l will not require admission to ED.

If blood glucose is now >4 mmol/l, follow up treatment as described on the left.

Glucagon may take up to 15 minutes to work and can be ineffective in the very young, older people, undernourished patients or those with hepatic disease.
In patients with renal/cardiac disease, use IV fluids with caution.
Avoid fruit juice in renal failure. **Note:** the carbohydrate content of some commercially available glucose-containing drinks varies – individual product labels should be checked. Diet drinks may not contain sugar.

Figure 3.10 – Hypoglycaemic emergencies algorithm.

Source: http://www.diabetologists-abcd.org.uk/JBDS/JBDS_HypoGuideline_FINAL_280218.pdf

normal after the acute illness has settled), or the patient may be taking medication that causes a rise in blood glucose, e.g. steroids, anti-retrovirals.[25] Patients should be advised to see their GP for an HbA1c test to determine their risk of Type 2 diabetes.

- If patients have no symptoms of diabetes yet a capillary glucose of >=11.1 mmol/l, they should be directed to their GP for confirmatory tests for diabetes.
- If patients have typical osmotic symptoms such as excessive thirst, polyuria, tiredness, weight loss, thrush or recurrent infections, with capillary glucose >=11.1 mmol/l, that is diagnostic of diabetes, in which case follow the guidance on hyperglycaemia below.
- The majority of children who develop diabetes have Type 1 diabetes, the diagnosis and treatment of which is a medical emergency. In order to prevent these children developing diabetic ketoacidosis, prompt diagnosis is necessary as DKA is the principal cause of death in children with diabetes. Clinicians should maintain a high index of suspicion when presented with any generally ill child with a blood glucose >11 mmol/l and convey immediately to ED/Paediatric Assessment Unit (PAU). If blood glucose is 7–10.9 mmol/l, diabetes or hyperglycaemia due to illness should be considered and referred to/discussed with the patient's GP.[26]
- Type 1 diabetes can occur even in infants. These children may have blood glucose levels that are particularly difficult to control and may be very difficult to manage.

5. Diabetic Ketoacidosis (DKA)

- A relative lack of circulating insulin means that cells cannot take up glucose from the blood and use it to provide energy. This forces the cells to provide energy for metabolism from other sources, such as fatty acids.
- Omissions or inadequate dosage of insulin or other hypoglycaemic therapy may also contribute or be responsible. Some medications, particularly steroids, may greatly exacerbate the situation.
- Ketones are produced as a by-product of fatty acid metabolism in the liver. Ketones are acidic chemicals whose accumulation leads to the development of a metabolic acidosis. Ketone production ceases with insulin therapy, which allows the body to convert from fat to its preferred fuel substrate, glucose. Insulin with IV fluids allow the body to stop ketone production and excrete ketones via the urine, which explains why urine ketostix tests remain positive even after DKA has resolved.
- New onset Type 1 diabetes may present with DKA. More frequently it complicates intercurrent illness in a person with diabetes. Infections, myocardial infarction (which may be silent) or a stroke may precipitate the condition.
- Patients may present with one or more signs and symptoms and this should alert the pre-hospital provider to the possibility of hyperglycaemia and DKA (refer to Table 3.52).
- Diabetic ketoacidosis (DKA) may occur relatively rapidly in children, sometimes without a long history of the classical symptoms. The absolute blood glucose level is not a good indicator of the presence of DKA – some children with blood glucose levels in the >20 range may appear quite well and not have DKA.
- Where available, ketone measurement (blood or urine) is useful in the diagnosis of DKA.
- Patients with diabetes may present with significant dehydration, resulting in reduced fluid in both the vascular and tissue compartments. Often this has taken time to develop and will take time to correct.
- In adults, dehydration is very common in association with DKA and usually requires IV fluid resuscitation in line with intravascular fluid therapy guidelines. Note that rapid fluid replacement into the vascular compartment can compromise the cardiovascular system, particularly where there is pre-existing cardiovascular disease and in the elderly. Gradual rehydration over hours rather than minutes is indicated.
- Children and young adults with DKA may also present with significant dehydration – however there is an increased risk of cerebral oedema associated with IV fluid therapy in this age group (refer to **Intravascular Fluid Therapy in Children**). Do not give children in DKA IV fluids unless they have clear evidence of hypovolaemic shock. Consider giving fluids when the time to get the patient to hospital is prolonged. Caution is advised in children, young adults and adults with a low BMI as there have been reports of cerebral oedema.
- Do not try to give oral fluids to children with DKA – they have a very high risk of aspiration.

6. Hyperosmolar Hyperglycaemic State (HHS) – previously Hyperglycaemic Hyperosmotic Non-Ketotic Coma (HONK)

- HHS is a complication of Type 2 diabetes and is defined by the presence of high blood glucose (>30 mmol/l) usually without the presence of ketones, with a resultant state of hyperosmolality.

Glycaemic Emergencies in Adults and Children

TABLE 3.52 – Signs and Symptoms of Hyperglycaemia and DKA	
Hyperglycaemia	**Diabetic ketoacidosis**
The symptoms of hyperglycaemia include: ● polyuria ● polydipsia ● weight loss ● lethargy ● recurrent infections especially thrush ● blurred vision ● fruity odour of ketones on the breath (resembling nail varnish remover) **NB** Not everyone can detect this odour. ● presence of ketones (measured) in the urine and/or blood ● hyperventilation	In addition to symptoms of hyperglycaemia, the patient presenting with DKA may also have: ● vomiting ● abdominal pain ● rapid breathing ● appear confused ● other autoimmune conditions are more common in Type 1 diabetes, e.g. Addison's disease which can predispose to DKA ● dehydration, dry mouth and possible circulatory failure due to hypovolaemia ● Kussmaul breathing
The signs of ketoacidosis may include: ● A – reduced conscious level/coma – check airway. ● B – rapid deep breathing (Kussmaul respiration). ● C – clinically dehydrated with possible circulatory failure due to hypovolaemia. ● D – conscious level may be reduced; check airway protected. Aspiration may be a risk. ● E – appear thin or exhibit signs of dramatic weight loss; there may be evidence of diabetes complications, e.g. previous toe/foot amputation or foot ulceration. Consider pregnancy in women of child-bearing age. The fetus is very sensitive to ketosis in the mother.	

TABLE 3.53 – ASSESSMENT and MANAGEMENT of: DKA in Adults and Children	
ASSESSMENT	**MANAGEMENT**
● Undertake ABCD assessment	● Start correcting ABC problems (refer to **Medical Emergencies in Adults – Overview** and **Medical Emergencies in Children – Overview**). ● Consider giving IV fluids if there is clear evidence of circulatory failure or dehydration **and in under age 18 no more than 10 ml/kg sodium chloride** (refer to **Intravascular Fluid Therapy** and/or **0.9% Sodium Chloride**). **This caution should also be extended to young adults with a low BMI who may also be at increased risk of cerebral oedema.**
● If the patient is **TIME CRITICAL**	● Correct life-threatening conditions, airway and breathing on scene. ● Then commence transfer to nearest suitable receiving hospital. **NB** These patients have a potentially life-threatening condition – they require urgent hospital treatment including insulin and fluid/electrolyte therapy.
● Consider and look for medical alert/information signs (alert bracelets, chains, tattoos and cards)	
● Assess for blood glucose level	● Measure and record blood glucose level.

(continued)

15. Eckert-Norton M, Kirk S. Non-diabetic hypoglycaemia. JCEM. 2013, 98(10): 39–40.
16. Graveling AJ et al. Impaired awareness of hypoglycaemia: A review. *Diabetes and Metabolism*, 36: S64–S74.
17. Frier BM. Impaired awareness of hypoglycaemia. In BM Frier and M Fisher (eds), *Hypoglycaemia in Clinical Diabetes*. Oxford: John Wiley and Sons, 2007: 141–170.
18. Gold AE, Macleod KM, Frier BM. Frequency of severe hypoglycemia in patients with Type I diabetes with impaired awareness of hypoglycaemia. *Diabetes Care*. 1994, 17(7): 697–703.
19. Cranston I, Lomas J, Amiel SA, Maran A, Macdonald I. Restoration of hypoglycaemia awareness in patients with long-duration insulin-dependent diabetes. *The Lancet*. 1994, 344(8918): 283–287.
20. Dagogo-Jack S, Rattarasarn C, Cryer PE. Reversal of hypoglycaemia unawareness, but not defective glucose counter-regulation, in IDDM. *Diabetes*. 1994, 43: 1426–1434.
21. Fanelli C, Pampanelli S, Epifano L, Rambotti AM, Vincenzo A et al. Long-term recovery from unawareness, deficient counterregulation and lack of cognitive dysfunction during hypoglycaemia, following institution of rational, intensive insulin therapy in IDDM. *Diabetologia*. 1994, 37: 1265–1267.
22. Geddes J, Schopman JE, Zammitt NN et al. Prevalence of impaired awareness of hypoglycaemia in adults with Type 1 diabetes. *Diabet Med*. 2008, 25: 501–504.
23. Hepburn DA, Patrick AW, Eadington DW et al. Unawareness of hypoglycaemia in insulin-treated diabetic patients: prevalence and relationship to autonomic neuropathy. *Diabet Med*. 1990, 7: 711–717.
24. Duncan EAS, Fitzpatrick D, Ikegwuonu T et al. Role and prevalence of impaired awareness of hypoglycaemia in ambulance service attendances to people who have had a severe hypoglycaemic emergency: a mixed-methods study. *BMJ Open*. 2018, 8: e019522.
25. Sampson M, Haq M, Hanley S. New diagnosis of diabetes in inpatients [JBDS Guideline 14 – forthcoming]. Available at: https://abcd.care/joint-british-diabetes-societies-jbds-inpatient-care-group.
26. South West Paediatric Diabetes Network. *Referral and Ongoing Care for Children with Suspected Diabetes*. 2014. Available at: http://rms.kernowccg.nhs.uk/content/Referral%20and%20Ongoing%20Care%20for%20Children%20with%20suspected%20Diabetes.pdf.
27. National Institute for Health and Care Excellence. *Diagnosis and Management of Type 1 Diabetes in Children, Young People and Adults* [CG15]. London: NICE, 2004. Available at: https://www.nice.org.uk/guidance/cg15
28. National Institute for Health and Care Excellence. *Diabetes in Pregnancy: Management from pre-conception to the postnatal period* [NG3]. London: NICE, 2015. Available at: https://www.nice.org.uk/guidance/ng3.
29. National Institute for Health and Care Excellence. *Diabetes (Type 1 and Type 2) in Children and Young People: Diagnosis and management* [NG18]. London: NICE 2015. Available at: https://www.nice.org.uk/guidance/ng18.
30. National Institute for Health and Care Excellence. *Type 2 Diabetes in Adults: Management* [NG28]. London: NICE, 2015. Available at: https://www.nice.org.uk/guidance/ng28.
31. BCT Field, R Nayar, A Kilvert, M Baxter, J Hickey et al. A retrospective observational study of people with Type 1 diabetes with self-reported severe hypoglycaemia reveals high level of ambulance attendance but low levels of therapy change and specialist intervention. *Diabet Med*. 2018. Available at: https://onlinelibrary.wiley.com/doi/pdf/10.1111/dme.13670.
32. Welsh Government. *Diabetes Delivery Plan for Wales 2016-2020*. Available at: https://gov.wales/topics/health/nhswales/plans/diabetes/?lang=en.
33. National Institute for Health and Care Excellence. *Sepsis: Recognition, diagnosis and early management* [NG51]. London: NICE 2016. Available at: https://www.nice.org.uk/guidance/ng51.
34. National Institute for Health and Care Excellence. *Fever in Under 5s: Assessment and initial management* [CG160]. London: NICE 2017. Available at: https://www.nice.org.uk/guidance/cg160.
35. Royal College of Paediatrics and Child Health. National Paediatric Diabetes Audit Report 2015–16. Available at: https://www.rcpch.ac.uk/work-we-do/quality-improvement-patient-safety/national-paediatrics-diabetes-audit.
36. Diabetes UK. *Do You Know the 4 Ts of Type 1 Diabetes?* Available at: https://www.diabetes.org.uk/Get_involved/Campaigning/4-Ts-campaign.
37. Joint British Diabetes Societies Inpatient Care Group. *The management of the hyperosmolar hyperglycaemic state (HHS) in adults with diabetes*. August 2012. Available at: http://www.diabetologists-abcd.org.uk/JBDS/JBDS_IP_HHS_Adults.pdf.
38. Stoner GD. Hyperosmolar Hyperglycemic State. *Am Fam Physician*. 171(9): 1723–1730.

Headache

1. Introduction

- Headache disorders are among the most common disorders of the nervous system and are a feature of both minor and major illness, which can prove challenging for a clinician.
- Most headaches are simple and not serious, but care must be taken to ensure that **TIME CRITICAL** conditions are not missed.
- A detailed history is vital when dealing with headache as the aetiology may go back hours, days, months or even years in relation to family history or childhood illness, e.g. tumours.

2. Incidence

- More than 10 million people in the UK suffer from headaches. Most headaches are not serious and can be treated with over-the counter medicines and lifestyle changes such as getting more rest and drinking enough fluids. However, there are red flags in both history and examination that may indicate more concerning causes.
- The severity of headaches varies from patient to patient in terms of the pain the patient experiences. Although the pain may be the primary concern of the patient, it may not be associated with the severity of the underlying cause.
- The outcome for a patient presenting to ambulance services for headache will be as varied as the cause of the headache: the clinical significance of the headache and the progression are all dependent on the presenting factors.

3. Types of Headache

- Headaches can be broadly defined as primary or secondary:
  - **Primary headaches** are those which occur spontaneously (simple headaches); occur in response to a lifelong condition (e.g. migraines); are 'tension-type' headaches (various aetiologies); or are severe, short-lasting headaches (cluster headaches). These should not be considered as being pathophysiological as that is normal for the patient.
  - **Secondary headaches** are secondary to illness or injury and are pathological in origin, for instance head trauma (skull fracture); infective origin (i.e. meningitis); intracranial haemorrhage (i.e. spontaneous subarachnoid bleed or subdural bleed following trauma); or vascular (i.e. temporal arteritis).
- It is difficult to accurately differentiate between a simple headache, which requires no treatment, and a potentially more serious condition. Table 3.55 lists **'red flag'** symptoms that require the patient to undergo hospital assessment. **NB** This does not mean that any patient presenting without these symptoms is safe to be left at home.
- Consideration should be given to transferring all first presentations of severe headache to the emergency department for further investigation.

TABLE 3.55 — Red Flag Signs and Symptoms
• Headache localised to the vertex, i.e. top of the head.
• Escalating headache of an unusual nature.
• Changed visual acuity.
• Meningeal irritation, i.e. neck stiffness and photophobia.
• Cranial nerve palsy.
• Worsening headache with fever.
• Sudden-onset or thunderclap headache reaching maximum intensity within five minutes.
• New-onset neurological deficit, i.e. loss of function or altered sensation.
• New-onset cognitive dysfunction.
• Change in personality.
• Impaired level of consciousness.
• Recent head trauma, typically within the past three months.
• Headache triggered by cough, Valsalva (trying to breathe out with nose and mouth blocked) or sneeze.
• Headache triggered by exercise.
• Orthostatic headache, i.e. a headache that changes with posture.
• Symptoms suggestive of giant cell arteritis, which could include pain and tenderness over the temples, jaw pain while eating or talking, or vision problems.
• Symptoms and signs of acute narrow-angle glaucoma, i.e. red eye.
• A substantial change in the characteristics of their headache.
• Vomiting without other obvious cause.
• Newly presenting ataxia, i.e. a neurological sign consisting of a lack of voluntary coordination of muscle movements.
• Any evidence of a rash.

3.1 Migraine

- A migraine is a severe headache felt as a throbbing pain that is usually unilateral and frontal, often accompanied by nausea and vomiting. Some people also have other symptoms, such as sensitivity to light. Migraine is a common health condition, affecting about 15% of adults in the UK.

Headache

TABLE 3.56 – ASSESSMENT and MANAGEMENT of: **Headache** *(continued)*	
– Blood pressure and fluids	● Measure and record blood pressure, if required administer fluids, refer to **Intravascular Fluid Therapy in Adults** and **Intravascular Fluid Therapy in Children**.
– Blood Glucose	● If appropriate, measure and record blood glucose for hypo/hyperglycaemia, refer to **Glycaemic Emergencies in Adults and Children.**
– Temperature	● Measure and record temperature.
– NEWS2	● These observations will enable you to calculate a NEWS2 Score, refer to **Sepsis**.
– Record pain score	● Assess the **SOCRATES** of the pain: **S**ite — where exactly is the pain? **O**nset — what was the patient doing when the pain came on? **C**haracter — what does the pain feel like? **R**adiates — where does the pain spread to? **A**ssociated symptoms — e.g. nausea, dizziness. **T**iming — how long has the patient had pain? **E**xacerbating/relieving factors — what makes it better or worse? **S**everity — obtain an initial pain score. ● Offer symptomatic pain relief for clinically benign headaches, using appropriate pain management drug therapy and taking into account the patient's preference, co-morbidities and risk of adverse events. ● Consideration should therefore be given to initial management with NSAID and/or paracetamol, combined with onward referral for consideration of additional therapies such as anti-emetics and triptans **EXCEPT** in cluster headaches where paracetamol, NSAIDs, opioids, ergots or oral triptans should **NOT** be offered for the acute treatment. In this instance, the patient should be referred to their GP for onward management. Beware of making the diagnosis of cluster headaches as it is very rare and other serious conditions may present in this way. ● Where medication overuse is the cause, advise the patient to stop taking all overused acute headache medication and see their GP. It is best to stop abruptly rather than gradually. It is important to note that headache symptoms are likely to get worse in the short term before they improve and that there may be associated withdrawal symptoms. ● **Avoid morphine** due to potential side effects, which could worsen the patient's condition and/or hinder further assessment.
● Assess for:	● Key questions for a patient with headache: – Is this the worst headache ever? – Is it different from your usual headache? – Is this a new headache?
● Assess for red flag symptoms (refer to Table 3.55)	● **Multiple red flags significantly increase the risk of serious pathology.** ● Undertake a **TIME CRITICAL** transfer to the nearest suitable receiving hospital. ● Provide an alert or information call.
● Documentation	● Complete documentation to include all clinical findings, advice from other clinicians, onward referral and worsening advice given.

Headache

KEY POINTS!

Headache

- **It is preferable to be cautious when dealing with patients with headaches as diagnosis can be challenging.**
- **Headaches with different or unusual characteristics are significant.**
- **Sufferers of migraines are at risk of serious intracranial events.**
- **With headache, blood pressure must be checked.**
- **Any headache is significant if it is persistent or if it is associated with altered conscious levels or unusual behaviour.**
- **Sinister headaches may or may not be accompanied by neurology. Do not exclude simply based on physical examination — HISTORY IS KEY.**

Bibliography

1. NHS Evidence. *Headache Assessment/Management: How should I assess someone presenting with a headache?* Clinical Knowledge Summaries. London: NHS Evidence, 2010.
2. Scottish Intercollegiate Guidelines Network. *Diagnosis and Management of Headache in Adults* (Guideline 107). Edinburgh: SIGN, 2008. Available from: http://www.sign.ac.uk/assets/sign107.pdf.
3. The Headache Classification Subcommittee of the International Headache Society. *The International Classification of Headache Disorders, 2nd Edition (ICHD-II),* 1st revision. The International Headache Society, 2005.
4. World Health Organization. *Headache Disorders* (Fact sheet 277). Available from: http://www.who.int/mediacentre/factsheets/fs277/en, 2004.

Heart Failure

- Right heart failure is primarily caused by left heart failure but can also be caused in isolation by lung disease, such as COPD or pulmonary embolism as well as valvular disease. An increase in pressure in the pulmonary vasculature causes an increase in right ventricular afterload, resulting in ventricular hypertrophy and subsequently leads to progressive dilation and eventual failure.
- This mechanism gives rise to the common signs and symptoms seen in a right-sided pathology – raised JVP, hepatomegaly, ascites and significant peripheral oedema.

4.1 Factors Triggering Acute Heart Failure

- An identifiable trigger/s causing the acute decompensation of heart failure can be found in two thirds of cases. This is relevant as you may need to address two or more acute conditions at once. Some triggers, such as ischaemia and pneumonia, are associated with increased mortality risk. The commonest triggers are:
  - myocardial infarction
  - acute coronary syndrome
  - tachyarrhythmia, e.g. atrial fibrillation or ventricular tachycardia
  - infection, e.g. pneumonia, infective endocarditis or sepsis
  - excessive rise in blood pressure
  - non-adherence to medications
  - bradyarrhythmia
  - toxic substances, e.g. alcohol or recreational drugs
  - drugs, e.g. NSAIDs, corticosteroids, negative inotropic substances or cardiotoxic chemotherapeutics
  - exacerbation of chronic obstructive pulmonary disease
  - pulmonary embolism.
- Chest trauma, cardiac intervention, acute native or prosthetic valve incompetence secondary to endocarditis, aortic dissection or thrombosis are also causes.

5. Assessment and Management

- It can be difficult to differentiate heart failure from other causes of breathlessness, such as exacerbation of COPD, pulmonary embolism or pneumonia. Acute heart failure is frequently mistaken for sepsis as both can present with collapse and hypotension. If the patient has a history of heart failure or valve disease, STOP and THINK before administering intravenous fluids, as these can be harmful, especially if given quickly and in large amounts. A thorough history and physical examination of the patient is required. Assessment should focus on signs and symptoms associated with heart failure.
- Red flag indicators for heart failure are:
  - **Orthopnoea**: increased breathlessness on lying down. The patient may have slept in the chair on preceding nights.
  - **Paroxysmal nocturnal dyspnoea (PND)**: waking up at night short of breath and relieved by sitting up.
  - **New dyspnoea** with a past history of myocardial infarction/hypertension/angina.
  - **New peripheral oedema**, accompanied by dyspnoea.
  - **Coughing up pink frothy sputum**.
- Patients with an existing diagnosis of chronic heart failure may be known to or currently under the care of a specialist multidisciplinary heart failure team. These teams often know the patients well and can offer advice on treatment. If the patient is sufficiently stable and there is time to do so, contact the team for advice. Not all chronic heart failure patients are palliative, and the majority should still be managed actively and conveyed to hospital. Good care plans, if available, should help decisions around need for conveyance to hospital.
- Patients with advanced disease may have a personal or anticipatory care plan/end of life plan in place. This may be available by contacting a locally agreed directory of service or accessible electronically. For these patients, try to follow the care plan or contact the team for advice before admission. Following the care plan may involve assisting or instructing patients to take prescribed anticipatory medications such as extra oral diuretics, i.e. furosemide, bumetanide, bendroflumethiazide or metolazone, or taking the next dose early, in conjunction with a care plan/ contact with community team.
- Currently, many more heart failure patients who are palliative or at the end of their life are cared for at home in their final days with the express wish to remain at home. Consider end of life plans and refer to **End of Life Care**.
- Some patients with advanced heart failure may have left ventricular assist devices (LVADs), a mechanical pump that is implanted inside a person's chest to augment the weakened heart (refer to **Management and Resuscitation of Patients with Left Ventricular Assist Devices (LVADs)**).
- Assessment and management of acute heart failure should focus on identifying the underlying cause, stabilisation and transport to the most appropriate facility (refer to Table 3.57 and Figure 3.12).
- If conveyance to hospital is necessary, the patient should be conveyed rapidly to the most appropriate receiving hospital as per local pathways, preferably to a site with a cardiology department and/or CCU/ICU. Recent data

Heart Failure

TABLE 3.57 – ASSESSMENT and MANAGEMENT of: Acute Heart Failure

ASSESSMENT	MANAGEMENT
• Undertake an **<C>ABCD** assessment	• Start correcting <C>ABC problems (refer to **Medical Emergencies in Adults**).
• If the patient is **TIME CRITICAL**	• Correct life-threatening conditions, airway and breathing on scene. • Then commence transfer to the nearest suitable receiving hospital. • If the patient is in the palliative care stage, refer to their end of life pathway or anticipatory care plans and medicines. Be aware that a number of heart failure patients will have community DNACPR forms. Ask if the patient has an active DNACPR form. • If the patient is stable and known to community heart failure services, consider contacting them for advice.
Appropriate history: • HF diagnosis • SOB/SOBOE • chest pain • COPD/asthma • orthopnoea • paroxysmal nocturnal dyspnoea	• Document history and review any existing care plans.
Examination: • heart rate • blood pressure • respiratory rate • SpO_2 • oedema • auscultation	• Non-invasive monitoring, including pulse oximetry, blood pressure, respiratory rate and a continuous ECG, should be instituted within minutes of patient contact and continued during transport to hospital. **Clinical indicators of potential heart failure**: • Symptoms include dyspnoea, worsening cough, waking at night gasping for breath, breathlessness on lying down and anxiousness/restlessness. • Fine crackling sounds (rales) are suggestive of pulmonary oedema, commonly heard in the lung bases, but may be heard over other lung fields as well. These crackles are often accompanied by expiratory wheeze. • Coughing up of frothy sputum, white or pink (blood stained) in colour in decompensated heart failure. • Although peripheral oedema is a common sign of heart failure, it is not specific to heart failure and may be a consequence of numerous pathologies. Peripheral oedema starts at the feet and extends up the body as the condition progresses. The patient may also have abdominal ascites and pleural effusion. People with venous insufficiency, obesity or lymphoedema may have chronic oedema. • JVP provides an estimation of right atrial filling pressure as there are no valves between the right atrium and the internal jugular vein. It is accepted that assessment of JVP can be challenging, particularly in the pre-hospital environment. Assessment of JVP may be undertaken but should not delay treatment.
• Oxygen	• Oxygen therapy is recommended for patients with acute heart failure. • Target saturations 94–98%. • Administer the initial oxygen dose until a reliable SpO_2 measurement is available, then adjust oxygen flow to aim for a target saturation within the range of 94–98% (refer to **Oxygen**).

(continued)

CPAP therapy, pressure remains constant through the inspiratory and expiratory phases.

- Prospective randomised controlled trials have demonstrated that CPAP improves survival to hospital discharge and decreases intubation rates.
- A systematic review of 8 pre-hospital randomised trials of CPAP and BiPAP suggested that CPAP is the most effective treatment in terms of mortality and intubation rate compared to standard care. The effect of BiPAP on mortality and intubation rate was uncertain.
- The objective of non-invasive positive pressure ventilation (CPAP) is two-fold. The first is to 'splint' open collapsing alveoli and increase intra-alveolar pressure. The increase in pressure helps shift fluid present in the alveoli back into the pulmonary capillaries, thereby reducing pulmonary oedema. The second is to raise intrathoracic pressure throughout the respiratory cycle. This increase in intrathoracic pressure increases pressure in the vena cavae, and consequently serves to reduce filling pressures. Combined, these two actions reduce congestion.

KEY POINTS!

Heart Failure

- **Acute heart failure is a life-threatening medical condition. For all new cases and all chronic cases, unless there is an advanced care plan or palliative management in place, a TIME CRITICAL transfer to hospital is required for urgent assessment and treatment, ideally at a hospital that has a coronary care unit.**
- **If the patient has a history of heart failure or valve disease, STOP and THINK before administering intravenous fluids, as these can be harmful, especially if given quickly and in large amounts.**
- **Consider administering furosemide and/or GTN.**
- **In patients with systolic BP <110 mmHg, or with symptomatic hypotension, GTN/nitrates should be avoided.**
- **CPAP should be utilised where equipment and suitably trained clinicians are available.**
- **Pulmonary oedema can be difficult to differentiate from other causes of breathlessness, such as exacerbation of COPD, pulmonary embolism or pneumonia; therefore, a thorough history and physical examination are needed.**
- **Establish if the patient has a personal care plan or end of life plan and if they are being managed by a specialist heart failure team. Follow plans or liaise with other healthcare professionals to manage the patient appropriately.**
- **Initial management depends on the clinical presentation: acute pulmonary oedema, peripheral oedema, respiratory distress or cardiogenic shock.**

Further Reading

Further important information and evidence in support of this guideline can be found in the Bibliography.[4,5,6,7,8,9]

Bibliography

1. Ponikowski P, Voors AA, Anker SD et al. 2016 ESC Guidelines for the diagnosis and treatment of acute and chronic heart failure: The Task Force for the diagnosis and treatment of acute and chronic heart failure of the European Society of Cardiology (ESC). *European Heart Journal*. 2016, 37(27): 2129–2200.
2. National Institute for Health and Care Excellence. *Acute Heart Failure: Diagnosis and management* [CG187]. Manchester: NICE, 2014. Available from: https://www.nice.org.uk/guidance/cg187
3. National Institute for Health and Care Excellence. *Chronic Heart Failure in Adults: Management* [CG108]. Manchester: NICE, 2010. Available from: https://www.nice.org.uk/guidance/cg108.
4. British Medical Association and the Royal Pharmaceutical Society. *British National Formulary 75 (BNF) March – September 2018*. London: The Pharmaceutical Press.

Heart Failure

5. Goodacre S, Stevens JW, Pandor A et al. Prehospital noninvasive ventilation for acute respiratory failure: Systematic review, network meta-analysis, and individual patient data meta-analysis. *Academic Emergency Medicine*. 2014, 21: 960–970.
6. Vital FMR, Saconato H, Ladeira MT, Sen A, Hawkes CA et al. Non-invasive positive pressure ventilation (CPAP or bilevel NPPV) for cardiogenic pulmonary edema (Review). Cochrane Database Systematic Review. 2013, CD005351.
7. Wakai A, McCabe A, Kidney R et al. Nitrates for acute heart failure syndromes. Cochrane Database Systematic Review. 2013, CD005151.
8. Peacock WF, Emerman C, Costanzo MR et al. Early vasoactive drugs improve heart failure outcomes. *Congest Heart Fail.* 2009, 15: 256–264.
9. Vaswani A, Khaw HJ, Dougherty S et al. *Cardiology in a Heartbeat*. 2016, Scion Publishing: Banbury.

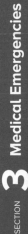

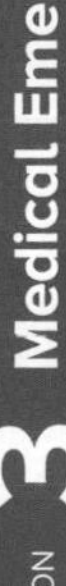

Heat Related Illness

1. Introduction

- Heat related illness is a relatively uncommon presenting condition to ambulance services but it can be life-threatening.
- Heat related illness can be **exogenous,** caused by environmental factors (e.g. the sun) or **endogenous** (e.g. drugs and exercise).
- Heat related illness is a continuum of heat related conditions (refer to Figure 3.13).

The management of heat related illness is supportive: refer to Table 3.61.

Heat stress

- Heat stress is a mild form of heat illness, characterised by the features below (refer to Table 3.58). This level of heat disorder is often self-managed, but if left untreated can progress to more serious conditions.

Heat exhaustion

- A less severe heat illness than heat stroke, lacking the defining neurological symptoms of this condition. Symptoms are mainly due to excess fluid loss and electrolyte imbalance.

Heat stroke

- A 'systemic inflammatory response' to a core body temperature >40°C in addition to a change in mental status and organ dysfunction (European Resuscitation Council Guidelines).

There are two types of heat stroke:

a. **Non-exertional heat stroke** due to very high external temperatures and/or high humidity; it tends to be more common in very hot climates. It tends to occur in the:
   - older person
   - very young
   - chronically ill.

b. **Exertional heat stroke** is due to excess heat production. This tends to occur in:
   - athletes including marathon and fun-runners
   - manual workers
   - firefighters
   - military recruits.

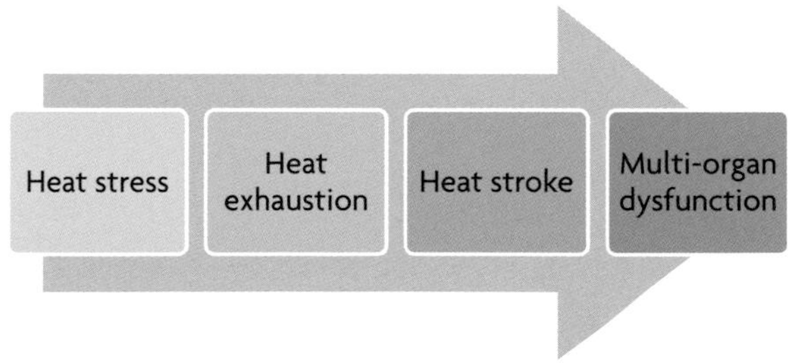

Heat stress → Heat exhaustion → Heat stroke → Multi-organ dysfunction

Figure 3.13 – Continuum of heat related illness.

TABLE 3.58 – Features of Heat Stress (European Resuscitation Council Guidelines)
Heat stress
• **Temperature:** normal or mildly elevated.
• **Heat oedema:** swelling of feet and ankles.
• **Heat syncope:** vasodilation and dehydration causing hypotension.
• **Heat cramps:** sodium depletion causing cramps.

2. Incidence

The exact incidence of heat stroke is unknown, with many sufferers self-managing their condition. Mortality, in the absence of a heat wave is relatively low; in the United Kingdom it is estimated to be 40 deaths per million annually.

TABLE 3.59 – Features of Heat Exhaustion (ERC)
Heat exhaustion
• Systemic reaction to prolonged heat exposure (hours to days).
• Temperature >37°C and <40°C.
• Headache, dizziness, nausea, vomiting, tachycardia.
• Hypotension, sweating, muscle pain, weakness and cramps.
• Haemoconcentration.
• Hyponatraemia or hypernatraemia.
• May progress rapidly to heat stroke.

TABLE 3.60 – Features of Heat Stroke (ERC)
Heat stroke
• Core temperature ≥40°C.
• Hot, dry skin (sweating is present in about 50% of cases of exertional heat stroke).
• Early signs and symptoms are extreme fatigue, headache, fainting, facial flushing, vomiting and diarrhoea.
• Cardiovascular dysfunction including arrhythmias and hypotension.
• Respiratory dysfunction including acute respiratory distress syndrome (ARDS).
• Central nervous system dysfunction including seizures and coma.
• Liver and renal failure.
• Coagulopathy.
• Rhabdomyolysis.

Heat Related Illness

A variety of medications may predispose to the development of heat illness. In addition, individuals who take drugs of abuse (e.g. cocaine, ecstasy, amphetamines) and then engage in vigorous dancing in crowded 'rave' settings may also develop heat illness.

3. Severity and Outcome

- Heat stroke is a life-threatening emergency that requires prompt appropriate treatment, with estimates of mortality of 10–50%. Recovery from heat stroke even after appropriate treatment and rehabilitation may be incomplete and leave patients with persistent functional impairment.
- **Systemic effects** – heat stroke can lead to a variety of life-threatening systemic conditions including: disseminated intravascular coagulation, rhabdomyolysis, renal failure, hepatic necrosis, metabolic acidosis and decreased tissue perfusion, in addition to cerebral and cerebellar damage.

4. Pathophysiology

- In heat illnesses there is an imbalance in the metabolic production and subsequent loss of heat by the body. This increase in core body temperature has multiple undesirable effects on many body systems. Systemically this increased temperature leads to swelling and degeneration at both cellular and tissue levels.
- **Cellular changes** – at increased temperatures cellular organelles swell and stop functioning properly. Cell membranes become distorted, leading to unwanted increased permeability and inappropriate movement of ions into and out of cells. Red blood cells also change shape at elevated temperatures and their capacity to carry oxygen is decreased. At higher temperatures cells will also undergo inappropriate apoptosis and die.

5. Assessment and Management

- For the assessment and management of heat related illness refer to Table 3.61.

TABLE 3.61 – ASSESSMENT and MANAGEMENT of: Heat Related Illness

ASSESSMENT	MANAGEMENT
• Assess <C>ABCD	• If any of the following **TIME CRITICAL** features are present: – major **<C>ABCD** problems, refer to **Medical Emergencies in Adults – Overview** and **Medical Emergencies in Children – Overview** – haemodynamic compromise – decreased level of consciousness, then: • Start correcting any **<C>ABCD** problems. • Undertake a **TIME CRITICAL** transfer to nearest appropriate receiving hospital. • Continue patient management en-route. • Provide an ATMIST information call.
• Assess	Undertake physical examination and assess for the presence of features of heat related illness (refer to Tables 3.58–3.59) • Remove the patient from the hot environment or remove cause if possible. • Remove to an air-conditioned vehicle where available. • Remove all clothing. • Commence cooling with fanning, tepid sponging, water misting or with a wet sheet loosely over the patient's body. **NB** Consider other potential causes (e.g. diabetes or cardiac problems).
• Temperature	Measure and record: • The patient's core temperature. • If possible and time allows measure the environmental temperature. **NB** The core temperature may or may not be elevated, but patients may be tachycardic, hypotensive and/or sweating excessively.

(continued)

Heat Related Illness

TABLE 3.61 – ASSESSMENT and MANAGEMENT of: Heat Related Illness *(continued)*	
● Heat stroke	Heat stroke is potentially fatal and the patient needs to be cooled as an emergency. ● If cold or iced water is used, massaging of the skin may be needed to overcome cold induced vasoconstriction and ensure effective heat loss. ● Apply ice packs, if available, wrapped in a thin cloth or towel to the patient's neck, axilla and groin. **NB** Ice packs applied directly to the skin can cause frostbite. ● Transfer the patient with air conditioning turned on or with windows open. **NB** Immersion in ice water is effective but usually not possible in the pre-hospital environment.
● Respiratory rate	● Measure and record respiratory rate.
● Pulse	● Measure and record pulse.
● Oxygen saturation	● Monitor the patient's SpO_2, administer oxygen to achieve saturations of >94% if the patient presents as hypoxemic on air, refer to **Oxygen**.
● Blood pressure and fluids	Measure and record blood pressure. If required, administer fluids. Refer to **Intravascular Fluid Therapy in Adults** and **Intravascular Fluid Therapy in Children**.
● Blood glucose	● Measure and record blood glucose for hypo/hyperglycaemia, refer to **Glycaemic Emergencies in Adults and Children**.
● NEWS2	● These observations will enable you to calculate a NEWS2 Score, refer to **Sepsis**.
● ECG	● If required, monitor and record 12-Lead ECG. Assess for abnormality, refer to **Cardiac Rhythm Disturbance**.
● Assess the patient's pain	● Where present, assess the **SOCRATES** of pain and record initial and subsequent pain scores. ● Consider analgesia if appropriate, refer to **Pain Management in Adults** and **Pain Management in Children**.
● Transfer	● Transfer patients to nearest appropriate receiving hospital.
● Documentation	● Complete documentation to include all clinical findings, advice from other clinicians, onward referral and worsening advice given.

SECTION 3 Medical Emergencies

KEY POINTS!

Heat Related Illness

- **Heat exhaustion/heat stroke occurs in high external temperatures, as a result of excess heat production and with certain drugs. The higher the level of activity the lower the environmental temperature required to produce heat stroke.**
- **Do not assume that collapse in an athlete is due to heat – check for other causes.**
- **In heat exhaustion the patient may present with flu-like symptoms, such as headache, nausea, dizziness, vomiting, and cramps; the temperature may not be elevated.**
- **In heat stroke the patient will have neurological symptoms such as decreased level of consciousness, ataxia and convulsions, and the temperature will usually be elevated, typically >40°C.**
- **Remove the patient from the hot environment or remove cause, if possible, remove clothing and cool.**

Heat Related Illness

Bibliography

1. Soar J, Perkins GD, Abbas G, Alfonzo A, Barelli A, Bierens JJLM, et al. European Resuscitation Council Guidelines for Resuscitation 2010 Section 8: Cardiac arrest in special circumstances: electrolyte abnormalities, poisoning, drowning, accidental hypothermia, hyperthermia, asthma, anaphylaxis, cardiac surgery, trauma, pregnancy, electrocution. *Resuscitation* 2010, 81(10): 1400–1433.
2. Bouchama A, Dehbi M, Mohamed G, Matthies F, Shoukri M, Menne B. Prognostic factors in heat wave related deaths: a meta-analysis. *Archives of Internal Medicine* 2007, 167(20): 2170–6.
3. Pease S, Bouadma L, Kermarrec N, Schortgen F, Regnier B, Wolff M. Early organ dysfunction course, cooling time and outcome in classic heatstroke. *Intensive Care Medicine* 2009, 35(8): 1454–8.
4. Allen A, Segal-Gidan F. Heat-related illness in the elderly. *Clinical Geriatrics* 2007, 15(7): 37–45.
5. Belmin J, Auffray J-C, Berbezier C, Boirin P, Mercier S, de Reviers B, et al. Level of dependency: a simple marker associated with mortality during the 2003 heatwave among French dependent elderly people living in the community or in institutions. *Age and Ageing* 2007, 36(3): 298–303.
6. Brody GM. Hyperthermia and hypothermia in the elderly. *Clinics in Geriatric Medicine* 1994, 10(1): 213–29.
7. Daniel V, Paladugu N, Fuentes G. Heat stroke and cocaine in an inner-city New York hospital. *Internet Journal of Emergency and Intensive Care Medicine* 2008, 11(1): doi 10.5580/157e.
8. de Galan BE, Hoekstra JBL. Extremely elevated body temperature: case report and review of classical heat stroke. *Netherlands Journal of Medicine* 1995, 47(6): 281–7.
9. Hausfater P, Megarbane B, Dautheville S, Patzak A, Andronikof M, Santin A, et al. Prognostic factors in non-exertional heatstroke. *Intensive Care Medicine* 2010, 36(2): 272–80.
10. Stafoggia M, Forastiere F, Agostini D, Biggeri A, Bisanti L, Cadum E, et al. Vulnerability to heat-related mortality: a multicity, population based, case-crossover analysis. *Epidemiology* 2006, 17(3): 315–23.
11. Vicario SJ, Okabajue R, Haltom T. Rapid cooling in classic heatstroke: effect on mortality rates. *American Journal of Emergency Medicine* 1986, 4(5): 394–8.
12. Bernardo LM, Crane PA, Veenema TG. Treatment and prevention of pediatric heat-related illnesses at mass gatherings and special events. *Dimensions of Critical Care Nursing* 2006, 25(4): 165–71.
13. Guard A, Gallagher SS. Heat related deaths to young children in parked cars: an analysis of 171 fatalities in the United States, 1995–2002. *Injury Prevention* 2005, 11(1): 33–7.
14. Gutierrez G. Solar injury and heat illness: treatment and prevention in children. *Physician and Sportsmedicine* 1995, 23(7): 43–8.
15. Krous HF, Nadeau JM, Fukumoto RI, Blackbourne BD, Byard RW. Environmental hyperthermic infant and early childhood death: circumstances, pathologic changes, and manner of death. *American Journal of Forensic Medicine and Pathology* 2001, 22(4): 374–82.
16. Ohshima T, Maeda H, Takayasu T, Fujioka Y, Nakaya T. An autopsy case of infant death due to heat stroke. *American Journal of Forensic Medicine and Pathology* 1992, 13(3): 217–21.
17. Rossi R. Emergency treatment of an infant with heatstroke. *Notfallmedizin* 1993, 19(3): 109–11.
18. Wagner C, Boyd K. Pediatric heatstroke. *Air Medical Journal* 2008, 27(3): 118–22.
19. Martinez M, Devenport L, Saussy J, Martinez J. Drug-associated heat stroke. *Southern Medical Journal* 2002, 95(8): 799–802.
20. Aarseth HP, Eide I, Skeie B, Thaulow E. Heat stroke in endurance exercise. *Acta Medica Scandinavica* 1986, 220(3): 279–83.
21. Armstrong LE, Crago AE, Adams R, Roberts WO, Maresh CM. Whole-body cooling of hyperthermic runners: comparison of two field therapies. *American Journal of Emergency Medicine* 1996, 14(4): 355–8.
22. Binkley HM, Beckett J, Casa DJ, Kleiner DM, Plummer PE. National Athletic Trainers' Association position statement: exertional heat illnesses. *Journal of Athletic Training* 2002, 37(3): 329–43.
23. Clapp AJ, Bishop PA, Muir I, Walker IL. Rapid cooling techniques in joggers experiencing heat strain. *Journal of Science and Medicine in Sport* 2001, 4(2): 160–7.
24. Hansen RD, Olds TS, Richards DA, Richards CR, Leelarthaepin B. Infrared thermometry in the diagnosis and treatment of heat exhaustion. *International Journal of Sports Medicine* 1996, 17(1): 66–70.
25. Hee-Nee P, Rupeng M, Lee VJ, Chua W-C, Seet B. Treatment of exertional heat injuries with portable body cooling unit in a mass endurance event. *American Journal of Emergency Medicine* 2010, 28(2): 246–8.
26. McDermott BP, Casa DJ, O'Connor FG, Adams WB, Armstrong LE, Brennan AH, et al. Cold-water dousing with ice massage to treat exertional heat stroke: a case series. *Aviation Space and Environmental Medicine* 2009, 80(8): 720–2.
27. Centers for Disease Control and Prevention. Heat-related deaths among crop workers: United States, 1992–2006. *Morbidity and Mortality Weekly Report* 2008, 57(24): 649–53.
28. Maeda T, Kaneko S-Y, Ohta M, Tanaka K, Sasaki A, Fukushima T. Risk factors for heatstroke among Japanese forestry workers. *Journal of Occupational Health* 2006, 48(4): 223–9.
29. Tranter M. An assessment of heat stress among laundry workers in a Far North Queensland hotel. *Journal of Occupational Health and Safety Australia and New Zealand* 1998, 14(1): 61–3.
30. Yoshino K, Takano K, Nagasaka A, Shigeta S. An experimental study on the prediction of heat stress of workers in a hot environment. With special reference to the relation between wearing suits, work load and environmental temperature. *Japanese Journal of Industrial Health* 1987, 29(6): 466–79.
31. Angerer P, Kadlez-Gebhardt S, Delius M, Raluca P, Nowak D. Comparison of cardiocirculatory and thermal strain of male firefighters during fire suppression to exercise stress test and aerobic exercise testing. *American Journal of Cardiology* 2008, 102(11): 1551–6.
32. Barr D, Gregson W, Reilly T. The thermal ergonomics of firefighting reviewed. *Applied Ergonomics* 2010, 41(1): 161–72.

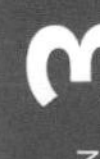

Hyperventilation Syndrome

1. Introduction

- Hyperventilation syndrome is defined as 'breathing in excess of metabolic requirements'.[1]
- It is characterised by an irregular and disorganised breathing pattern with an increased rate and depth of respirations, known as tachypnoea.[2]
- Hyperventilation has many causes, including a number of life-threatening conditions such as:
  - myocardial infarction
  - pulmonary embolism
  - diabetic ketoacidosis
  - asthma
  - sepsis.
- This guideline focuses on acute episodes of primary or idiopathic hyperventilation, which means there is no underlying cause.[3,4] This condition was initially termed Hyperventilation Syndrome (HVS), but more recently the term HVS has slowly disappeared in favour of:
  - Panic/anxiety attack
  - Panic/anxiety disorder
  - Dysfunctional breathing
  - Breathing pattern disorder.[5,6,7,8,9]

2. Incidence

- It is estimated that 6–10% of the general adult population may suffer from some form of HVS. The condition is more common in women.[6,7] Within UK ambulance services the prevalence of HVS is estimated to be 1%, which is comparable to estimates for emergency departments, which range from 0.3%–6%.[10,11,3,12]
- HVS is rare in children, where the most likely cause is physical illness.
- Patients with HVS use a significant amount of hospital and emergency service resources because they frequently seek care in the emergency department or from paramedics due to fearing they are experiencing life-threatening emergencies.[13,11]

3. Severity and Outcome

- As per its definition, HVS has no organic cause and is self-limiting. No organic cause means that there is no underlying physical change to the patient's cells, tissues or organs, which could account for the experienced symptoms. The signs and symptoms of HVS may be distressing for the patient but these will subside once a good respiratory pattern is established.
- Within the literature there are case study reports of apnoeic episodes following HVS, but these are rare.[14]
- **A diagnosis of HVS must be a diagnosis of exclusion of organic causes for hyperventilation.** This is due to the differential diagnoses of HVS including many life-threatening conditions with poor prognosis if the correct treatment is withheld. Potential differential diagnoses are listed in Table 3.62.

4. Pathophysiology

- The basic rhythm of respiration is controlled subconsciously by the medullary respiratory centre.[19] The automatic control of respiration can be overridden by anxiety, which causes central stimulation of the medullary respiratory centre's inspiratory area, leading to an increased rate and depth of respiration.[20]
- An increased rate and depth of respiration results in faster elimination of carbon dioxide through exhalation, causing a decrease in alveolar and arterial carbon dioxide known as hypocapnia.[18] Hypocapnia reduces the formation of hydrogen ions and bicarbonate ions in the blood causing a rise in pH levels known as respiratory alkalosis.[21]
- Hypocapnia also causes constriction of cerebral arteries, thereby increasing vascular resistance and reducing blood flow to the brain.[18] This diminished cerebral perfusion may explain some of the neurological symptoms associated with HVS.[22]
- The physiological mechanisms by which many of the other HVS symptoms occur are not entirely clear, but they must nonetheless be seen as genuine consequences of physiological imbalances rather than figments of patients' imagination.[23]
- Signs and symptoms of HVS are wide-ranging, vague and can vary between patients. Experiencing the frightening symptoms of HVS may exacerbate patients' anxiety which promotes further hyperventilation resulting in HVS symptoms entering a vicious cycle.

Assessment and Management

For the assessment and management of hyperventilation syndrome refer to Table 3.64 and Figure 3.14.

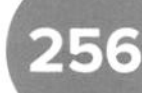

Hyperventilation Syndrome

TABLE 3.62 – Differential Diagnoses of HVS by body system[15,16,17,18]

Body System	Differential Diagnoses	
Cardiovascular	• Angina • Aortic aneurysm • Coronary artery disease • Tachyarrhythmia	• Myocardial infarction • Pericarditis • Heart failure
Neurological	• Brain stem lesions • Encephalitis • Head trauma • Mèniére's disease	• Meningitis • Stroke • Vertigo
Respiratory	• Asthma • Chronic obstructive pulmonary disease • Cystic fibrosis • Interstitial lung disease	• Lung tumour • Pneumonia • Pneumothorax • Pulmonary embolism • Pleural effusion
Gastrointestinal	• Cholecystitis • Liver failure • Hiatus hernia	• Liver cirrhosis • Peptic ulcer
Endocrine	• Diabetic ketoacidosis • Pheochromocytoma	• Thyrotoxicosis
Renal	• Kidney failure	
Environmental	• Heat or altitude acclimatisation	• Carbon monoxide poisoning
Other	• Anaemia • Drug intoxication • Drugs or caffeine (withdrawal) • Pain	• Hypokalaemia • Sepsis • Serious aspirin overdoses • Pregnancy

TABLE 3.63 – Signs and symptoms of HVS by body system[22,20,2,4]

Body System	Signs and Symptoms
Cardiovascular	Palpitations, tachycardia, arrhythmias, chest pain, blotchy flushing
Neurological	Paraesthesia (numbness and tingling of the mouth/lips/extremities), dizziness/unsteadiness/light-headedness, syncope, headache, blurred or tunnel vision, impaired concentration and memory
Respiratory	Tachypnoea, shortness of breath, tightness in chest/throat, frequent sighing, yawning, feeling of suffocation/choking
Gastrointestinal	Globus, dysphagia, epigastric discomfort, excessive air swallowing, dry mouth, belching, flatulence, nausea
Musculoskeletal	Aching of the muscles of the chest, tremors, weakness, tetany of hands or feet (e.g. carpopedal spasm)
Psychological	Tension, anxiety, panic, feelings of unreality or disorientation, fear of dying, fear of losing control or going crazy, hallucinations, phobias
General	Fatigue, exhaustion, sleep disturbance, sweating, weakness, chills or heat sensations

Hyperventilation Syndrome

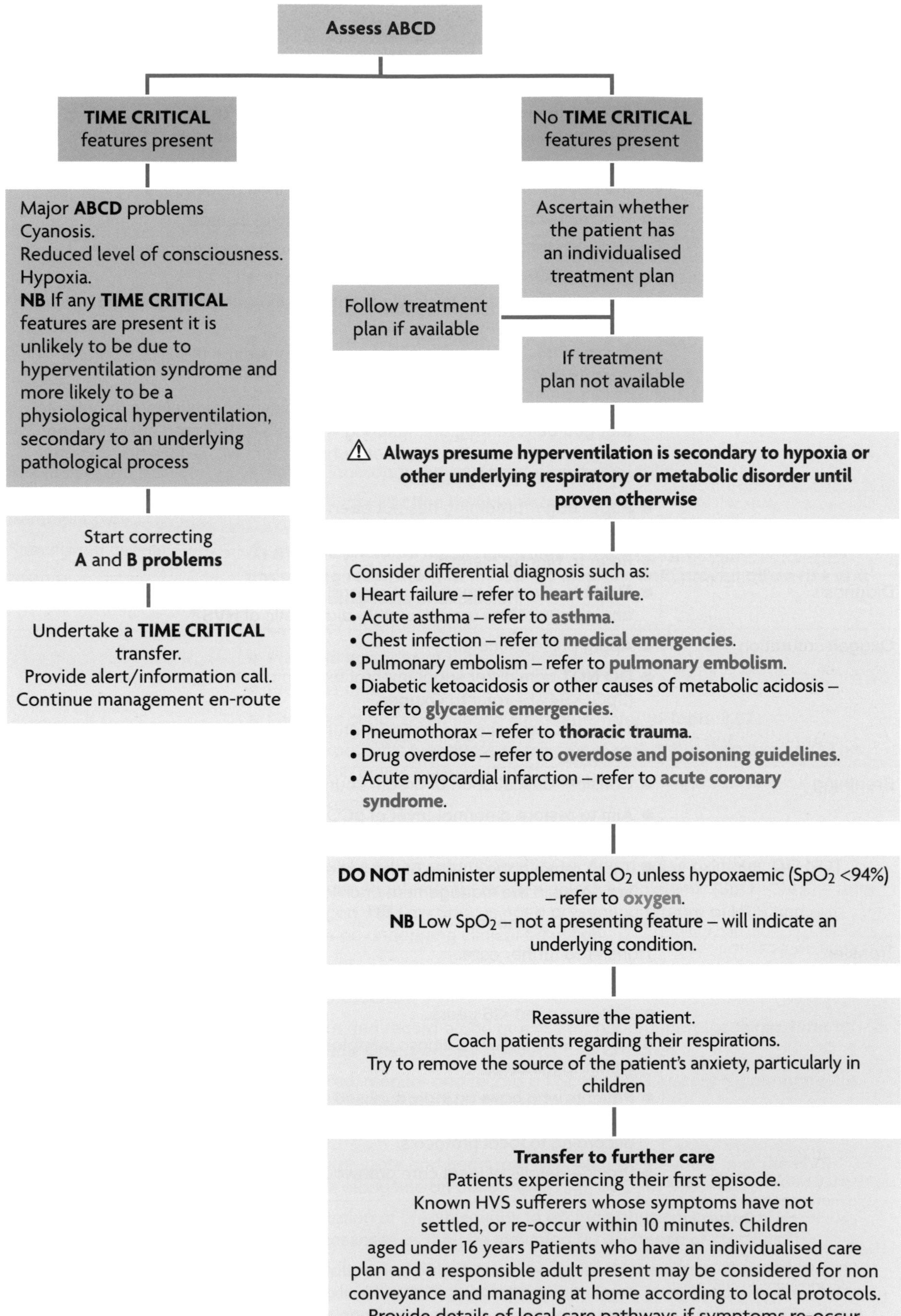

Assess ABCD
TIME CRITICAL features present
No TIME CRITICAL features present
Major ABCD problems
Cyanosis.
Reduced level of consciousness.
Hypoxia.
NB If any TIME CRITICAL features are present it is unlikely to be due to hyperventilation syndrome and more likely to be a physiological hyperventilation, secondary to an underlying pathological process
Start correcting A and B problems
Undertake a TIME CRITICAL transfer.
Provide alert/information call.
Continue management en-route
Ascertain whether the patient has an individualised treatment plan
Follow treatment plan if available
If treatment plan not available
Always presume hyperventilation is secondary to hypoxia or other underlying respiratory or metabolic disorder until proven otherwise
Consider differential diagnosis such as:
• Heart failure – refer to heart failure.
• Acute asthma – refer to asthma.
• Chest infection – refer to medical emergencies.
• Pulmonary embolism – refer to pulmonary embolism.
• Diabetic ketoacidosis or other causes of metabolic acidosis – refer to glycaemic emergencies.
• Pneumothorax – refer to thoracic trauma.
• Drug overdose – refer to overdose and poisoning guidelines.
• Acute myocardial infarction – refer to acute coronary syndrome.
DO NOT administer supplemental O_2 unless hypoxaemic (SpO_2 <94%) – refer to oxygen.
NB Low SpO_2 – not a presenting feature – will indicate an underlying condition.
Reassure the patient.
Coach patients regarding their respirations.
Try to remove the source of the patient's anxiety, particularly in children
Transfer to further care
Patients experiencing their first episode.
Known HVS sufferers whose symptoms have not settled, or re-occur within 10 minutes. Children aged under 16 years Patients who have an individualised care plan and a responsible adult present may be considered for non conveyance and managing at home according to local protocols.
Provide details of local care pathways if symptoms re-occur

Figure 3.14 – Assessment and management of hyperventilation syndrome algorithm.

Hyperventilation Syndrome

KEY POINTS!

Hyperventilation Syndrome

- **HVS is a diagnosis of exclusion.**
- **Differential diagnosis: Many life-threatening medical conditions can cause hyperventilation.**
- **In children a medical cause is more likely than anxiety.**
- **Administer supplemental oxygen if hypoxaemic (SpO_2 <94%).**
- **Reassure the patient and coach their breathing.**

Further Reading

Further important information and evidence in support of this guideline can be found in the Bibliography.[29,30,31,32,33,34,35,36,37,38,39,40,41,42]

Bibliography

1. Gardner WN. Hyperventilation: a practical guide. *Medicine* 2003, 31(11): 7–8.
2. Caroline N. *Emergency Care in the Streets, 7th edition* Burlington, MA: Jones and Bartlett, 2016.
3. Pfortmueller CA, Pauchard-Neuwerth SE, Leichtle AB, Fiedler GM, Exadaktylos AK, et al. Primary Hyperventilation in the Emergency Department: A First Overview. *PLOS ONE* 2015, 10(6).
4. Clarke V, Townsend P. Respiratory assessment. In: Blaber AY, Harris G. *Assessment skills for paramedics, 2nd ed* . Maidenhead: Open University Press, 2016: 14–46.
5. Kerr WJ, Gliebe PA, Dalton JW. 1938. Physical phenomena associated with anxiety states: the hyperventilation syndrome. *Cal West Med* 1938, 48(1):12–6.
6. Thomas M, McKinley RK, Freeman E, Foy C. Prevalence of dysfunctional breathing in patients treated for asthma in primary care. *BMJ* 2001, 322(7294):1098–100.
7. Thomas M, McKinley RK, Freeman E, Foy C, Price D. The prevalence of dysfunctional breathing in adults in the community with and without asthma. *Prim Care Respir J* 2005, 14(2):78–82.
8. Warburton CJ, Jack S. Can you diagnose hyperventilation? *Chron Respir Dis* 2006, 3(3):113–5.
9. Todd S, Walsted ES, Grillo L, Livingston R, Menzies-Gow A, Hull JH. Novel assessment tool to detect breathing pattern disorder in patients with refractory asthma. *Respirology* 2017, 23:284–290.
10. Wilson C, Harley C, Steels S. PP09 Pre-hospital diagnostic accuracy for hyperventilation syndrome. *Emerg Med J* 2017: 34:e3.
11. Coley KC, Saul MI, Seybert AL. Economic burden of not recognizing panic disorder in the emergency department. *J Emerg Med* 2009, 36(1):3–7.
12. Greenslade JH, Hawkins T, Parsonage W, Cullen L. Panic disorder in patients presenting to the emergency department with chest pain: prevalence and presenting symptoms. *Heart Lung Circ* 2017, 26(12):1310–6.
13. Katerndahl DA, Realini JP. Where do panic attack sufferers seek care? *J Fam Pract* 1995, 40(3):237–43.
14. Munemoto T, Masuda A, Nagai N, Tanaka M, Yuji S. Prolonged post-hyperventilation apnea in two young adults with hyperventilation syndrome. *BioPsychoSocial medicine* 2013, 7(1). 9.
15. Pfeffer JM. The aetiology of the hyperventilation syndrome. *Psychother Psychosom* 1978, 30(1):47–55.
16. Ong JR, Hou SW, Shu HT, Chen HT, Chong CF. Diagnostic pitfall: carbon monoxide poisoning mimicking hyperventilation syndrome. *Am J Emerg Med* 2005, 23(7):903-4.
17. Brashear RE. Hyperventilation syndrome *Lung* 1983, 161(1):257–73.
18. Pizzorno JE, Murray MT, Joiner-Bey H. *The clinician's handbook of natural medicine, 3rd ed* . St Louis: Elsevier, 2016.
19. Aehlert B *Paramedic practice today: Above and beyond.* Burlington, MA: Jones and Bartlett, 2011.
20. Porth CM, Litwack K. Disorders of acid-base balance. In: Porth CM, Matfin G. *Pathophysiology: Concepts of altered health states, 8th ed.* Philadelphia: Lippinkott Williams & Wilkins, 2009: 805–25.
21. Khurana I. *Medical physiology for undergraduate students.* New Delhi: Elsevier, 2012.
22. Evans RW. Unilateral paresthesias due to hyperventilation syndrome. *Pract Neurol* June 2005: 65–68.
23. Chapman S, Robinson G, Stradling J, West S. *Oxford Handbook of Respiratory Medicine.* Oxford: Oxford University Press, 2009.
24. National Institute for Health and Care Excellence. *Breathlessness* Clinical Knowledge Summaries. Available from: https://cks.nice.org.uk/breathlessness, 2017.
25. O'Driscoll BR, Howard LS, Earis J on behalf of the British Thoracic Society Emergency Oxygen Guideline Group. BTS guideline for oxygen use in adults in healthcare and emergency settings. *Thorax* 2017, 72:ii1–ii90.
26. Michaelides AP, Liakos CI, Antoniades C, Tsiachris DL, Soulis D, Dilaveris PE, Tsioufis KP, Stefanadis CI. ST-segment depression in hyperventilation indicates a false positive exercise test in patients with mitral valve

SECTION 3 Medical Emergencies

Hypothermia

4. Severity and Outcome

The severity of hypothermia can be classified into mild, moderate and severe depending on the patient's core body temperature (refer to Figure 3.15).

- However, in the pre-hospital environment, where appropriate thermometers and the skills to use them are often unavailable, it may be better to define the severity clinically (refer to Table 3.66).

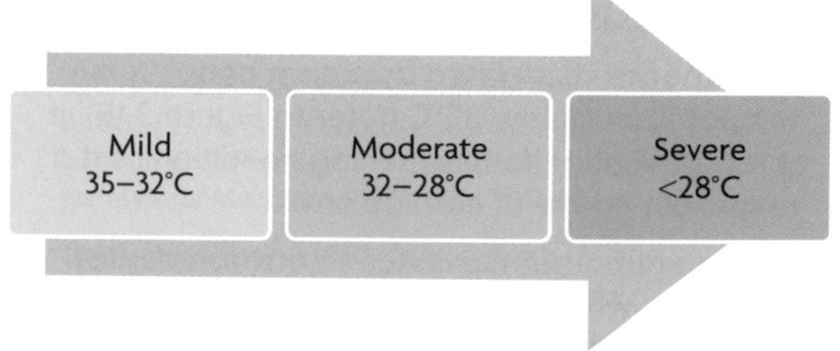

Figure 3.15 – Severity of hypothermia.

5. Assessment and Management

For the assessment and management of hypothermia refer to Table 3.67.

TABLE 3.66 – Clinical Stages of Hypothermia

Stage	Clinical Signs
I	Conscious and shivering.
II	Reduced conscious level; may or may not be shivering.
III	Unconscious; vital signs present.
IV	Apparent death; vital signs absent.

TABLE 3.67 – ASSESSMENT and MANAGEMENT of: Hypothermia

ASSESSMENT	MANAGEMENT
● Assess <C>ABCD	● If any of the following **TIME CRITICAL** features are present: – major **<C>ABCD** problems, refer to **Medical Emergencies in Adults – Overview** and **Medical Emergencies in Children – Overview**. – Haemodynamic compromise. – Decreased level of consciousness. – Cardiac arrest, then: ● Start correcting any **<C>ABCD** problems. ● Undertake a **TIME CRITICAL** transfer to nearest appropriate receiving hospital or consider transfer to a hospital that provides extracorporeal life support (ECLS), as per local pathways. ● Continue patient management en-route. ● Provide an ATMIST information call.
● Assess	Undertake physical examination and assess for the presence of features of hypothermia (refer to Table 3.66): symptoms are often non-specific and can include ataxia, slurred speech, apathy, irrational behaviour, and decrease in the level of consciousness (refer to **Altered Level of Consciousness**), heart rate and rhythm, and respiratory rate.
● Temperature	Measure and record the patient's core temperature – temperature measurement in the field is difficult, therefore it is important to suspect and treat hypothermia from the history and circumstances of the situation. Shivering peaks around 34°C and is minimal or stopped by 31-32°C. Shivering is a very effective way of raising body temperature BUT there must be adequate energy stores to fuel it.
● Warming	**PREVENT FURTHER HEAT LOSS** as in the mildly hypothermic patient, preventing further heat loss will enable the patient to warm up by their own metabolism. ● Place in vehicle. ● Consider using foil blankets. Foil blankets work by reflecting radiated heat so are only useful in mild hypothermia. In severe hypothermia, minimal heat is radiated. ● Some foil blankets may only have one reflective surface so must be placed the right way round.

TABLE 3.67 – ASSESSMENT and MANAGEMENT of: Hypothermia *(continued)*	
	• If the patient is conscious provide a hot drink/food if available and appropriate. • **DO NOT** rub the patient's skin as this causes vasodilatation and may increase heat loss. • **DO NOT** give the patient alcohol as this causes vasodilatation and may increase heat loss. • Manage co-existing trauma or medical conditions as they arise (refer to appropriate **trauma/medical** guidelines).
• Resuscitation	**BEWARE:** Severely hypothermic patients may initially appear to be dead but frequently have a very slow and weak pulse, very slow and shallow respirations, fixed dilated pupils and increased muscle tone. Dilated pupils can be seen in hypothermia and therefore should not be used as a sign of death. • Rough handling can invoke cardiac arrhythmias (including VF and pulseless VT) so handle patients carefully. • Airway – clear the airway. • Ventilation – if there are no signs of respiration, ventilate with high concentrations of oxygen, but do NOT hyperventilate. A respiratory rate and tidal volume appropriate in normothermia is inappropriate in hypothermia, refer to **appropriate Resuscitation guidelines.** • Signs of life – look for signs of life (palpate central artery, ECG monitoring etc) for up to 1 minute. • Cardiac arrest – refer to **appropriate Resuscitation guidelines** and additional information below. Remember that the rules for normothermic arrest must not be extrapolated completely to hypothermic arrest. • Cardiac arrythmias (except VF) will usually revert spontaneously with re-warming and do not need treatment unless they persist after re-warming.
• Respiratory rate	• Measure and record respiratory rate.
• Pulse	• Measure and record pulse.
• Oxygen	• It is unlikely that SpO_2 can be reliably measured using a finger probe in a hypothermic patient. Oxygen should be given in all cases, and particularly if the patient is shivering and has co-morbidities, as the metabolic demand of intense shivering puts an extra burden on the heart. Administer 15 litres per minute until a reliable SpO_2 measurement can be obtained and then adjust oxygen flow to aim for target saturation within the range of 94–98% refer to **Oxygen**.
• Blood pressure and fluids	• Measure and record blood pressure. If required, administer fluids (preferably warmed fluids). Refer to **Intravascular Fluid Therapy in Adults** and **Intravascular Fluid Therapy in Children**.
• Blood glucose	• Measure and record blood glucose for hypo/hyperglycaemia, refer to **Glycaemic Emergencies in Adults and Children**.
• NEWS2	• These observations will enable you to calculate a NEWS2 Score, refer to **Sepsis**.
• ECG	• Monitor and record 12-Lead ECG. Assess for abnormality, refer to **Cardiac Rhythm Disturbance**.
• Assess the patient's pain	• Where present, assess the **SOCRATES** of pain and record initial and subsequent pain scores. • Consider analgesia if appropriate, refer to **Pain Management in Adults** and **Pain Management in Children**.

(continued)

Implantable Cardioverter Defibrillator

1. Introduction

The implantable cardioverter defibrillator (ICD) has revolutionised the management of patients at risk of developing a life-threatening ventricular arrhythmia. Several clinical trials have testified to their effectiveness in reducing deaths from sudden cardiac arrest in selected patients, and the devices are implanted with increasing frequency.

ICDs are used in both children and adults.

ICD systems consist of a generator connected to electrodes placed transvenously into cardiac chambers (the ventricle, and sometimes the right atrium and/or the coronary sinus) (refer to Figure 3.16). The electrodes serve a dual function allowing the monitoring of cardiac rhythm and the administration of electrical pacing, defibrillation and cardioversion therapy. Modern ICDs are slightly larger than a pacemaker and are usually implanted in the left subclavicular area (refer to Figure 3.16). The ICD generator contains the battery and sophisticated electronic circuitry that monitors the cardiac rhythm, determines the need for electrical therapy, delivers treatment, monitors the response and determines the need for further therapy.

The available therapies include:

- Conventional programmable pacing for the treatment of bradycardia.
- Anti-tachycardia pacing (ATP) for ventricular tachycardia (VT).
- Delivery of biphasic shocks for the treatment of ventricular tachycardia and ventricular fibrillation (VF).
- Cardiac resynchronisation therapy (CRT) (biventricular pacing) for the treatment of heart failure.

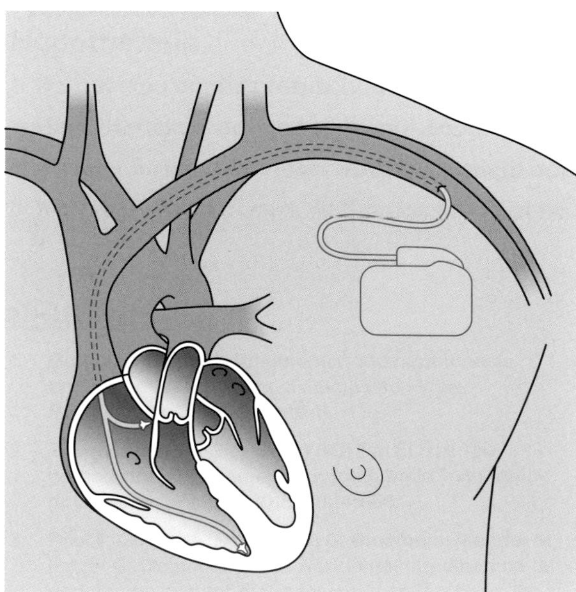

Figure 3.16 – Usual location of an ICD.

These treatment modalities and specifications are programmable and capable of considerable sophistication to suit the requirements of individual patients. The implantation and programming of devices is carried out in specialised centres. The patient should carry a card or documentation which identifies their ICD centre and may also have been given emergency instructions.

The personnel caring for such patients in emergency situations are not usually experts in arrhythmia management or familiar with the details of the sophisticated treatment regimes offered by modern ICDs. Moreover, the technology is complex and evolving rapidly. In an emergency patients will often present to the ambulance service or emergency department (ED) and the purpose of this guidance is to help those responsible for the initial management of these patients.

2. General Principles

Some important points should be made at the outset.

On detecting VF/VT the ICD will usually discharge a maximum of eight times before shutting down. However, a new episode of VF/VT will result in the recommencing of its discharge sequence. A patient with a fractured ICD lead may suffer repeated internal defibrillation as the electrical noise is misinterpreted as a shockable rhythm.

These patients are likely to be conscious with a relatively normal ECG rate.

When confronted with a patient in cardiac arrest the usual management guidelines are still appropriate (refer to **cardiac arrest** and **arrhythmia** guidelines). If the ICD is not responding to VF or VT, or if shocks are ineffective, external defibrillation/cardioversion should be carried out. Avoid placing the defibrillator electrodes/pads/paddles close to or on top of the ICD; ensure a minimum distance of 8 cm between the edge of the defibrillator paddle pad/electrode and the ICD site. Most ICDs are implanted in the left sub-clavicular position (refer to Figure 3.16) and are usually readily apparent on examination; the conventional (apical/right subclavicular) electrode position will then be appropriate. The anterior/posterior position may also be used, particularly if the ICD is right sided.

Whenever possible, record a 12-lead electrocardiogram (ECG) and record the patient's rhythm (with any shocks). Make sure this is printed out and stored electronically (where available) for future reference. Where an external defibrillator with an electronic memory is used (whether for monitoring or for therapy) ensure that the ECG report is printed and handed to appropriate staff. Again, whenever possible, ensure that the record is archived for future reference. Record the rhythm during any therapeutic measure (whether by drugs or electricity). All these records may provide vital information for the ICD centre that may greatly influence the patient's subsequent management.

Implantable Cardioverter Defibrillator

The energy levels of the shocks administered by ICDs (up to 40 Joules) are much lower than those delivered with external defibrillators (120–360 J). **Personnel in contact with the patient when an ICD discharges are unlikely to be harmed, but it is prudent to minimise contact with the patient while the ICD is firing.** Chest compression and ventilation can be carried out as normal and protective examination gloves should be worn as usual.

Placing a ring magnet over the ICD generator can temporarily disable the shock capability of an ICD. The magnet does not disable the pacing capability for treating bradycardia. The magnet may be kept in position with adhesive tape if required. Removing the magnet returns the ICD to the status present before application. The ECG rhythm should be monitored at all times when the device is disabled. An ICD should only be disabled when the rhythm for which shocks are being delivered has been recorded. If that rhythm is VT or VF, external cardioversion/defibrillation must be available. With some models it is possible to programme the ICD so that a magnet does not disable the shock capabilities of the device. This is usually done only in exceptional circumstances, and consequently, such patients are rare.

The manufacturers of the ICDs also supply the ring magnets. Many implantation centres provide each patient with a ring magnet and stress that it should be readily available in case of emergency. With the increasing prevalence of ICDs in the community it becomes increasingly important that emergency workers have this magnet available to them when attending these patients.

Decisions to apply a Do Not Attempt Cardio Pulmonary Resuscitation (DNACPR) order will not be made in the emergency situation by the personnel to whom this guidance is directed. Where such an order does exist it should not be necessary to disable an ICD to enable the implementation of such an order.

Many problems with ICDs can only be dealt with permanently by using the programmer available at the ICD centre.

The guidelines should be read from the perspective of your position and role in the management of such patients. For example, the recommendation to 'arrange further assessment' will mean that the ambulance clinician should transport the patient to hospital. For ED staff, however, this might mean referral to the medical admitting team or local ICD centre.

Coincident conditions that may contribute to the development of arrhythmia (e.g., acute ischaemia worsening heart failure) should be managed as appropriate according to usual practice.

Maintain oxygen saturations above 94%.

Receiving ICD therapy may be unpleasant 'like a firm kick in the chest', and psychological consequences may also arise. It is important to be aware of these, and help should be available from implantation centres. An emergency telephone helpline may be available.

3. Management

The following should be read in conjunction with the treatment table (refer to Table 3.68) and algorithm (refer to Figure 3.17). Approach and assess the patient and perform basic life support according to current BLS guidelines.

Monitor the ECG	
3.1	If the patient is in cardiac arrest.
3.1.1	Perform basic life support in accordance with current BLS guidelines. Standard airway management techniques and methods for gaining IV/IO access (as appropriate) should be established.
3.1.2	If a shockable rhythm is present (VF or pulseless VT) but the ICD is not detecting it, perform external defibrillation and other resuscitation procedures according to current resuscitation guidelines.
3.1.3	If the ICD is delivering therapy (whether by anti-tachycardia pacing or shocks) but is failing to convert the arrhythmia, then external defibrillation should be provided, as per current guidelines.
3.1.4	If a non-shockable rhythm is present manage the patient according to current guidelines. If the rhythm is converted to a shockable one, assess the response of the ICD, performing external defibrillation as required.
3.1.5	If a shockable rhythm is converted to one associated with effective cardiac output (whether by the ICD or by external defibrillation), manage the patient as usual and arrange further treatment and assessment.
3.2	If the patient is not in cardiac arrest.
3.2.1	Determine whether an arrhythmia is present.

Implantable Cardioverter Defibrillator

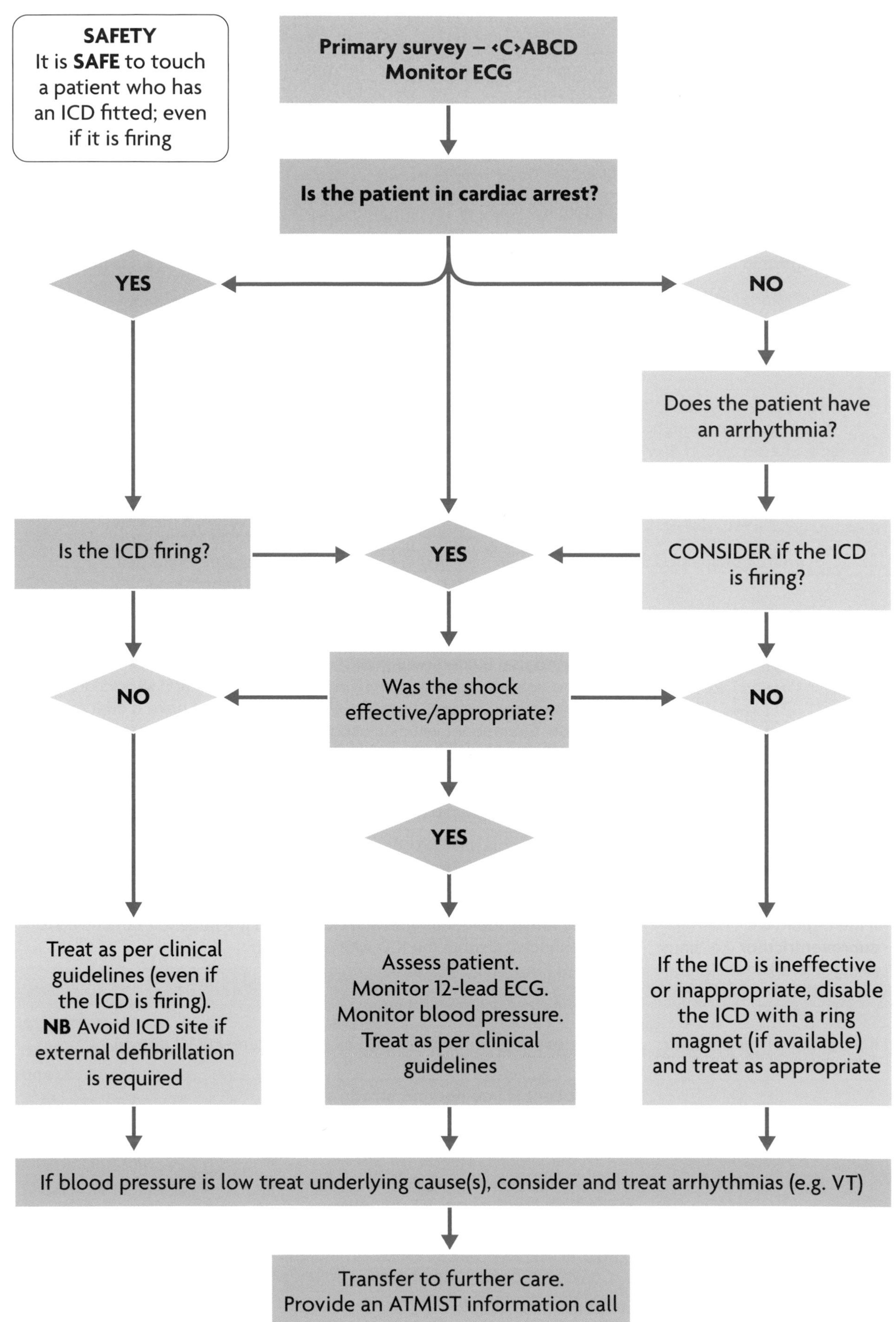

Figure 3.17 – Implantable cardioverter defibrillator algorithm.

Implantable Cardioverter Defibrillator

KEY POINTS!

Implantable Cardioverter Defibrillators (ICDs)

- **ICDs deliver therapy with bradycardia pacing, ATP and shocks for VT not responding to ATP or VF.**
- **ECG records, especially at the time that shocks are given, can be vital in subsequent patient management. A recording should always be made if circumstances allow.**
- **Cardiac arrest should be managed according to normal guidelines.**
- **Avoid placing the defibrillator electrode over or within 8 cm of the ICD box.**
- **A discharging ICD is unlikely to harm a rescuer touching the patient or performing CPR.**
- **An inappropriately discharging ICD can be temporarily disabled by placing a ring magnet directly over the ICD box.**

Bibliography

1. Deakin CD, Nolan JP, Soar J, Sunde K, Koster RW, Smith GB, et al. European Resuscitation Council Guidelines for Resuscitation 2010 Section 4: Adult advanced life support. *Resuscitation* 2010, 81(10): 1305–1352.
2. Koster RW, Baubin MA, Bossaert LL, Caballero A, Cassan P, Castren M, et al. European Resuscitation Council Guidelines for Resuscitation 2010 Section 2: Adult basic life support and use of automated external defibrillators. *Resuscitation* 2010, 81(10): 1277–1292.
3. Nolan JP, Soar J, Zideman DA, Biarent D, Bossaert LL, Deakin C, et al. European Resuscitation Council Guidelines for Resuscitation 2010 Section 1: Executive summary. *Resuscitation* 2010, 81(10): 1219–76.
4. Deakin CD, Nolan JP, Sunde K, Koster RW. European Resuscitation Council Guidelines for Resuscitation 2010 Section 3: Electrical therapies: automated external defibrillators, defibrillation, cardioversion and pacing. *Resuscitation* 2010, 81(10): 1293–1304.
5. Deakin CD, Morrison LJ, Morley PT, Callaway CW, Kerber RE, Kronick SL, et al. Part 8: Advanced life support: 2010 International Consensus on Cardiopulmonary Resuscitation and Emergency Cardiovascular Care Science with Treatment Recommendations. *Resuscitation* 2010, 81(1): e93–174.
6. Sunde K, Jacobs I, Deakin CD, Hazinski MF, Kerber RE, Koster RW, et al. Part 6: Defibrillation: 2010 International Consensus on Cardiopulmonary Resuscitation and Emergency Cardiovascular Care Science with Treatment Recommendations. *Resuscitation* 2010, 81(1): e71–85.

through the non-functional LVAD13 and systemic anticoagulation. In a patient who is critically ill or in circulatory arrest, the balance of risk and benefit favours restarting a non-functioning LVAD. If LVAD non-function is suspected in a patient who is not severely compromised, immediate advice should be sought from the VAD centre (see section 7 for contact details).

2.1 Assessment of Airway and Breathing

- The assessment starts with a rapid evaluation of the patient's responsiveness and breathing. In an unresponsive patient who is not breathing normally despite an open airway, that is, not breathing or giving only infrequent 'agonal' gasps (the features usually used to identify cardiac arrest),[23] ambulance clinicians should consider that a likely cause is that the LVAD has stopped and should proceed to the assessment of circulation. In the patient who is breathing normally, administration of oxygen and assessment to identify other respiratory conditions should follow standard guidelines.

2.2 Assessment of Circulation

- This part of the assessment starts by determining if the LVAD is running. Unresponsiveness and absence of normal breathing usually implies circulatory arrest.
- In an LVAD recipient, sudden failure of the LVAD is the cause most likely to be corrected by prompt, appropriate intervention.
- Sudden LVAD failure does not always cause circulatory arrest, so in an LVAD patient who is very ill but breathing, it is still important to check at this stage whether the LVAD is running.
- Clinicians should minimise delay by avoiding futile repeated attempts to palpate a pulse and record the arterial BP and oxygen saturation, as these may be difficult or impossible to detect in compromised LVAD recipients.
- A loud alarm coming from the controller is likely to indicate a stopped LVAD, unless its display shows another explanation.
- If no alarm is sounding, LVAD failure is still a possibility (due to alarm battery depletion or alarm failure), so a stethoscope should be placed over the apex of the heart to listen for a humming sound. Absence of a humming sound indicates that the LVAD is not working. If a loud alarm is sounding (with no other cause shown) or the pump is inaudible via stethoscope, the clinician is directed to Algorithm 2 (LVAD troubleshooting) (refer to Figure 3.20).

2.3 LVAD Troubleshooting

- If the LVAD has stopped, the most effective resuscitation manoeuvre is to restart it without delay. Operation of the LVAD is dependent on:

1 secure connection of an external controller to the percutaneous cable (driveline) of the implanted blood pump

AND

2 the supply of power to the external controller, either via a rechargeable battery or via mains power.

- The percutaneous driveline usually exits the skin over the abdomen to the right of the umbilicus.
- All adult LVADs in use in the UK have two power connections to the controller, both of which are usually connected, although only a single working power source is needed for the LVAD to operate. This allows replacement of one power source, without interrupting LVAD operation.
- The controller and batteries may be carried in a bag, contained within pockets of the patient's clothing or belt-mounted.
- If the LVAD is not running, first, check the external components of the LVAD. The clinician should open the LVAD bag containing the controller and batteries to expose the contents, and check that all connections to the controller are fully engaged and secure.
- Next, check the battery charge by pressing a button on the battery that illuminates a display similar to a fuel gauge. If the battery charge level is low, the power source must be changed. Depleted batteries should be replaced with charged ones or with a mains power supply. If a mains power supply is in use and potentially defective, the device should be switched to a charged battery.
- If these measures fail to restart the LVAD, it is presumed that the controller is defective. The spare controller (carried by the patient at all times) should be connected to a charged battery (or mains power). Then, the driveline should be disconnected from the presumed-defective controller and connected to the replacement controller whereupon the LVAD should restart.
- If these actions do not restart the LVAD, the possibility of cable fracture within the driveline causing loss of electrical continuity should be considered. If this is suspected, gentle manipulation of the driveline may restore LVAD operation, in which case the driveline should be stabilised (using tape).
- If the LVAD cannot be restarted, or in the unlikely event that an LVAD patient is found in an unconscious state with a non-functioning LVAD that cannot be restarted and no spare equipment, the clinician should proceed to Algorithm 3 (Figure 3.21) and the VAD centre should be contacted using a telephone number located:
  - on an identification card or bracelet
  - on an Immediate Action Notice, in an envelope in the bag with the controller in use

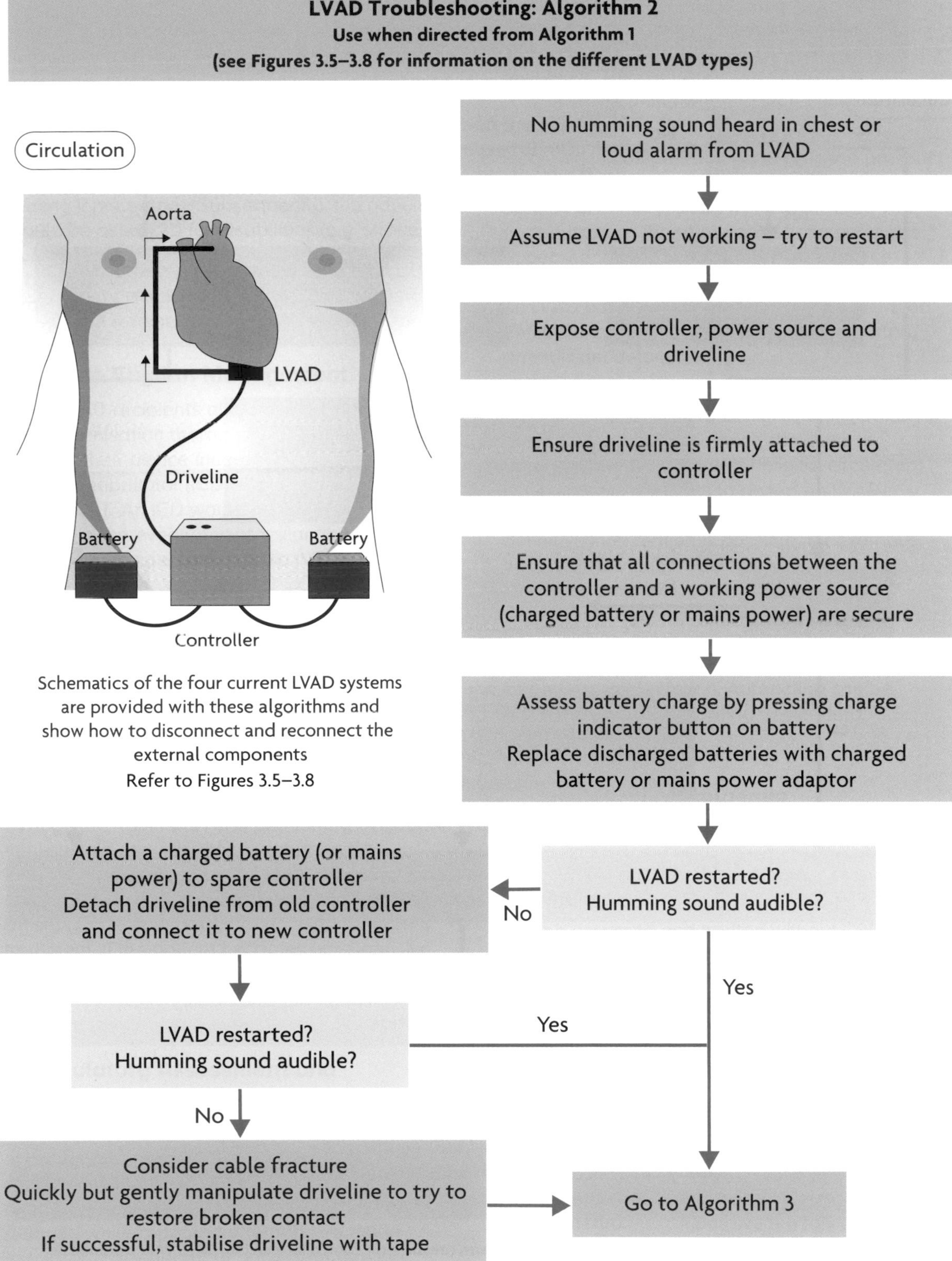
LVAD Troubleshooting: Algorithm 2
Use when directed from Algorithm 1
(see Figures 3.5–3.8 for information on the different LVAD types)
Circulation
Aorta
LVAD
Driveline
Battery
Battery
Controller
Schematics of the four current LVAD systems are provided with these algorithms and show how to disconnect and reconnect the external components
Refer to Figures 3.5–3.8
No humming sound heard in chest or loud alarm from LVAD
Assume LVAD not working – try to restart
Expose controller, power source and driveline
Ensure driveline is firmly attached to controller
Ensure that all connections between the controller and a working power source (charged battery or mains power) are secure
Assess battery charge by pressing charge indicator button on battery
Replace discharged batteries with charged battery or mains power adaptor
LVAD restarted?
Humming sound audible?
No
Attach a charged battery (or mains power) to spare controller
Detach driveline from old controller and connect it to new controller
Yes
LVAD restarted?
Humming sound audible?
Yes
No
Consider cable fracture
Quickly but gently manipulate driveline to try to restore broken contact
If successful, stabilise driveline with tape
Go to Algorithm 3

Figure 3.20 – Algorithm 2 – LVAD troubleshooting.

  – on the LVAD controller itself
  – in an emergency bag carried separately by the patient.
- Where the specific VAD centre cannot be contacted, the ambulance crew should contact the operations centre and attempts can be made to contact the local VAD centre for further advice and support. **If the clinician cannot rapidly establish which VAD centre the patient is from, they should call the nearest VAD centre for further advice and support.**

Management and Resuscitation of Patients with Left Ventricular Assist Devices (LVADs)

4. Transfer to Hospital

- Whether a patient should be transported to the local ED or to the VAD centre should be determined by dialogue with the VAD centre. This decision will depend on the patient's clinical condition and logistical considerations.
- Appropriately trained caregivers should be encouraged to accompany the patient during ambulance transfer to hospital.
- It is of paramount importance that all emergency LVAD equipment (including the spare controller, rechargeable batteries, mains power adapter and battery charger) is transferred to hospital with the patient, as sustained LVAD function is dependent on the availability of these components.
- It is important to monitor the patient continuously during transfers as clinical deterioration can be sudden.

5. Advance Decisions to Refuse Treatment and Do-Not-Attempt-CPR Decisions

- There is evidence of sporadic initiation of advance statements (living wills) or Advance Decisions to Refuse Treatment (England and Wales) (ADRTs) in UK LVAD outpatients. More frequently, do-not-attempt-CPR (DNACPR) decisions have been recorded by healthcare professionals for LVAD inpatients, typically with participation of the patient in the decision-making process if they have the capacity, otherwise their family or authorised representative.[31] The increasing international use of LVADs for destination therapy in more elderly patients has focused debate on end-of life care planning, with more patients preferring to die in their home rather than in hospital.[32]
- It is recommended that the existence and location of advance statements, ADRTs and recommendations about CPR and/or other life-sustaining treatments should be recorded in the PSP. Unless there is a valid and applicable advance statement, ADRT or other recommendations warranting a different response in a community setting, the measures recommended in these guidelines may be assumed to be appropriate for any critically ill LVAD recipient.

6. Schematics of LVAD Types

Four different types of LVADs are implanted in the UK. Schematics of these different devices are included for reference purposes.

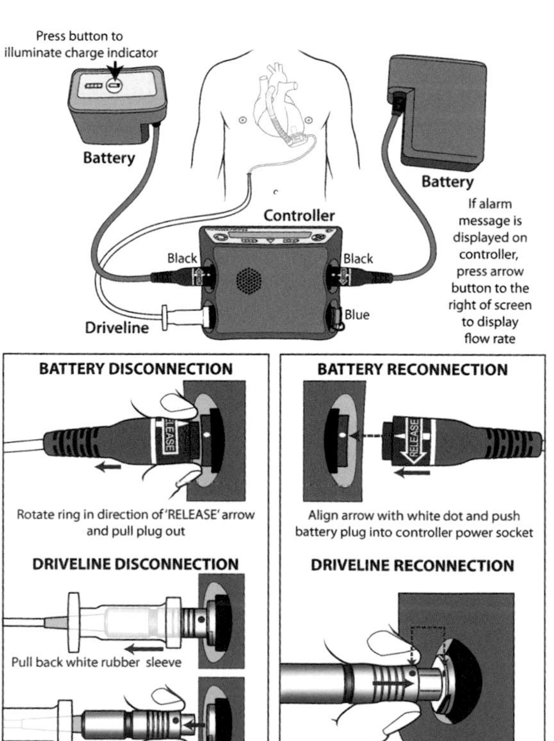

Figure 3.22 – Medtronic Inc. (formerly Heartware Inc.) HVAD

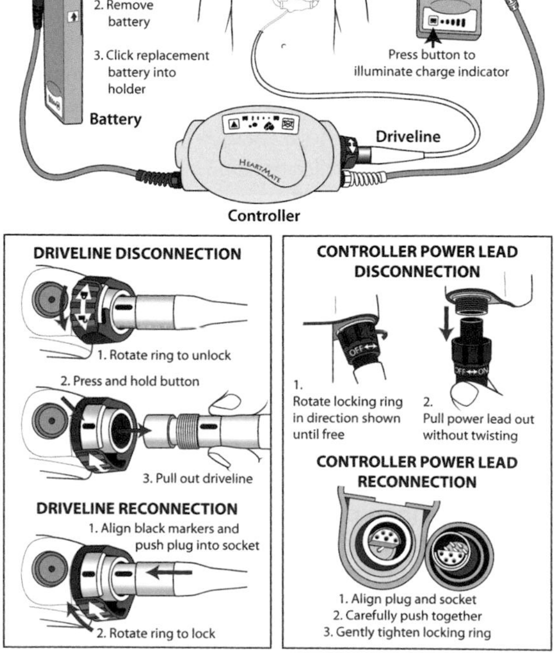

Figure 3.23 – LVAD type - Abbott Inc. (formerly Thoratec Inc.) HeartMate II, original version

Management and Resuscitation of Patients with Left Ventricular Assist Devices (LVADs)

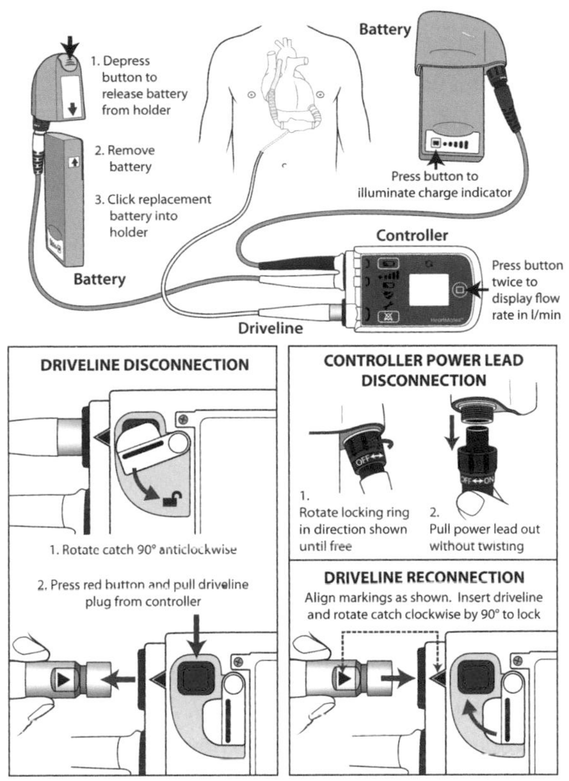

Figure 3.24 – LVAD type - Abbott Inc. (formerly Thoratec Inc.) HeartMate II, pocket controller version

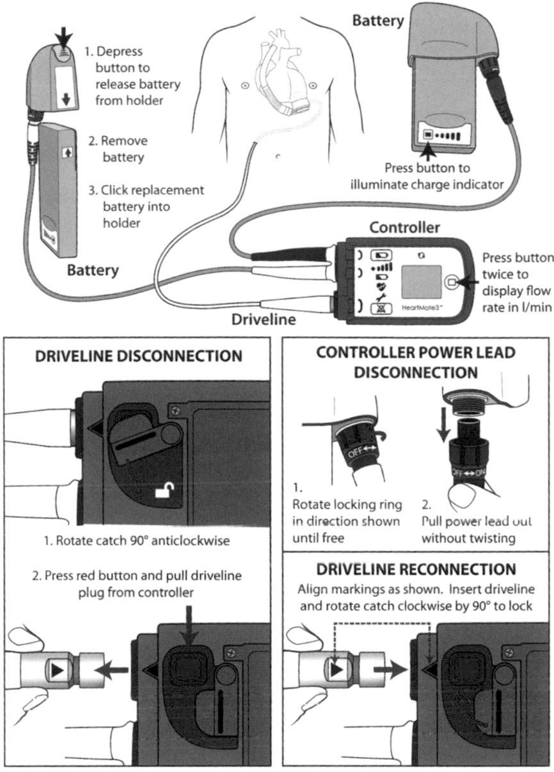

Figure 3.25 – LVAD type - Abbott Inc. (formerly Thoratec Inc.) HeartMate 3

7. Contact Details for Ventricular Assist Device Implantation Centres

Centre	Service	Emergency Number	Hospital Switchboard
Birmingham, QEII	Adult	07787570692	0121 627 2000
Cambridge, Royal Papworth	Adult	01480 830541 and ask for the transplant coordinator	01480 830541
Glasgow, Golder Jubilee	Adult	0141 951 5784	0141 951 5000
London, Great Ormond Street	Paediatric	Mon to Friday 08.00 to 16.00: 0207 405 9200 ext. 5807 Out of hours: Cardiology ext. 1632	0207 405 9200
London, Harefield	Adult	07805768819	01895 823737
Manchester, Wythenshawe	Adult	0161 998 7070 and ask for the VAD coordinator on call	0161 998 7070
Newcastle, Freeman	Adult	0191 244 8444	0191 233 6161
Newcastle, Freeman	Paediatric	0191 244 8961	0191 233 6161

Ambulance services should use the emergency number in the first instance and, if there is no response, should ring the hospital switchboard and ask for the VAD coordinator, or alternative speciality, as detailed.

Meningococcal Meningitis and Septicaemia

1. Introduction

- Meningococcal disease is the leading cause of death by infection in children and young adults and can kill a healthy person of any age within hours of their first symptoms.

2. Incidence

- In England and Wales, the incidence of meningococcal disease is falling with around 750 cases being reported each year (decreased incidence attributed to the efficacy of Men C and Men B vaccines).

3. Pathophysiology

- Two clinical categories are described, although they often overlap:
  1) meningitis.
  2) septicaemia.
- In meningitis, the meninges covering the brain and spinal cord are infected by bacteria causing inflammation.
- In septicaemia, bacteria invade the bloodstream, releasing toxins and producing a clinical picture of shock and circulatory collapse. Deterioration can be rapid and may be irreversible, with treatment becoming less effective by the minute. Early recognition and prompt treatment improves clinical outcomes.
- A minority of patients will have pure septicaemia and it is these patients who carry the worse prognosis.

4. Severity and Outcome

- The mortality from septicaemia can be up to 40% but if recognised early, resuscitated aggressively and managed on ITU, mortalities of less than 5% can be achieved.

5. Assessment and Management

- These presentations should be managed in the same way as any other form of severe sepsis with a <C>ABCD approach, and a **TIME CRITICAL** transfer to hospital with an ATMIST pre-alert. Refer to **Sepsis**.

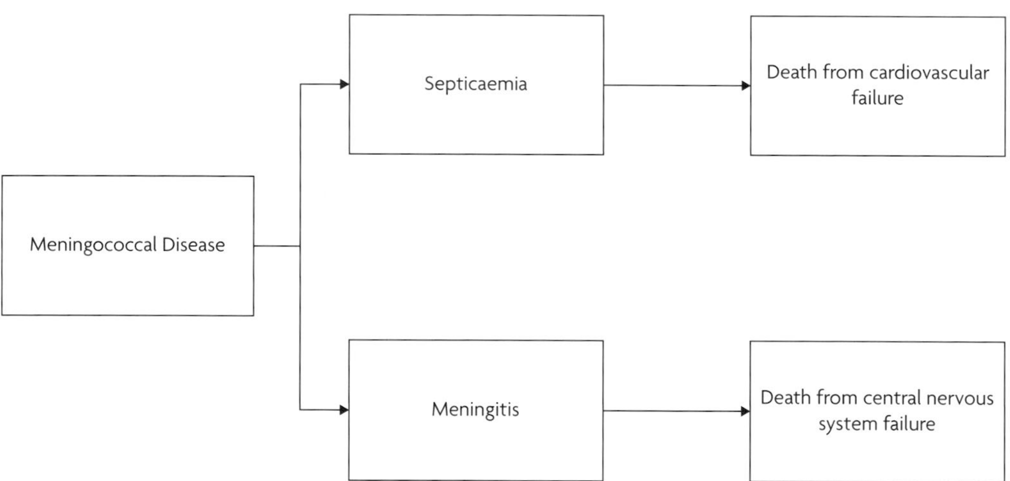

Figure 3.26 – Meningococcal Meningitis and Septicaemia

TABLE 3.69 – ASSESSMENT and MANAGEMENT Of Meningococcal Meningitis And Septicaemia

ASSESSMENT	MANAGEMENT
• Assess <C>ABCD:	• If any of the following **TIME CRITICAL** features are present: – Major **<C>ABCD** problems refer to **Medical Emergencies Overview**. – Seizures. – Rash – progressive petechial rash becoming purpuric – like a bruise or blood-blister. – Start correcting any **<C>ABCD** problems. • Undertake a **TIME CRITICAL** transfer to nearest appropriate receiving hospital. • Continue patient management en route. • Provide an ATMIST information call.

Meningococcal Meningitis and Septicaemia

TABLE 3.69 – ASSESSMENT AND MANAGEMENT of Meningococcal Meningitis and Septicaemia *(continued)*	
• Clinical findings	• The patient may have been previously unwell with non-specific symptoms, for example: – Irritability. – Pyrexia. – 'Flu-like' symptoms. • The patient may be 'unwell' and deteriorate rapidly. In some individuals the meningococcal bacteria cross the blood-brain barrier, producing inflammation and swelling in the meninges and the brain tissue itself. This causes raised intracranial pressure, which can lead to neurological damage and death. • The main symptoms of meningitis are due to central nervous system dysfunction. They may be very hard to assess and parents' anxieties about their child's condition must always be taken seriously. • 'Classic' features (neck stiffness, photophobia and haemorrhagic rash) should be sought and can help you make the diagnosis when present. However, an absence of these signs should not be taken as evidence that meningococcal disease has been excluded. Do not be falsely reassured! • Clinical features include: – Fever (may be masked by peripheral shutdown or antipyretics). – Cold, mottled skin (especially extremities). The skin may rarely be warm and flushed; features of 'warm shock'. – Raised respiratory rate and effort. – O_2 saturations – reduced or unrecordable (poor perfusion). – Raised heart rate. – Capillary refill time >2 seconds. – Pain in joints, muscles and limbs. – Rash – progressive petechial rash becoming purpuric – like a bruise or blood-blister. **NB** these rashes are often not present at presentation. – Headache. – Vomiting, abdominal pain and diarrhoea. – Drowsiness/confusion. – Rigors. – Seizures. – Photophobia (less common in young children). – Neck stiffness (less common in young children).
• The rash	• The classic description of a haemorrhagic, non-blanching rash (may be petechial or purpuric) is only seen in approximately 40% of infected children. • In pigmented skin it can be helpful to look at the conjunctiva under the lower eyelid. • Early signs and symptoms are often subtle. • Septicaemia: rashes do not necessarily develop at the same rate as the septicaemia. • The rapidly-evolving, haemorrhagic rash described in textbooks may be a very late sign – by time this rash is present, resuscitative attempts may be too late. • Up to 30% of cases start with a blanching pink rash, which fades with pressure, before becoming purpuric later. • The rash may be absent. **The 'glass' or 'tumbler' test** • A petechial or purpuric rash does not blanch/fade when pressed with a glass tumbler. • **NB** If the 'glass' test is negative, do not assume that meningococcal disease has been excluded.

(continued)

Meningococcal Meningitis and Septicaemia

TABLE 3.69 – ASSESSMENT AND MANAGEMENT of Meningococcal Meningitis and Septicaemia *(continued)*	
• Specific clinical features	• Neck stiffness is rarely seen (but is more common in older children, teenagers and adults, being quite rare in pre-school children – the age group most at risk of infection). Small children often present with non-specific signs such as nausea, vomiting, loss of appetite, sore throat and coryzal symptoms – features that might otherwise suggest a diagnosis of viral illness.
• Benzylpenicillin	• Where the patient meets the indication for administration of **Benzylpenicillin**, and where the clinician has a high index of suspicion of bacterial meningococcal septicaemia, even without the presence of a rash, benzylpenicillin should be administered. • **NB** Meningococcal septicaemia can progress rapidly – early antibiotic administration is associated with better outcomes. • Withhold benzylpenicillin only when there is a clear history of anaphylaxis after a previous dose; a history of a rash following penicillin is not a contraindication. • In the unlikely event of an allergic reaction following administration of benzylpenicillin, manage according to **Allergic Reactions including Anaphylaxis**. • Administer benzylpenicillin en-route to further care.
• Respiratory rate	• Measure and record respiratory rate.
• Pulse	• Measure and record pulse.
• Oxygen saturation	• Monitor the patient's SpO_2, administer oxygen to achieve saturations of >94% if the patient presents as hypoxemic on air, refer to **Oxygen**.
• Blood pressure and fluids	• Measure and record blood pressure, if required administer fluids, refer to **Intravascular Fluid Therapy in Adults** and **Intravascular Fluid Therapy in Children**. • Hypovolaemia complicating meningococcal septicaemia will require fluid resuscitation. • **DO NOT** delay at scene for fluid replacement; cannulate and give fluid en-route to hospital wherever possible.
• Blood glucose	• If appropriate, measure and record blood glucose for hypo/hyperglycaemia, refer to **Glycaemic Emergencies in Adults and Children**.
• Temperature	• Measure and record temperature.
• NEWS2	• These observations will enable you to calculate a NEWS2 Score, refer to **Sepsis**. A National Paediatric Early Warning Score is still in development.
• ECG	• If required, monitor and record 12-Lead ECG. Assess for abnormality, refer to **Cardiac Rhythm Disturbance**.
• Assess the patient's pain	• Assess the **SOCRATES** of pain and record initial and subsequent pain scores. • Consider analgesia if appropriate, refer to **Pain Management in Adults** and **Pain Management in Children**.
• Documentation	• Complete documentation to include all clinical findings, advice from other clinicians and onward referral.

6. Risk of Infection to Ambulance Personnel

- Meningococcal bacteria do not survive outside the nose and throat.
- Ambulance personnel directly exposed to large respiratory particles, droplets or secretions from patients with meningococcal disease should be offered preventative antibiotics. Such exposure is unlikely to occur unless working in very close proximity to the patient (e.g. inhaling droplets coughed or sneezed by the patient, or when undertaking airway management).
- Public Health will provide post-exposure antibiotics for meningococcal contacts who may otherwise be at increased risk of infection.

Meningococcal Meningitis and Septicaemia

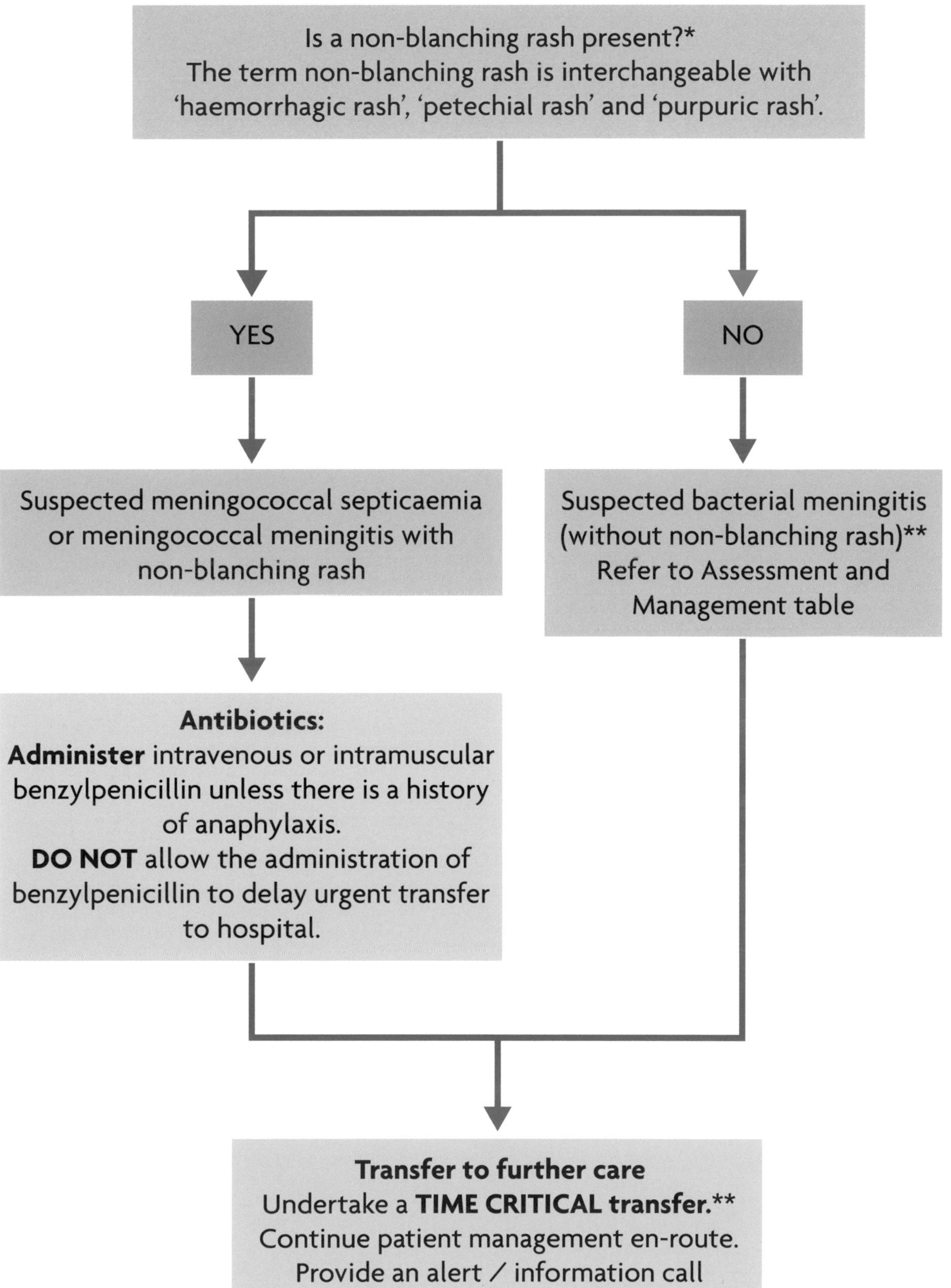

Is a non-blanching rash present?*
The term non-blanching rash is interchangeable with 'haemorrhagic rash', 'petechial rash' and 'purpuric rash'.
YES
NO
Suspected meningococcal septicaemia or meningococcal meningitis with non-blanching rash
Suspected bacterial meningitis (without non-blanching rash)**
Refer to Assessment and Management table
Antibiotics:
Administer intravenous or intramuscular benzylpenicillin unless there is a history of anaphylaxis.
DO NOT allow the administration of benzylpenicillin to delay urgent transfer to hospital.
Transfer to further care
Undertake a TIME CRITICAL transfer.**
Continue patient management en-route.
Provide an alert / information call

Figure 3.27 – Management algorithm for patients with suspected meningococcal disease.

* The term non-blanching rash is interchangeable with 'haemorrhagic rash', 'petechial rash' and 'purpuric rash'.

** If bacterial meningitis is suspected and urgent transfer is not possible, administer antibiotics even in the absence of a non-blanching rash.

Meningococcal Meningitis and Septicaemia

KEY POINTS!

Meningococcal Meningitis and Septicaemia

- **Meningococcal disease is the leading cause of death from infection in children and young adults. It can kill a healthy person of any age within hours of their first symptoms.**
- **Two clinical categories are described – meningitis and septicaemia – although they often overlap.**
- **Non-specific symptoms, such as pyrexia or a 'flu-like' illness may be the only clinical features at first presentation.**
- **A non-blanching rash should be sought, suggestive of meningococcal septicaemia (not universally present).**
- **A TIME CRITICAL transfer should be undertaken whenever meningococcal disease is suspected (irrespective of the presence or absence of a rash).**
- **Administer benzylpenicillin if septicaemia is suspected. The illness progresses rapidly and early antibiotics can improve outcomes.**

Bibliography

1. National Institute for Health and Clinical Excellence. Feverish Illness in Children: Assessment and Initial Management in children younger than five years. NICE, 2013. Available from: https://www.nice.org.uk/guidance/cg160
2. National Institute for Health and Clinical Excellence. *Meningitis - bacterial meningitis and meningococcal disease*. London: NICE, 2019. Available from: https://cks.nice.org.uk/meningitis-bacterial-meningitis-and-meningococcal-disease.
3. Meningitis Research Foundation. *Lessons from research for doctors in training: recognition and early management of meningococcal disease in children and young people*. Bristol: MRF, 2004. Available from: https://www.meningitis.org/healthcare-professionals/resources.
4. National Collaborating Centre for Women's and Children's Health. *Bacterial Meningitis and Meningococcal Septicaemia: Management of bacterial meningitis and meningococcal septicaemia in children and young people younger than 16 years in primary and secondary care* (CG102). London: National Institute for Health and Clinical Excellence, 2010. Available from: https://www.nice.org.uk/guidance/cg102.
5. Thompson MJ, Ninis N, Perera R, Mayon-White R, Phillips C, Bailey L, et al. Clinical recognition of meningococcal disease in children and adolescents. *The Lancet* 2006, 367(9508): 397–403.
6. Strang JR, Pugh EJ. Meningococcal infections: reducing the case fatality rate by giving penicillin before admission to hospital. *British Medical Journal* 1992, 305(6846): 141–3.
7. Riordan FA, Thomson AP, Sills JA, Hart CA. Who spots the spots? Diagnosis and treatment of early meningococcal disease in children. *British Medical Journal* 1996, 313(7067): 1255–6.
8. Scottish Intercollegiate Guidelines Network. *Management of Invasive Meningococcal Disease in Children and Young People* (Guideline 102). Edinburgh: SIGN, 2008.
9. Chief Medical Officer. *Meningococcal infection* (letter, PL/CMO/99/1). London: Department of Health, 1999.
10. Hart CA, Thomson AP. Meningococcal disease and its management in children. *British Medical Journal* 2006, 333(7570): 685–90.
11. Hahne SJ, Charlett A, Purcell B, Samuelsson S, Camaroni I, Ehrhard I, et al. Effectiveness of antibiotics given before admission in reducing mortality from meningococcal disease: systematic review. *British Medical Journal* 2006, 332(7553): 1299–303.
12. Meningitis Research Foundation. *Meningococcal Septicaemia: Identification & management for ambulance personnel*, second edition. Bristol/Edinburgh/Belfast: Meningitis Research Foundation, 2008.
13. Cartwright K, Reilly S, White D, Stuart J. Early treatment with parenteral penicillin in meningococcal disease. *British Medical Journal* 1992, 305(6846): 143–7.
14. Booy R, Habibi P, Nadel S, de Munter C, Britto J, Morrison A, et al. Reduction in case fatality rate from meningococcal disease associated with improved healthcare delivery. *Archives of Disease in Childhood* 2001, 85(5): 386–90.
15. Pollard AJ, Cloke A, Glennie L, Faust SN, Haines C, Heath PT, et al. *Management of Meningococcal Disease in Children and Young People*, seventh edition. Bristol/Edinburgh/Belfast: Meningitis Research Foundation, 2010. Incorporates NICE *Bacterial Meningitis and Meningococcal Septicaemia* (CG102). Distributed in partnership with NICE.
16. Health Protection Agency. *Meningococcal Reference Unit Isolates of Neisseria Meningitidis: England and Wales, by region, age group & epidemiological year, 2000–2001 to 2009–2010*. London: HPA, 2010.
17. Surtees SJ, Stockton MG, Gietzen TW. Allergy to penicillin: fable or fact? *British Medical Journal* 1991, 302(6784): 1051–2.
18. Carcillo JA, Davis AL, Zaritsky A. Role of early fluid resuscitation in pediatric septic shock. *Journal of the American Medical Association* 1991, 266(9): 1242–5.

Mental Health Presentation: Crisis, Distress and Disordered Behaviour

1. Introduction

An ambulance clinician is often faced with behaviour that has made carers or bystanders concerned. Problematic behaviour is not in itself diagnostic of mental illness. There are three common problematic behaviours which may have multiple causes:

1 Violence and aggression, which has many underlying causes ranging from conflict, criminal intent, head injury, intoxication, metabolic disturbance, hypoxia and major mental illness.[1]

2 Treatment refusal and leaving against professional advice: this can seem counterintuitive and may be a decision made with or without capacity. Assessing a person's capacity to make decisions likely to lead to a clinical decline or even death in these circumstances can be difficult, as they may not be engaging in the decision-making process.[2]

3 Self-harm and suicidality: these may seem the most obvious behaviours linked to mental illness but equally occur acutely in previously well people in high stress or distress situations, in people with autism and intellectual disability or as part of drug, alcohol or gambling use disorders.[3]

It is therefore important that ambulance clinicians do not leap to the conclusion that the problematic behaviour is due to mental illness and assume that the pathway of care should be by way of the Health Based Place of Safety. It is important to consider that intoxication by alcohol and/or drugs is a more common cause of both problematic behaviour and psychotic presentation.

Medical and trauma conditions need to be excluded and access to the right care, including appropriate investigations, arranged.

People with severe and enduring mental disorders will most often be known to their primary care and specialist mental health services, have a care plan that includes information on their **'relapse signature'** (the usual signs and symptoms each person has when relapsing) and statements about the care and treatment that works for them when presenting in crisis.

2. Management in the Pre-hospital Emergency Care Setting

- Ambulance clinicians may well be the first contact that a person with a mental health problem has with health services; we need to recognise the importance of our role. Patients will present in a variety of ways, but they will almost all be experiencing significant distress at the time. Successfully managing the distress (however this is displayed) will be key to ensuring a safe and satisfactory outcome for the patient.
- Whatever underlying mental health condition a patient may have, when in distress it is likely to manifest as an emotional response – it is this emotion that the ambulance clinician has to manage in order to establish a rapport and provide good-quality care for the patient.
- Understanding the basic components of an emotion will help to identify possible reasons for certain behaviours, and facilitate appropriate ways of managing them – for example, to reduce anxiety or anger. Being able to understand why a person is behaving in a certain way will make it easier to manage the situation safely and professionally.
- In 2011, Richards and Whyte outlined the ABC Model of Emotion,[4] which describes what an emotion is by breaking it down into three constituent parts – **autonomic, behavioural** and **cognitive** – that interact and influence each other.

3. Transporting Patients Detained Under the MHA

- Detained patients being transferred by ambulance (from a public or private place) should have an escort (this is **not** usually the approved mental health professional), along with authority to convey and completed 'Section' papers.

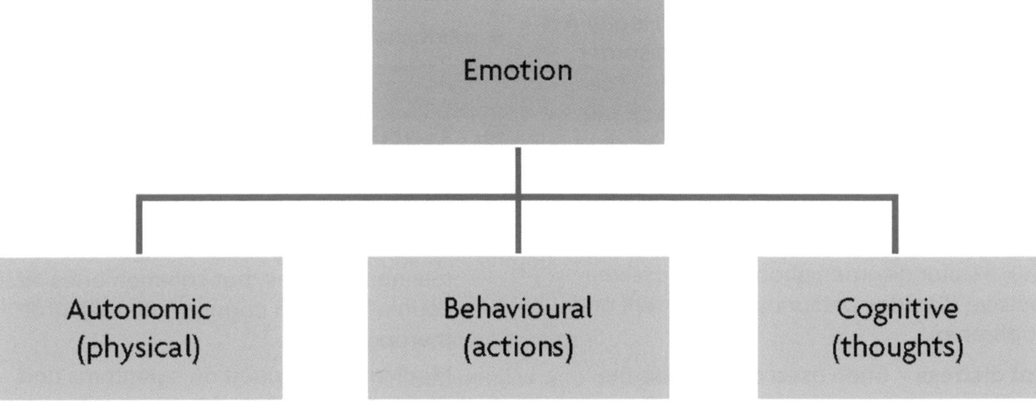

Figure 3.28 – ABC model of emotion (based on Richards and Whyte, 2011).

Mental Health Presentation: Crisis, Distress and Disordered Behaviour

Key Aspects to Note During Assessment

- Does the patient have capacity to make specific decisions regarding their current situation (e.g. consent/withholding consent for proposed intervention or treatment)? If there are any doubts, an ambulance mental capacity assessment should be completed in line with local policy.
- A patient **HAS** capacity only if they can:
  1 understand information about the decision to be made
  2 retain that information in their mind
  3 use or weigh-up the information as part of the decision-making process
  4 communicate their decision (in whatever way they usually communicate).
- If a person lacks capacity in any of these areas, then (on the balance of probabilities) this represents a lack of capacity.[10]
- Are there any safeguarding issues (e.g. suicidal patient, patient is single parent, patient is frail elderly)? Remember that people in distress are vulnerable to abuse from others. Complete a safeguarding referral in line with local policy.

8. Common Causes of Mental Distress

Anxiety

- Anxiety is a normal feeling, usually experienced temporarily in a situation that is threatening or difficult. Recurrent/persistent episodes of anxiety for no apparent reason become a problem, interfere with life and can damage physical health.[11]
- During an episode of heightened anxiety, simple strategies include:
  - staying with the person
  - encouraging them to sit
  - reassuring the person
  - demonstrating control of the situation; being firm but caring
  - encouraging the person to breathe in and out slowly
  - considering the environment; how much is noise and external stimulation influencing the anxiety? Can this be reduced?
  - ascertaining if this has happened previously, in which case does the patient have any appropriate coping skills? If so, encourage the patient to use them.
  - considering separation if there is an audience or relative/carer adding to the distress.

Depression

- Most people have periods of low mood from time to time, but these usually resolve spontaneously. Persistent low mood over a prolonged period of time is often indicative of an underlying depression.
- Depression is very common; one person in every five will experience an episode of depression during the course of their lifetime, ranging from mild (low mood, but not severe enough to impact on normal activities of daily living) to severe and life-threatening (making the person feel suicidal and worthless). Some people with severe depression will experience psychotic episodes.[12]
- During an episode of depression, simple strategies include:
  - being patient
  - adopting a non-judgemental approach

TABLE 3.72 – ABC of Anxiety

A – Autonomic	B – Behavioural	C – Cognitive
• Increased respiration. • Increased heart rate/palpitations. • Sweating. • Nausea/gastrointestinal disturbance. • Frequency of micturition/urgency. • Shaking/tremor. • Dry mouth.	• Rubbing palms/hands. • Pacing/restlessness. • Shouting. • Withdrawn. • Avoidance. • Increased consumption of alcohol and/or recreational drugs. • **NB** Not all 'behaviours' are within the control of the patient while in a heightened emotional state.	• Fear (of the unknown) – 'What's happening?' • Panic – 'Something awful is going to happen.' • Inability to concentrate. • Not in control – 'I can't control this.' • 'I'm dying.' • Unable to focus on their current situation.
Things which happen automatically and are not within control of the person.	Actions/behaviours which the person may exhibit.	Thoughts experienced by the person.
This is not an exhaustive list. It has been used to briefly illustrate the ABC Model of Emotion.		

Mental Health Presentation: Crisis, Distress and Disordered Behaviour

TABLE 3.73 – ABC of Depression

A – Autonomic	B – Behavioural	C – Cognitive
• Decreased appetite. • Increased sensitivity to pain. • Reduced/weakened immune system. • Insomnia; or sleeping more than usual. • Tearful for no apparent reason.	• Anxious, upset. • Withdrawn. • Poor eye contact. • Changes in normal sleep pattern.	• Poor concentration. • Low self-esteem and confidence. • Reduced motivation. • Feeling worthless. • Difficulty making decisions. • Suicidal ideation (not in all cases). • Pessimism. • Impaired memory.
This is not an exhaustive list. It has been used to briefly illustrate the ABC Model of Emotion.		

TABLE 3.74 – Tips on talking to someone about self-harm[14]

Do ...	Don't ...
• Actively listen. • Provide support and reassurance. • Encourage the use of any positive coping strategies. • Treat the patient with dignity and respect.	• Minimise the person's feelings or problems. • Use statements that don't take the patient's pain seriously (such as 'but you've got a great life' or 'things aren't that bad'). • Try to solve the patient's problems for them. • Touch (e.g. hug or hold the patient's hand/arm) without their permission. • Use terms such as 'self-mutilator', 'self-injurer' or 'cutter' to refer to the patient. • Accuse the patient of attention seeking. • Make the patient feel guilty about the effect their self-injuring is having on others. • Set goals or pacts.

  - gaining an understanding of the person's situation
  - listening carefully to what the patient is saying
  - taking any threats or warnings of suicide seriously.

Self-harm

- Definition: self-poisoning or self-injury, irrespective of the apparent purpose of the act.[13]
- Self-harm is **NOT** classified as a specific mental disorder; however, a history of self-harm can be a strong predictor for repeated self-harm and completion of suicide. It is more commonly used as a way for a person to cope with life, rather than a failed attempt to end it; and there are many reasons why a person self-harms. Some examples are listed below:
  - release or catharsis
  - making an emotional pain a 'real' physical pain
  - having control when feeling out of control
  - as a self-punishment.
- A large part of the work for the ambulance clinician is likely to be centred on the physical nature of the self-harm. However, talking about the self-harm is vital as part of the assessment; it acknowledges what has happened and with this it communicates to the person that you are not rejecting them. This often helps reduce feelings of shame and stigma, which can help maintain self-harm.
- When working with someone who has self-harmed it is important that these factors are addressed:
  - What led up to it? (i.e. what was the trigger – interpersonal stressors and/or situational aspects?)
  - What was the intent of the act?
  - What was the motivation?
  - Was it planned or impulsive?
  - Are there practical protective factors in place to reduce the risk of harm occurring? (see IPAP Tool)
- These questions may overlap somewhat with a suicide risk assessment; but ambulance clinicians should be aware to separate these two aspects and to treat each accordingly.

Mental Health Presentation: Crisis, Distress and Disordered Behaviour

Risk Management

Risk management is a statement of plans and allocation of responsibility (where appropriate) to support, contain or respond to the risk(s) identified.

Formulating and agreeing a plan of action provides challenges and opportunities for both the clinician and patient. Consent and collaboration need to be at the heart of the decision making process.

The components of the plan of action should include:

- The immediacy and severity of the risk.
- Service options – what the ambulance service can provide. What mental health specific services are available in the area?
- What the patient wants.
- Duty of care – particularly with issues of confidentiality. Professionals have a duty of care to balance confidentiality with the need to know, particularly regarding colleagues from other agencies. The issue of confidentiality is further clouded by the duty of care you hold to others, to pass on information to (or about) a third party you know to be at risk.

Some strategies to help care for a suicidal patient are:

- Ask directly about suicide e.g. are you thinking about suicide – don't use euphemisms like 'harm yourself, or 'do something stupid'
- Your primary role is to listen intently – not at this stage to direct or to make plans for the person
- Ask the person to tell you their story. Listen carefully and without distraction – they will often talk about positives in their life as well as the crisis situation they are in today
- When someone mentions positive things e.g. relationships, pets, plans for tomorrow, reflect these things back, amplify these things and highlight that there are things or moments when they have been happy
- Ask the person if they would be prepared to think about how they could keep themselves safe for now – and what it would take to help them to keep safe
- Try to focus on the here and now
- Think about resources around the person – neighbours, friends, family, connections and supports that can help to keep the person safe
- Write the safety plan down with the person and ask them to keep adding ideas on how they might keep themselves safe
- Make the environment safe – people will often tell you about the means of suicide they are contemplating, and may be willing for you to remove the means from their home e.g. medications
- Work with the person to identify what helps to soothe them e.g. music, baths, walks, talking to others
- Identify people who might be able to offer immediate support and who can help to implement the safety plan.

Mania

- Definition: unusually happy with exaggerated thoughts, feelings and behaviours affecting many aspects of life.[16]
- Common reasons for mania include substance abuse, bipolar disorder, schizoaffective disorder or an organic condition.
- During an episode of mania, simple strategies include:
  - remaining calm; avoid raising your voice or speaking fast
  - avoiding sudden/abrupt movements
  - trying not to restrict the patient's movements unless essential for safety
  - not responding in a challenging manner to the patient
  - considering the environment, how much noise and external stimulation may be influencing the situation – can this be reduced?

Acute Psychosis

- The term acute psychosis is used to describe symptoms or experiences that happen together. Each person will have different symptoms; the common feature is that they are not experiencing reality like most other people.[17]
- Common reasons include substance abuse, schizophrenia, bipolar disorder and psychotic depression.
- During an episode of acute psychosis, simple strategies include:
  - remaining calm; avoid raising your voice or speaking fast
  - reassuring the patient that you want to help them
  - avoiding sudden/abrupt movements
  - accepting that any hallucinations or delusions are very real to the patient
  - trying not to restrict the patient's movements unless essential for safety
  - not responding in a challenging manner to the patient
  - remembering it is the patient's symptoms that cause the fear/suspicion/paranoia, and doing all you can to reduce these and reassure the patient
  - taking any threats or warnings seriously, particularly if the patient believes they are being persecuted.[18]

Mental Health Presentation: Crisis, Distress and Disordered Behaviour

TABLE 3.76 – ABC of Mania

A – Autonomic	B – Behavioural	C – Cognitive
• Increased respiration. • Increased heart rate/ palpitations. • Sweating. • Nausea/gastrointestinal disturbance. • Dilated pupils. • Flushed face.	• Rubbing palms/hands. • Pacing/restlessness. • Shouting. • Short tempered/irritable. • Aggressive. • Speaking very quickly and changing the subject frequently. • Laughing inappropriately. • Unwilling/unable to sleep. • Agitated. • Unable to relax. • Increase in consumption of alcohol or recreational drugs. • Over familiarity. • Increased sexual activity. • Overspending.	• Very happy and excited. • Feeling more important than usual. • Feeling full of energy. • Auditory hallucinations. • Belief that they have special powers. • Racing thoughts.
This is not an exhaustive list. It has been used to briefly illustrate the ABC Model of Emotion.		

TABLE 3.77 – ABC of Acute Psychosis

A – Autonomic	B – Behavioural	C – Cognitive
• Increased respiration. • Increased heart rate/palpitations. • Sweating. • Dilated pupils. • Flushed face.	• Aggressive/suspicious/pre-occupied. • Hyperactive. • Very intense eye contact – or no eye contact at all. • Intrusive conduct. • May be extremely withdrawn. • Shouting/swearing/laughing inappropriately. • Placing hands over ears. • Evidence (and/or self-reports) of hallucinations. • Increase in consumption of alcohol or recreational drugs.	• Appears pre-occupied. • Obsessive or disordered thinking. • Sudden loss of train of thought, resulting in an abrupt pause in conversation or activity. • Displaying unusual beliefs or delusional, (unrealistic) ideas about themselves, others or the world in general (e.g. that there is a special/secret meaning in TV programmes/ vehicles passing on a road/printed documents, or that someone is trying to poison/control them). • Altered perception of reality – unable to distinguish their thoughts and ideas from reality. • Believes that their thoughts can be read, changed or removed from their minds.
This is not an exhaustive list. It has been used to briefly illustrate the ABC Model of Emotion.		

Personality Disorders

- The Royal College of Psychiatrists (RCPsychs) describes 'personality' as a collection of characteristics – or traits – that individuals develop as they mature from children to adults.[19] These are unique and include ways that each individual thinks, feels and behaves in response to any given situation.
- An individual's personality is usually fully developed by the late teens or early 20s and will remain consistent throughout the rest of life. An important aspect of a developed personality is the ability to get on with other people (this requires empathy and self-awareness), but for some this does not happen, and certain personality traits make life difficult – both for the person and those around them.

- Several personality 'disorders' have been described and, according to the RCPsychs, research suggests that they tend to fall into three groups, according to their emotional 'flavour':
  - **Cluster A** – odd or eccentric.
  - **Cluster B** – dramatic, emotional or erratic.
  - **Cluster C** – anxious or fearful.[20]
- People with any type of personality disorder can be stigmatised because of their diagnosis. They can attract fear, anger and disapproval rather than compassion, support and understanding. This is both unfair and unhelpful.[21]

Emotionally Unstable Personality Disorder

- One of the most common types of personality disorder that ambulance clinicians encounter is from Cluster B – emotionally unstable personality disorder (often referred to as EUPD).
- People diagnosed with this condition:
  - are impulsive
  - find it hard to control their emotions
  - feel bad about themselves
  - often self-harm and/or attempt suicide
  - describe feeling 'empty'
  - make relationships quickly, but easily lose them
  - can be very demanding
  - can feel paranoid or depressed
  - may hear noises or voices when stressed.
- Treatment for EUPD may involve individual or group psychotherapy, usually carried out by specially trained professionals within a community mental health setting. If required, appropriate medication may be prescribed for any specific symptoms associated with the condition (e.g. antipsychotics for auditory hallucinations).
- Treatment in an emergency situation will depend entirely on the presenting symptoms of the patient at the time.

Hints and Tips When Caring for Someone with EUPD

- Remain calm and non-judgemental.
- Use the ABC Model of Emotion to manage emotional aspects of the patient's presentation.
- Remember that EUPD is a diagnosed condition and your patient is unwell – not 'just' being manipulative and 'wasting' your time.
- The person with EUPD may not be able to verbalise how they are feeling, so won't be able to explain to you why they are feeling, or behaving, a certain way.
- Remember that the person with EUPD is responsible for his or her own actions and behaviours.
- Stick to professional boundaries and those outlined in a care plan if available. People with EUPD respond better to clear – and firm – boundaries.
- Do not engage in bargaining.
- Refer to a recent care plan if available.
- Consult with a specialist mental health professional if available.
- Use a locally agreed alternative care pathway if available (and necessary).
- Simple strategies include:
  - listening actively
  - focusing on the emotions, not the words
  - remaining calm
  - validating the patient's experience.
- As with any patient presenting with mental distress, clear communication is essential in achieving a safe and effective outcome for your patient.

Dementia

- Dementia is the name given to a group of diseases that affect the brain and share a common set of symptoms. Dementia is a progressive illness that can affect any area of the brain and have a significant impact upon the lives of a patient and their relatives and carers.
- There is currently no known cure for dementia; however, there are a number of medications that are used to alleviate symptoms and prolong the quality and length of the patient's life.
- Dementia is a growing issue in the UK with numbers of sufferers expected to be in excess of 1 million by 2025. The rate of 'early onset dementia' in those under the age of 65 is also increasing.[22]
- The most commonly encountered forms of dementia include Alzheimer's disease and vascular dementia.
- Other types of dementia include Lewy body dementia, fronto-temporal lobe dementia, Creutzfeldt–Jakob disease, HIV-related cognitive impairment, Parkinson's related dementia and young onset dementia.[23]
- **Korsakoff's or alcohol related brain damage** – Although sharing many common symptoms with dementia and often used in the same context, Korsakoff's is not a type of dementia. Brain damage can be caused by consistent alcohol misuse resulting in many of the symptoms similar to dementia. If diagnosed early and managed well, progression can sometimes be halted, unlike dementia.[24]

Dementia and Mental Capacity

- Patients with dementia generally experience a decline in their abilities over time. Therefore, the need to take into consideration a patient's capacity should not be underestimated (refer to **Mental Capacity Act 2005 (England and Wales)**).

- A diagnosis of dementia does not mean that the patient lacks capacity, and all measures must be taken to ensure correct assessment and treatment. Check for the presence of an advance directive or living will, power of attorney, end of life plan, ReSPECT form or check if the patient is currently subject to a section of the Mental Health Act or a deprivation of liberty order.
- Any visit to hospital can be distressing and unpleasant, but in the case of a person with dementia, it can be significantly more distressing. Consider whether the patient needs to be conveyed to hospital and, if so, what specific issues and concerns they may have. Refer to local pathways, GPs and community care services when possible to avoid hospital attendances.
- When thinking about admission to hospital for a person living with severe dementia, carry out an assessment that balances their current medical needs with the additional harms they may face in hospital, for example:
  - disorientation
  - a longer length of stay
  - increased mortality
  - increased morbidity on discharge
  - delirium
  - the effects of being in an impersonal or institutional environment.
- When thinking about admission to hospital for a person living with dementia, take into account:
  - any advance care and support plans
  - the value of keeping them in a familiar environment.

TABLE 3.78 – Common Medications for Dementia

• Treatment of cognitive symptoms	• Acetylcholinesterase inhibitors (or cholinesterase inhibitors) act to slow or reduce the progression of symptoms. • Donepezil hydrochloride, rivastigmine and galantamine.
• Reduction of symptom progression and severity	• NMDA receptor antagonists (N-methyl-D-aspartate receptor antagonist). • Memantine hydrochloride.
• Treatment of non-cognitive symptoms (e.g. aggression, hallucinations, depression)	• Antipsychotic medications and benzodiazepines (used with caution due to side effects). • Antidepressants, hypnotics.

Communication

- Dementia causes damage to the areas of the brain that affect an individual's ability to communicate, retain information, make decisions or problem solve, eventually even on a very basic level. This can, and often does, lead to anxiety, frustration and fear. Communicating effectively with someone who has dementia is a skill that, if used properly, can make a considerable difference to experience and outcome for patients.
- Each patient with dementia must be treated as an individual with their own specific set of needs. Ensure patients are included, informed and consent is gained whenever possible to reduce their anxiety and fears.
- Care home staff, family, carers and friends should be asked to help provide a detailed history and can determine the changes in a patient from their normal state. Those who know the patient best should be asked to help you with assessing, moving and handling, treating and helping a patient to understand what is happening.

Safeguarding

- Safeguarding issues should be considered for every encounter with a patient with dementia. Patients who live alone or who depend upon carers/relatives may be at a greater risk of abuse or neglect.
- Carers and families may also be at risk themselves and require additional support.

Early Intervention and Diagnosis

- Ambulance clinicians can often be the first to recognise the signs and symptoms of dementia before diagnosis or referral has taken place. Early diagnosis and intervention is shown to slow the progression of a number of symptoms.
- Assessment tools could be considered such as the Mini-Mental State Examination for the clinician to consider the need for a full assessment. Therefore, all clinicians should consider making a referral or signposting patients with potential undiagnosed dementia using local pathways.[25]

9. Pregnancy and Mental Health

- During pregnancy the mind changes as well as the body. It is important to consider that mothers during and after pregnancy may be particularly at risk of mental health illness. This includes mothers with pre-existing mental health problems, or those whose mental health illness is a result of pregnancy. Post-natal depression affects 10–15% of women who have recently given birth.
- The 2015 report: MBRRACE-UK: Mothers and Babies: Reducing Risk through Audits and Confidential Enquiries across the UK showed that

TABLE 3.79 – Tips for Communicating with Patients with Dementia

- Consider the potential barriers to effective communication.
- Consider carefully what language and questions can be used to minimise confusion and worry.
- Ask simple questions one at a time and wait for an answer appropriately.
- Reduce distractions such as noise and activity.
- Use non-verbal communication such as tone of voice, posture and body position making sure you appear approachable and non-threatening.
- Using the person's name, make eye contact and appropriate touch.
- Encourage the person to focus upon and communicate with you.
- Take your time, try not to rush conversation.
- Do not finish their sentence or presume you already know the answer.
- Create a friendly and respectful rapport and environment.
- Don't become frustrated.

TABLE 3.80 – Post-natal Depression: Red Flag Signs

- Recent significant change in mental state or emergence of new symptoms
- New thoughts or acts of violent self-harm
- New and persistent expressions of incompetency as a mother or estrangement from the infant.

almost a quarter of women who died between 6 weeks and 1 year after pregnancy died from mental health related causes. One in seven women died from suicide.

- Women who present with any of the 'Red Flag' presentations described in Table 3.80 **MUST** be referred urgently to a specialist perinatal mental health team.[10] Refer to **Safeguarding Adults at Risk**.

Refer to local pathways and consider the need for conveyance to ED or an alternative care facility. Consider safeguarding issues and referral.

10. Pathways for Referral

It is recommended that providers of pre-hospital care have clear policies and procedures that set out the routes for onward referral to other agencies within their locality, such as:

- Direct consultation with a mental health professional – via Ambulance Trust Clinical Contact Centre (or equivalent), or locally agreed referral routes with statutory mental health service providers. This may include:
  - community mental health teams (usually during normal working hours)
  - crisis or other out-of-hours teams (outside of normal working hours)
  - hospital mental health liaison services.
- Locally agreed alternative care pathways – to avoid use of emergency departments where other clinical pathways would be more appropriate.

If the patient is already known to local mental health services:

- Ask to see a copy of their care plan and follow the recommendations/advice, as appropriate.
- Contact their care co-ordinator (during normal office hours).

11. Physical Interventions/Safe Holding

It is beyond the scope of this guidance to prescribe fidelity to any particular training model for physical interventions/safe holding, or to mandate the depth and degree of training that each trust must adopt to safely discharge its duties to protect patients, staff and the public. This must be determined locally based on current national guidance, a training needs analysis and assessment of risk.

Physical interventions broadly fall into three areas, these being:

1 Disengagement techniques often referred to as breakaway techniques which are skills designed to effect physical disengagement and escape from an assailant.

2 Physical restraint techniques often described as safe holding, which are manual holds and interventions to restrict the movement of an individual who may present a risk to self or others. These techniques will require a minimum of two staff to deploy safely.

3 Mechanical restraint, which describes techniques to restrict movement, using implements designed for the purpose, e.g. cuffs used by law enforcement agencies. The use of mechanical restraints is not appropriate for ambulance services.

These techniques are all potential interventions that should only be deployed when verbal de-escalation techniques have proved ineffective, and where restraint techniques are deployed, following formal assessment under the guidance of the Mental Capacity Act (MCA) or Mental Health Act.

Where staff training in these areas is considered appropriate, the following guidelines should be regarded as mandatory.

1 All training programmes must be accredited and delivered by a certified physical interventions

tutor, who has attended the requisite refresher training to continue practice.

2 Training programmes must include training in verbal de-escalation skills and interventions.

3 Training must form part of a rolling programme where appropriate refresher training intervals are mandated.

4 Training programmes and interventions must follow the guiding principles of NICE guideline NG10 and ideally BILD accreditation.

5 It is important to distinguish that physical intervention skills training in the ambulance service is primarily related to decisionmaking under the mental capacity act where the threshold is a risk of serious harm or a life-threatening condition. Physical restraint is only occasionally a consideration under the Mental Health Act and where safe to do so following a risk assessment.

6 Any planned intervention needs to be assessed considering risk and the consequence of doing nothing, and the risk of the least restrictive physical intervention.

Ambulance staff are obliged under the MCA to act in the best interests of/for patients who lack capacity, even when the patient refuses treatment or is abusive, threatening or violent.

The MCA also protects carers from liability when 'reasonable force' is required to ensure that patients lacking capacity receive care that is in their best interests; or to protect them from further harm. As stated previously, Section 6 of the Act defines restraint as the use, or threat, of force where an incapacitated person resists, and any restriction of liberty or movement, whether or not the person resists.

Ambulance staff have limited training in this aspect. Minimal restraint (now known as 'safer-holding') can be used in cases where patients lack capacity, and there is no perceived risk of harm to the ambulance crew. If the behaviour of the patient exceeds what the crew can safely manage then assistance must be requested in line with local policy (this does not necessarily have to be police).

A Dynamic Risk Assessment should always be completed prior to the use of any form of safer-holding and these decisions and actions must be recorded in the Patient Clinical Record.

Ambulance staff should always monitor the physical well-being of the patient and should be familiar with ambulance service information related to Acute Behavioural Disturbance and safer-holding.

Conclusion

- Fundamental to the management of any mental health incident is the approach taken by the health professional involved. Often what patients remember is not the advice tendered, but the warmth, empathy and concern of the healthcare professional who looked after them at a time of distress. These qualitative aspects of the intervention are particularly important when supporting patients with mental health concerns.
- Staff who are able to establish rapport, manage distress, and provide reassurance, are more likely to elicit true expressions of feelings and worries from the patient, and this facilitates an effective assessment to formulate a safe outcome.

12. Traffic Light Tool for Assessing Mental Health

Low Mood

Persistent low mood may be an indicator of underlying depression (RCPsychs, 2017).

TABLE 3.81 – Traffic Light Assessment Tool for Low Mood

	Green Low risk	**Amber** Medium risk	**Red** High risk
Behaviour Verbal and non-verbal signs	**Calm, relaxed. Appropriate eye contact, body language and conduct.**	**Anxious, upset. Tearful for no apparent reason. Withdrawn. Poor eye contact. Reduced motivation. Changes in normal sleep pattern.**	**Withdrawn. Little or no eye contact. No motivation. Extremely tired.**
Appearance	**Attire is functional and appropriate to situation. No recent self-harm.**	**Evidence of reduced self-care. Signs of recent self-harm.**	**Attire may be appropriate or inappropriate to situation. Unkempt, evidence of poor hygiene. Recent self-harm.**

(continued)

Mental Health Presentation: Crisis, Distress and Disordered Behaviour

TABLE 3.81 – Traffic Light Assessment Tool for Low Mood *(continued)*

	Green Low risk	**Amber** Medium risk	**Red** High risk
Speech and rapport with others	**Appropriate. Able to follow the flow of conversation. Positive attitude towards others. Normal rate and volume of speech. Spontaneous conversation.**	**Mild/minor difficulties following flow of conversation. Slower rate/ lower volume of speech. Limited spontaneous conversation but able to answer questions using full sentences.**	**Poor. Unable to follow the flow of conversation. Negative attitude towards self and others. Unable to articulate thoughts clearly. Altered rate and/or volume of speech. Monosyllabic answers to questions.**
Mood	**Low/flat. Noticed some impact on daily life.**	**Continuous low mood/ sadness. Blunted. Flat. Varies, inappropriate to the situation at times. Lost interest in things previously enjoyed. Anxious. Significant impact on daily life.**	**Feels numb. Flat. Hopeless. Helpless. Low self-esteem. Irritable and intolerant of others. Finds it impossible to cope with daily life.**
Cognition	**Orientated to time, place and person. Short term memory intact (able to retain and recall information). Able to concentrate and follow simple instructions.**	**Orientated to time, place and person. Difficulty retaining and recalling information. Some difficulty following simple instructions or making decisions. Future appears bleak.**	**Orientated to time, place and person. Unable to concentrate or follow simple instructions. Difficulty making any decision. Can see no future.**
Thoughts	No evidence (or self-reports) of suicidal thoughts.	Occasional/fleeting thoughts of suicide.	Appears pre-occupied. Frequent, recurring thoughts of suicide. Feeling guilt ridden.
Insight	Understands and accepts their current situation and the need to receive further assessment/ treatment.	Some understanding of their current situation. Unsure about need for further assessment/treatment.	Does not understand their current situation and the need to receive further assessment/treatment. Feels like nothing will help.
Risk to self/ others People diagnosed with severe depression are much more likely to attempt suicide than the general population *(NHS Choices, 2016).*	None apparent. No previous history of mental disorder/self-harm/suicide attempt.	Moderate risk to self (suicide/self-harm). Previous history of mental disorder/ self-harm/suicide attempt.	Evidence of risk to self and/ or others, e.g. threats to harm self/others. Previous history of mental disorder, self-harm or suicide attempts. History of alcohol, drug misuse or dependence. Recent significant life event.
Recommended intervention:	No further action required. Routine appointment with GP. Contact 111 or GP if symptoms deteriorate.	Complete IPAP Suicide Risk Assessment. Urgent psychiatric assessment. Contact care coordinator if known to local services, or GP if not known. OOH GP.	Complete IPAP Suicide Risk Assessment. Urgent psychiatric assessment. Contact care coordinator if known to local services, or GP if not known. Consider an OOH GP.

Mental Health Presentation: Crisis, Distress and Disordered Behaviour

Anxiety

'Anxiety is a normal feeling, usually experienced temporarily in a situation that is threatening or difficult. Recurrent/persistent episodes of anxiety for no apparent reason become a problem, interfere with life and can damage physical health' (RCPsychs, 2017).

Common triggers for anxiety: Saying something that could offend someone. Getting stuck on public transport/in a lift. Arriving somewhere late. Fearing something could go wrong. Forgetting to do something important. Not being able to control what's happening now or in the future. Wondering if loved ones are upset with you. Making a mistake at work that will result in being judged by others. Looking stupid in a social setting. Feeling anxious about being anxious.

TABLE 3.82 – Traffic Light Assessment Tool for Anxiety

	Green Low risk	**Amber** Medium risk	**Red** High risk
Behaviour Verbal and non-verbal signs	Calm, relaxed. Appropriate eye contact, body language and conduct.	Anxious, upset. Tearful for no apparent reason. Withdrawn. Poor eye contact. Reduced motivation. Changes in normal sleep pattern.	Withdrawn. Little or no eye contact. No motivation. Extremely tired.
Appearance	Attire is functional and appropriate to situation. No recent self-harm.	Evidence of reduced self-care. Signs of recent self-harm.	Attire may be appropriate or inappropriate to situation. Unkempt, evidence of poor hygiene. Recent self-harm.
Speech and rapport	Appropriate. Able to follow the flow of conversation. Positive attitude towards others. Normal rate and volume of speech. Spontaneous conversation.	Mild/minor difficulties following flow of conversation. Slower rate/ lower volume of speech. Limited spontaneous conversation but able to answer questions using full sentences.	Poor. Unable to follow the flow of conversation. Negative attitude towards self and others. Unable to articulate thoughts clearly. Altered rate/volume of speech. Monosyllabic answer to questions.
Mood/Affect	Low/flat. Noticed some impact on daily life.	Continuous low mood/ sadness. Blunted. Flat. Varies, inappropriate to the situation at times. Lost interest in things previously enjoyed. Anxious. Significant impact on daily life.	Feels numb. Flat. Hopeless. Helpless. Low self-esteem. Irritable and intolerant of others. Finds it impossible to cope with daily life.
Cognition	Orientated to time, place and person. Short term memory intact (able to retain and recall information). Able to concentrate and follow simple instructions.	Orientated to time, place and person. Difficulty retaining and recalling information. Some difficulty following simple instructions or making decisions. Future appears bleak.	Orientated to time, place and person. Unable to concentrate or follow simple instructions. Difficulty making any decision. Can see no future.
Thoughts	No evidence (or self-reports) of suicidal thoughts.	Occasional/fleeting thoughts of suicide.	Appears pre-occupied. Frequent, recurring thoughts of suicide. Feeling guilt ridden.
Insight	Understands and accepts their current situation and the need to receive further assessment/treatment.	Some understanding of their current situation. Unsure about need for further assessment/treatment.	Does not understand their current situation and the need to receive further assessment/treatment. Feels like nothing will help.

(continued)

TABLE 3.82 – Traffic Light Assessment Tool for Anxiety *(continued)*			
	Green Low risk	**Amber** Medium risk	**Red** High risk
Risk to self/ others People diagnosed with severe depression are much more likely to attempt suicide than the general population *(NHS Choices, 2016)*.	None apparent. No previous history of mental disorder/self-harm/suicide attempt.	Moderate risk to self (suicide/self-harm). Previous history of mental disorder/ self-harm/suicide attempt.	Evidence of risk to self and/or others (e.g. threats to harm self/others). Previous history of mental disorder/self-harm/ suicide attempt. History of alcohol/drug misuse/ dependence. Recent significant life event.
Recommended intervention:	**No further action required. Routine appointment with GP. Contact 111 or GP if symptoms deteriorate.**	**Complete IPAP Suicide Risk Assessment. Urgent psychiatric assessment. Care coordinator if known to local services. GP if not known. OOH GP.**	**Complete IPAP Suicide Risk Assessment. Emergency psychiatric assessment. Local Crisis Resolution/Home Treatment Team. ED as a last resort or when treatment for medical condition is required.**

Mania

Unusually happy with exaggerated thoughts, feelings, and behaviours affecting many aspects of life (RCPsychs, 2017). Common reasons include: substance induced, bipolar disorder, schizoaffective disorder or an organic condition.

TABLE 3.83 – Traffic Light Assessment Tool for Mania			
	Green Low risk	**Amber** Medium risk	**Red** High risk
Behaviour Verbal and non-verbal signs	Calm, relaxed. Appropriate eye contact, body language and conduct.	Unable to sit still for long. Pacing.	Agitated. Pacing. Unable to relax. Increase in consumption of alcohol or recreational drugs.
Appearance	Attire is functional and appropriate to situation. No recent self-harm.	Evidence of reduced self-care. Signs of recent self-harm.	Attire may be appropriate or inappropriate to situation. Unkempt, evidence of poor hygiene. Recent self-harm.
Speech and rapport	Appropriate. Able to follow the flow of conversation. Positive attitude towards others. Normal rate and volume of speech. Spontaneous conversation.	Mild/minor difficulties following flow of conversation. Faster rate of speech than normal. Very 'chatty'.	Unable to follow the flow of conversation. Intolerant/threatening attitude towards others. Unable to articulate thoughts clearly. Altered rate/volume of speech. Speaking very quickly, frequently switching from one topic of conversation to another without any clear link.
Mood/Affect	Happy/euphoric. Noticed some impact on daily life.	Persistent happiness. Increased energy. Decreased need for sleep/food. Significant impact on daily life.	Feeling very happy, elated or overjoyed most of the time. Feeling full of energy/ self-important/full of great new ideas and having important plans. Easily distracted. Easily irritated or agitated. Impatient with others. Impossible to cope with daily life.

Mental Health Presentation: Crisis, Distress and Disordered Behaviour

TABLE 3.83 – Traffic Light Assessment Tool for Mania *(continued)*

	Green Low risk	**Amber** Medium risk	**Red** High risk
Cognition	Orientated to time, place and person. Short term memory intact (able to retain and recall information). Able to concentrate and follow simple instructions.	Orientated to time, place and person. Difficulty retaining and recalling information. Some difficulty following simple instructions or making decisions.	Not orientated to time, place and person. Unable to concentrate or follow simple instructions.
Thoughts	No evidence (or self-reports) of suicidal thoughts or disordered thinking/perception of reality.	Racing. Full of important plans.	Easily distracted. Obsessive, or disordered, thinking. Flight of ideas (racing thoughts, switching from one aspect to another very quickly with no clear links evident). Unusual beliefs or delusional, (unrealistic) ideas about themselves, others, or the world in general (e.g. that they have special powers, are a celebrity or a very important public figure). Altered perception of reality - unable to distinguish their own thoughts and ideas from reality.
Hallucinations/ Delusions			Being delusional, having hallucinations and disturbed or illogical thinking
Insight	Understands and accepts their current situation and the need to receive further assessment/treatment.	Some understanding of their current situation. Unsure about need for further assessment/ treatment.	Does not understand their current situation and the need to receive further assessment/treatment.
Risk to self/ others People diagnosed with bipolar disorder are 20 times more likely to attempt suicide than the general population (NHS Choices, 2016).	None apparent. No previous history of mental disorder/self-harm/suicide attempt.	Moderate risk to self (suicide/self-harm). Previous history of mental disorder/self-harm/ suicide attempt.	Doing things that often have disastrous consequences – such as spending large sums of money on expensive and sometimes unaffordable items. Making decisions or saying things that are out of character and that others see as being risky or harmful.
Recommended intervention:	**No further action required. Routine appointment with GP. Contact 111 or GP if symptoms deteriorate.**	**Complete IPAP Suicide Risk Assessment if suicidal ideation present. Urgent psychiatric assessment. Care coordinator if known to local services. GP if not known. OOH GP.**	**Complete IPAP Suicide Risk Assessment if suicidal ideation present. Emergency psychiatric assessment. Local Crisis Resolution/ Home Treatment Team. ED as a last resort or when treatment for medical condition is required.**

Mental Health Presentation: Crisis, Distress and Disordered Behaviour

Psychosis

Term used to describe symptoms or experiences that happen together. Each person will have different symptoms; the common feature is that they are not experiencing reality like most other people (RCPsychs, 2017).

Common reasons include: substance induced, schizophrenia, bipolar disorder and psychotic depression.

TABLE 3.84 – Traffic Light Assessment Tool for Psychosis

	Green Low risk	**Amber** Medium risk	**Red** High risk
Behaviour Verbal and non-verbal signs	Calm, relaxed. Appropriate eye contact, body language and conduct.	Anxious, upset, unable to settle. Inappropriate body language. May be withdrawn. Increase in consumption of alcohol or recreational drugs.	Aggressive/suspicious/pre-occupied. Hyperactive. Too intense eye contact – or no eye contact at all. Intrusive conduct. May be extremely withdrawn. Shouting/swearing/ laughing inappropriately.
Appearance	Attire is functional and appropriate to situation. No recent self-harm.	Evidence of reduced self-care. Signs of recent self-harm.	Attire is inappropriate to situation. Unkempt, evidence of poor hygiene. Recent self-harm.
Speech and rapport	Appropriate. Able to follow the flow of conversation. Positive attitude towards others. Normal rate and volume of speech. Spontaneous conversation.	Mild/minor difficulties following flow of conversation. Ambivalent attitude towards others – may be fearful/suspicious of certain people. Altered rate/volume of speech (e.g. too fast or too slow).	Poor. Unable to follow the flow of conversation. Negative/suspicious/threatening attitude towards others. Unable to articulate thoughts clearly. Altered rate/volume of speech (e.g. too fast or too slow). Frequent changes to the topic of conversation, to unrelated topics or to whatever they observe in front of them. Using nonsense words or very mixed up sentences ('word salad').
Mood/Affect	Altered. Noticed some impact on daily life.	Incongruous. Blunted. Varies, inappropriate to the situation at times. Significant impact on daily life.	Flat. Labile. Euphoric. Inappropriate to the situation most of the time. Impossible to cope with daily life.
Cognition	Orientated to time, place and person. Short term memory intact (able to retain and recall information). Able to concentrate and follow simple instructions.	Orientated to time, place and person. Difficulty retaining and recalling information. Some difficulty following simple instructions.	Not orientated to time, place and person. Unable to concentrate or follow simple instructions.

TABLE 3.84 – Traffic Light Assessment Tool for Psychosis *(continued)*

	Green Low risk	**Amber** Medium risk	**Red** High risk
Thoughts	No evidence (or self-reports) of disordered thinking or unusual beliefs.	Evidence of some disordered thinking and/or unusual beliefs. Some suspicion about certain things, or people, may be evident.	Appears pre-occupied. Have obsessive, or disordered, thinking. Sudden loss in their train of thought, resulting in an abrupt pause in conversation or activity. Display unusual beliefs or delusional (unrealistic) ideas about themselves, others, or the world in general (e.g. that there is a special/secret meaning in TV programmes/ vehicles passing on a road/printed documents, or that someone is trying to poison/control them). Altered perception of reality - unable to distinguish their own thoughts and ideas from reality.
Hallucinations/ Delusions	No evidence (or self-reports) of hallucinations/ delusions.	Previous history of hallucinations/ delusions. Patient may feel that they themselves are not real or that the situation they are in is not real.	Evidence (and/or self reports) of hallucinations. Visual/auditory hallucinations are the most common (individual to the patient). Patient believes that their thoughts can be read, changed or removed from their minds.
Insight	Understands and accepts their current situation and the need to receive further assessment/treatment. Understands how their behaviour impacts on others.	Some understanding of their current situation. Unsure/ suspicious about need for further assessment/treatment.	Does not understand their current situation and the need to receive further assessment/treatment; nor how their behaviour impacts on others.
Risk to self/ others As 1 in 10 people with psychosis die by suicide, it is important not to miss any symptoms of depression *(RCPsychs, 2017).*	None apparent.	Moderate risk to self (suicide/self-harm).	Evidence of risk to self and/or others (e.g. threats to harm self/others).
Recommended intervention:	**No further action required. Contact 111 or GP if symptoms deteriorate.**	**Complete IPAP Suicide Risk Assessment if suicidal ideation present. Urgent psychiatric assessment. Care coordinator if known to local services. GP if not known. OOH GP.**	**Complete IPAP Suicide Risk Assessment if suicidal ideation present. Emergency psychiatric assessment. Local Crisis Resolution/Home Treatment Team. ED as a last resort or when treatment for medical condition is required.**

Mental Health Presentation: Crisis, Distress and Disordered Behaviour

Bibliography

1. eLearning for Health. *Violence and Aggression.* Leeds: Health Education England, 2016. Available from: http://portal.e-lfh.org.uk/Component/Details/432728.
2. eLearning for Health. *Suicide and Self-Harm.* Leeds: Health Education England, 2016. Available from: https://portal.e-lfh.org.uk/Component/Details/448052.
3. eLearning for Health. *Abscond and Treatment Refusal.* Leeds: Health Education England, 2016. Available from: http://portal.e-lfh.org.uk/Component/Details/439829.
4. Richards D, Whyte M. Reach Out. *National Programme Student Materials to Support the Delivery of Training for Psychological Wellbeing Practitioners Delivering Low Intensity Interventions.* London: Rethink Mental Illness, 2011.
5. World Health Organization. *Promoting Mental Health: Concepts, emerging evidence, practice (Summary Report).* Geneva: WHO, 2004.
6. Parliament of the United Kingdom. *The Mental Health Act 1983 (amended 2007).* London: The Stationery Office, 2007.
7. McManus S, Meltzer H, Brugha TS, Bebbington PE, Jenkins R. *Adult Psychiatric Morbidity in England, 2007: Results of a household survey.* London: The NHS Information Centre for Health and Social Care, 2009.
8. McManus S, Bebbington P, Jenkins R, Brugha T (eds). *Mental Health and Wellbeing in England: Adult psychiatric morbidity survey 2014.* Leeds: NHS Digital, 2016.
9. Scowcroft E. *Samaritans Suicide Statistics Report 2017.* Surrey: Samaritans, 2017, p. 6.
10. Ministry of Justice. *The Mental Capacity Act 2005 Code of Practice 2007.* London: The Stationery Office, 2005. Available from: https://www.gov.uk/government/publications/mental-capacity-act-code-of-practice.
11. Royal College of Psychiatrists. *Anxiety, Panic and Phobias – information leaflet.* London: RCPsychs, 2018.
12. Royal College of Psychiatrists. *Depression: Key facts.* London: RCPsychs, 2015.
13. National Institute for Health and Care Excellence. *Clinical Practice Guideline No 23: self-harm.* The British Psychological Society & the Royal College of Psychiatrists. London: NICE, 2004.
14. Mental Health First Aid. *Self-injury First Aid Guideline.* Melbourne: MHFA, 2014.
15. Mental Health First Aid. *Suicide First Aid Guideline.* Melbourne: MHFA, 2014.
16. Royal College of Psychiatrists. *Bi-Polar Disorder – information leaflet.* London: RCPsychs, 2015.
17. Royal College of Psychiatrists. *Psychosis – information leaflet.* London: RCPsychs, 2017.
18. Mental Health First Aid. *Psychosis First Aid Guideline.* Melbourne: MHFA, 2008.
19. Royal College of Psychiatrists. *Personality Disorder.* London: RCPsychs, 2018.
20. Royal College of Psychiatrists. *Personality Disorder: Key facts.* London: RCPsychs, 2016.
21. eLearning for Health. *Personality Disorder.* Leeds: Health Education England, 2016. Available from: http://portal.e-lfh.org.uk/Component/Details/421730.
22. Alzheimers Research UK. *Dementia Symptoms.* Cambridge: Alzheimers Research UK, 2018. Available from: https://www.alzheimersresearchuk.org/about-dementia/types-of-dementia/frontotemporal-dementia/symptoms/.
23. National Institute for Health and Care Excellence. *Dementia: Assessment, management and support for people living with dementia and their carers* [NG97]. London: NICE, 2018.
24. Alzheimers Research UK. *Frontotemporal Dementia.* Cambridge: Alzheimers Research UK, 2018. Available from: https://www.alzheimersresearchuk.org/about-dementia/types-of-dementia/frontotemporal-dementia/symptoms/.
25. PAR Inc. *Mini-Mental State Examination.* Florida: PAR Inc, 2009. Available from: https://www.parinc.com/products/pkey/237.

Mental Capacity Act 2005

1. Introduction

The Mental Capacity Act 2005 (MCA) was implemented in England and Wales to provide protection and powers to individuals aged 16 years and over who may lack capacity to make some (or all) decisions for themselves. It is also for people working with, or caring for them. It applies to public and private locations.

2. What is the MCA?

The MCA empowers individuals to make their own decisions where possible and protects the rights of those who lack capacity. Where an individual lacks capacity to make a specific decision at a particular time, the MCA provides a legal framework for others to act and make that decision on their behalf, in their best interest. This include decisions about their care and/or treatment.

3. What is Mental Capacity?

'Capacity' is "the ability of an individual to make decisions regarding specific elements of their life" (MCA, 2005) and it is crucial within the pre-hospital emergency care environment since everything done to/for a conscious patient requires their consent. Patients must have mental capacity in order to give (or withhold) consent and, apart from situations where the Mental Health Act 1983 (MHA) applies, mental capacity is central to determining whether treatment and care can be given to someone who refuses.

For the person's wishes to be overridden there must be evidence that some impairment or disturbance of mental functioning exists, rendering the person unable to make an informed decision at the time it needs to be made. In simple terms 'capacity' is the ability to a make a decision at the time it needs to be made. In order to demonstrate capacity a person must be able to:

- Understand information relevant to the decision.
- Retain the information relevant to the decision.
- Consider all the factors involved i.e. weigh up the pros and cons.
- Communicate their decision.

4. Responsibilities Under the Act

Ambulance staff have a formal duty of regard to the Act and the Code of Practice; and every Ambulance Trust should as best practice have a formal process (i.e. a policy/protocol) for establishing the capacity of patients to give, or withhold, consent for assessment, treatment and/or being transported for further care, when required.

There must always be a presumption of capacity. In every situation, staff must assume that a person can make their own decision(s) unless it is found, on balance of probabilities, that they are unable to do so.

Doubts about mental capacity may arise for many reasons including the person's behaviour, circumstances, or concerns raised by someone else. Approximately two million people in England and Wales may lack capacity to make decisions for themselves because of:

- Dementia.
- Learning disabilities.
- Mental health problems.
- Stroke and brain injuries.
- Temporary impairment due to medication, intoxication, injury or illness.

Staff must always act in the best interests of any person who lacks capacity; but if the impairment is temporary you should consider if it is safe to wait until the patient regains capacity before acting on their behalf.

5. Legal Context

The MCA has five Key Principles which emphasise the fundamental concepts and core values of the Act. These must be considered and applied when you are working with, or providing care or treatment for, people who lack capacity.

They are:

Every adult has the right to make decisions and must be assumed to have capacity to do so unless it is proved otherwise.

- This means that you cannot assume that someone is unable to make a decision for themselves just because they have a particular medical/neurological condition, disability or because of their age.

People must be supported as much as possible to make a decision before anyone concludes that they cannot make their own decision.

- This means that you should make every effort to encourage and support the person to make the decision for themselves. If a lack of capacity is established, it is still important that you involve the person as much as possible in making decisions.

People have the right to make what others might regard as an unwise or eccentric decision.

- This means that capacity should not be confused with an assessment of the reasonableness of the person's decision. A person is entitled to make a decision which others might perceive to be unwise, eccentric or irrational, *as long as they have the capacity to do so.*
- However, it is important to note that when an apparently irrational decision is based on a misperception of reality (e.g. someone experiencing hallucinations/delusions/ disordered thinking), rather than a different *value system* to that held by the assessor, then the patient may not truly be able to understand. This would lead to doubts about their ability to make a decision and an assessment should be completed.

Apply best interest principles.

- This means that anything done for, or on behalf of, a person who lacks mental capacity must be done in their best interests.

Anything done for, or on behalf of, people without capacity should be the least restrictive of their basic rights and freedoms.

- This means that you must choose the option that interferes least with their rights and freedom of action. Make sure that whatever you do, you do not limit their freedom of movement any more than is absolutely necessary. Always use the least restrictive intervention.

6. Helping People to Make Decisions for Themselves

When a person in your care needs to make a decision you must start from the assumption that the person has capacity to make the decision in question (Principle 1). You should make every effort to encourage and support the person to make the decision themselves (Principle 2) and you will have to consider a number of factors to assist in the decision making process.

These could include:

- Does the person have all the relevant information needed to make the decision? If there is a choice, has all the information been given on the alternatives?
- Could the information be explained or presented in a way that is easier for the person to understand? Help should be given to communicate information wherever necessary. For example, a person with a learning disability might find it easier to communicate using pictures, photographs, or sign language.
- Are there particular times of the day when a person's understanding is better, or is there a particular place where they feel more at ease and able to make a decision? For example, if a person becomes drowsy soon after they have taken their medication this would not be a good time for them to make a decision.
- Can anyone else help or support the person to understand information or make a choice? For example, a relative, carer, friend or advocate.

When there is reason to believe that a person lacks capacity to make a decision you should consider the following:

- Has everything been done to help and support the person make the decision?
- Does the decision need to be made without delay?
- If not, is it possible to wait until the person does have the capacity to make the decision for him/herself?

7. Assessing Capacity

There are two questions to consider when you are assessing a person's capacity:

- Is there an impairment of, or disturbance in the functioning of, the person's mind or brain (this can be temporary or permanent)?
- Is the impairment or disturbance sufficient to cause the person to be unable to make that particular decision at the relevant time?

And, if so:

A person may be mentally incapable of making the decision in question either because of a long-term mental disability or because of temporary factors such as unconsciousness, confusion or the effects of fatigue, shock, pain, anxiety, anger, alcohol or drugs (or drug withdrawal). When possible, attempts should be made to enhance capacity by, for example, pain management.

Assessments of capacity are 'functional', and are related to the individual decision that needs to be made - at the time it needs to be made (i.e. can the person complete the functions required to make the decision, thus demonstrating they have capacity?). The more serious or complex the decision, the greater the level of capacity required. If an adult is mentally capable of making the decision, then his or her decision about whether to receive treatment or care must be respected; even if a refusal may risk permanent injury to that person's health or even lead to premature death (unless he or she is mentally disordered and can be treated under the MHA). Refusals of treatment can vary in importance. Some may involve a risk to life or of irreparable damage to health; others may not. What matters is whether, at the time in question, the patient has capacity to make that decision.

When consent is refused by a competent adult the least you should do is:

- Respect the patient's refusal as much as you would their consent.
- Make sure that the patient is fully informed of the implications of refusal.
- Involve other members of the health care team (as appropriate).
- Ensure this is clearly and fully documented in the patient's records.

Local policy may require additional elements.
If there is uncertainty as to the consequences of the act of self-harm, then it should be assumed that the consequences will be serious.

When an individual is reasonably believed to lack capacity to make the decision required, ambulance staff have a legal duty to act in that person's best interests – unless a valid and applicable Advance Decision to Refuse Treatment (ADRT) is in place.

Mental Capacity Act 2005

The following flowchart outlines the assessment process. Assessors must be able to show how their assessment was completed if required later on and details must be included in the patient's clinical record.

Remember that an unwise decision made by a person does not itself indicate a lack of capacity. Most people will be able to make most decisions, even when they have a diagnosis that may seem to imply that they cannot. This is a general principle that cannot be over-emphasised. The more complex the decision is, the greater the level of capacity required to make it.

ALCOHOL

When determining if there is an impairment of the mind or brain, the consumption of alcohol is often a complicating factor. This does not necessarily mean that the patient is not aware of their behaviour, or aware of the decisions they make, but it may mean that they are less aware/concerned about the consequences than they would otherwise be. Judging capacity in such circumstances is difficult and subjective, but the patient's safety is paramount, so consideration should be given to balancing the risk of getting the determination of capacity wrong against the clinical risk of non-intervention.

SELF HARM

The NICE Clinical Guideline 16 'Factors that can affect capacity' states:

"If the mental capacity of a person who has self-harmed has been impaired by the effects of alcohol or drugs, or by that person's emotional distress, staff must be satisfied that these temporary factors are operating to such a degree that the assumption of mental capacity is overridden. In such a case, where incapacity is temporary, staff should decide whether it is safe to defer treatment decisions until capacity is regained.

If a person appears to be calm but refuses potentially life-saving treatment, or expresses the wish to die by suicide, the assumption of capacity could be rebutted by evidence that the person does not truly comprehend the consequences of his or her decision, that the person is acting under the undue influence of another, that the person's emotional distress associated with the stated reason for wishing to be dead is impairing his or her judgement, or that the person's behaviour shows that he or she is deeply ambivalent about the decision (for example if the person initially sought help for the effects of the self-harm)."

Once again, careful consideration should be given to balancing the risk of getting the determination

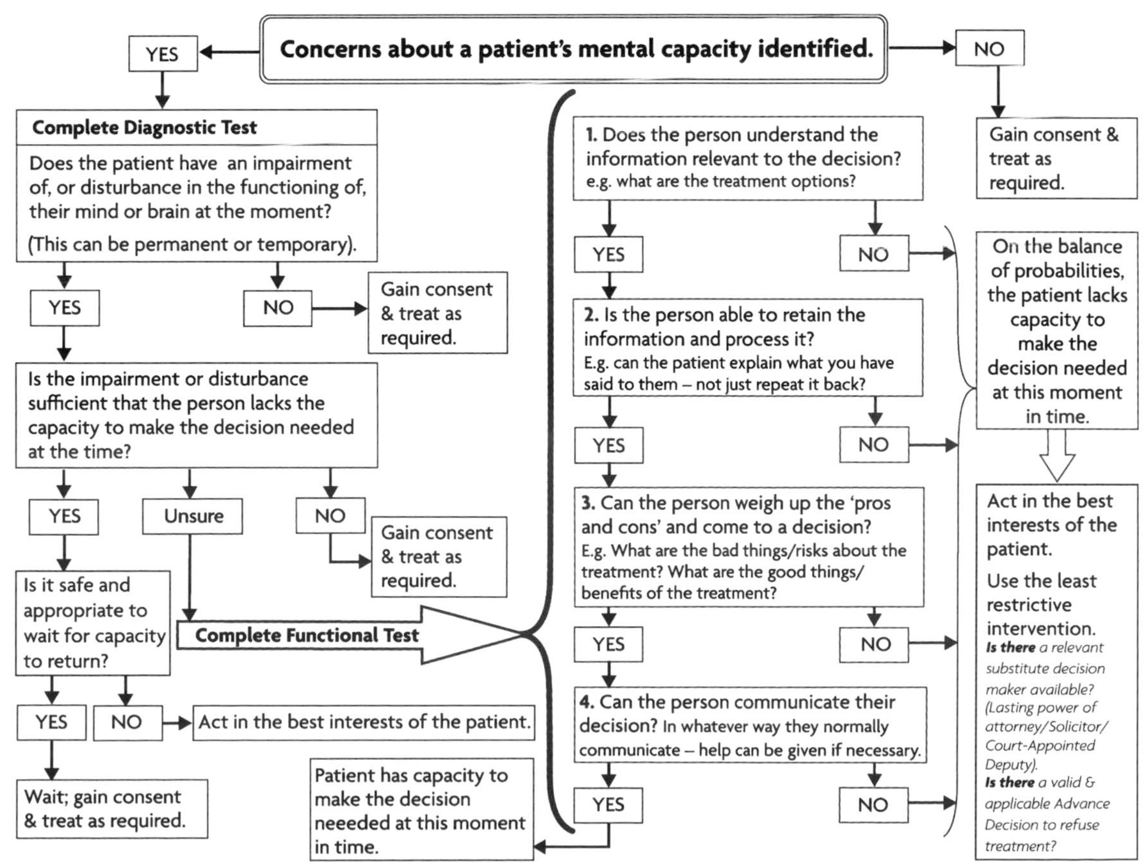

Figure 3.30 – Flow chart outlining MCA assessment for ambulance staff.

Reproduced with permission of S Putman.

of capacity wrong against the clinical risk of non-intervention.

Section 5 of the MCA Code of Practice (CoP) outlines specific actions taken by ambulance staff (and others) which will be protected from liability and includes the following:

- Carrying out diagnostic examinations and tests (to identify an illness, condition or other problem).
- Providing professional medical, dental and similar treatment.
- Giving medication.
- Taking someone to hospital for assessment or treatment.
- Providing nursing care (whether in hospital or the community).
- Carrying out any other necessary medical procedures (e.g. taking a blood sample) or therapies (e.g. physiotherapy or chiropody).
- Providing care in an emergency.

8. Best Interests

If a person has been assessed as lacking capacity then any action taken, or any decision made for - or on behalf of - that person, must be made in their best interests (Principle 4).

'Best Interest Assessors' (BIA) are appointed to assist making complex decisions for those who are unable to do so for themselves (e.g. when deciding on long term treatment for a medical condition, or on where to live).

There is a significant difference between making a "best interest" decision involving a BIA and making a decision which is in the best interest of the patient in an emergency. BIAs are required to consider a wide range of elements when making such a decision on someone else's behalf. In emergencies, where there is limited or no information available, it will often be in a patient's best interests for urgent treatment to be provided without delay.

Key factors which you must consider when working out what is in the best interests of a person who lacks capacity (whenever possible) include:

Identify all relevant circumstances.

Try to identify all the things that the person would take into account if they were making the decision or acting for themselves.

Find out the person's views.

Try to find out the views of the person who lacks capacity, including:

- Their past and present wishes and feelings – these may have been expressed verbally, in writing or through behaviour or habits (e.g.an ADRT).
- Any beliefs and values (e.g. religious, cultural, moral or political) that would be likely to influence the decision in question.
- Any other factors the person themselves would be likely to consider if they were making the decision or acting for themselves.

Relatives/friends/carers may be able to assist with this.

Avoid discrimination.

- Do not make assumptions about someone's best interests simply on the basis of the person's age, appearance, condition or behaviour.

Assess whether the person might regain capacity.

- Consider whether the person is likely to regain capacity. (If so, can the decision wait until then? It may be that the person lacks capacity to make a decision to accept initial treatment but, having received that treatment, regains capacity to refuse further treatment/intervention (including transport to hospital).

If the decision concerns life-sustaining treatment.

- This should not be motivated in any way by a desire to bring about the person's death.
- Always check for an advance decision to refuse treatment – if the person has previously made arrangements for withholding life sustaining treatment (when they had capacity to do so) this should be recorded in an ADRT. If a **valid and applicable** ADRT is found, it must be respected and treatment withheld.

Consult others.

- As far as possible the decision maker must consult other people (e.g. family, friends, carers, Lasting Power of Attorney) if it is appropriate to do so, and take into account their views as to what would be in the best interests of the patient lacking capacity.

Avoid restricting the person's rights.

- Use the least restrictive intervention.

Take all of this into account.

- Whenever possible, weigh up all of these factors in order to work out what is in the person's best interests.

9. Record Keeping

Decision-makers should ensure that where a capacity assessment is undertaken, this is recorded in the individual's care and treatment record in line with local policy. If the person was restrained the following should also be recorded:

- Why restraint was required.
- How the person was restrained.
- Who was involved?
- How long was restraint required?

It is recognised that it may not be possible to complete full details in an emergency situation but do remember that it is not sufficient to say a patient does not have capacity, without detailing how that decision was reached. A written record of the ambulance crew assessment and outcome must be made at the earliest opportunity.

10. Deprivation of Liberty/ Restraint

Deprivation of Liberty Safeguards (DoLS) exist to protect the human rights of people who lack capacity to consent to arrangements for their care or treatment, and who might need to be deprived of their liberty. E.g. a person who has dementia may need to have doors locked to prevent them walking away from where they live and getting lost, or coming to harm, as a result.

Deprivation of liberty without lawful justification is prohibited under Article 5 of the European Convention on Human Rights. There is a distinction between restraining or *restricting* an individual's movements, and depriving that individual of their liberty.

Restraint is defined in Section 6 of the MCA as:

- the use, or threat, of force where an incapacitated person resists, and any restriction of liberty or movement, whether or not the person resists.

Restraint, or restrictions, on an incapacitate individual's liberty can be justified under the MCA provided:

- The person lacks capacity and restraint is in their best interest.
- Restraint is used to prevent harm to the person.
- It is proportionate to the seriousness of the harm.

The least restrictive method must be used for the shortest amount of time.

Any power to restrain a person as a result of the MCA does not interfere with any other existing powers of arrest for criminal offences or powers under the Mental Health Act 1983.

However, the distinctions between restraining or restricting an individual, and depriving them of their liberty, are not always easy to identify. For example, it is possible to 'deprive' someone of their liberty not just by physical confinement, but also by virtue of the level of control exercised over an individual's movements. It is important to note however, that DoLS are highly unlikely to be a required for conveying patients.

The concepts of restraint, restriction, and deprivation of liberty are best understood as existing on the same continuum; with deprivation of liberty involving a higher degree or intensity, of restrictions over that individual. Ultimately, the concept is one to be interpreted in view of the specific circumstances of that individual at the time.

In simple terms - any person who is subject to regular and recurrent restrictions of their liberty should be considered for DoLS. Under this process safeguards are put in place to keep the person safe, this includes regular review of the need for restriction. DoLS only apply to an individual at a stated location (address). If the person moves to another address (e.g. goes into hospital) then a new DoLS application will be required by the agency caring for them; DoLS authority will not be required during transit from one place to another.

11. Use of Restraint by Ambulance Staff

Ambulance staff are obliged under the MCA to act in the best interests of/for patients who lack capacity, even when the patient refuses treatment or is abusive, threatening or violent.

The MCA also protects carers from liability when "reasonable force" is required to ensure that patients lacking capacity receive care that is in their best interests; or to protect them from further harm. As stated previously, Section 6 of the Act defines restraint as the use or threat of force where an incapacitated person resists, and any restriction of liberty or movement, whether or not the person resists.

Ambulance staff have limited training in this aspect. Minimal restraint (i.e. reasonable force) can be used in cases where patients lack capacity, and there is no perceived risk of harm to the ambulance crew. If the behaviour of the patient exceeds what the crew can safely manage then assistance must be requested in line with local policy (this does not necessarily have to be police).

A Dynamic Risk Assessment should always be completed prior to the use of any form of restraint; recording decisions and actions in the Patient Clinical Record.

Ambulance staff should always monitor the physical well-being of the patient and should be familiar with the information elsewhere in this guidance pertaining to Acute Behavioural Disturbance, which may result after prolonged forcible restraint.

12. Transfer and Continuing Care of the Patient

Ambulance staff must complete a clinical record (in line with local policy) with the normal clinical information including, full details of the capacity assessment, risk factors, and - where relevant - actions agreed with others such as the transport method and a description of any restraint applied by either ambulance staff or others.

Consider if a pre-alert to the receiving hospital/unit is required, and complete if necessary.

Ambulance staff must provide a full clinical handover at hospital and a copy of the completed patient clinical record. Emergency Department (ED) staff must be informed that the patient has been brought to ED using the provisions of the MCA. ED staff may need to re-assess the patient's capacity to make a decision regarding staying for further care, assessment and/or treatment.

13. Other Mental Capacity Act Safeguards

The MCA includes other safeguards to protect vulnerable people who have reduced capacity, and those using the Act to care for them.

Briefly, these include (amongst others):

- **Lasting Power of Attorney (LPA)** – An individual can give another person the authority to make a decision on their behalf if/when they become unable to do so. This is achieved by establishing a Lasting Power of Attorney. Once activated, the LPA can make decisions that are as valid as one made by the person. There are two types – Health and Wellbeing and Property and Financial Affairs. The LPA should always act in the best interest of the person.
- **Advance Decisions to Refuse Treatment.**

Allow people to refuse treatment, providing that the decision to do so was made when the person had capacity.

To make a valid ADRT the person must:

- Be at least 18 years of age
- Have capacity to make the decision.
- Make a decision that is specific and able to be complied with (i.e. outline in detail what they want to refuse and the circumstances in which it can be refused).

The ADRT doesn't need to be in writing, unless it relates to life sustaining treatment – in which case it must be in writing and witnessed.

An ADRT is only valid and applicable when all of the conditions described are met, and the person lacks capacity to make the decision themselves.

If ambulance staff are not aware of an ADRTs existence, when caring for someone who lacks capacity, then they should continue to act in the best interest of the patient.

- **Court of Protection.**

Makes decisions on financial or welfare matters for people who can't make decisions at the time they need to be made, and have no one appropriate to do this for them. Most cases are heard by district judges and a senior judge but can sometimes be heard by High Court judges.

- **Court Deputies.**

People who are appointed by the Court of Protection to act on behalf a person with reduced capacity when there is no LPA. Court Deputies have similar powers to that of an LPA.

- **Independent Mental Capacity Advocates (IMCAs).**

IMCAs are a legal right for people over 16 who lack capacity and do not have an appropriate family member or friend to represent their views. An IMCA can be used to assist with decisions regarding serious medical treatment or a change of accommodation.

The position taken in this guideline is that staff of the ambulance services should refer to their employers any questions or concerns that they might have as regards gaining lawful consent from their patients, application of the relevant legislation (and associated codes of practice) that apply in the jurisdiction in which they work for assessing, caring for and treating apparently incapacitous persons.

Readers should be aware that there are different laws relating to capacity and consent, and different mental health primary and secondary legislation in England and Wales, Northern Ireland, and Scotland. This guideline cannot cover in detail any of that legislation, the associated codes of practice and governmental guidance. Therefore, this guideline provides a very brief overview of some facets of the process in England and Wales.

Bibliography

1. Department of Constitutional Affairs. *The Mental Capacity Act 2005*. London: The Stationery Office, 2005.
2. Parliament of the United Kingdom. *The Mental Health Act 1983 (amended 2007)*. London: The Stationery Office, 2007.
3. Department of Constitutional Affairs*Mental Capacity Act Code of Practice*. London: The Stationery Office, 2007.
4. Department of Health *Reference guide to consent for examination or treatment. Second edition*. London: The Stationery Office, 2009.
5. S Willis, R Dalrymple. *Fundamentals of Paramedic Practice: A Systems Approach*. Oxford: Wiley-Blackwell, 2015.
6. National Collaborating Centre for Mental Health. *Self-Harm: The Short-Term Physical and Psychological Management and Secondary Prevention of Self-Harm in Primary and Secondary Care*. Leicester: British Psychological Society, 2004.
7. Department of Health*Positive and Proactive Care: reducing the need for restrictive interventions*. London: The Stationery Office, 2014.
8. Ministry of Justice *The Human Rights Act 1998*. London: The Stationery Office, 1998.
9. Ministry of Justice *Mental Capacity Act 2005: Deprivation of liberty safeguards – Code of Practice to supplement the main Mental Capacity Act 2005 Code of Practice*. London: The Stationery Office, 2008.

Respiratory Illness in Children

1. Introduction

- Children should not be viewed simply as 'little adults'. The assessment and management of paediatric patients may include potential pitfalls for the unwary and inexperienced and present healthcare providers with significant challenges wherever the setting.
- There are many important differences between children and adults in their anatomy, their physiology and their immunity. There may also be differences in the types of illnesses they encounter, as well as the ways in which these conditions present, develop and progress.
- Children may have difficulties verbalising and communicating their condition, presenting an additional challenge to clinicians.

'Major' and 'minor' illnesses

- Before considering 'minor' illnesses in children, it is crucial to both appreciate and understand that 'major' childhood illnesses (including life-threatening conditions such as meningococcal disease) rarely present in extremis, but more commonly present with relatively innocent features that can easily be mistaken for minor illnesses.
- Children with advanced major illness (or significant injury) typically have deranged vital signs that are usually readily detected. Earlier in their illness, these children may well have had normal physiology and appeared relatively well. If they were assessed early in their illness, there is a risk they might be misdiagnosed with only a minor illness.

This guideline on childhood respiratory illnesses includes:

1 Asthma.

2 Bronchiolitis.

3 Croup.

4 URTIs (tonsillitis, otitis media).

5 Pneumonia.

For the management of mild, moderate, severe and life-threatening asthma refer to **Asthma**.

2. Bronchiolitis

2.1 Introduction

Bronchiolitis is an acute, self-limiting respiratory infection that is usually caused by respiratory syncytial virus (RSV) and occurs predominantly in the autumn and winter months. It is characterised by inflammation of the bronchioles.

It is more prevalent during the winter months, peaking over a 6-8 week period, and is the most common lower respiratory tract infection during the first year of life.

Most children will recover without intervention. However, some may have difficulty breathing and need more input, especially very young babies.

2.2 Assessment

Bronchiolitis is commonly preceded by coryzal prodrome (upper respiratory infection, characterised by a non-specific cough, rhinorrhea, and fever) for 1 to 3 days.

- Clinical presentation: a coryzal baby (peak age 2–5 months) with their first wheezy episode.
- Irregular breathing and apnoeas are frequently reported.
- During the first 72 hours, bronchiolitic infants may deteriorate clinically, before symptomatic improvements are seen.
- The baby's parents and siblings often have concurrent respiratory illnesses and may report sore throats or dry coughs.

Signs and symptoms
↓ oxygen saturations
↑ respiratory rate
recession
fine, bilateral inspiratory crackles
high-pitched expiratory wheezes
low grade fever
rhinorrhoea (runny nose)
cough
poor Feeding
vomiting
pyrexia
apnoea
cyanosis

- Consider bronchiolitis as the provisional diagnosis if **all** of the following symptoms are present:
  - persistent cough
  - either tachypnoea or chest recession (or both)
  - either wheeze or crackles on chest auscultation (or both).
- When diagnosing bronchiolitis, take into account that the following symptoms are common in children with this disease:
  - fever (in around 30% of cases, usually of less than 39°C)
  - poor feeding (typically after 3 to 5 days of illness)
  - young infants may present with apnoea without other clinical signs.
- **NB** Consider a diagnosis of pneumonia if the child has high fever (over 39°C) and/or persistently focal crackles.

2.3 Management

- Give oxygen supplementation to children with bronchiolitis if their oxygen saturation is persistently less than 94%.
- Treatments aim to provide respiratory support and support feeding/hydration.
- Antivirals, antibiotics, steroids, nebulisers, physiotherapy, steam treatments, nasal decongestants, homeopathy and complementary therapies have not been shown to be effective.
- Acute bronchiolitis lasts approximately two weeks from its onset, but can last up to four weeks.
- Ongoing cough and persisting wheeze are not uncommon after the initial illness has passed but should prompt further medical assessment.
- Generally, management of bronchiolitis will be conservative with oxygen being the only drug administered in the pre-hospital environment. In most cases, medication is not needed to manage bronchiolitis because it is usually self-limiting (i.e., it settles without the need for treatment).
- Helping parents and carers to understand this can increase their confidence in caring for their child at home. It can also help them understand why medicines are not being administered en route to hospital.
- Clinicians should be aware of the increased need for hospital admission in infants fulfilling the following criteria:
  - pre-existing lung disease, congenital heart disease, neuromuscular weakness, immunodeficiency
  - age under 3 months
  - prematurity
  - family anxiety
  - re-attendance or re-contact for the same presentation
  - duration of illness is less than 3 days.
- Premature babies, those with chronic lung disease, children with congenital heart disease, cystic fibrosis, congenital or acquired immune deficiency (HIV), and those either aged <2 months or having apnoeas are at highest risk and must be transferred to further care.
- Previously well babies with diminished feeding, irregular breathing, hypoxia (O_2 saturations <94% on air), tachypnoea or tachycardia should also be transferred to further care where they will receive respiratory support and help with feeding/hydration.
- If the patient is managed on scene, robust safety netting advice should be provided on how to recognise developing red flag symptoms such as:
  - worsening work of breathing such as grunting, nasal flaring, marked chest recession
  - fluid intake is 50–75% of normal or no wet nappy for 12 hours
  - apnoea or cyanosis
  - exhaustion (e.g., not responding normally to social cues; wakes only with prolonged stimulation).
- Safety netting advice should also include:
  - advice that people should not smoke in the child's home because it increases the risk of more severe symptoms in bronchiolitis
  - instructions on how to get immediate help from an appropriate professional should any red flag symptoms develop.

3. Croup

3.1 Introduction

- Croup is a common, acute, respiratory illness of gradual onset, characterised by stridor that typically is mild and self-limiting.
- Viral infections can spread to the larynx and trachea, causing inflammation and therefore compromise of the airway in severe cases.
- Croup is less common in older children who are more likely to have epiglottis, a more serious condition, and need to be admitted.

3.2 Incidence

- Croup mostly affects children between the ages of 6 months and 3 years, presenting most commonly in the second year of life.[11] However, children up to 15 years of age may be affected.
- It can occur all year round but peaks are seen in both spring and autumn.

3.3 Pathophysiology

- Croup results from viral infections, most commonly parainfluenza, but also RSV, influenza A and B, as well as *Mycoplasma pneumoniae*.
- Stridor, hoarseness and a barking 'seal-like' cough result from inflammation and narrowing around the subglottic region of larynx. (This is the narrowest point of the paediatric airway).

NB Stridor is also seen in epiglottitis, bacterial tracheitis, retropharyngeal abscesses, foreign body ingestion, anaphylaxis and angio-oedema, blunt trauma, glandular fever, hot gases inhalation and diphtheria – all children with any of these conditions should be transferred to further care.

3.4 Assessment

- Croup commonly has a gradual onset. Initial symptoms include a mild fever and a runny nose. This progresses to a sore throat and a barking cough, typical of the condition. Young children have smaller air passages and inflammation in the voice box leads to a narrowing of the gap between the vocal cords.

- Croup develops over a period of one or two days; the severity varies over that period but it is normally worse on the second night of the cough.
- Stridor associated with croup can also be caused by other conditions. Clinicians should consider differential diagnoses, such as:
  - epiglottitis
  - bacterial tracheitis
  - foreign bodies
  - anaphylaxis
  - angio-oedema
  - glandular fever
  - blunt trauma
  - retropharyngeal abscesses
  - inhalation of hot gases
  - diphtheria.
- All children with these conditions should be transferred to further care.
- The Modified Taussig Score is a simple clinical tool that can be used to determine the severity of croup and the most appropriate way to manage the patient. Score the stridor and recession elements, and then add the scores together. Mild croup is defined as a score of 1-2, moderate 3-4 and severe/life-threatening 5-6 (Table 3.85).
- The child with croup may have mild clinical features in keeping with a simple, upper respiratory tract infection although they can present with more worrying features including respiratory distress, respiratory failure and respiratory arrest.
- The features of respiratory distress – increased respiration rate, increased work of breathing, recession, nasal flaring, grunting, use of accessory muscles and stridor – are described in the **medical emergencies in children** guideline.

TABLE 3.85 – Modified Taussig Croup Score

		Score Mild: 1–2; Moderate: 3–4; Severe: 5–6
Stridor	None	0
	Only on crying, exertion	1
	At rest	2
	Severe (biphasic)	3
Recession	None	0
	Only on crying, exertion	1
	At rest	2
	Severe (biphasic)	3

3.5 Management

- Keep the child in a position of comfort, sat upright and supported on a parent's lap – children often 'know' how to maintain their own airways in an optimal position (they often adopt a so-called 'tripod' posture).
- A calm approach is to be encouraged at all times. Any intervention likely to upset the child – examining their ears, nose or throat, blood sugar measurement, cannulation and even nebulisation (see below) – must be avoided, as distressing procedures can precipitate acute deterioration and complete airway obstruction. This is of particular importance in the pre-hospital environment where skills for expert airway intervention are not readily available.
- Steroids are the mainstay of treatment – usually oral dexamethasone (nebulised budesonide may be used as an alternative but may distress the child, adversely worsening their symptoms) – and work by relieving subglottic inflammation.
- Children with mild, moderate or severe croup (Modified Taussig Score >1), may benefit from early steroid treatment.
- Oral dexamethasone (refer to **dexamethasone** guideline) is preferred to nebulised budesonide, as nebulisation frequently distresses small children, producing further airway narrowing.

3.6 Referral Pathway

As above, irrespective of whether steroids are given, all children with stridor must still be transferred to further care for subsequent observation, even if clinical improvements are noted at home.

- All children under the age of 2 with croup must be conveyed to hospital
- All children with a respiratory rate above 40 breaths/min with croup must be conveyed to hospital.

If the patient is to be discharged on scene, it is important to give parents/guardians appropriate advice:

- Explain that croup is self-limiting and symptoms usually resolve within 48 hours, although occasionally they may last for up to a week. Resolution of croup symptoms is usually followed by symptoms of upper respiratory tract infection.
- Advise the use of paracetamol or ibuprofen to control fever and pain/distress.
  - do not over or under dress a child with fever
  - tepid sponging is not recommended
  - do not routinely give antipyretic drugs to a child with fever with the sole aim of reducing body temperature.
- Explain that cough medicines, decongestants, and short-acting beta-agonists are not effective. Croup is usually a viral illness and antibiotics are not needed.

- Ensure an adequate fluid intake.
- Do not advise humidified air (e.g. steam inhalation).
- Arrange for a clinician to review the child within a few hours, either by face-to-face consultation or by telephone. Advise parents to seek urgent medical advice if:
  - There is progression from mild to moderate airways obstruction, such as development of intermittent stridor at rest or increased effort of breathing (chest and suprasternal in-drawing), as the child may need to be observed in hospital.
  - If the child becomes toxic (pale, very high fever, tachycardic) as this may mean the child has an alternative diagnosis (e.g. bacterial tracheitis or epiglottitis).
- Advise the parents to call 999 or take the patient immediately to the emergency department if the child:
  - Becomes cyanosed.
  - Is unusually sleepy.
  - Is struggling to breathe and cannot be calmed down quickly.
  - Is restless, agitated or upset.
  - Or if stridor can be heard continually and recession is seen (the skin between the ribs is pulling in with every breath).
  - Is very pale, blue, or grey (includes blue lips) for more than a few seconds.
  - Is not responding.
  - Is having a lot of trouble breathing (e.g., the belly is sinking in while breathing, or the skin between the ribs or over the windpipe is pulling in with each breath; the nostrils may also be flaring in and out).
  - Wants to sit instead of lie down.
  - Cannot talk.
  - Drooling.
  - Is having trouble swallowing.

Ensure that there is a communication to the patient's registered GP to inform then about the episode, the outcomes reached and any treatment given.

4. Upper Respiratory Tract Infections (URTIs) e.g. tonsillitis (sore throat, acute pharyngitis, acute exudative tonsillitis), otitis media, etc.

4.1 Introduction

Upper respiratory tract infections (URTIs) are one of the commonest reasons for paediatric presentation, especially during the winter months.

4.2 Incidence

25% of all under five year olds will see their GPs each year for tonsillitis.

4.3 Assessment

- Children with URTIs frequently complain of:
  - sore throat
  - cough
  - fever
  - headache
  - earache
  - systemic illness
  - anorexia and lethargy.
- Physical examination may reveal:
  - cervical lymphadenopathy
  - offensive breath
  - inflamed, purulent tonsils.

Breathing may also be compromised by either stridor or respiratory distress. In these circumstances, avoid attempts to examine the throat (see croup guidance above) and transfer urgently to further care.

The child's hydration status should be estimated as fluid intake can be significantly decreased.

4.4 Management

URTIs are usually self-limiting. Parents should be offered simple advice about managing their child's symptoms (rest, extra fluids, analgesia, antipyretics etc) and informed about the likely duration of their child's illness (refer to Table 3.86).

Antibiotics are not prescribed routinely. Most URTIs are viral and do not respond to antibiotics. Bacteria (e.g. streptococci) also cause URTIs but even in these cases antibiotics are rarely needed; they don't improve the child's symptoms and they can often cause diarrhoea, vomiting and rashes.

GPs tend to use one of three antibiotic strategies:

1 No antibiotics are needed where the URTI is thought likely to be self-limiting.

2 Delayed antibiotics are useful when symptoms fail to improve or worsen.

TABLE 3.86 – Typical Duration of Acute Respiratory Illnesses

Condition	Duration
acute otitis media	4 days
acute sore throat/pharyngitis/ tonsillitis	1 week
common cold	1½ weeks
acute rhinosinusitis	2½ weeks
acute cough/bronchitis	3 weeks

3 Immediate antibiotic prescriptions are reserved for the most severe cases, including:

- Under twos with acute bilateral otitis media.
- Children with acute otitis media and otorrhoea (ear discharge).
- Children with acute streptococcal URTIs (no cough but fever, pustular tonsils and tender lymph nodes).

Antibiotics are also prescribed for children who are:

- Systemically very unwell.
- At high risk of serious complications because of pre-existing illnesses (heart, lung, renal, liver or neuromuscular disease, diabetes, cystic fibrosis, prematurity, immunosuppression or previous hospitalisations).

Over-the-counter cough and cold preparations often contain sedatives and antihistamines that are dangerous if taken accidentally by small children in overdose. As a result, these medicines are no longer available for children aged two years or under. Children in this age group with colds and fever should now only be offered paracetamol or ibuprofen to manage their temperature, if needed.

Simple cough syrups containing glycerol, and honey and lemon may still be given, as well as vapour rubs and inhalant decongestants (see individual labelling).

4.5 Referral pathway

Hospital admission may also be indicated when:

- There is diminished fluid intake (e.g. young child with severe tonsillitis and teenagers with glandular fever).
- Where concerns regarding the diagnosis persist (**NB** early meningococcal disease is frequently misdiagnosed as an URTI in small children – where this diagnosis cannot be excluded, arrangements for an urgent medical opinion should be made). Refer to **Febrile Illness in Children**.
- Children with 'muffled' voices – they sound as if they have something hot in their mouths. These children must be transferred to further care to exclude quinsy (peritonsillar abscess).
- Tenderness behind the ear (over their mastoid process) in a child with otitis media, whose ear may/may not be starting to 'stick out' suggests mastoiditis (a dangerous infection of the bone around the ear) and must be transferred to further care.

4.6 Management in the community

As when managing the febrile child, if a decision not to transfer a child to further care has been reached, a clinically justifiable reason should be present and properly documented. Refer to **febrile illness in children** guideline.

'Safety netting,' with written advice, should again be encouraged and follow-up arrangements should be provided.

Where doubts persist seek senior advice or review.

5. Pneumonia (lower respiratory tract infections, 'chest infections')

Children with pneumonia are likely to have the following signs and symptoms:

- Fever.
- Cough.
- Tachypnoea.
  - RR > 60 breaths/min, age 0–5 months
  - RR > 50 breaths/min, age 6–12 months
  - RR > 40 breaths/min, age > 12 months
- Nasal flaring.
- Chest indrawing.
- Oxygen saturations <95%.
- Crackles in the chest.
- Cyanosis.

Such children are likely to require antibiotics and additional oxygen and should be seen by either their GP or a paediatrician.

Table 3.87 indicates severity of disease by age of the patient. This should be used to determine whether urgent referral in the community is appropriate or transfer to the Emergency Department. Children with severe symptoms (oxygen saturations <92% or where auscultation demonstrates absent breath sounds or percussion presents as dull) should be transferred to the Emergency Department.

Respiratory Illness in Children

TABLE 3.87 – Severity Assessment		
	Mild to moderate	**Severe**
Infants	Temperature <38.5°C Respiratory rate <50 breaths/min Mild recession Taking full feeds	Temperature >38.5°C Respiratory rate >70 breaths/min Moderate to severe recession Nasal flaring Cyanosis Intermittent apnoea Grunting respiration Not feeding Tachycardia* Capillary refill time ≥2s
Older children	Temperature <38.5°C Respiratory rate <50 breaths/min Mild breathlessness No vomiting	Temperature >38.5°C Respiratory rate >50 breaths/min Severe difficulty in breathing Nasal flaring Cyanosis Grunting respiration Signs of dehydration Tachycardia* Capillary refill time ≥2s
*Values To Define Tachycardia Vary With Age And With Temperature		

KEY POINTS!

Respiratory Illness

- **Childhood respiratory illnesses are common and usually self-limiting.**
- **Antibiotics are rarely indicated.**
- **Children with underlying conditions (e.g. prematurity, chronic lung disease, congenital heart disease, cystic fibrosis, congenital or acquired immune deficiency (HIV), cerebral palsy), are especially vulnerable and must be seen either by their GP or a paediatrician in hospital.**
- **Tachypnoea is a feature in all respiratory illnesses.**
- **Respiratory distress causes increased respiratory rate, increased work of breathing, recession, nasal flaring, grunting, use of accessory muscles and stridor.**
- **Exhaustion suggests respiratory failure and respiratory arrest may rapidly follow.**
- **Stridor can progress rapidly to complete upper airway obstruction and respiratory arrest.**
- **Approach a child with stridor calmly and gently. Sit them upright, in a position of comfort and avoid painful/distressing procedures.**
- **Transfer all children with stridor for further medical assessment and observation.**
- **Steroids (dexamethasone) are frequently used to treat croup.**
- **Children with pneumonia require antibiotics and possibly oxygen therapy. They should be seen by either their GP or a paediatrician.**
- **Whilst URTIs are very common, early meningococcal disease can easily be misdiagnosed as an URTI. (When unable to exclude this diagnosis, make arrangements for an urgent second opinion.)**
- **Provide a 'safety net' (with written information) for all children with respiratory illness not transferred to hospital.**
- **If uncertain, seek advice from either the child's GP or the out-of-hours doctor.**

Respiratory Illness in Children

Bibliography

1. Godden CW, Campbell MJ, Hussey M, Cogswell JJ. Double blind placebo controlled trial of nebulised budesonide for croup. *Archives of Disease in Childhood* 1997, 76(2): 155–8.
2. Russell KF, Liang Y, O'Gorman K, Johnson DW, Klassen TP. Glucocorticoids for croup. *Cochrane Database of Systematic Reviews* 2011(1): CD001955.
3. Scottish Intercollegiate Guidelines Network. *Management of Sore Throat and Indications for Tonsillectomy* (Guideline 117). Edinburgh: SIGN, 2010. Available from: https://www.sign.ac.uk/sign-117-management-of-sore-throat-and-indications-for-tonsillectomy.html.
4. Sparrow A, Geelhoed G. Prednisolone versus dexamethasone in croup: a randomised equivalence trial. *Archives of Disease in Childhood* 2006, 91(7): 580–3.
5. Baumer JH. Glucocorticoid treatment in croup. *Archives of Disease in Childhood Education and Practice Edition* 2006, 91(2): ep58–60.
6. Sandell JM, Charman SC. Can age-based estimates of weight be safely used when resuscitating children? *Emergency Medicine Journal* 2009, 26(1): 43–7.
7. Taussig LM, Castro O, Beaudry PH, Fox WW, Bureau M. Treatment of laryngotracheobronchitis (croup): use of intermittent positive-pressure breathing and racemic epinephrine. *American Journal of Diseases of Children* 1975, 129(7): 790–3.
8. Centre for Clinical Practice at the National Institute for Health and Clinical Excellence. *Acutely Ill Patients in Hospital: Recognition of and response to acute illness in adults in hospital* (CG50). London: NICE, 2007. Available from: https://www.nice.org.uk/guidance/cg50.
9. National Institute for Health and Clinical Excellence. *Respiratory Tract Infections – Antibiotic Prescribing: Prescribing of antibiotics for self-limiting respiratory tract infections in adults and children in primary care* (CG 69). London: NICE, 2008. Available from: https://www.nice.org.uk/guidance/cg69.
10. National Institute for Health and Care Excellence. *Bronchiolitis in children: diagnosis and management.* Available from: https://www.nice.org.uk/guidance/ng9, 2015.
11. National Institute for Health and Clinical Excellence. *Croup. NICE Clinical Knowledge Summaries* London: NICE, 2012. Available from: https://cks.nice.org.uk.

Sickle Cell Crisis

1. Introduction

- Sickle cell disease is a hereditary condition affecting the haemoglobin contained within red blood cells.
- A previous history of sickle cell disease and sickle cell crisis will be present in most cases, with the patient almost always being aware of their condition.
- The signs and symptoms include (**any of those listed below may apply**):
  - severe pain, most commonly in the long bones and/or joints of the arms and legs, but also in the back and abdomen
  - high temperature
  - difficulty in breathing
  - Reduced oxygen (O_2) saturation
  - Cough
  - Chest pain
  - pallor
  - tiredness/weakness
  - dehydration
  - headache
  - priapism.

2. Incidence

- There are different types of sickle cell disease found mainly in people of African or Afro-Caribbean origin, but these can also affect people of Mediterranean, Middle Eastern and Asian origin. In the United Kingdom it is estimated that 15,000 adults and children suffer from sickle cell disease with 1 in every 2,000 babies born with the condition.

3. Severity and Outcome

- These painful crises can result in damage to the patient's lungs, kidneys, liver, bones, other organs and tissues. The recurrent nature of these acute episodes is the most disabling feature of sickle cell disease, and many chronic problems can result, including leg ulcers, blindness and stroke.
- **Acute chest syndrome** is the leading cause of death amongst sickle cell patients. This is a common and potentially life-threatening complication of painful crises and is often precipitated by a chest infection. The patient becomes breathless, hypoxic and tachypnoeic/tachycardic over a short period of time. Chest pain is often present, and the hypoxia responds poorly to inhaled oxygen. Crackles are often present in the lung bases and will ascend rapidly to involve the whole lung fields in severe cases.
- Radiological changes follow late and patients may be critically ill with near normal radiology.
- If a chest crisis is suspected, treatment should be initiated with inhaled oxygen and intravenous fluids. In hospital, intravenous antibiotics and urgent exchange transfusion are likely to be instituted after discussion with the haematology team. Intensive care and mechanical ventilation may be required in some cases.
- Pulmonary embolus is an important differential diagnosis.

4. Pathophysiology

- The red cells of patients with sickle cell disease are prone to assuming a permanently sickled shape when exposed to a variety of factors including hypoxia, cold or dehydration. These cells are prone to mechanical damage, hence haemolytic anaemia in this group of patients. This can lead to occlusion of the microvasculature resulting in tissue hypoxia, pain and end organ damage.
- A crisis may follow as a result of an infection, during pregnancy, following surgery or a variety of other causes including physiological and psychological stress.

5. Assessment and Management

For the assessment and management of patients with sickle cell crisis refer to Table 3.88 or Figure 3.31.

Sickle Cell Crisis

TABLE 3.88 – ASSESSMENT and MANAGEMENT of: Sickle Cell Crisis

ASSESSMENT	MANAGEMENT
• Assess <C>ABCD	• If any of the following **TIME CRITICAL** features present: – major **<C>ABCD** problems, refer to **Medical Emergencies in Adults – Overview** and **Medical Emergencies in Children – Overview** – acute chest syndrome, then: • Start correcting **<C>ABCD** problems. • Undertake a **TIME CRITICAL** transfer to nearest receiving hospital. • Continue patient management en-route. • Provide an ATMIST information call.
• Ask the patient if they have an individualised treatment plan	• Be aware that the patient may have a treatment plan and follow this if it is available. • Patient's with long term conditions will often be able to guide their care. • Follow **Medical Emergencies in Adults – Overview** and **Medical Emergencies in Children – Overview** in addition to the specific management detailed below.
• Pulse	• Measure and record pulse rate.
• Respiratory rate	• Measure and record respiratory rate.
• Oxygen	• Administer supplemental oxygen to **ALL** patients including those with chronic sickle lung disease; oxygen helps to counter tissue hypoxia and reduce cell clumping. • Administer high levels of supplemental oxygen via an appropriate mask/nasal cannula until a reliable SpO_2 measurement is available; then adjust the oxygen flow to aim for target saturation within the range of 94–98%. Refer to **Oxygen**. **NB** It is safer to over-oxygenate until a reliable SpO_2 measurement is available.
• Blood glucose	• If appropriate, measure and record blood glucose for hypo/hyperglycaemia, refer to **Glycaemic Emergencies in Adults and Children**.
• Temperature	• Measure and record temperature.
• NEWS2	• These observations will enable you to calculate a NEWS2 Score, refer to **Sepsis**.
• ECG	• If required, monitor and record 12-Lead ECG. Assess for abnormality, refer to **Cardiac Rhythm Disturbance**.
• Blood pressure and fluids	• Patients with a sickle cell crisis will not have acute fluid loss but may present with dehydration if they have been ill for an extended period of time. • Measure and record blood pressure, if required administer fluids, refer to **Intravascular Fluid Therapy in Adults** and **Intravascular Fluid Therapy in Children**.

(continued)

Sickle Cell Crisis

TABLE 3.88 – ASSESSMENT and MANAGEMENT of: Sickle Cell Crisis *(continued)*	
• Pain management	• Where present, assess the **SOCRATES** of pain and record initial and subsequent pain scores. Offer **ALL** patients pain relief. • **Entonox** – administer initially but do not administer for extended periods, refer to **Entonox**. • **Opiate analgesia** – administer orally or subcutaneously rather than intravenously if possible (refer to **Morphine Sulfate**). The dose should be guided by the patient's individualised treatment plan if available, otherwise refer to **Pain Management in Adults** and **Pain Management in Children**.
• Conveyance to hospital	• Consider conveying direct to specialist unit where the patient is usually treated, as per local pathways. • Patients should not walk to the ambulance as this will exacerbate the effects of hypoxia in the tissues.
• Consider conveyance to hospital for patients with:	• A temperature >38°C as there is a risk of rapid deterioration. • Chest symptoms, as acute chest syndrome may develop quickly. • Unmanageable pain. • Severe vomiting/diarrhoea.
• Consider management in the community or referral to other services for:	• Adult patients who are well and have only mild or moderate pain and a temperature of <38°C. • Paediatric patients who are well, have only mild or moderate pain and do not have an increased temperature. Consider referral in line with local pathways. • Admission is not necessarily required if the source of infection is obvious (such as a viral illness) and can be managed in the community.
• Appropriate advice	• Make sure that patients are aware of chest symptoms and/or their parents/carers understand the importance of seeking urgent medical advice if their clinical condition deteriorates, especially if breathing becomes faster or more laboured. • Advice to be given includes: – Increase fluid intake, as dehydration will prolong a painful episode. – Avoid other factors that may trigger acute painful crisis, such as cold weather and excessive physical activity. – For pain management, use distraction techniques, such as games, computers, and television. • If the patient has no individualised treatment plan for pain, advise over the counter analgesia techniques, such as Paracetamol, Ibuprofen and Codeine. **NB** Avoid Ibuprofen if the patient has renal impairment. • Advise the patient and/or their parents/carer to seek urgent medical advice or go straight to hospital, if they: – Become unwell or develop a fever with a temperature greater than 38°C (or any increased temperature in a child). – Develop acute chest syndrome symptoms, such as breathlessness. – Have severe vomiting or diarrhoea, due to the risk of dehydration.
• Documentation	• Complete documentation to include all clinical findings, advice from other clinicians, onward referral and worsening advice given.

Sickle Cell Crisis

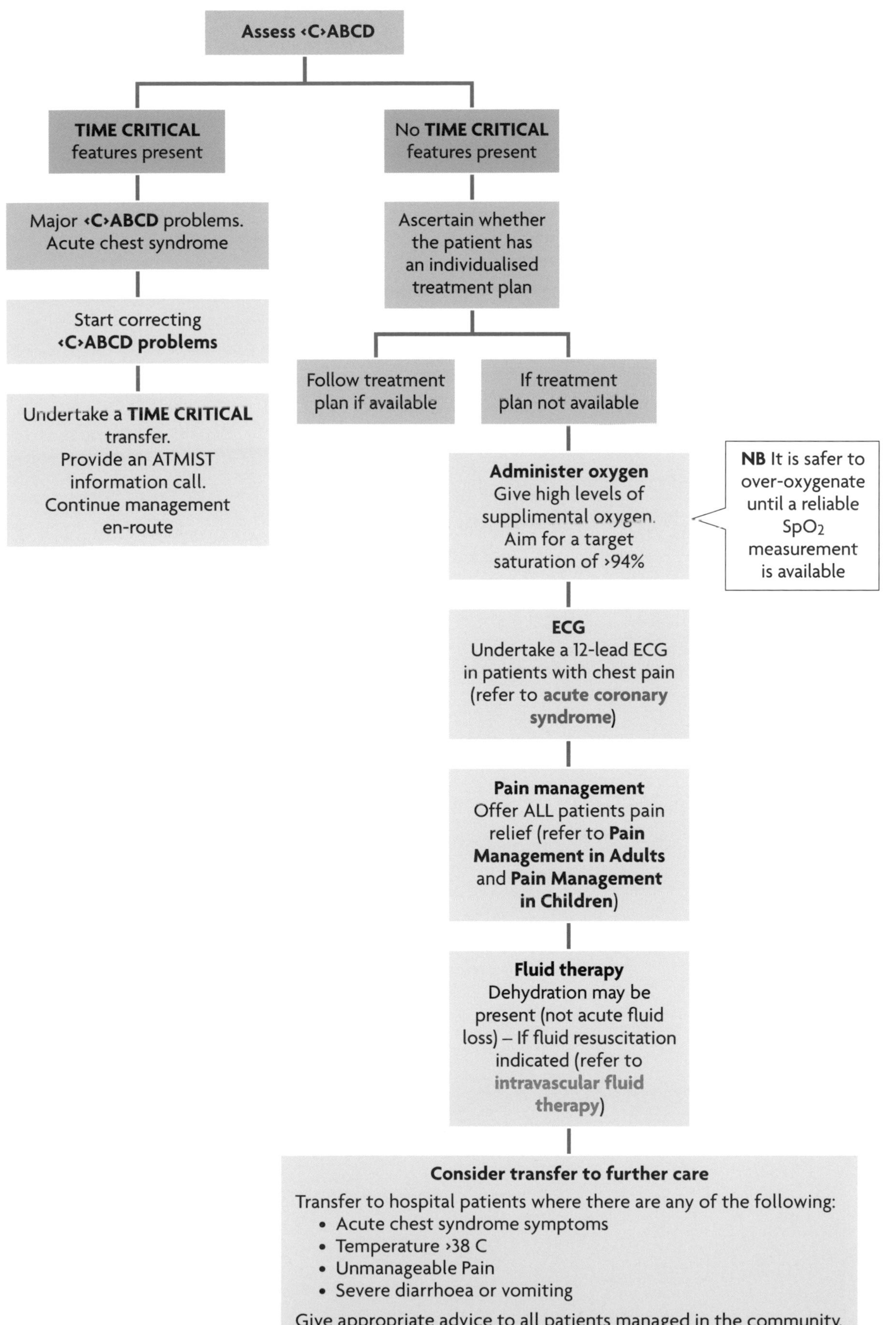

Assess ‹C›ABCD
TIME CRITICAL features present
No TIME CRITICAL features present
Major ‹C›ABCD problems. Acute chest syndrome
Start correcting ‹C›ABCD problems
Undertake a TIME CRITICAL transfer. Provide an ATMIST information call. Continue management en-route
Ascertain whether the patient has an individualised treatment plan
Follow treatment plan if available
If treatment plan not available
Administer oxygen Give high levels of supplimental oxygen. Aim for a target saturation of ›94%
NB It is safer to over-oxygenate until a reliable SpO2 measurement is available
ECG Undertake a 12-lead ECG in patients with chest pain (refer to acute coronary syndrome)
Pain management Offer ALL patients pain relief (refer to Pain Management in Adults and Pain Management in Children)
Fluid therapy Dehydration may be present (not acute fluid loss) – If fluid resuscitation indicated (refer to intravascular fluid therapy)
Consider transfer to further care
Transfer to hospital patients where there are any of the following:
• Acute chest syndrome symptoms
• Temperature ›38 C
• Unmanageable Pain
• Severe diarrhoea or vomiting
Give appropriate advice to all patients managed in the community.
Refer to Assessment and Management Table.

Figure 3.31 – Assessment and management algorithm for sickle cell crisis.

Sickle Cell Crisis

KEY POINTS!

Sickle Cell Crisis

- **Sickle cell disease is a hereditary condition affecting the haemoglobin contained within red blood cells; the cells are irregular in shape and occlude the microvasculature leading to tissue ischaemia.**
- **Sickle cell crises can result in damage to the lungs, kidneys, liver, bones, other organs and tissues.**
- **Sickle cell crises can be very painful and patients should be offered pain relief.**
- **In sickle cell crisis and acute chest syndrome, aim for an oxygen saturation of 94–98% or the saturation level that is usual for the individual patient.**
- **Patients with sickle cell disease can be dangerously unwell but in no pain (e.g. aplastic crisis, stroke, hepatic sequestration, PE, etc).**
- **Acute chest syndrome is a leading cause of death amongst sickle cell patients and is characterised by hypoxia and tachypnoea.**

Bibliography

1. Johnson AG. *Report of a Working Party of the Standing Medical Advisory Committee on Sickle Cell, Thalassaemia and other Haemoglobinopathies: Policy in confidence*. London: HMSO, 1993.
2. Maxwell K, Streetly A, Bevan D. Experiences of hospital care and treatment-seeking behavior for pain from sickle cell disease: qualitative study. *Western Journal of Medicine* 1999, 171(5–6): 306–13.
3. Vichinsky EP, Neumayr LD, Earles AN, Williams R, Lennette ET, Dean D, et al. Causes and outcomes of the acute chest syndrome in sickle cell disease. National Acute Chest Syndrome Study Group. *The New England Journal of Medicine* 2000, 342(25): 1855–65.
4. Yale SH, Nagib N, Guthrie T. Acute chest syndrome in sickle cell disease: crucial considerations in adolescents and adults. *Postgraduate Medicine* 2000, 107(1): 215–22.
5. National Institute for Health and Care Excellence. *Sickle cell disease* Clinical Knowledge Summaries. Available from: https://cks.nice.org.uk/sickle-cell-disease#!references/1381889, 2016.

Sepsis

1. Introduction

1.1 Terminology

- Suspected sepsis is not a specific illness but rather a syndrome encompassing a pathophysiology of which understanding is changing on a yearly basis. It is identified by a constellation of clinical signs and symptoms in a sick patient with an infection.
- The final diagnosis of sepsis is usually only confirmed at the end of an admission, when all the evidence becomes available.
- National Early Warning Scores (NEWS) are the best physiological scoring system for assessing sepsis and all causes of deterioration.
- A NEWS2 score greater than or equal to 5 highlights a sick patient who needs urgent clinical review; it does not represent a diagnosis, only a patient at significant risk.

1.2 Clinical Judgement

- Clinical judgement in determining what is or is not suspected sepsis is critical.
- Clinicians can rule out suspected sepsis in mimic conditions (e.g. asthma, diabetic ketoacidosis, mental health crisis), and rule in suspected sepsis when they are concerned.
- Over 70% of cases arise in the community, and ambulance clinicians are often the first point of contact for these patients.
- If left untreated, sepsis can lead to shock, multi-organ failure and death.
- Ambulance clinicians can help improve the outcomes by recognising sepsis early and providing a pre-alert and time critical transfer to the ED. Management should include (if indicated) high-flow oxygen, fluid resuscitation and benzylpenicillin if meningitis or meningococcal septicaemia is suspected.
- **Suspect sepsis in:**
  - anyone that presents with fever/feeling unwell
  - **and** NEWS2 greater than or equal to 5
  - **and/or** looks unwell with a history of infection.

2. Sepsis Definitions

2.1 Surviving Sepsis Campaign (2016)

- Sepsis is defined as life-threatening organ dysfunction caused by a dysregulated host response to infection.[1]

2.2 NICE (2016)

- Sepsis is a clinical syndrome caused by the body's immune and coagulation systems being switched on by an infection. Sepsis with shock is a life-threatening condition that is characterised by low blood pressure despite adequate fluid replacement, and organ dysfunction or failure.

3. Incidence

- There are an estimated 150,000 cases of sepsis each year in the UK with approximately 44,000 deaths attributed to sepsis. Half of ED sepsis patients arrive by ambulance.[2,3] Sepsis patients arriving at the ED by ambulance are 'sicker' than patients arriving by other means.[4,5,6] Of patients admitted to ITU from the ED, 80–90% will have arrived by ambulance.[7,8]

4. Severity and Outcome

- Sepsis has a high mortality rate and this can be as high as 50% in some patients.[9]
- Sepsis cases are responsible for 27% of all intensive care unit beds in England and Wales, and costs the NHS an estimated £2.5 billion per year.[10]
- Having a high index of suspicion, early recognition and rapid transport to hospital ensures early treatment with antibiotics and access to expert-led care.
- Survivors can suffer from long-term physical and psychological problems, resulting in significantly reduced quality of life.[1]
- Each hour of delay in giving antibiotics to a patient with septic shock has an increased mortality rate of 7.6%.[11] Treatment within one hour is considered best practice.

5. Pathophysiology

Sepsis is a multifaceted host response to the invasion of normally sterile tissue by pathogenic, or potentially pathogenic, micro-organisms.[1,12,13] The clinical manifestations of sepsis are highly variable between individuals due to age, underlying co-morbidities, the causative pathogen and medications.[1,14] Small amounts of cytokines are released into the circulation, leading to recruitment of inflammatory cells and an acute-phase response normally limited by anti-inflammatory mediators. In sepsis, there is a failure to control the inflammatory cascade, leading to a loss of capillary integrity, maldistribution of microvascular blood flow and stimulation of nitric oxide production, all leading towards organ injury and dysfunction.[12,13]

6. Risk Factors for Sepsis[10]

The following groups of patients are at higher risk of developing sepsis:

- The very young (under 1 year) and older people (over 75 years) or people who are very frail.
- People who have impaired immune systems because of illness or drugs, including those:
  - being treated for cancer with chemotherapy (refer to Section 7 below on neutropaenic sepsis)
  - who have impaired immune function (for example, people with diabetes, people who

have had a splenectomy, or people with sickle cell disease)
  - taking long-term steroids
  - taking immunosuppressant drugs to treat non-malignant disorders, such as rheumatoid arthritis.
- People who have had surgery, or other invasive procedures, in the past 6 weeks.
- People with any breach of skin integrity (for example, cuts, burns, blisters or skin infections).
- People who misuse drugs intravenously.
- People with indwelling lines or catheters.
- Pregnant women (refer to Section 8 below).

Take into account the following risk factors for sepsis in a newborn baby:

- History of maternal fever during labour or in the 24 hours before and after birth or maternal treatment with intravenous antibiotics for suspected infection.
- History of previous baby with sepsis during the newborn period.
- History of ruptured membranes before labour.
- Preterm birth following spontaneous labour (before 37 weeks gestation).
- Suspected or confirmed sepsis in another baby in the case of a multiple pregnancy.

7. Neutropaenic Sepsis

- Neutropaenic sepsis is a potentially fatal complication of cancer treatments, such as chemotherapy. Mortality rates as high as 21% have been reported in adults.[15] Patients can have neutropaenia as a result of the cancer therapy, which increases their risk of developing severe infections. Cancer patients can become neutropaenic, and not develop severe infections or sepsis. If a patient is neutropaenic and not showing signs of infection but is unwell, this should be taken seriously. Many patients develop this serious complication; therefore, always suspect neutropaenic sepsis in patients having cancer treatment who become unwell.
- Patients may have been given an advice line number to ring by their oncology service. Consider ringing advice lines such as this in line with your local procedures, as it may inform the appropriate destination or care pathway for the patient.
- Any of the following features could indicate that a neutropaenic patient has an infection and is at risk of sepsis:
  - tachypnoea
  - tachycardia
  - hypotension
  - temperature greater than 37.5°C
  - pleuritic chest pain
  - shivering episodes
  - flu-like symptoms
  - catheter site infections.
- Note that neutropaenic patients are unable to produce the pus normally associated with skin infections.
- A neutropaenic patient at risk of sepsis can look deceptively well and can deteriorate rapidly. A high index of suspicion is necessary, particularly if a patient who has recently undergone chemotherapy has an increased temperature. Patients who have received treatment within 6–8 weeks are at risk and at higher risk within the first 10 days after treatment.
- Neutropaenic sepsis is a medical emergency and all patients should be transported to the nearest emergency department or locally agreed pathway (oncology) with a hospital pre-alert.

8. Women and Pregnancy

- Have a very high index of suspicion for pregnant women who are unwell and have signs of infection.
- Take into account that women who are pregnant, have given birth or had a termination of pregnancy or miscarriage in the past 6 weeks are in a high-risk group for sepsis.[10] In particular, women who:
  - have impaired immune systems because of illness or drugs
  - have gestational diabetes, diabetes or other co-morbidities
  - needed invasive procedures (for example, caesarean section, forceps delivery, removal of retained products of conception)
  - had prolonged rupture of membranes
  - have or have been in close contact with people with group A streptococcal infection, for example, scarlet fever
  - have continued vaginal bleeding or an offensive vaginal discharge.
- Note that the baseline heart rate in pregnancy is 10–15 beats per minute more than normal and there may be a decrease in systolic and diastolic blood pressure by an average of 10–15 mmHg. Therefore, this should be taken into account when considering sepsis, and rapid transport to definitive care is the priority and not extended on-scene times.
- These physiological changes in pregnancy can mask signs of significant sepsis and shock. Therefore, a strong index of suspicion must be maintained and transfer to hospital considered when underlying sepsis is suspected during or after pregnancy.
- Refer to **Maternity Care** for other changes in pregnancy.

9. Assessment

- Assess **ABCD** (refer to **Medical Emergencies in Adults – Overview** and **Medical Emergencies in Children – Overview**).
- Take extra care if the patient cannot provide a reliable history.
- Consider sepsis in all patients with non-specific, non-localised presentations, for example feeling very unwell, with a low or high temperature.
- Think about potential infection causing general deterioration, particularly in older patients presenting with new confusion (delirium), falls or new immobility.
- Pay particular attention if concerns are expressed by the patient, or their family/carers, regarding changes in behaviour.
- Examine people with suspected sepsis for mottled or ashen appearance, cyanosis of the skin, lips or tongue, non-blanching rash of the skin, any breach of skin integrity (for example, cuts, burns or skin infections) or other rash indicating potential infection.
- If possible, try to identify a source of infection.
- Be highly suspicious of neutropaenic sepsis in patients having cancer treatment who become unwell.
- Use a structured screening tool and NEWS2 score to stratify risk if sepsis is suspected.

10. Signs of Infection

Look for signs of infection by conducting a systems assessment, with particular regard for the areas covered in Table 3.89.

11. Respiratory Rate

- An increased respiratory rate is an early indicator of illness, and can be one of the first clinical observations to become abnormal. Therefore, accurately measuring respiratory rate (e.g. over 30 seconds) is essential. The respiratory rate will increase due to a compensatory mechanism to reduce metabolic acidosis, a consequence of sepsis. Development of sepsis screening tools has demonstrated that respiration rate will be higher in septic patients compared to non-septic patients.[16,17]
- Respiratory rate is particularly important in children, and is a very early sign of illness. It is recommended that children presenting with signs and symptoms of an infection have an accurate respiration rate measured as it can be an important marker for serious illness.[18]
- Always refer to the relevant 'Page for Age' for vital signs of normal parameters.

12. Oxygen Saturation in Suspected Sepsis

- Take into account that if peripheral oxygen saturation is difficult to measure in a person with suspected sepsis, this may indicate poor peripheral circulation because of shock.
- In some groups of patients, pulse oximetry may be difficult, for example in children, or those with existing chronic respiratory disease, due to lack of appropriate or suitable equipment, chronic low saturations or patient compliance.

TABLE 3.89 – Signs of Infection

The review of systems should cover the following areas:	
• General	• Lethargy, fever/rigors.
• Neurological system	• Severe headaches, new confusion. • Signs of meningitis or encephalitis (neck stiffness/photophobia).
• Cardiovascular	• Shortness of breath, shortness of breath on exertion.
• Respiratory	• Pleurisy, shortness of breath, shortness of breath on exertion, cough, sputum, haemoptysis, increased respiratory rate or effort.
• Gastrointestinal	• Abdominal pain/distension, diarrhoea/vomiting
• Genito-urinary	• UTI symptoms (offensive urine, frequency, dysuria), reduced urine output, abdominal, flank and back pain.
• Musculoskeletal	• Hot painful joint, non-weight bearing.
• Skin	• Rapidly progressive cellulitis, diabetic foot and ulcers, burns, purpuric rash/mottling.
• Other	• Dental problems, foreign travel, exposure to other unwell contacts.
NB This is not an exhaustive list and clinical judgement should be used when considering whether a sign or symptom of a serious bacterial infection is present.	

13. Heart Rate in Suspected Sepsis[10]

Interpret the heart rate of a person with suspected sepsis in context, taking into account that:

- baseline heart rate may be lower in young people and adults who are fit
- older people with an infection may not develop an increased heart rate
- older people may develop a new arrhythmia in response to infection rather than an increased heart rate
- heart rate response may be affected by medicines, such as beta-blockers.

Always refer to the children's 'Page for Age' for vital signs of normal parameters.

14. Blood Pressure in Suspected Sepsis[10]

- Interpret blood pressure in the context of a person's usual blood pressure, if known.
- Patients may present with a normal BP but still have sepsis, particularly children and young people.

15. Confusion, Mental State and Cognitive State in Suspected Sepsis[10]

- Interpret a person's mental state in the context of their normal function and treat changes as being significant.
- Be aware that changes in cognitive function may be subtle and assessment should include history from the patient and family or carers.
- Changes in cognitive function may present as changes in behaviour or irritability in both children and in adults with dementia.
- Changes in cognitive function in older people may present as acute changes in functional abilities.

16. Temperature in Suspected Sepsis[10]

- Do not use a person's temperature as the sole predictor of sepsis.
- Do not rely on fever or hypothermia to rule sepsis either in or out.
- Ask the person with suspected sepsis and their family or carers about any recent fever or rigors.
- Take into account that some groups of people with sepsis may not develop a raised temperature. These include:
  - people who are older or very frail
  - people having treatment for cancer
  - people deteriorating with sepsis
  - infants or young children.

Do not ignore a high temperature or symptoms of fever/rigors as they are useful in highlighting patients with infection.

17. Pre-hospital Sepsis Screening Tools

- Exclusion or diagnosis of sepsis is only possible by obtaining complete blood test results from a laboratory or after urine output monitoring.
- Several pre-hospital sepsis screening tools have been proposed/developed; however, none have been validated in pre-hospital clinical practice.
- JRCALC recommends using tools that have been agreed locally in your own organisation, or across a network or region, and use of a NEWS2 score.
- Several additional screening tools have been proposed internationally, the PreSep score, PRESS score, and BAS 90-30-90 score have been proposed specifically to identify sepsis in the pre-hospital environment, but none have been validated clinically.[16,19,20] The Critical Illness Score was developed to identify all critically ill patients attended by EMS (not just sepsis patients). Again, this score has not been validated clinically.[21]

18. National Early Warning Score (NEWS2)

- NEWS2 should be undertaken for all patients who are ill, including suspected sepsis.
- NEWS2 is designed as a system to help to identify a seriously ill or deteriorating patient in a standardised way across the NHS. It is not designed to identify the cause of the clinical deterioration. Its strength is its simplicity and pragmatism – using routine physiological measurements.
- NEWS2 allows healthcare workers to communicate in a common language.
- With regard to sepsis, a NEWS2 score of 5 or more predicts at least a twofold increase in the risk of adverse outcomes, **BUT** NEWS2 does not diagnose sepsis – it simply identifies sick patients who need urgent senior medical review and intervention. The nature of the intervention requires confirmation of the diagnosis.
- NEWS2 is the first step in a two-step process: (1) identification of the sick and/or deteriorating patient, and (2) a timely and competent clinical response.
- NEWS2 scores may be masked in patients who are taking beta-blockers and/or steroids.

Sepsis

Physiological parameter	Score 3	2	1	0	1	2	3
Respiration rate (per minute)	≤8		9–11	12–20		21–24	≥25
SpO_2 Scale 1 (%)	≤91	92–93	94–95	≥96			
SpO_2 Scale 2 (%)	≤83	84–85	86–87	88–92 ≥93 on air	93–94 on oxygen	95–96 on oxygen	≥97 on oxygen
Air or oxygen?		Oxygen		Air			
Systolic blood pressure (mmHg)	≤90	91–100	101–110	111–219			≥220
Pulse (per minute)	≤40		41–50	51–90	91–110	111–130	≥131
Consciousness				Alert			CVPU
Temperature (°C)	≤35.0		35.1–36.0	36.1–38.0	38.1–39.0	≥39.1	

Figure 3.32 – NEWS2 chart. Reproduced from: Royal College of Physicians. *National Early Warning Score (NEWS) 2: Standardising the assessment of acute-illness severity in the NHS*. Updated report of a working party. London: RCP, 2017. Available at: https://www.rcplondon.ac.uk/projects/outputs/national-early-warning-score-news-2

National Early Warning Score (NEWS2)

Suspect sepsis in:

anyone that presents with fever/feeling unwell

- **and**

NEWS2 greater than or equal to 5

and/or looks unwell with history of infection.

19. Children and Sepsis

Suspect sepsis in:

- children <12 years that present with fever/feeling unwell
- **OR**
- children with abnormal observations
- **OR**
- children with very worried parents/carers.

TABLE 3.90 – Adult 'Red Flag' Sepsis – Time Critical Emergency
The following markers are suggestive of 'red flag' sepsis:
Responds only to voice or pain/is unresponsive.
Systolic BP ≤90 mmHg (or drop ≥40 from normal) or mean arterial pressure less than 65 mmHg.
Heart rate ≥130 per minute.
Respiratory rate ≥25 per minute.
Needs oxygen to keep SpO_2 ≥92%.
Non-blanching rash, mottled/ashen/cyanotic.
Not passed urine in last 18 hours.
Recent chemotherapy (in past 6 weeks).

TABLE 3.91 – Adult 'Amber Suspect' Sepsis –
The following are markers to indicate sepsis is likely:
History from friend/family of new altered mental behaviour/state.
Impaired immune system.
Trauma/surgery in past 6 weeks.
Respiration rate 21–24 per minute or increased work of breathing.
Heart rate 91–130 per minute.
Systolic BP 91–100 mmHg.
Not passed urine in the last 12–18 hours.
Tympanic temperature <36°C/axillary temperature <35°C.
Signs of potential infection at wound (increased redness/discharge).

Sepsis

TABLE 3.92 – Child 'Red Flag' Sepsis – Time Critical Emergency	
High risk criteria suspect 'Red flag' sepsis:	
Colour	• Pale/mottled/ashen/blue.
Activity	• No response to social cues. • Appears very ill to a healthcare professional. • Does not wake or, if roused, does not stay awake. • Weak, high-pitched or continuous cry.
Respiratory	• Grunting. • Severe tachypnoea. • Moderate or severe chest indrawing. • Oxygen saturations ≤90% on air.
Hydration	• Reduced skin turgor. • Severe tachycardia (see below). • Bradycardia <60. • Not passed urine/no wet nappies in last 18 hours.
Other	• Temperature <36°C. • Non-blanching rash. • Bulging fontanelle. • Neck stiffness. • Status epilepticus. • Focal neurological signs. • Focal seizures.

TABLE 3.93 – Child 'Amber Suspect' Sepsis –	
Sepsis likely/intermediate risk for sepsis (if history suggestive of infection):	
Colour	• Pallor reported by parent/carer.
Activity	• Not responding normally to social cues/not wanting to play. • Wakes only with prolonged stimulation. • Significantly decreased activity. • No smile.
Respiratory	• Nasal flaring. • Moderate tachypnoea (see below). • Oxygen saturations ≤92% on air. • Crackles.
Hydration	• Dry mucous membranes. • Moderate tachycardia (see below). • Poor feeding in infants. • CRT ≥3 seconds. • Reduced urine output. • Cold feet or hands.
Other	• Age 0–3 months ≥38°C. • Age 3–6 months ≥39°C. • Fever for ≥5 days. • Rigors. • Swelling of a limb or joint. • Leg pain. • Non-weight bearing/not using an extremity.

TABLE 3.94 – Child Low Risk for Sepsis	
• **Colour**	• Normal colour of skin, lips and tongue.
• **Activity**	• Responds normally to social cues. • Content/smiles. • Stays awake or awakens quickly. • Strong normal cry/not crying.
• **Hydration**	• Normal skin and eyes. • Moist mucous membranes.
• **Other**	• Child >2 years.

Clinical observations in children <12 years with suspected sepsis:

- Assess temperature, heart rate, respiratory rate, level of consciousness, oxygen saturation and capillary refill time.
- Only measure blood pressure in children <12 years in community settings if facilities to measure blood pressure, including a correctly-sized cuff, are available and taking a measurement does not cause a delay in assessment or treatment.

Sepsis

TABLE 3.95 – Sepsis Risk in Children in Relation to Respiratory and Heart Rates

AGE	TACHYPNOEA		TACHYCARDIA	
	Moderate	Severe	Moderate	Severe
1 year	50–59	≥60	150–159	≥160
1–2 years	40–49	≥50	140–149	≥150
3–4 years	35–39	≥40	130–139	≥140
5 years	27–28	≥29	120–129	≥130
6–7 years	24–26	≥27	110–119	≥120
8–11 years	22–24	≥25	105–114	≥115

TABLE 3.96 – MANAGEMENT of: Sepsis

Oxygen therapy	Sepsis is categorised as critical illness and requires supplemental oxygen regardless of initial oxygen saturation reading (SpO_2). Give oxygen to achieve a target saturation of 94-98% for adult patients or 88-92% for those at risk of hypercapnic respiratory failure (e.g. COPD) where the conscious level or respiratory rates fall at the higher saturation levels. Oxygen should be given to children with suspected sepsis who have signs of shock or oxygen saturation (SpO_2) of less than 91% when breathing air. Treatment with oxygen should also be considered for children with an SpO_2 of greater than 92%, as clinically indicated.[14]
• **Fluid therapy**	• The choice of fluid is crystalloid. • For adults and children aged ≥12 years with suspected sepsis and systolic blood pressure less than 90 mmHg or mean arterial pressure (MAP) less than 65 mmHg, give an intravenous fluid bolus of 500 ml over 15 minutes and monitor response. • Regularly reassess the patient after completion of the intravenous fluid bolus, and titrate response up to a maximum of 2000 ml if the systolic blood pressure remains below 90 mmHg and MAP below 65. • IV fluids should be given to children if haemodynamically shocked or unresponsive. • Give a bolus of 20 ml/kg over less than 10 minutes up to a maximum of 40 ml/kg. Assess response to fluids. Take into account pre-existing conditions (for example, cardiac disease or kidney disease), because smaller fluid volumes may be needed.
• **Rapid transport to hospital with pre-alert**	• Keep on-scene times to a minimum. • Make a **TIME CRITICAL** transfer. • Provide a pre-alert and NEWS2 score to the receiving hospital – 'patient has suspected sepsis' – in line with local arrangements. • Handover to hospital using local handover tools, such as SBAR, and give a NEWS2 score: • **S** – Situation • **B** – Background • **A** – Assessment • **R** – Recommendation.

20. Management

20.1 Further Management Considerations

Antibiotic Therapy

- If meningococcal disease is specifically suspected (fever and purpuric rash) give appropriate doses of parenteral benzylpenicillin and refer to **Meningococcal Meningitis and Septicaemia**.
- Any organisation considering pre-hospital antibiotic therapy for sepsis, particularly where journey times to hospital are more than one hour, should seek agreement from their relevant clinical networks.

Sepsis

- Early studies suggested significant survival benefit from early antibiotic administration in sepsis.[11] However, more recent studies fail to demonstrate such significant benefit. A recent meta-analysis indicated no survival benefit for antibiotics within the first hour of severe sepsis and septic shock.[22]
- Very few studies addressing pre-hospital antibiotic therapy have been undertaken. Some studies have also failed to demonstrate any survival benefit.[23] A recent study suggests that each hour of delay in giving antibiotics to a patient with septic shock increases mortality[24,25,26] At present there is insufficient evidence to make a robust recommendation in favour of, or against, pre-hospital antibiotic therapy.

Paracetamol

- Paracetamol should not to be given solely for reducing a high temperature but may be considered if the patient is in pain or to relieve distressing symptoms such as rigors.
- Paracetamol should be given intravenously only if the patient is unable to take anything orally or is in severe pain, otherwise oral paracetamol remains the first-line choice.
- Anti-pyretics such as paracetamol are often used in ICUs to manage fever in critically unwell patients by reducing the physiological stress fever causes; however, there is limited evidence to show any improvement in mortality.[27,28,29] Paracetamol is not part of any agreed sepsis pathway,[30] therefore may not be beneficial and does not improve outcomes in septic patients.[28,31]
- It should be noted that paracetamol may mask the abnormal physiology and therefore treatment opportunities for sepsis may be missed in hospital due to dampening of the sepsis signs.
- If paracetamol is used it should be highlighted in the SBAR handover at hospital.

Measurement of Lactate

- Currently there is insufficient evidence to make a robust recommendation in favour of changing current practice to include pre-hospital lactate measurement.
- NICE have not recommended measuring pre-hospital lactate for suspected sepsis so at this time we do not recommend it for pre-hospital use.
- Lactate itself is not a predictor of sepsis. Lactate may be elevated in a number of clinical conditions, and indeed may be normal in cases of septic shock.

SECTION 3 Medical Emergencies

KEY POINTS!

Sepsis

- **Suspect sepsis in:**
  - **anyone that presents with fever/feeling unwell**
  - **and NEWS2 greater than or equal to 5**
  - **and/or looks unwell with a history of infection.**
- **NEWS2 does not diagnose sepsis – it simply identifies sick patients who need urgent senior medical review and intervention.**
- **Keep on-scene times to a minimum.**
- **Provide a pre-alert and NEWS2 score to the receiving hospital – 'patient has suspected sepsis' – in line with local arrangements.**

Further Reading

Further important information and evidence in support of this guideline can be found in the Bibliography.[32,33,34,35] Other useful resources include:

http://sepsistrust.org/

https://www.nice.org.uk/guidance/ng51

Bibliography

1. Singer M, Deutschman CS, Seymour CW, Shankar-Hari M, Annane D, Bauer M, Bellomo R et al. The Third International Consensus definitions for sepsis and septic shock (Sepsis-3). *JAMA* 2016, **315:** 801–810.
2. Wang HE, Weaver MD, Shapiro NI, Yealy DM. Opportunities for emergency medical services care of sepsis. *Resuscitation* 2010, **81:** 193–197.
3. Guerra WF, Mayfield TR, Meyers MS, Clouatre AE, Riccio JC. Early detection and treatment of patients with severe sepsis by prehospital personnel. *Journal of Emergency Medicine* 2013, **44:** 1116–1125.
4. Van der Wekken LC, Alam N, Holleman F, Van Exter P, Kramer MH, Nanayakkara PW. Epidemiology of sepsis and its recognition by emergency medical services personnel in the Netherlands. *Prehosp Emerg Care* 2016, 20(1): 90–96.
5. Groenewoudt M, Roest AA, Leijten FMM, Stassen PM. Septic patients arriving with emergency medical

services: A seriously ill population. *European Journal of Emergency* Medicine 2014, 21: 330–335.

6. Roest AA, Stoffers J, Pijpers E, Jansen J, Stassen PM. Ambulance patients with nondocumented sepsis have a high mortality risk: a retrospective study. *Eur J Emerg Med* 2017, 24(1): 36–43.

7. Gray A, Ward K, Lees F, Dewar C, Dickie S, McGuffie C, Committee SS. The epidemiology of adults with severe sepsis and septic shock in Scottish emergency departments. *Emergency Medicine Journal* 2013, 30: 397–401.

8. Ibrahim I, Jacobs IG. Can the characteristics of emergency department attendances predict poor hospital outcomes in patients with sepsis? *Singapore Med J* 2013, 54: 634–638.

9. Martin GS, Mannino DM, Eaton S, Moss M. The epidemiology of sepsis in the United States from 1979 through 2000. *N Engl J Med* 2003, 348(16): 1546–1554.

10. National Institute for Health and Clinical Excellence. *Sepsis: Recognition, Diagnosis and Early Management* (NG51). London: NICE, 2017.

11. Liu VX, Fielding-Singh V, Greene JD, Baker JM, Iwashyna TJ, Bhattacharya J, Escobar GJ. The timing of early antibiotics and hospital mortality in sepsis. *American Journal of Respiratory and Critical Care Medicine*, 2017. Available from: http://atsjournals.org/doi/abs/10.1164/rccm.201609-1848OC.

12. Bone RC, Balk RA, Cerra FB, Dellinger RP, Fein AM, Knaus WA, Schein RM, Sibbald WJ. Definitions for sepsis and organ failure and guidelines for the use of innovative therapies in sepsis. The ACCP/SCCM Consensus Conference Committee. American College of Chest Physicians/Society of Critical Care Medicine. *Chest* 1992, 101: 1644–1655.

13. Bone RC, Sibbald WJ, Sprung CL. The ACCP-SCCM consensus conference on sepsis and organ failure. *Chest* 1992, 101: 1481–1483.

14. Angus DC, Van der Poll T. Severe sepsis and septic shock. *N Engl J Med* 2013, 369: 2063.

15. Herbst C, Naumann F, Kruse EB, Monsef I, Bohlius J, Schulz H, Engert A. Prophylactic antibiotics or G-CSF for the prevention of infections and improvement of survival in cancer patients undergoing chemotherapy, *Cochrane Database Syst Rev* 2009, 21(1): CD007107.

16. Polito CC, Isakov A, Yancey AH, Wilson DK, Anderson BA, Bloom I, Martin GS, Sevransky JE. Prehospital recognition of severe sepsis: development and validation of a novel emergency medical services screening tool. *Am J Emerg Med* 2015, 33(9):1119–1125.

17. Goerlich CE, Wade CE, McCarthy JJ, Holcomb JB, Moore LJ. Validation of sepsis screening tool using StO_2 in emergency department patients. *J Surg Res* 2014, 190: 270–275.

18. Davis T. NICE guideline: feverish illness in children--assessment and initial management in children younger than 5 years. *Arch Dis Child Educ Pract Ed* 2013, 98: 232–235.

19. Bayer O, Schwarzkopf D, Stumme C, Stacke A, Hartog CS, Hohenstein C, Kabisch B, Reichel J, Reinhart K, Winning J. An early warning scoring system to identify septic patients in the prehospital setting: The PRESEP Score. *Acad Emerg Med* 2015, 22: 868–871.

20. Wallgren UM, Castren M, Svensson AE, Kurland L. Identification of adult septic patients in the prehospital setting: a comparison of two screening tools and clinical judgment. *Eur J Emerg Med* 2014, 21: 260–265.

21. Seymour CW, Kahn JM, Cooke CR, Watkins TR, Heckbert SR, Rea TD. Prediction of critical illness during out-of-hospital emergency care. *JAMA* 2010, 304: 747–754.

22. Sterling SA, Miller WR, Pryor J, Puskarich MA, Jones AE. The impact of timing of antibiotics on outcomes in severe sepsis and septic shock: A systematic review and meta-analysis. *Crit Care Med* 2015, 43: 1907–1915.

23. Band RA, Gaieski DF, Hylton JH, Shofer FS, Goyal M, Meisel ZF. Arriving by emergency medical services improves time to treatment endpoints for patients with severe sepsis or septic shock. *Academic Emergency Medicine* 2011, 18: 934–940.

24. Seymour CW, Gesten F, Prescott HC, Friedrich ME, Iwashyna TJ, Phillips GS et al. Time to treatment and mortality during mandated emergency care for sepsis. New England Journal of Medicine, 21 May, 2017. Available from: http://www.nejm.org/doi/full/10.1056/NEJMoa1703058?query=featured_home#t=articleTop.

25. Shaw J, Fothergill RT, Clark S, Moore F. Can the prehospital National Early Warning Score identify patients most at risk from subsequent deterioration? *EMJ Online First*, 13 May, 2017.

26. Jarvis S, Kovacs C, Briggs J, Meredith P, Schmidt PE, Featherstone PI et al. Aggregate National Early Warning Score (NEWS) values are more important than high scores for a single vital signs parameter for discriminating the risk of adverse outcomes. *Resuscitation* 2015, 87: 75–80.

27. Anderson HA, Young J, Marrelli D, Black R, Lambreghts K, Twa MD. Training students with patient actors improves communication: a pilot study. *Optom Vis Sci* 2014, 91: 121–128.

28. Lee BH, Inui D, Suh GY, Kim JY, Kwon JY, Park J, Tada K et al. Association of body temperature and antipyretic treatments with mortality of critically ill patients with and without sepsis: multi-centered prospective observational study. *Crit Care* 2012, 16: R33.

29. Janz DR, Bastarache JA, Rice TW, Bernard GR, Warren MA, Wickersham N, Sills G et al. Randomized, placebo-controlled trial of acetaminophen for the reduction of oxidative injury in severe sepsis: the Acetaminophen for the Reduction of Oxidative Injury in Severe Sepsis trial. *Crit Care Med* 2015, 43: 534–541.

30. Daniels R, Nutbeam T, McNamara G, Galvin C. The sepsis six and the severe sepsis resuscitation bundle: a prospective observational cohort study. *Emerg Med J* 2011, 28: 507–512.

31. Young P. Acetaminophen to treat fever in intensive care unit patients with likely infection: a response from the author of the HEAT trial. *J Thorac Dis* 2016, 8: E631–632.

32. Boland LL, Hokanson JS, Fernstrom KM, Kinzy TG, Lick CJ, Satterlee PA, Lacroix BK. Prehospital lactate measurement by emergency medical services in patients meeting sepsis criteria. *West J Emerg Med* 2016, 17: 648–655.

33. Brown AFT, Cadogan MD. *Emergency Medicine: Diagnosis and Management*. London: Hodder Arnold, 2001.

34. Chamberlain D. Prehospital administered intravenous antimicrobial protocol for septic shock: A prospective randomized clinical trial. *Critical Care* 2009, 13: S130–S131.

35. Tobias AZ, Guyette FX, Seymour CW, Suffoletto BP, Martin-Gill C, Quintero J, Kristan J, Callaway CW, Yealy DM. Pre-resuscitation lactate and hospital mortality in prehospital patients. *Prehosp Emerg Care* 2014, 18: 321–327.

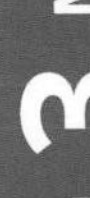

Stroke/Transient Ischaemic Attack (TIA)

1. Introduction

- Stroke is a major health problem in the UK. Improving care for patients with stroke and transient ischaemic attack (TIA) is a key national priority. The most recent national clinical guideline for stroke was developed by the Intercollegiate Stroke Guideline Working Party and published by the Royal College of Physicians in 2016, under a process accredited by the National Institute for Health and Care Excellence (NICE). The JRCALC guidelines draw heavily on these. The 2008 NICE guidelines for stroke and TIA are currently being reviewed and a focused update is expected to be published in May 2019.
- The Intercollegiate Stroke Guideline Working Party (2016) and JRCALC acknowledge the paucity of evidence for pre-hospital assessment and management of patients with suspected stroke. Many recommendations are therefore based on expert consensus and accepted practice. Ambulance services are increasingly engaging with stroke specialists and academic partners on high-quality research to help develop the evidence to inform future guidelines and practice.

Pathophysiology

1.1 Acute stroke

- Stroke is defined as a clinical syndrome, of presumed vascular origin, typified by rapidly developing signs of focal or global disturbance of cerebral functions lasting more than 24 hours or leading to death. Cerebrovascular disease is the third leading cause of disability in the UK. Approximately, 85% of strokes are caused by cerebral infarction resulting from ischaemic stroke, 10% by primary intracerebral haemorrhage (ICH) and 5% by subarachnoid haemorrhage. The risk of recurrent stroke is 26% within 5 years of a first stroke and 39% by 10 years.
- Acute stroke is a TIME CRITICAL medical emergency. For eligible patients with ischaemic stroke, treatment with thrombolytic therapy with alteplase is highly time dependent. Data from the Sentinel Stroke National Audit Programme (SSNAP) shows that in 2017-18 only 11.5% of all UK stroke patients received thrombolysis. In order to determine suitability for treatment, patients must undergo a brain scan; therefore, patients need to be transferred to an appropriate hospital as rapidly as possible once the diagnosis is suspected. As an additional treatment for a specific cohort of selected patients, interventional therapy is available. Mechanical Intra-Arterial Thrombectomy (IAT) is becoming increasingly available in specialist centres and may extend the time window of treatment for stroke patients beyond the current thrombolysis window.
- According to the Intercollegiate Stroke Working Party (2016):

  There is strong evidence that specialised stroke unit care initiated as soon as possible after the onset of stroke provides effective treatments that reduce long-term brain damage, disability and healthcare costs.
- The vast majority (95%) of people with stroke present in the community setting. Public information campaigns, notably the Stroke Association's FAST campaign, have raised awareness of stroke symptoms and encourage early call for help using the 999 system. Research has helped to inform procedures in ambulance Emergency Operations Centres to recognise stroke as early and accurately as possible to facilitate an appropriate emergency response. Reducing time from symptom onset by calling for help, and by speeding up pre-hospital assessment and reducing on-scene time, can expedite admission to an appropriate hospital. This reduces overall time to treatment and helps improve patient outcomes.
- **The most sensitive features associated with diagnosing stroke in the pre-hospital setting are unilateral facial weakness, arm or leg weakness, and speech disturbance.**

It is important to remember that thrombolysis is not the only management proven to benefit stroke patients. Admission to a stroke unit for early specialist care is known to be life saving and to reduce disability, even if thrombolysis is not indicated.

- Other symptoms and signs may include:
  - complete paralysis of one side of the body
  - sudden visual loss or blurring of vision
  - dizziness/vertigo
  - vomiting
  - confusion
  - difficulty understanding what others are saying
  - an inability to speak
  - problems with balance and co-ordination (ataxia)
  - difficulty swallowing, known as dysphagia
  - a sudden and very severe headache resulting in a blinding pain unlike anything experienced before (unlike their usual pattern of headaches)
  - reduced level of consciousness
  - locked-in syndrome (full body paralysis below the neck)
  - acute focal neurological deficit
  - new onset focal seizures
  - altered mental status including transient loss of consciousness or behavioural changes
  - sudden onset of neck pain or neck stiffness
  - witnessed acute focal neurological deficit which has since resolved.

- Be aware that the following non-specific symptoms can be present in a child presenting with stroke:
  - nausea or vomiting
  - fever
  - acute focal neurological signs may be absent, and that attention should be given to parental or young person concerns about the presentation of unusual symptoms.
- However, there may be other causes for these symptoms, referred to as 'stroke mimics':
  - seizures
  - syncope
  - sepsis
  - hypoglycaemia
  - migraine
  - decompensation of previous stroke
  - functional disorders.

1.2 TIA

- TIA is defined as an acute loss of focal cerebral or ocular function with symptoms lasting less than 24 hours. It is thought to be caused by inadequate cerebral or ocular blood supply as a result of low blood flow, thrombosis or embolism associated with diseases of the blood vessels, heart or blood. TIA is associated with a very high risk of stroke in the first month and up to one year after the event. A suspected cerebrovascular event needs to be urgently followed up with investigation and treatment at a timely TIA specialised clinic.
- During the first few hours of a patient's symptoms it is not possible to differentiate between a TIA or stroke. **Therefore, patients presenting with any ongoing facial weakness, arm weakness, speech impairment, loss of focal cerebral or ocular function should immediately be taken to hospital and treated as suspected stroke.**

1.3 Intracerebral and Subarachnoid Haemorrhage

- Haemorrhagic strokes are generally more severe and are associated with a considerably higher risk of dying within the first three months and beyond when compared to ischaemic strokes. Around 1 in 10 patients who have a haemorrhagic stroke die before reaching hospital.
- Intracerebral haemorrhage (ICH) is the most devastating and disabling type of stroke where due to an often spontaneous rupture of a vessel, blood will fill within the brain itself. Uncontrolled hypertension (HTN) is the most common risk factor for spontaneous ICH.
- Subarachnoid haemorrhage (SAH) is a haemorrhage from a cerebral blood vessel, aneurysm or vascular malformation into the subarachnoid space, which is the space surrounding the brain where blood vessels lie between the arachnoid and pia mater. The presentation of SAH is usually different from other types of stroke as it typically presents with the sudden onset of severe headache and vomiting, and with non-focal neurological signs that may include loss of consciousness and neck stiffness. Refer to **Headache** guideline.

2. Incidence

Stroke

- According to the State of the Nation report published by the Stroke Association in 2018 there are more than 100,000 strokes in the UK each year. That is calculated at approximately one stroke every 5 minutes. The Burden of Stroke in Europe report published by King's College, London using 2015 data highlighted 39.3 strokes per 100,000 inhabitants annually within the UK. There are over 1.2 million stroke survivors residing within the UK. Stroke is the fourth biggest killer in England and Wales, and the third biggest killer in Scotland and Northern Ireland.

Childhood Stroke

- There are over 400 childhood strokes a year in the UK, which is more than one child every day. Anyone of any age can have a stroke, including babies and children. The causes of stroke in children are very different from those in adults, although the risk of stroke in healthy children is extremely low; the risk of a thrombotic stroke is six times higher following a recent illness, such as cold/flu or chickenpox. For children having had none or only some of their routine vaccinations, the risk of a thrombotic stroke is eight times higher compared to those who've had all of their routine vaccinations. The risk of stroke in children is 19 times higher in children with congenital heart disease.

TIA

- The estimated incidence of first-ever TIA in the UK is 50 people per 100,000 population each year. This is likely to be an underestimate. 1 in 12 people (8%) will have a full stroke within a week of having a TIA.

Haemorrhage

- SAH incidence is 6–12 people per 100,000 population each year in the UK. Approximately, 85% of patients bleed from an intracranial aneurysm, 10% from a non-aneurysmal peri-mesencephalic haemorrhage and 5% from other vascular abnormalities including arteriovenous malformation.

Stroke/Transient Ischaemic Attack (TIA)

2.1 Severity and Outcome

- The case fatality of ischaemic stroke in adults aged 45 or older is estimated at 10.4 per 100 discharges, suggesting 53,004 deaths due to stroke each year, 41.5 deaths per 100,000 inhabitants annually.

3. Assessment and Management

In a suspected acute stroke patient a positive FAST test should be considered a **TIME CRITICAL** condition. Perform a brief secondary survey but keep on scene times to a minimum.

These components make up the **FAST** (face, arms, speech & time) assessment tool that should be used and carried out on **ALL** patients with suspected stroke/TIA. A deficit in any one of the face, arms or speech domains is sufficient for the patient to be identified as 'FAST positive'.

- The FAST test is well established in UK practice for both clinicians and the general public. FAST will not identify all patients with stroke, such as those with sudden-onset visual disturbance/lateralising cerebellar dysfunction. The Intercollegiate Working Party (2016) recommends clinicians should continue to treat a person as having a suspected stroke if they are suspicious of the diagnosis despite a negative FAST test.
- The Recognition Of Stroke In the Emergency Room (ROSIER) tool has been shown to be superior to the FAST test in identifying strokes in emergency departments, but was not better than the FAST test for pre-hospital recognition of stroke in a study undertaken by London Ambulance Service. ROSIER is not, therefore, recommended for pre-hospital use at this time.
- The majority of strokes are ischaemic. Distinguishing between ischaemic and haemorrhagic strokes is not currently feasible in the pre-hospital setting. Pre-hospital brain imaging is being evaluated in other countries (and in one UK centre) but the evidence is not

TABLE 3.97 – FAST Test

Facial weakness	Ask the patient to smile or show teeth. Look for **NEW** lack of symmetry.
Arm weakness	Ask the patient to lift their arms together and hold for five seconds. Does one arm drift or fall down? The arm with motor weakness will drift downwards compared to the unaffected limb.
Speech	Ask the patient to repeat a phrase. Assess for slurring or difficulty with the words or sentence, hesitation or even an inability to speak at all.
Time	Note the time of onset, if known, and pass this to the hospital as this has been shown to expedite time to CT scan.

TABLE 3.98 – Assessment and Management of Stroke/TIA

• Assess <C>ABCD	• If any of the following **TIME CRITICAL** features are present: – Major **<C>ABCD** problems refer to **Medical Emergencies in Adults – Overview** and **Medical Emergencies in Children – Overview**. – Fast positive or suspected stroke, convey to specialist stroke centre. – May have airway and breathing problems (refer to **Airway and Breathing Management**). – Level of consciousness may vary (refer to **Altered Level of Consciousness**). – Assess blood glucose level, as hypoglycaemia may mimic a stroke. • Start correcting any **<C>ABCD** problems. • Undertake a **TIME CRITICAL** transfer to nearest appropriate receiving hospital. Continue patient management en-route. • Provide an ATMIST pre-alert call including time of onset of symptoms, if known. **NB** A UK study (Sheppard et al) reported that providing a hospital pre-alert message is the most influential pre-hospital factor in facilitating timely assessment for acute stroke patients upon arrival in hospital and confirms in a UK setting the findings of previous work elsewhere. However, patients were only pre-alerted where stroke was recognised and symptom onset time recorded.

Stroke/Transient Ischaemic Attack (TIA)

TABLE 3.98 – Assessment and Management of Stroke/TIA *(continued)*	
• GCS	• Assess Glasgow Coma Scale (GCS) on unaffected side – eye and motor assessments may be more readily assessed if speech is badly affected.
• Respiratory rate	• Measure and record respiratory rate.
• Pulse	• Measure and record pulse.
• Oxygen saturation	• Monitor the patient's SpO_2, administer oxygen to achieve saturations of >94% if the patient presents as hypoxemic on air, refer to **Oxygen**. **NB** Among non-hypoxic patients with acute stroke, the prophylactic use of low-dose oxygen supplementation does not reduce death or disability at 3 months. Oxygen therapy is not recommended unless the patient is hypoxic.
• Blood pressure and fluids	• Measure and record blood pressure, if required administer fluids, refer to **Intravascular Fluid Therapy in Adults** and **Intravascular Fluid Therapy in Children**. **NB** The BP will be used as a baseline in hospital. **NB** Intravenous access is not essential unless the patient requires specific interventions, and may delay transport to hospital.
• Blood glucose	• Measure and record blood glucose for hypo/hyperglycaemia, refer to **Glycaemic Emergencies in Adults and Children**. **NB** Hypoglycaemia may mimic a stroke.
• Temperature	• Measure and record temperature.
• NEWS2	• These observations will enable you to calculate a NEWS2 Score, refer to **Sepsis**.
• ECG	• Do not delay transport to hospital to record a 12-Lead ECG. **NB** Although the prevalence of electrocardiogram abnormalities was found in a systematic review to be common in hospitalised patients, and atrial fibrillation was found in 25% of pre-hospital stroke patients in one study, the recording of a pre-hospital 12-lead ECG has been associated with delay and worse outcomes in stroke patients. Do not delay transport to hospital to record a 12 lead ECG. Patients should have continuous (e.g. 3-lead) cardiac monitoring en route to capture arrhythmias and specifically Atrial Fibrillation (AF) which increases a patients chance of developing a stroke fivefold. This valuable information will help during any subsequent specialist assessment.
• Assess the patient's pain	• Where present, assess the **SOCRATES** of pain and record initial and subsequent pain scores. • Consider analgesia if appropriate, refer to **Pain Management in Adults** and **Pain Management in Children**.
• Transfer	• The destination hospital will depend on local commissioning arrangements. For example, bypassing local hospitals for a 'hyper acute' centre may require patients in some networks to meet specific criteria. • Pre alert the receiving hospital for all FAST positive patients within locally agreed treatment windows of care. • Conscious patients should be conveyed in the most comfortable position for them. A large international randomised trial of hospitalised stroke patients reported that outcomes after acute stroke did not differ significantly between patients assigned to a lying-flat position and those assigned to a sitting-up position with the head elevated. • Patients with suspected acute stroke should remain nil by mouth until they have a swallowing assessment in hospital. • Where possible, a witness should be asked to accompany the patient to hospital, to assist with further assessment.
• Documentation	• Complete documentation to include all clinical findings, advice from other clinicians, onward referral and worsening advice given.

sufficient to recommend wider implementation at this time.

NB Use of a risk score (such as ABCD2) to determine stroke risk following suspected TIA is not recommended. All patients with suspected TIA should be considered at increased risk of stroke. Local pathways will determine where patients should be taken. A recent scoping review found that paramedic protocols for TIA referral have not been formally assessed, and a survey of UK ambulance services reported a minority had introduced such pathways.

4. Audit Information

- Ambulance services are required to monitor aspects of stroke care through the National Ambulance Quality Indicators. Careful documentation of your assessment and management, including accurate timings, is essential to improving care for this group of patients.
- SSNAP are currently working with NHS England on an ambulance-linkage project to complement and extend the current dataset, incorporating pre-hospital data.

KEY POINTS!

Stroke and Transient Ischaemic Attack

- **Time is of the essence in suspected acute stroke. Time is brain and 1.9-2.0 million neurons die every minute in an untreated stroke.**
- **Record time of onset if known or last seen well time and pre-alert the appropriate hospital.**
- **Stroke is common and may be due to either cerebral infarction or haemorrhage.**
- **Mechanical Intra-Arterial Thrombectomy (IAT) is becoming increasingly available in specialist centres and may extend the time window of treatment for stroke patients beyond the current thrombolysis window.**
- **The most sensitive features associated with diagnosing stroke in the pre-hospital setting are facial weakness, arm and leg weakness, and speech disturbance — the FAST test.**
- **The FAST test should be carried out on ALL patients with suspected stroke or TIA.**
- **Patients with TIA may be at high risk of stroke and require urgent specialist assessment based on locally agreed pathways of care.**

Bibliography

1. Royal College of Physicians. *National Clinical Guideline for Stroke, 5th ed.* London: RCP, 2016. Available from: https://www.rcplondon.ac.uk/guidelines-policy/stroke-guidelines.
2. National Institute for Health and Clinical Excellence. Stroke: The diagnosis and initial management of acute stroke and transient ischaemic attack (CG68). London: NICE, 2008. Available from: https://www.nice.org.uk/guidance/conditions-and-diseases/cardiovascular-conditions/stroke-and-transient-ischaemic-attack
3. Pre-hospital care concise stroke guide for stroke 2016. Available from: https://www.strokeaudit.org/SupportFiles/Documents/Guidelines/Profession-Specific-Guides/5-Pre-Hospital.aspx
4. Kobayashi A1,2,3, Czlonkowska A3,4, Ford GA5, Fonseca AC6, Luijckx GJ7, Korv J8, de la Ossa NP9, Price C10, Russell D11, Tsiskaridze A12, Messmer-Wullen M13,14, De Keyser J7,15. European Academy of Neurology and European Stroke Organization consensus statement and practical guidance for pre-hospital management of stroke. Eur J Neurol 2018, 25(3): 425–433. Available from: https://onlinelibrary.wiley.com/doi/epdf/10.1111/ene.13539
5. State of the nation: stroke statistics 2018 Available from: https://www.stroke.org.uk/resources/state-nation-stroke-statistics.
6. Burden of stroke in Europe. Available from: http://strokeeurope.eu/data-comparison/results/?country1=United+Kingdom&country2=Belgium&criteria=StrokeEpidemilogy
7. Sentinel Stroke National Audit Programme. Available from: https://www.strokeaudit.org/
8. Watkins CL, Jones SP, Leathley MJ, Ford GA, Quinn T, McAdam JJ, Gibson JME, Mackway-Jones KC, Durham S, Britt D, Morris S, O'Donnell M, Emsley HCA, Punekar S, Sharma A, Sutton CJ. *Emergency Stroke Calls: Obtaining Rapid Telephone Triage (ESCORTT) — a programme of research to facilitate recognition of stroke by emergency medical dispatchers*. Southampton (UK): NIHR Journals Library, 2014. Available from: https://www.ncbi.nlm.nih.gov/books/NBK262723/
9. Nor AM, McAllister C, Louw SJ, Dyker AG, Davis M, Jenkinson D, et al. Agreement between ambulance paramedic- and physician-recorded neurological signs with Face Arm Speech Test (FAST) in acute stroke patients. *Stroke: A Journal of Cerebral Circulation* 2004, 35(6): 1355–9.
10. Harbison J, Hossain O, Jenkinson D, Davis J, Louw SJ, Ford GA. Diagnostic accuracy of stroke referrals from primary care, emergency room physicians, and ambulance staff using the face arm speech test. *Stroke: A Journal of Cerebral Circulation* 2003, 34(1): 71–6.

11. Wilson C, Harley C, Steels S Systematic review and meta-analysis of pre-hospital diagnostic accuracy studies. *Emerg Med J* 2018, 35: 757–764. Available from: https://emj.bmj.com/content/35/12/757.long

12. McClelland G, Rodgers H, Flynn D, Price C.The frequency, characteristics and aetiology of stroke mimic presentations: a narrative review. *Eur J Emerg Med* 2019, 26(1): 2–8. Available from: https://insights.ovid.com/pubmed?pmid=29727304

13. Neves Briard J, Zewude RT, Kate MP, Rowe BH, Buck B, Butcher K, Gioia LC. Stroke Mimics Transported by Emergency Medical Services to a Comprehensive Stroke Center: The Magnitude of the Problem. *J Stroke Cerebrovasc Dis*. 2018, 27(10): 2738–2745. Available from: https://www.strokejournal.org/article/S1052-3057(18)30293-3/fulltext

14. Fothergill RT, Williams J, Edwards MJ, Russell IT, Gompertz P. Does use of the recognition of stroke in the emergency room stroke assessment tool enhance stroke recognition by ambulance clinicians? *Stroke* 2013, 44(11): 3007–12.

15. Morris S, Hunter RM, Ramsay AI, Boaden R, McKevitt C, Perry C, Pursani N, Rudd AG, Schwamm LH, Turner SJ, Tyrrell PJ, Wolfe CD, Fulop NJ. Impact of centralising acute stroke services in English metropolitan areas on mortality and length of hospital stay: difference-in-differences analysis. *BMJ* 2014, 349: g4757.

16. Ramsay AI, Morris S, Hoffman A, Hunter RM, Boaden R, McKevitt C, Perry C, Pursani N, Rudd AG, Turner SJ, Tyrrell PJ, Wolfe CD, Fulop NJ. Effects of Centralizing Acute Stroke Services on Stroke Care Provision in Two Large Metropolitan Areas in England. *Stroke* 2015, 46(8): 2244–51.

17. Rodrigues FB, Neves JB, Caldeira D, Ferro JM, Ferreira JJ, Costa J. Endovascular treatment versus medical care alone for ischaemic stroke: systematic review and meta-analysis. *BMJ* 2016, 353: i1754.

18. Zerna C, Thomalla G, Campbell BCV, Rha JH, Hill MD. Current practice and future directions in the diagnosis and acute treatment of ischaemic stroke. *Lancet* 2018, 392(10154): 1247–1256. Available from: https://www.thelancet.com/journals/lancet/article/PIIS0140-6736(18)31874-9/fulltext

19. Evans BA, Ali K, Bulger J, Ford GA, Jones M, Moore C, Porter A, Pryce AD, Quinn T, Seagrove AC, Snooks H, Whitman S, Rees N; TIER Trial Research Management Group. Referral pathways for patients with TIA avoiding hospital admission: a scoping review. Available from: https://bmjopen.bmj.com/content/7/2/e013443.long

20. Bulger JK, Ali K, Edwards A, Ford G, Hampton C, Jones C, Moore C, Porter A, Quinn T, Seagrove A, Snooks H, Rees N. Care pathways for low-risk transient ischaemic attack. *Journal of Paramedic Practice* 2018,10 (6).

21. Roffe C, Nevatte T, Sim J, Bishop J, Ives N, Ferdinand P, Gray R; Stroke Oxygen Study Investigators and the Stroke OxygenStudy Collaborative Group. Effect of Routine Low-Dose Oxygen Supplementation on Death and Disability in Adults With Acute Stroke: The Stroke Oxygen Study Randomized Clinical Trial. *JAMA* 2017, 318(12): 1125–1135. Available from: https://jamanetwork.com/journals/jama/fullarticle/2654819

22. Munro SF, Cooke D, Kiln-Barfoot V, Quinn T. The use and impact of 12-lead electrocardiograms in acute stroke patients: A systematic review. *Eur Heart J Acute Cardiovasc Care* 2018, 7(3): 257–263. Available from: https://journals.sagepub.com/doi/full/10.1177/2048872615620893?url_ver=Z39.88-2003&rfr_id=ori%3Arid%3Acrossref.org&rfr_dat=cr_pub%3Dpubmed

23. Bobinger T, Kallmünzer B, Kopp M, Kurka N, Arnold M, Heider S, Schwab S, Köhrmann M. Diagnostic value of prehospital ECG in acute stroke patients. *Neurology* 2017, 88(20): 1894–1898. Available from: http://n.neurology.org/content/88/20/1894.long

24. Anderson CS, Arima H, Lavados P, Billot L, Hackett ML, Olavarría VV, Muñoz Venturelli P, Brunser A, Peng B, Cui L, Song L, Rogers K, Middleton S, Lim JY, Forshaw D, Lightbody CE, Woodward M, Pontes Neto O, De Silva HA, Lin RT, Lee TH, Pandian JD, Mead GE, Robinson T, Watkins C; HeadPoST Investigators and Coordinators. Cluster-Randomized, Crossover Trial of Head Positioning in Acute Stroke. *N Engl J Med* 2017, 376(25): 2437–2447. Available from: https://www.nejm.org/doi/10.1056/NEJMoa1615715?url_ver=Z39.88-2003&rfr_id=ori:rid:crossref.org&rfr_dat=cr_pub%3dwww.ncbi.nlm.nih.gov

25. Royal College of Paediatrics and Child Health. *Stroke in Childhood - clinical guideline for diagnosis, management and rehabilitation*. London: Royal College of Paediatrics and Child Health, 2017. Available from: https://www.rcpch.ac.uk/resources/stroke-childhood-clinical-guideline-diagnosis-management-rehabilitation

26. Royal College of Paediatrics and Child Health. *Management of children and young people with an acute decrease in conscious level - clinical guideline*. London, Royal College of Paediatrics and Child Health, 2016. Available from: https://www.rcpch.ac.uk/resources/management-children-young-people-acute-decrease-conscious-level-clinical-guideline

Non-Traumatic Chest Pain/Discomfort

1. Introduction

- Chest pain is one of the most common symptoms of acute coronary syndrome (ACS).
- It is also a common feature in many other conditions such as aortic dissection, chest infection with pleuritic pain, pulmonary embolus, reflux oesophagitis, indigestion, and musculoskeletal chest pain.
- There must be a high index of suspicion that any chest pain is cardiac in origin.
- There are a number of specific factors that may help in reaching a reasoned working diagnosis, and applying appropriate management measures to the patient.
- ACS cannot be excluded on clinical examination alone (refer to **Acute Coronary Syndrome**).
- Do not assess symptoms differently in women and men or patients from different ethnic groups.

2. Assessment and Management

Assessing the type of pain is particularly important in the management of non-traumatic chest pain. For the types of pain typical for each cause refer to Table 3.99.

For the assessment and management of non-traumatic chest pain/discomfort refer to Table 3.100.

TABLE 3.99 – Descriptions of Non-Traumatic Chest Pain
Features which suggest a diagnosis of myocardial ischaemia include: • Central chest pain. • Crushing or constricting in nature. • Persists for >15 minutes. • Pain may also present in: – the shoulders – upper abdomen – referred to the neck, jaws or arms.
Features which suggest a diagnosis of stable angina include: • Pain is typically related to exertion and tends to last minutes but should it persist for >15 minutes, or despite usual treatment, ACS is more likely.
Features of pleuritic type pain: • Stabbing. • Generally one-sided. • Worse on breathing in. • Usually associated with a cough and sputum. • Raised temperature (>37.5°C) indicative of infection.
Features of indigestion type pain: • Central. • Related to ingestion of food. • May be associated with belching and a burning sensation. **NB** Some patients with ACS may also suffer indigestion type pain and belching.
Features of muscular type pain: • Sharp/stabbing. • Worse on movement. • Often associated with tenderness on palpation.
Features of aneurysm type pain: • Sudden, severe pain. • Pulsing sensation in the abdomen (like a heartbeat). • Sudden, intense and persistent abdominal or back pain, which can be described as a tearing sensation. • Pain that radiates to the back or legs.

Non-Traumatic Chest Pain/Discomfort

TABLE 3.100 – ASSESSMENT and MANAGEMENT of: Non-Traumatic Chest Pain/Discomfort	
NB A defibrillator must always be taken at the earliest opportunity to patients with symptoms suggestive of a myocardial infarction and remain with the patient until hand-over to hospital staff.	
ASSESSMENT	**MANAGEMENT**
• Assess **<C>ABCD**	If any of the following **TIME CRITICAL** features are present: • Major <C>ABCD problems, refer to **Medical Emergencies in Adults – Overview** and **Medical Emergencies in Children – Overview**. • Suspected acute coronary syndrome especially ST-segment-elevation myocardial infarction (STEMI) (refer to **Acute Coronary Syndrome**). • Aortic dissection. Start correcting any **<C>ABCD** problems. Undertake a **TIME CRITICAL** transfer to the nearest appropriate receiving hospital. Continue management en-route. Provide an ATMIST information call.
• ECG	Monitor and record 12-Lead ECG. Assess for abnormality, refer to **Cardiac Rhythm Disturbance**. **NB** For non-traumatic chest pain, an ECG should be taken as soon as practically possible to diagnose a STEMI requiring immediate conveyance to a centre able to provide Primary Percutaneous Coronary Intervention. **NB** DO NOT exclude an acute coronary syndrome when the patient has a normal 12-lead ECG.
• Assess for specific accompanying features	• Nausea/vomiting. • Sweating. • Pallor. • Cough. • Breathlessness – **NB** If breathlessness is a predominant symptom/sign with tightness in the chest, then causes of breathlessness must also be considered, refer to **Dyspnoea**.
• Undertake a clinical assessment specifically for:	• Heart failure. • Cardiogenic shock. • Ask the patient if they have a previous history of coronary heart disease.
• Other conditions	• If clinical examination and a 12-lead ECG make a diagnosis of ACS less likely, assess for other acute conditions such as: – pulmonary embolism, refer to **Pulmonary Embolism**. – aortic dissection – pneumonia, refer to **Medical Emergencies in Adults – Overview** and **Medical Emergencies in Children – Overview**.
• Respiratory rate	• Measure and record respiratory rate.
• Oxygen saturation	• Monitor the patient's SpO_2, administer oxygen to achieve saturations of >94% if the patient presents as hypoxemic on air, refer to **Oxygen**.
• Blood pressure and fluids	• Measure and record blood pressure, if required administer fluids, refer to **Intravascular Fluid Therapy in Adults** and **Intravascular Fluid Therapy in Children**.
• Blood glucose	• If appropriate, measure and record blood glucose for hypo/hyperglycaemia, refer to **Glycaemic Emergencies in Adults and Children**.
• Temperature	• Measure and record temperature.
• NEWS2	• These observations will enable you to calculate a NEWS2 Score, refer to **Sepsis**.

(continued)

Non-Traumatic Chest Pain/Discomfort

TABLE 3.100 – ASSESSMENT and MANAGEMENT of: Non-Traumatic Chest Pain/Discomfort *(continued)*	
• Assess patient's pain	• For the features of specific types of pain refer to Table 3.99. • Where present, assess the **SOCRATES** of pain and record initial and subsequent pain scores. • Consider analgesia if appropriate, refer to **Pain Management in Adults** and **Pain Management in Children**.
• Documentation	• Complete documentation to include all clinical findings, advice from other clinicians, onward referral and worsening advice given.

KEY POINTS!

Non-Traumatic Chest Pain/Discomfort

- **Most chest pain is not acute coronary syndrome – but this possibility needs to be excluded rapidly.**
- **Always consider another life-threatening cause (e.g. aortic dissection).**
- **Have a low threshold for recording a 12-lead ECG.**
- **A normal ECG cannot reliably exclude ACS.**

SECTION 3 Medical Emergencies

Bibliography

1. National Institute for Health and Clinical Excellence. *Chest Pain of Recent Onset: Assessment and diagnosis of recent onset chest pain or discomfort of suspected cardiac origin* (CG95). London: NICE, 2010. Available from: https://www.nice.org.uk/guidance/cg95.
2. Porter A, Snooks H, Youren A, Gaze S, Whitfield R, Rapport F et al. 'Covering our backs': ambulance crews' attitudes towards clinical documentation when emergency (999) patients are not conveyed to hospital. *Emergency Medicine Journal* 2008, 25(5): 292–295.
3. NHS. *Abdominal aortic aneurysm.* London: NHS, 2017. Available from: https://www.nhs.uk/conditions/abdominal-aortic-aneurysm.

Overdose and Poisoning in Adults and Children

1. Introduction

Overdose and poisoning is a common cause of calls to the ambulance service. When dealing with overdose and poisoning, advice is available online from TOXBASE®: https://www.toxbase.org. Consult your local procedures on how to use TOXBASE. An app containing searchable, offline access to the TOXBASE® database is available free to NHS users. A 24-hour, seven-day telephone advice line is also available from the National Poisons Information Service: 0344 892 0111.

1.1 Overdose and Poisoning

Exposure may occur by ingestion, inhalation, topical absorption, injection, inoculation or radiation of a quantity of a substance(s) and may result in mortality or morbidity.

Common agents include:

- Consumer products, for example washing powders, washing-up liquids and fabric cleaning liquid/tablets, bleaches, hand gels and screen-washes, anti-freeze and de-icers, silica gel, batteries, petroleum distillates, white spirit (e.g. paints and varnishes), descalers and glues. Exposure in children generally occurs as a result of ingestion but can arise from eye and skin contact; exposure can arise via multiple routes.
- Pharmaceutics, for example paracetamol, ibuprofen, co-codamol, aspirin, tricyclic antidepressants, selective serotonin uptake inhibitors (SSRIs), beta-blockers (atenolol, sotalol, propranolol), calcium channel blockers, benzodiazepines, opioids, iron tablets, cocaine and amphetamines.
- Naturally occurring poisons, toxins and venoms, for example snake envenomation and poisonous plants, including foxglove, laburnum, laurel, iris, castor oil plant and *Amanita phalloides*. For further details of poisonous plants refer to TOXBASE®.
- Alcohol.
- Chemicals (refer to **Major, Complex and High Risk Incidents**).
- Cosmetics.

Exposure may be:

- Accidental – This typically occurs in young children aged under 5 years, and ingestion of tablets and household products is most common, although almost anything, however unpalatable, may be ingested. Fortunately, the vast majority of ingestions and exposures in young children result in no or very mild symptoms. Many common ingestions involve low toxicity substances. Exploratory ingestion may raise the possibility of safeguarding concerns, as a result of either inadequate supervision or the nature of the ingested substance, even in the absence of a toxic effect on the child. If suspected this must be reported (refer to **Safeguarding Children** and **Safeguarding Adults at Risk**).
- Intentional – Attempted poisoning as an act of deliberate self-harm. Over-the-counter medicine (e.g. paracetamol) or prescribed drugs are commonly used, although deliberate exposure to any substance, irrespective of actual toxicity, with the expectation or intent of self-harm is significant. Poisoning may also result from intentional exploratory risk-taking behaviour, for example with alcohol or recreational drugs, or as a result of solvent misuse. The expectation of effect is important. The patient does not need to be unwell for this to be a concern.
- Non-accidental (or deliberate) by a third party – This type of poisoning is extremely unlikely to be detected by the Ambulance Service, but if it is suspected it must be reported (refer to **Safeguarding Adults at Risk** and **Safeguarding Children**).

2. Incidence

- It is difficult to estimate the exact number of overdose and poisoning incidents that occur, as not all cases are reported. In 2016/2017 there were 43,611 poison-related telephone queries involving patients to the National Poisons Information Service. Approximately one-third of those concerned children under the age of five. Most of these incidents were accidental and occurred in the home.

3. Severity and Outcome

- There are a number of factors that affect severity and outcome following exposure, in particular, age and weight of the patient, toxicity of the agent, quantity, route of exposure and co-morbidities or physical injury.
- In patients that self-harm, death commonly results from airway obstruction and respiratory arrest, secondary to a decreased level of consciousness.

4. Pathophysiology

- The toxic effect following exposure will depend primarily on the individual substance. For details of the effects of specific substances refer to TOXBASE®.

5. Assessment and Management

For the assessment and management of overdose and poisoning, refer to Tables 3.101 and 3.102.

TABLE 3.101 – ASSESSMENT and MANAGEMENT of: Overdose and Poisoning in Adults and Children *(continued)*	
• Transfer to further care	• For certain patients, urgent transfer to further care may be appropriate, for example: – deliberate self-poisoning – patients who are symptomatic – patients who have ingested poisons with a delayed action such as aspirin, iron, paracetamol, tricyclic antidepressants, co-phenotrope and all modified-release preparations – where the type of poison is not known – all children and young people who have or may have been exposed to a potentially toxic substance – all patients suffering an opioid overdose whether or not they have responded to naloxone – the effects of respiratory depression opioid overdose can last 4–5 hours and may be further prolonged in cases involving a sustained release preparation or a long acting opiate, such as methadone. • Methadone has a longer half-life, which can be greater than 24 hours in regular users, and this should be considered when assessing patients and advising on whether to attend hospital. • In cases of self-harm, even if the substance (or amount of substance) is considered harmless, if the patient does not require emergency treatment, but a mental health assessment may be required, consider alternative pathways (e.g. specialist mental health service) as per local protocol. **NB This decision should take into account the patient's preferences, and the views of the receiving service.** • Following an exploratory ingestion some **patients may be considered safe to be left at home if:** – the substance is verified by TOXBASE®/NPIS as harmless – the incident is/was accidental – there is a responsible adult present and there are no safeguarding concerns – advice is given to seek medical advice if the patient becomes unwell – arrangements have been made to inform the health visitor or GP. **NB Seek further advice should there be any doubt.** • In adults that refuse to go to hospital the reason for refusal should be determined and information about the potential consequences of not receiving further care provided. • If the person still refuses care that is felt to be in their best interests, an assessment of their mental capacity may be required (refer to **Mental Capacity Act 2005**) and consideration given to whether an assessment for compulsory admission under the Mental Health Act is needed (refer to **Mental Health Presentation: Crisis, Distress and Disordered Behaviour**). • If necessary, seek medical advice and inform the patient's GP – follow local protocol.

6. Specific Substance Management

The clinical features, signs and symptoms listed below are not exhaustive, especially if there have been multiple drug exposures. The lists of common or street names for drugs are similarly non-exhaustive. Visit www.talktofrank.com for an A-to-Z glossary of street names.

Overdose and Poisoning in Adults and Children

TABLE 3.102 – Specific Substance Management	
Alcohol Ethanol	
• Signs and symptoms	• Nausea, vomiting, slurred speech, confusion, ataxia, convulsions, unconsciousness, hypotension.
• Description	• Alcohol intoxication is a common emergency, especially in young adults, and is usually a transient problem. Alcohol poisoning follows the consumption of excessive amounts of alcohol. It can be fatal, so should be taken seriously. It is not uncommon in teenagers.
• Effects	• Can cause severe hypoglycaemia, even in teenagers. • Adulteration of ethanol with toxic alcohols, such as ethylene glycol or methanol, may occur.
• Management	• Alcohol intoxication may cause alcohol-induced hypoglycaemia. Correct the blood glucose level (refer to **Glycaemic Emergencies in Adults and Children**). Other relevant guidelines are **Glucose 10%** and **Glucagon**, although glucagon is often not effective in overdoses. **ALWAYS** check the blood glucose levels in any child or young person with a decreased conscious level, especially in children and young adults who are 'drunk', as hypoglycaemia (blood glucose <4.0 mmol/l) is common and requires treatment with oral glucose or glucose 10% IV (refer to **Glycaemic Emergencies in Adults and Children**). • When alcohol is combined with drugs in overdose, it may pose a major problem. For example, when combined with opiate drugs or sedatives, it will further decrease the level of consciousness with increased risk of respiratory depression and aspiration of vomit. In combination with paracetamol, chronic alcohol excess increases the risk of liver damage.
Amphetamines Methamphetamine. Street names: Bennies and Billy Whizz.	
• Signs and symptoms	• Mood swings, extreme hunger, sleeplessness and hyperactivity.
• Description	• Amphetamines were developed in the 1930s and have been medically prescribed in the past for diet control and as a stimulant. • Administration: – They can be swallowed, sniffed or, rarely, injected. Onset approximately 30 minutes. Lasts for several hours. Used with other drugs or alcohol, the effects are magnified.
• Effects	Increases energy levels, confidence and sociability. **Cardiovascular** • Tachycardia can lead to heart failure even in healthy individuals (refer to **Cardiac Rhythm Disturbance**). • Hypertension can produce pinpoint haemorrhages in skin, especially on the face, and even lead to stroke. **Central nervous system** • 'High' feelings, panic, paranoia which can lead to mental ill health in the long term, poor sleep and hyperpyrexia. **Gastrointestinal** • Liver failure.

(continued)

SECTION **3** Medical Emergencies

Overdose and Poisoning in Adults and Children

TABLE 3.102 – Specific Substance Management *(continued)*	
• Effects	• Induces a sense of exhilaration, euphoria, excitement and reduced hunger in the user primarily by blocking the re-uptake of the neurotransmitter dopamine in the midbrain, which blocks noradrenaline uptake causing vasoconstriction and hypertension. **NB** Crack cocaine is pure and therefore more potent than street cocaine; it enters the bloodstream more quickly and in higher concentrations. Because it is smoked, crack cocaine's effects are felt more quickly and they are more intense than those of powder cocaine. However, the effects of smoked crack are shorter lived than the effects of snorted powder cocaine. It is highly addictive even after only one use. • The symptoms of a cocaine overdose are intense and generally short lived. Although uncommon, people do die from cocaine or crack overdose, particularly following ingestion (often associated with swallowing 'evidence'). • All forms of cocaine/crack use can cause coronary artery spasm, myocardial infarction and accelerated ischaemic heart disease, even in young people. • Various doses of cocaine can also produce other neurological and behavioural effects such as: – dizziness – headache – movement problems – anxiety – insomnia – depression – hallucinations. • The unwanted effects of cocaine or crack overdose may include some or all of the following: – tremors – dangerous or fatal rise in body temperature – delirium – hypertension – tachycardia and dysrhythmia – myocardial infarction – cardiac arrest – seizures including status epilepticus – stroke – kidney failure.
• Management	• Transfer patient rapidly to hospital. • Administer supplemental oxygen (refer to **Oxygen**). • Consider assisted ventilation at a rate of 12–20 breaths per minute if: – SpO_2 is <90% on high concentration O_2 – respiratory rate is >30 breaths per minute – expansion is inadequate. • Undertake a 12-lead ECG – if the patient has a 12-lead ECG suggestive of myocardial infarction and a history of recent cocaine use, administer nitrates but do not administer thrombolysis. • Administer aspirin and GTN if the patient complains of chest pain (refer to **Aspirin** and **Glyceryl Trinitrate (GTN)**). • **Chest pain** – Administer diazepam if the patient has severe chest pain (refer to **Diazepam**). In symptomatic cocaine toxicity, titrate diazepam slowly to response. • **Convulsions** (refer to **Convulsions in Adults** and **Convulsions in Children**) – In cases of seizures due to cocaine toxicity, administer the full dose of diazepam (refer to **Diazepam**).

TABLE 3.102 – Specific Substance Management *(continued)*	
	● **Hypertension** – If systolic BP >220 and diastolic BP >140 mmHg in the absence of longstanding hypertension, seek medical advice. ● **Hyperthermia** – Actively cool if the body temperature is elevated. **NB** Swallowed crack cocaine represents a severe medical emergency and needs **URGENT** transportation to hospital **EVEN IF ASYMPTOMATIC**.
Corrosive injuries[2]	
● Mechanism of injury	● Corrosives can injure any biological surface that they meet. The corrosive effects are a function of both the oxidizing capacity and the pH of the solution.
● Signs and symptoms	● Either strong acids or strong alkalis may cause pain, blistering, penetrating necrosis and coagulating burns. Cardiovascular collapse and metabolic acidosis may occur secondary to an extensive corrosive injury.
● Management	● **Ingestion** of a corrosive should by managed by an urgent assessment of the airway and the cardiovascular system. If there is evidence of oedema of the upper airway, early intubation or tracheotomy should be considered. ● **Inhalation** may occur directly in the presence of a volatile corrosive or indirectly through the aspiration of gastric contents. The upper airway should be assessed for potential injury. If there is evidence of oedema of the upper airway, early intubation or tracheotomy should be considered. Injury to the lower airway may result in a pneumonitis or acute respiratory distress syndrome. ● **Skin** contact with a corrosive should be treated by urgent irrigation with water for 10 – 15 minutes and be assessed and treated as a thermal burn. Any contaminated clothing should be removed. Personal protective equipment should be worn. ● **Eye** contact with a corrosive should be treated with urgent irrigation with water or normal saline for 10 – 15 minutes.
Cyanide	
● Signs and symptoms	● Confusion, drowsiness, decreased level of consciousness, dizziness, headache, convulsions.
● Management	● Cyanide poisoning requires specific treatment – seek medical advice. Provide full supportive therapy and transfer immediately to hospital. Provide an alert/information call. ● Cyanide poisoning can occur in patients exposed to smoke in a confined space (e.g. house fire). Remove the patient from the source and administer continuous supplemental oxygen in as high a concentration as possible. If there are signs of decreased levels of consciousness transfer immediately to hospital. Provide an alert/information call. ● In cases of CBRNE the HART/SORT team will provide guidance. ● Poisoning may occur in certain industrial settings. Cyanide 'kits' should be available, and the kit should be taken to hospital with the patient. The patient requires injection with dicobalt edetate or administration of the drug hydroxycobalamin.
Foreign bodies	
● Description	● The majority of swallowed objects are low risk objects and can be managed conservatively.
● Effects	● Large objects (>6 cm long or 2.5 cm wide) may obstruct the gut – these children should be transferred to hospital.
● Management	● There is no need for transfer to hospital for patients who: – give a reliable history of ingestion of a small, low risk object – look well and are pain free – have no respiratory distress – can eat and drink – have no significant past medical history.

(continued)

TABLE 3.102 – Specific Substance Management *(continued)*	
	• Depression, panic and anxiety may also occur. **Liver and kidney injury** • Liver failure and severe kidney damage may occur. **Other** • Cystitis and heavy periods may occur in females who use 'E'.
• Management	• Agitation can be challenging and difficult to manage, and there are a number of options, including safe holding techniques or the use of appropriate medications. Advanced/specialist paramedics may have received additional training in this area. Refer to local procedures. • Treat convulsions with diazepam (refer to **Diazepam**). • If the systolic BP >220 and diastolic >140 mmHg in the absence of longstanding hypertension, seek medical advice. • Correct hypotension by raising the foot of the bed and/or by giving fluids as per medical emergencies (refer to **Intravascular Fluid Therapy in Adults** and **Intravascular Fluid Therapy in Children**). • Active cooling measures (refer to **Heat Related Illness**) may be helpful but should not delay transfer to further care.
Mephedrone Street names: MCAT, M-CAT, M kat, M-Cat, MD3, meow, meow meow, meph. Meth, M-Cat, White Magic, Meow Meow.	
• Signs and symptoms	• Agitation.
• Description	• Amphetamine-based drug of misuse. • Administration: sniffed or, rarely, injected.
• Effects	Psychoactive stimulant. **Cardiovascular** • Tachycardia can lead to heart failure even in healthy individuals (refer to **Cardiac Rhythm Disturbance**). • Hypertension can produce pinpoint haemorrhages in skin, especially on the face, and even lead to stroke. **Central nervous system** – Agitation, confusion, hyperpyrexia.
• Management	• **Vital signs** – Monitor pulse, blood pressure, cardiac rhythm. • **Agitation** – Agitation can be challenging and difficult to manage and there are a number of options, including safe holding techniques or the use of appropriate medications. Advanced/specialist paramedics may have received additional training in this area. Refer to local procedures. • **Convulsions** (refer to **Convulsions**). • **Cardiac rhythm disturbance** – Narrow-complex tachycardia with cardiac output is best left untreated. • **Hypertension** – If systolic BP >220 and diastolic BP >140 mmHg in the absence of longstanding hypertension, seek medical advice. • **Hypotension** – Correct hypotension by raising the foot of the trolley and/or by the administration of intravascular fluid (refer to **Intravascular Fluid Therapy in Adults** and **Intravascular Fluid Therapy in Children**). • **Hyperthermia** – Rapid transfer to hospital; active cooling measures may be undertaken en-route (refer to **Heat Related Illness**).

Overdose and Poisoning in Adults and Children

TABLE 3.102 – Specific Substance Management *(continued)*	
Novel Psychoactive Substances (NPS)[3,4] Commonly known as 'illegal highs'	
	• Novel psychoactive substances (NPS) is the name given to drugs that are newly synthesised or newly available. They include a multitude of substances, a diverse group of chemicals and have many different effects. • There is often little correlation between the drug a misuser believes they have taken and the actual chemical identity of the substance. NPS include substances with primarily stimulant effects, those with primarily hallucinogenic effects, as well as some central nervous system depressants and synthetic cannabinoids.
Opioids Heroin, Diamorphine, Amidone, Dolophine, Methadone, Fentanyl.	
• Signs and symptoms	• Drowsiness, nausea, vomiting, small pupils, respiratory depression, cyanosis, decreased level of consciousness, convulsions, non-cardiac pulmonary oedema.
• Description	• There are a wide variety of opioids, both naturally derived and synthetic. • Administration: injected, snorted or smoked.
• Effects	• Central nervous system and respiratory depression associated with pinpoint pupils. • Withdrawal symptoms may also occur: sweating, shivering, muscle cramps, lacrimation. • Reduced physical and psychological pain – relieving anxiety. The effects of methadone are less intense but may be prolonged. **Side effects:** • Cardiovascular system – Damage to veins and lungs, infection.
• Management	• Ensure the airway is open – administer supplemental oxygen (refer to **Oxygen**). • Profound respiratory depression can be reversed with naloxone (refer to **Naloxone Hydrochloride**). • Methadone is extremely dangerous for young children and its effects may take several hours to become apparent.
Orthochlorobenzalmalononitrile CS gas	
• Signs and symptoms	• Lacrimation, burning sensation of the eyes, excessive mucus production, nausea and vomiting.
• Effects	• Carried by police forces for defensive purposes. CS spray is aerosolised fine powder, which irritates the eyes ('tear gas') and respiratory tract.
• Management	• **AVOID** contact with the gas, which is given off from patient's clothing. Where possible keep two metres, **up-wind**, from the patient and give them self-care instructions. Symptoms normally resolve in 15 minutes but may potentiate or exacerbate existing respiratory conditions. If symptoms are present: • Remove the patient to a well-ventilated area. • Remove contaminated clothes and place them in a sealed bag. • If possible, remove contact lenses. • **DO NOT** irrigate the eyes as CS gas particles may dissolve and exacerbate irritation. If irrigation is required use copious amounts of saline. • Patients with severe respiratory problems should be immediately transported to hospital (refer to **Airway and Breathing Management**). • Ensure good ventilation of the vehicle during transfer to further care.

(continued)

Overdose and Poisoning in Adults and Children

TABLE 3.102 – Specific Substance Management *(continued)*	
Paracetamol and paracetamol-containing compound drugs	
• Signs and symptoms	• Nausea, vomiting, malaise, right upper quadrant abdominal pain, jaundice, confusion, drowsiness – unconsciousness may develop later. **NB** Frequently asymptomatic, symptoms are unreliable.
• Effects	• Paracetamol, even in modest doses, is **dangerous** and can induce severe liver and kidney damage. Initially there are no clinical features to suggest this, which may lull the patient and ambulance clinicians into a false sense of security. It frequently takes 24–48 hours for the effects of paracetamol damage to become apparent and urgent blood paracetamol levels are required to assess the patient's level of risk. • Patients who are malnourished, have been fasting, take enzyme inducing drugs, or regularly drink alcohol to excess are at higher risk of liver damage.
• Management	• Codeine and dextropropoxyphene are both derived from opioid drugs. This in overdose, especially if alcohol is involved, may well produce profound respiratory depression. This can be reversed with naloxone (refer to **Naloxone Hydrochloride**). • There are a number of analgesic drugs that contain paracetamol and a combination of codeine or dextropropoxyphene. Patients are not always aware that a medicine contains paracetamol. Always ask what medicines they have taken rather than just focusing on how much paracetamol they have taken. • Consider **Activated Charcoal**.
Synthetic Cannabinoid Receptor Agonists (SCRAs) Street names: Spice, JWH-015, 5F-ADBICA, 5F-AKB48, X, Hawaiian Haze, Bombay Blue, Black Mamba.	
• Signs and symptoms	• Agitation, confusion, hallucinations, psychosis, syncope, tachycardia, hypertension, hypotension, chest pain, acute kidney injury and muscle rigidity.
• Description	• Potent agonists of the cannabinoid-1 (CB_1) receptor, unlike Δ^9-tetrahydrocannabinoid the active alkaloid found in *Cannabis sativa*, which is a partial agonist at the CB_1 receptor. • Administration: the active chemical is usually impregnated onto plant matter and then smoked.
• Effects	• Disassociative with greater central nervous system and cardiovascular effects compared with cannabis.
• Management	• Agitation can be challenging and difficult to manage and there are a number of options, including safe holding techniques or the use of appropriate medications. Advanced/specialist paramedics may have received additional training in this area. Refer to local procedures. • Treat convulsions with diazepam (refer to **Diazepam**). • If the systolic BP >220 and diastolic >140 mmHg in the absence of longstanding hypertension, seek medical advice. • Correct hypotension by raising the foot of the bed and/or by giving fluids as per medical emergencies (refer to **Intravascular Fluid Therapy**).
Tricyclic antidepressants	
• Signs and symptoms	• Central nervous system: excitability, confusion, blurred vision, dry mouth, fever, pupil dilation, convulsions, decreased level of consciousness, arrhythmias, hypotension, tachycardia, respiratory depression; physical condition can rapidly change.
• Effects	• Poisoning with tricyclic antidepressants may cause impaired consciousness, profound hypotension and cardiac arrhythmias. They are a common treatment for patients who are already depressed. Newer antidepressants, such as fluoxetine (Prozac) and paroxetine (Seroxat), have different effects. • These medicines can be extremely dangerous to young children.

TABLE 3.102 – Specific Substance Management *(continued)*	
• Management	• Continuous ECG monitoring. • Obtain IV access. • Arrhythmias (refer to **Cardiac Rhythm Disturbance**). • The likelihood of convulsions is high (refer to **Convulsions**). • Monitor closely as the patient's physical condition can rapidly change. • Consider **Activated Charcoal**.

TABLE 3.103 – Signs and Symptoms of Carbon Monoxide Poisoning

Acute low-level exposure	Acute high-level exposure	Chronic low-level exposure
• Headache • Dizziness • Nausea • Vomiting • General lethargy	• Headache • Dizziness • Nausea • Vomiting • Lethargy • Muscle ataxia • Confusion • Chest pains • Shortness of breath/difficulty in breathing • Neurological deficit • Coma	• Headache • Dizziness • Nausea • Vomiting • General lethargy • Flu-like symptoms • Neurological decline • Visual problems

TABLE 3.104 – Questions to Be Asked in Cases of Carbon Monoxide Poisoning[5,6]	
Cohabitants/ companions	Does anyone else feel unwell? Are any pets behaving abnormally?
Outdoors	Do you feel better if you go outside or when you are away from the property for a prolonged time?
Maintenance	Are any heating appliances properly maintained?
Alarms	Do you have a working CO alarm? Has it activated?

7. Duty of Care

- It is not uncommon to find patients who have or claim to have taken an overdose and subsequently refuse treatment or admission to hospital. An assessment of their mental health state, capacity and suicide risk should be made (refer to **Mental Health Presentation: Crisis, Distress and Disordered Behaviour** and **Mental Capacity Act 2005**). If, despite reasonable persuasion, the patient refuses treatment, it is not acceptable to leave them in a potentially dangerous situation without any access to care.
- Assistance may be obtained from the medical/clinical director or a member of the clinical team and a judgement must be made to seek appropriate advice. Attendance of the police or local mental health team may be required, especially if the safety of the patient or others is at risk.

Overdose and Poisoning in Adults and Children

KEY POINTS!

- **Establish the event, drug or substance involved, the quantity, mode of poisoning and any alcohol consumed.**
- **NEVER induce vomiting.**
- **Bring the substance or substances and any containers for inspection at hospital, if it is safe to do so.**
- **Anyone with deliberate overdose must be transferred to hospital or referred to an appropriate mental health service.**
- **After confirmed exposure to a low toxicity substance, some patients may be considered for home management.**
- **Consider exposure to carbon monoxide.**
- **Agitation can be challenging and difficult to manage and there are a number of options, including safe holding techniques or the use of appropriate medications. Advanced/specialist paramedics may have received additional training in this area. Refer to local procedures.**

Bibliography

1. Coulson JM, Thompson JP. Investigation and management of the poisoned patient. *Clin Med* (Lond) 2008. 8(1): 89–91.
2. Bateman N, Jefferson R, Thomas S, Thompson J. Vale A (eds). *Oxford Desk Reference: Toxicology*. Oxford: OUP, 2014.
3. Dargan P, Wood D (eds). *Novel Psychoactive Substances: Classification, pharmacology and toxicology*. Cambridge, MA: Academic Press, 2013.
4. Novel Psychoactive Treatment UK Network (NEPTUNE). *Guidance on the Clinical Management of Acute and Chronic Harms of Club Drugs and Novel Psychoactive Substances*. London: NEPTUNE, 2015. Available from: https://www.drugsandalcohol.ie/24292
5. Department of Health. *Carbon Monoxide Poisoning: Recognise the symptoms and tackle the cause*. London: DOH, 2013.
6. Public Health England. *Diagnosing Poisoning: Carbon monoxide (CO)*. London: HMSO, 2015.
7. Soar J, Perkins GD, Abbas G, Alfonzo A, Barelli A, Bierens JJLM, et al. European Resuscitation Council Guidelines for Resuscitation 2010 Section 8: Cardiac arrest in special circumstances: electrolyte abnormalities, poisoning, drowning, accidental hypothermia, hyperthermia, asthma, anaphylaxis, cardiac surgery, trauma, pregnancy, electrocution. *Resuscitation* 2010, 81(10): 1400–1433.
8. The British National Formulary for Children. *Emergency Treatment of Poisoning*. Available from: https://www.evidence.nhs.uk/formulary/bnfc/current/emergency-treatment-of-poisoning, 2012–2013.
9. National Institute for Health and Clinical Excellence. *Self-harm in over 8s: short-term management and prevention of recurrence* (CG16). London: NICE, 2004. Available from: http://www.nice.org.uk/CG16.
10. Gunnell D, Bennewith O, Peters TJ, House A, Hawton K. The epidemiology and management of self-harm amongst adults in England. *Journal of Public Health* 2005, 27(1): 67–73.
11. Gwini SM, Shaw D, Iqbal M, Spaight A, Siriwardena AN. Exploratory study of factors associated with adverse clinical features in patients presenting with non-fatal drug overdose/self-poisoning to the ambulance service. *Emergency Medicine Journal* 2011, 28(10): 892–894.
12. Health Protection Agency, Centre for Radiation, Chemical and Environmental Hazards. *National Poisons Information Service Annual Report 2010/2011*. London: The Stationery Office, 2010.
13. Health Protection Agency, Centre for Radiation, Chemical and Environmental Hazards. *Current Awareness in Clinical Toxicology*. London: The Stationery Office, 2012.
14. Health Protection Agency, Centre for Radiation, Chemical and Environmental Hazards. *Chemicals & Poisons A–Z and Compendium*. London: The Stationery Office, 2012.
15. Health Protection Agency, Centre for Radiation, Chemical and Environmental Hazards. *Chemicals and Poisons*. London: The Stationery Office, 2012.
16. National Poisons Information Service. *TOXBASE*. Available from: http://www.npis.org/toxbase.html, 2012.
17. National Poisons Information Service. Available from: http://www.npis.org/index.html, 2012.
18. The British National Formulary. Emergency treatment of poisoning. *BNF 63*. London: Royal Pharmaceutical Society, 2012.
19. The British National Formulary. Medicines information services. *BNF 63*. London: Royal Pharmaceutical Society, 2012.

Paediatric Gastroenteritis

1. Introduction

- Every year 10% of the UK's under-5s will have an episode of infective gastroenteritis.
- Characteristically they present with sudden onset of diarrhoea (with or without vomiting), which usually resolves without any specific treatment.
- When severe, dehydration can occur, which can be life-threatening. Younger children are most at risk of dehydration.
- Children should not simply be viewed as 'little adults'. They pose many pitfalls for the unwary and inexperienced and present healthcare providers with significant challenges wherever the setting.
- Children display important differences in their anatomy, their physiology, their immunity and the illnesses they encounter, as well as the ways in which these conditions present, develop and progress.
- Difficulties verbalising and communicating their condition further add to these challenges.

'Major' and 'minor' illnesses

- Before considering 'minor' illnesses in children, it is crucial to both appreciate and understand that 'major' childhood illnesses – including life-threatening conditions such as meningococcal disease – rarely present in extremis, but more commonly present with relatively innocent features that can easily be mistaken for minor illnesses.
- Children with advanced major illness (or significant injury) typically have deranged vital signs that are usually readily detected. Earlier in their illness, these children may well have had normal physiology and appeared relatively well – if assessed early in their illness, these children might be misdiagnosed as only having a minor illness.

2. Severity and Outcome

In children with gastroenteritis:

- vomiting usually lasts 1–2 days, and stops within 3 days.
- diarrhoea usually lasts 5–7 days, and stops within 2 weeks.

3. Pathophysiology

- Many viruses, bacteria or other microbes can cause gastroenteritis. However, the most common cause in children is the Rotavirus. This virus can be spread easily through close contact as it is passed out in an infected person's diarrhoea.
- Once exposed to the virus, the incubation period is approximately 48 hours before symptoms start to show. It is thought that almost every child in the UK suffers a rotavirus infection at some point before they turn 5 years old. However, it is most common in children aged 6 months to 2 years old.
- In the UK, 18,000 children each year present at a hospital with a rotavirus infection. Ten per cent will need admission due to dehydration.
- Other causes include bacterial infection such as Escherichia Coli (E. coli), Salmonella and Campylobacter bacteria, that produce toxins that the food we eat. Once exposed to the virus, normally immunity is developed; hence it is uncommon in adults.

Escherichia coli 0157:H7 infection

- *E. coli* 0157:H7 is a bacterium found in the intestines of healthy cattle that can cause serious human infections especially in the young and older people.
- It often leads to bloody diarrhoea and occasionally kidney failure (referred to as haemolytic uraemic syndrome or HUS). Outbreaks have occurred following school farm visits or following consumption of undercooked, contaminated beef. (Beef burgers are notorious as the meat comes from many animals.)
- When *Escherichia coli* 0157:H7 infection is suspected (e.g. contact with a confirmed case), urgent specialist advice must be sought.

4. Assessment

- Gastroenteritis is diagnosed on clinical findings and should be suspected where there is a sudden change in stool consistency to loose or watery stools and/or a sudden onset of vomiting.

History: consider the diagnosis when the child has had:

- recent contact with someone with acute diarrhoea and/or vomiting
- exposure to a known source of enteric infection (farm visits, contaminated water or food – see *Escherichia coli* 0157 infection above)
- recent overseas travel.

Differential diagnosis

Apart from gastroenteritis, alternative diagnoses must be considered when the following features are found and a more experienced paediatric assessment should be sought:

- Fever:
  - temp ≥38°C in child <3 months old
  - temp ≥39°C in child ≥3 months old.
- Shortness of breath or tachypnoea.
- Altered consciousness.
- Neck stiffness.
- Bulging fontanelle in infants.
- Non-blanching rash.
- Blood and/or mucus in stool.

Paediatric Gastroenteritis

- Bilious (green) vomit.
- Severe or localised abdominal pain.
- Abdominal distension or rebound tenderness.
- History/suspicion of poisoning
- History of head injury.
- Appears systemically unwell.

Examination: clinical assessment for dehydration and shock

- Establish whether the child is red, amber or green on the traffic light system in Table 3.105.

Children most at risk of dehydration include:

- Infants of low birth weight (i.e. <2.5 kg).
- Children <1 year, especially those aged <6 months.
- >5 diarrhoeal stools in the previous 24 hours.
- >2 vomits in the previous 24 hours.
- Those who have not been offered/not been able to tolerate oral fluids.
- Breastfed infants who have stopped feeding.
- Malnourished children.

5. Management

Most children with gastroenteritis can be managed at home with oral fluids, although dehydrated children require NG or IV fluid replacement and those in shock may require urgent intravenous fluid resuscitation. Fluid losses can be replaced either via the oral route, via a nasogastric tube or intravenously.

TABLE 3.105 – Traffic Light System for Clinical Dehydration and Shock

	Green **Low Risk**	**Amber** **Intermediate Risk**	**Red** **High Risk**
Activity	• Responds normally to social cues • Content/smiling • Stays awake/awakens quickly • Strong normal cry/not crying	• Aged less than 1 year old • Altered response to social cues • Decreased activity • No smile	• Not responding normally to or no response to social cues • Appears ill to a healthcare professional • Unable to rouse or if roused does not stay awake • Weak, high-pitched or continuous cry
Skin	• Normal skin colour • Normal turgor	• Warm extremities	• Pale/mottled/ashen/blue • Cold extremities • Reduced skin turgor
Respiratory	• Normal breathing		• Tachypnoeic, refer to **Page for Age**
Hydration	• CRT≤ 2 secs • Moist mucous membranes • Normal urine	• CRT 2–3 secs • Dry mucous membranes (except after a drink) • Reduced urine output • Clinically dehydrated, refer to **Table 3.106**	• CRT >3 seconds • Clinically shocked, refer to **Table 3.106**
Pulses/Heart Rate	• Heart rate normal, refer to **Page for Age** • Peripheral pulses normal		• Tachycardic, refer to **Page for Age** • Peripheral pulses weak
Blood Pressure	• Normal, refer to **Page for Age**		• Hypotensive, refer to **Page for Age**
Eyes	• Normal eyes	• Sunken eyes	
Other		• At risk of dehydration	

Paediatric Gastroenteritis

TABLE 3.106 – Symptoms and Signs of Clinical Dehydration and Shock

Increasing severity of dehydration →		
Symptoms **No clinically detectable dehydration**	**Clinically dehydrated**	**Clinically shocked**
Appears well	Appears to be unwell or deteriorating	–
Alert and responsive	Altered responsiveness (e.g. irritable, lethargic)	Decreased level of consciousness
Normal urine output	Decreased urine output. Output often decreased in those with normal hydration as a compensatory mechanism Unreliable in those in nappies with diarrhoea	–
Skin colour unchanged	Skin colour unchanged	Pale or mottled skin
Warm extremities	Warm extremities	Cold extremities
Signs **No clinically detectable dehydration**	**Clinically dehydrated**	**Clinically shocked**
Alert and responsive	Altered responsiveness (e.g., irritable, lethargic)	Decreased level of consciousness
Skin colour unchanged	Skin colour unchanged	Pale or mottled skin
Warm extremities	Warm extremities	Cold extremities
Eyes not sunken	Sunken eyes	–
Moist mucous membranes (except after a drink)	Dry mucous membranes (except for 'mouth breather')	–
Normal heart rate	Tachycardia	Tachycardia
Normal breathing pattern	Tachypnoea	Tachypnoea
gns.Normal peripheral pulses	Normal peripheral pulses	Weak peripheral pulses
Normal capillary refill time	Normal capillary refill time	Prolonged capillary refill time
Normal skin turgor	Reduced skin turgor	–
Normal blood pressure	Normal blood pressure	Hypotension (decompensated shock)

NB Rectal examinations should never be performed in the pre-hospital assessment of the paediatric acute abdomen.

Consider dehydration risk factors when interpreting symptoms and signs.

Within the category of 'clinical dehydration' there is a spectrum of severity indicated by increasingly numerous and more pronounced symptoms and signs.

Within the category of 'clinical shock' one or more of the symptoms and/or signs listed would be expected to be present.

Dashes (–) indicate that these clinical features do not specifically indicate shock but may still be present. Symptoms and signs with red flags may help to identify children at increased risk of progression to shock.

If uncertain, manage as if the child has those red flag symptoms and/or signs.

SECTION 3 Medical Emergencies

Paediatric Gastroenteritis

- Oral (and nasogastric) fluids:
  - oral rehydration salt solutions (ORS) are given orally or via a nasogastric (NG) tube.
  - they should be given as small, frequent volumes.
  - response to oral rehydration must be monitored by regular clinical assessment.
  - Over the counter (OTC) commercially available ORS solutions include Dioralyte, Dioralyte Relief, Electrolade and Rapolyte.
- Intravenous interventions (IV):
  - IV fluids are required when shock is suspected or confirmed and requires urgent hospital transfer.
  - when intravenous access cannot be established, intraosseous fluids may be required.
- Other treatments:
  - antibiotics, antidiarrhoeals and anti-emetics are not routinely used in the management of gastroenteritis.

Consider the outcome for the child identified by clinical assessment

In those children who can be managed in the community:

- fluid intake should be actively encouraged (e.g. milk, water, squash) – under fives need approximately 10 ml of fluid every 10 minutes.
- in infants, breastfeeding and other milk feeds should be continued.
- in older children, fruit juices and fizzy drinks must be stopped.
- oral rehydration salt (ORS) solutions should be offered to those at increased risk of dehydration as supplemental fluids, although toddlers and small children frequently refuse ORS because of the taste!
- if oral intake is insufficient or if the child is persistently vomiting, they should be transferred to secondary care for NG or IV fluid replacement. (Inpatient management often includes a trial of ORS or NG fluids prior to IV fluid replacement.)

Any child found to be **in shock** must be taken to hospital (refer to red flag system, see Table 3.105). They will need additional fluids to not just **maintain** their normal body water but also to replace their fluid losses.

Clinically shocked children require intravenous fluid resuscitation and urgent hospital transfer:

- a rapid 20 ml/kg IV of infusion sodium chloride 0.9% may be given but should not delay hospital transfer.
- clinical response to fluid boluses must be monitored.
- if shock persists, this infusion should be repeated and other causes of shock considered – refer to **0.9% Sodium Chloride**.

Stool samples are not normally required but should be obtained in certain situations:

- Diarrhoea ≥7 days.
- Recent overseas travel.
- Possible septicaemia.
- Blood/mucus in stool.
- Immunocompromise.
- Persisting diagnostic uncertainty.
- Contact the GP or out-of-hours service where this is thought to be necessary.

See Figure 3.33 for a decision support tool.

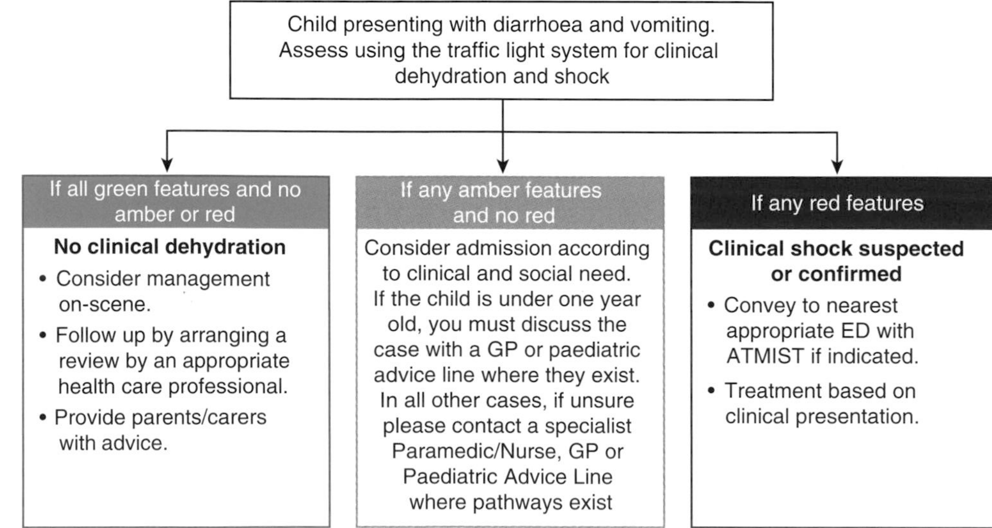

Figure 3.33 – Decision Support Tool for the Assessment of Children with Gastroenteritis

6. Referral Pathway

Children with gastroenteritis that are not dehydrated or shocked can initially be managed at home; if their condition progresses seek an additional medical opinion (GP, OOH, emergency department, Paediatrician) (see 'Safety netting' below).

Hospital transfer is required if:

- Oral intake is insufficient.
- The child is persistently vomiting.
- A child is found to be clinically dehydrated.
- A child is found to be clinically shocked (Emergency Transfer).
- A child requires intravenous therapy.
- Suspicion of an alternative cause for the child's symptoms e.g. UTI, meningococcal disease.
- Additionally some children's social circumstances will dictate additional/continued involvement of healthcare professionals.

Give the following advice for non-dehydrated children managed at home.

Nutritional considerations

During rehydration:

- Continue breastfeeding.
- Give full-strength milk straight away.
- Continue the child's usual solid food.
- Avoid fruit juices and fizzy drinks until the diarrhoea has stopped.
- Consider giving an extra 5 ml/kg of ORS solution after each large watery stool in children at increased risk of dehydration.
- If dehydration recurs after rehydration, restart oral rehydration therapy.

'**Safety Netting**' should be provided for children who do not require referral, giving written information to parents and carers on how to:

- Recognise developing red flag symptoms (refer to Table 3.106), and get immediate help from an appropriate healthcare professional if red flag symptoms develop and, if necessary, make arrangements for follow-up at a specified time and place, that is face-to-face assessment.

Information and advice for parents and carers

Advise parents, carers and children that:

- good handwashing is essential to prevent the spread of gastroenteritis to themselves and other family members; use soap (liquid if possible) in warm, running water followed by careful drying.
- wash hands after going to the toilet (children) or changing nappies (parents/carers) and before preparing, serving or eating food.
- infected children should not share towels.
- children should not go to school or other childcare facility while they have diarrhoea or vomiting caused by gastroenteritis and must stay away for at least 48 hours after the last episode of diarrhoea or vomiting.
- children should not swim in swimming pools for 2 weeks after the last episode of diarrhoea.

KEY POINTS!

Gastroenteritis

- **Gastroenteritis is common, frequently viral and usually self-limiting.**
- **When severe, shock and life-threatening dehydration can occur.**
- **Clinical assessment determines whether dehydration or shock is present (seek Red Flag symptoms and signs).**
- **Non-dehydrated children can frequently be managed at home with oral fluids or ORS.**
- **Failed oral rehydration requires either NG or IV fluid replacement in secondary care.**
- **Shocked children need urgent hospital treatment.**
- **Early meningococcal disease is known to mimic gastroenteritis in small children. An urgent second opinion should be sought if meningococcal disease cannot be excluded.**
- **Provide a 'safety net,' with written information, for all children with gastroenteritis not transferred to hospital.**
- **If uncertain, seek advice from the child's GP, an out-of-hours doctor or specialist advice line where available.**

Pulmonary Embolism

2. Incidence

- Pulmonary embolism is a relatively common cardiovascular condition affecting approximately 21 per 10,000 per annum.

3. Severity and Outcome

- Pulmonary embolism can be life-threatening leading to death in approximately 7–11% of cases; however, treatment is effective if given early.
- Patients with a previous episode(s) of PE are three times more likely to experience a recurrence.

4. Pathophysiology

- The development of a pulmonary embolism occurs when a blood clot (thrombus), comprising red cells, platelets, and fibrin, forms in a vein, subsequently dislodges (embolism) and travels in the circulation. This is known as venous thromboembolism (VTE). If the embolism is small it may be filtered in the pulmonary capillary bed, but if the embolism is large it may occlude pulmonary blood vessels. The development of a VTE can also lead to deep vein thrombosis.
- The haemodynamic problems occur when >30–50% of the pulmonary arterial bed is occluded.
- The probability of a PE can be assessed using a clinical predication tool such as the Wells Criteria (refer to Table 3.109). However, a low probability cannot rule out PE.

5. Assessment and Management

For the assessment and management of pulmonary embolism refer to Table 3.110 and Figure 3.34.

TABLE 3.109 – Wells Criteria for PE

Item		**Score**
Clinical signs and symptoms of DVT (leg swelling and pain with palpation of the deep veins).		3
An alternative diagnosis is less likely than pulmonary embolism.		3
Pulse rate >100 beats per minute.		1.5
Immobilisation or surgery in the previous 4 weeks.		1.5
Previous DVT/pulmonary embolism.		1.5
Haemoptysys.		1
Malignancy (treatment ongoing or within previous 6 months or palliative).		1
Clinical Probability of PE		**Total**
high	>6 points	
moderate	2–6 points	
low	<2 points	

TABLE 3.110 – ASSESSMENT and MANAGEMENT of: Pulmonary Embolism

ASSESSMENT	**MANAGEMENT**
• Assess <C>ABCD	• If any of the following **TIME CRITICAL** features are present: – major **<C>ABCD** problems – extreme breathing difficulty – cyanosis – severe hypoxia (SpO_2) <90% – unresponsive to oxygen. • Start correcting any **<C>ABCD** problems. • Undertake a **TIME CRITICAL** transfer to nearest appropriate receiving hospital. • Continue patient management en-route. • Provide an ATMIST information call.
• Specifically assess:	• Respiratory rate and effort. • Signs and symptoms combined with predisposing factors. • Lower limbs for unilateral swelling; may also be warm and red. • Calf tenderness/pain may be present – extensive leg clots may also lead to femoral tenderness. • Differential diagnoses include pleurisy, pneumothorax or cardiac chest pain.

TABLE 3.110 – ASSESSMENT and MANAGEMENT of: Pulmonary Embolism *(continued)*	
• Position	• Position patient for comfort and ease of respiration – often sitting forwards – but be aware of potential hypotension.
• Respiratory rate	• Measure and record respiratory rate.
• Oxygen saturation	• Monitor the patient's SpO_2, administer oxygen to achieve saturations of >94% if the patient presents as hypoxaemic on air, refer to **Oxygen**.
• Ventilation	• Consider assisted ventilation if indicated – refer to **Airway and Breathing Management**.
• Pulse	• Measure and record pulse.
• Blood pressure and fluids	• Measure and record blood pressure, if required administer fluids, refer to **Intravascular Fluid Therapy in Adults** and **Intravascular Fluid Therapy in Children**.
• Blood glucose	• If appropriate, measure and record blood glucose for hypo/ hyperglycaemia, refer to **Glycaemic Emergencies in Adults and Children**.
• Temperature	• Measure and record temperature.
• NEWS2	• These observations will enable you to calculate a NEWS2 Score, refer to **Sepsis**.
• ECG	• Monitor and record 12-Lead ECG – be aware that the classic S1 Q3 T3 12-lead ECG presentation is often NOT present, even during massive PE. The most common finding is a sinus tachycardia, refer to **Cardiac Rhythm Disturbance**.
• Assess the patient's pain	• Where present, assess the **SOCRATES** of pain and record initial and subsequent pain scores. • Consider analgesia if appropriate, refer to **Pain Management in Adults** and **Pain Management in Children**.
• Documentation	• Complete documentation to include all clinical findings, advice from other clinicians, onward referral and worsening advice given.
• Transfer to further care	• Transfer rapidly to nearest appropriate hospital. • Provide an alert/information call. • Continue patient management en-route.
	ADDITIONAL INFORMATION Whilst there is no specific pre-hospital treatment available, there may be a window of opportunity to manage massive PE before the patient progresses to cardiac arrest. Other in-hospital treatments may be effective including: haemodynamic and respiratory support, thrombolysis, surgical pulmonary embolectomy, percutaneous catheter embolectomy and fragmentation, and anticoagulation.

Pulmonary Embolism

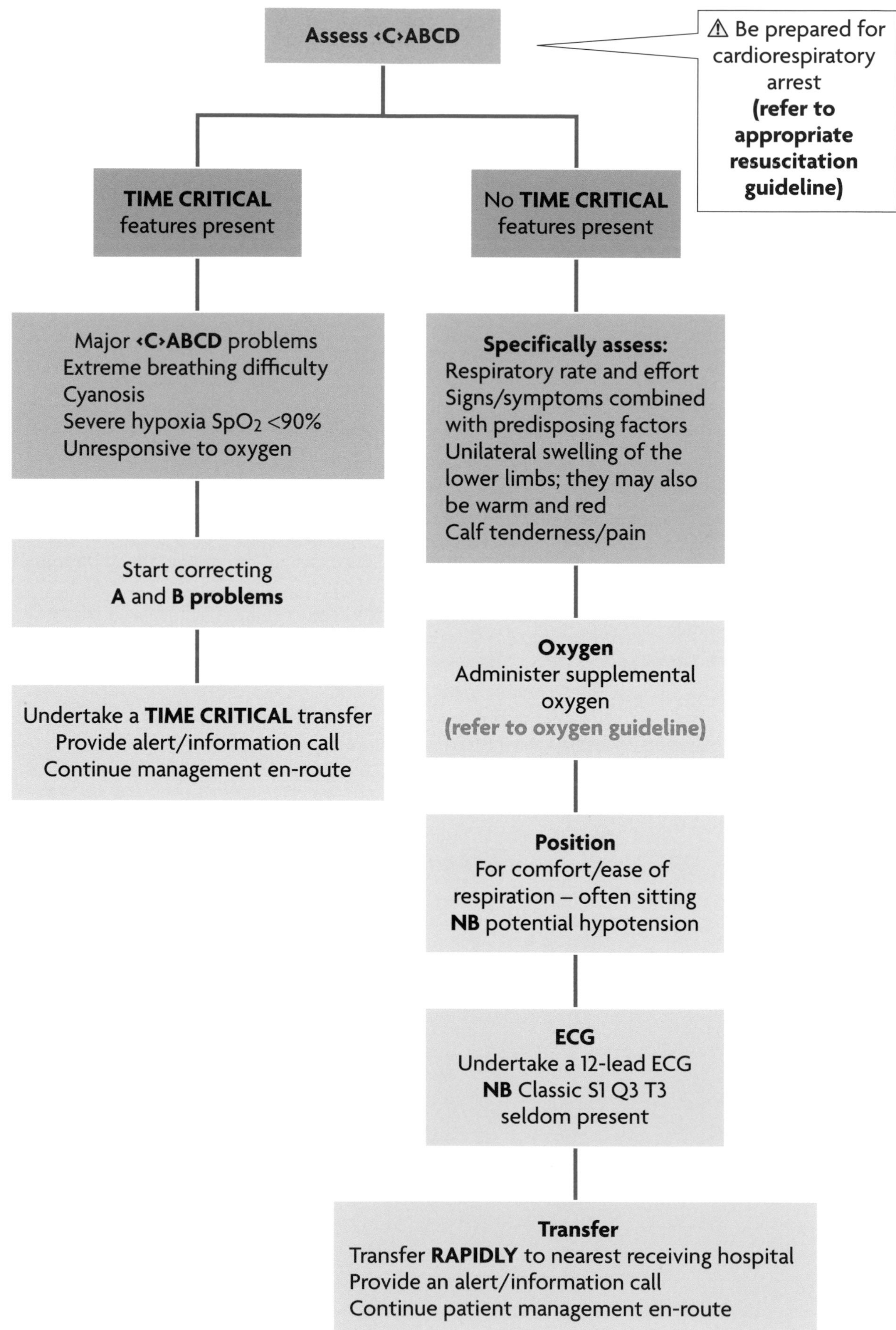

Figure 3.34 – Assessment and management algorithm of pulmonary embolism.

Pulmonary Embolism

KEY POINTS!

Pulmonary Embolism

- **Common symptoms of PE are dyspnoea, tachypnoea, pleuritic pain, apprehension, tachycardia, cough, haemoptysis, leg pain/clinical DVT.**
- **Risk factors may be identifiable from the history.**
- **Ensure ABCD assessment and apply a pulse oximetry monitor early.**
- **Patients may present with unilateral swelling of the lower limbs; they may also be warm and red.**
- **Apply oxygen and if in respiratory distress, transfer to further care as a medical emergency.**

Bibliography

1. Soar J, Perkins GD, Abbas G, Alfonzo A, Barelli A, Bierens JJLM, et al. European Resuscitation Council Guidelines for Resuscitation 2010 Section 8: Cardiac arrest in special circumstances: electrolyte abnormalities, poisoning, drowning, accidental hypothermia, hyperthermia, asthma, anaphylaxis, cardiac surgery, trauma, pregnancy, electrocution. *Resuscitation* 2010, 81(10): 1400–1433.
2. National Institute for Health and Clinical Excellence. *Venous Thromboembolism: Reducing the risk. Reducing the risk of venous thromboembolism (deep vein thrombosis and pulmonary embolism) in patients admitted to hospital* (CG 92). London: NICE, 2010. Available from: https://www.nice.org.uk/guidance/cg92.
3. Torbicki A, Perrier A, Konstantinides S, Agnelli G, Galie N, Pruszczyk P, et al. Guidelines on the diagnosis and management of acute pulmonary embolism. *European Heart Journal* 2008, 29(18): 2276–315.
4. Wells PS, Anderson DR, Rodger M, Ginsberg JS, Kearon C, Gent M. Derivation of a simple clinical model to categorize patients' probability of pulmonary embolism: increasing the models utility with the SimpliRED D-dimer. *Thrombosis and Haemostasis* 2000, 83: 416–20.
5. Cohen AT, Agnelli G, Anderson FA, Arcelus JI, Bergqvist D, Brecht JG, et al. Venous thromboembolism (VTE) in Europe: the number of VTE events and associated morbidity and mortality. *Thrombosis and Haemostasis* 2007, 98(4): 756–64.
6. Farmer RDT, Lawrenson RA, Todd JC, Williams TJ, MacRae KD, Tyrer F, et al. A comparison of the risks of venous thromboembolic disease in association with different combined oral contraceptives. *British Journal of Clinical Pharmacology* 2000, 49 (6): 580–90.
7. Goldhaber SZ, Morrison RB. Pulmonary embolism and deep vein thrombosis. *Circulation* 2002, 106(12): 1436–8.
8. Meyer G, Roy P-M, Gilberg S, Perrier A. Pulmonary embolism. *British Medical Journal* 2010, 340: c1421.
9. White RH. The epidemiology of venous thromboembolism. *Circulation* 2003, 107: I-4–8.
10. Wolf SJ, McCubbin T, Feldhaus KM, Faragher JP, Adcock DM. Prospective validation of Wells Criteria in the evaluation of patients with suspected pulmonary embolism. *Annals of Emergency Medicine* 2004, 44(5): 503–10.

4

Trauma

Trauma Emergencies In Adults – Overview

For references refer to individual trauma guidelines

1. Introduction

- Trauma is a leading cause of death in the UK. The wide range of traumatic injuries encountered in pre-hospital care can present a complex challenge. Research suggests that assessing and managing patients in a systematic way can lead to improved outcomes.
- This overview will outline the process of assessment and management of trauma patients. This guideline supports the following related guidelines:
  - abdominal trauma
  - head trauma
  - limb trauma
  - spinal injury and spinal cord injury
  - major pelvic trauma
  - thoracic trauma
  - trauma in pregnancy
  - traumatic cardiac arrest
  - airway management
  - burns and scalds
  - electrical injuries
  - fluid therapy
  - oxygen therapy
  - pain management.

This guideline uses mechanism of injury (MOI) and primary survey as the basis of care for all trauma patients.

2. Incidence

- In England it is estimated that there are approximately 20,000 cases of major trauma annually. Road traffic collisions (RTC) are the most common cause.

3. Severity and Outcome

- In England major trauma accounts for approximately 5,400 deaths each year, with many more cases leading to significant short- and long-term morbidity. In Scotland (1992–2002) there were 5,847 deaths resulting from trauma. Major trauma is the leading cause of death in patients under 45 years of age.

4. Incident Management

- Overall control of the incident allows paramedics to concentrate on patient assessment and management and it is recommended that a model, such as SCENE, is used to assess the initial trauma scene so that it can be managed effectively (refer to Table 4.1).

5. Patient Assessment

A primary survey should be undertaken for **ALL** patients as this will rapidly identify patients with actual or potential **TIME CRITICAL** injuries (refer to Table 4.3).

A secondary survey is a more thorough 'head-to-toe' assessment of the patient. It should be undertaken following completion of the primary survey, where time permits. The secondary survey will usually be undertaken during transfer to further care; however, in some patients with time critical trauma, it may not be possible to undertake the secondary survey before arrival at further care (refer to Table 4.4).

5.1 Primary survey

- The primary survey should take no more than 60–90 seconds and follow the **<C>ABCDE** approach. Document the vital signs and the time they were taken.

TABLE 4.1 – SCENE	
S	**Safety** Perform a dynamic risk assessment: are there any dangers now or will there be any that become apparent during the incident? This needs to be continually re-assessed throughout the incident. Appropriate personal protective equipment should be utilised according to local guidelines.
C	**Cause including MOI** Establish the events leading up to the incident. Is this consistent with your findings?
E	**Environment** Are there any environmental factors that need to be taken into consideration? These can include problems with access or egress, weather conditions or time of day.
N	**Number of patients** Establish exactly how many patients there are during the initial assessment of the scene.
E	**Extra resources needed** Additional resources should be mobilised now. These can include additional ambulances, helicopter or senior medical support. Liaise with the major trauma advisor according to local protocols.

Trauma Emergencies in Adults – Overview

- Consider mechanism of injury and the possible injury patterns that may result; but be aware that mechanism alone cannot predict or exclude injury and physiological signs should be utilised as well.
- Assessment and management should proceed in a '**stepwise**' manner and life-threatening injuries should be managed as they are encountered, i.e. do not move onto breathing and circulation until the airway is secured. Every time an intervention has been carried out, re-assess the patient.
- As soon as a life-threatening injury is identified and managed, it is recommended that transport should be immediately instigated to the appropriate trauma facility according to local procedures.
- If immediate transfer is not possible, consider mobilising senior clinical support if not already done during the SCENE assessment.

TABLE 4.2 – ATMIST

A	**A**ge
T	**T**ime of incident
M	**M**echanism
I	**I**njuries
S	**S**igns and symptoms
T	**T**reatment given/immediate needs

MANAGEMENT OVERVIEW

If the patient has a life-threatening condition start immediate transfer to an appropriate trauma facility according to local procedures with treatment undertaken en-route to hospital.

- Provide an alert/information call.
- Continue patient re-assessment and management.
- If a patient requires IV fluids and fulfils the criteria in steps 1 or 2 of the Pre-Hospital Major Trauma Triage Tool (Appendix) then they should receive a bolus of tranexamic acid if available (refer to **Tranexamic Acid**).
- **Pain management** – if analgesia is indicated refer to **Pain Management in Adults**.
- Hand-over – it is recommended that the patient is handed over to receiving clinicians using the ATMIST format (refer to Table 4.2).

If the patient is **NON-TIME CRITICAL** undertake a secondary survey (refer to Table 4.4).

5.2 Secondary survey

- A secondary survey should only commence after the primary survey has been completed and in critical patients only during transport.
- The secondary survey is a more thorough 'head-to-toe' survey of the patient; however, it is important to monitor the patient's vital signs during the survey.

TABLE 4.3 – ASSESSMENT and MANAGEMENT of: Trauma Emergencies

• All stages should be considered but some may be omitted if not considered appropriate. **• To reduce clot disruption avoid unnecessary movements.** **• When available administer tranexamic acid to all patients who require TIME CRITICAL transfer, except isolated head injuries.**		**At each stage consider the need for:** **• TIME CRITICAL – transfer to nearest appropriate hospital as per local trauma care pathway.** **• Early senior clinical support.**
STAGE	**ASSESSMENT**	**MANAGEMENT**
<C>	**CATASTROPHIC HAEMORRHAGE** – assess for the presence of **LIFE-THREATENING EXTERNAL BLEEDING**	Follow the management in Figure 4.1 and 4.2.
A	**AIRWAY** – assess the airway and **AT ALL TIMES** consider C-spine injury and the need to immobilise (refer to **Spinal Injury and Spinal Cord Injury**). **Look for** obvious obstructions (e.g. teeth/dentures, foreign bodies, vomit, blood, trauma, soot/burns/oedema in burn patients). **Listen for** noisy airflow (e.g. snoring, gurgling or no airflow). **Feel for** air movement.	Correct any airway problems immediately by: • Jaw thrust, chin lift (no neck extension). • Suction (if appropriate). • Nasopharyngeal airway. • Oropharyngeal airway. • Laryngeal mask airway (if appropriate). • Endotracheal intubation (only if waveform capnography available). • Needle cricothyroidotomy.

(continued)

SECTION 4 Trauma

Trauma Emergencies in Adults – Overview

TABLE 4.3 – ASSESSMENT and MANAGEMENT of: Trauma Emergencies *(continued)*

B	Assess rate, depth and quality of respiration Grade breathing 1–5: 1 patient not breathing 2 slow <12 per min 3 normal 12–20 but check depth 4 fast 20–30 observe very closely 5 very fast >30 Feel for depth and equality of chest movement, any instability of chest wall. Look for obvious chest injuries, wounds, bruising or flail segment. Auscultate lung fields assessing air entry on each side. Percuss the chest wall checking the pitch of the percussion note. In addition assess the chest and neck for the following using the mnemonic **TWELVE**: ● **T**racheal deviation ● **W**ounds, bruising or swelling ● **E**mphysema (surgical) ● **L**aryngeal crepitus ● **V**enous engorgement ● **E**xcluding open/tension pneumothorax, flail segment, massive haemothorax.	Administer 100% O_2 in all patients with critical trauma to target O_2 sats of 94–98%, even if there are risk factors such as COPD. ● Breathing graded at 1,2 should receive O_2 via BVM as should grade 5 if clinically appropriate. ● Breathing graded at 3,4 should receive supplemental 100% O_2 but be monitored very closely. ● Apply non-occlusive dressing to sucking chest wounds (refer to **Thoracic Trauma**). ● Decompress a tension pneumothorax (refer to **Thoracic Trauma**). ● Flail segments should not be splinted (refer to **Thoracic Trauma**). **NB Restraint (POSITIONAL) asphyxia** – If the patient is required to be physically restrained (e.g. by police officers) in order to prevent them injuring themselves or others, or for the purpose of being detained under the Mental Health Act, then it is paramount that the method of restraint allows both for a patent airway and adequate respiratory volume. **Under these circumstances it is essential to ensure that the patient's airway and breathing are adequate at all times.**
C	If massive external haemorrhage was controlled at start of assessment re-assess this now. Assess for radial and carotid pulses noting rate, rhythm and volume, assess central and peripheral capillary refill time, note skin colour, texture and temperature. Remain alert to the possibility of internal bleeding and assess for signs of blood loss in five places (blood on the floor and four more): 1 External 2 Chest (already done during breathing assessment) 3 Abdomen by palpation and observation of bruising or external marks 4 Pelvis – do not manipulate the pelvis – MOI may suggest a fracture 5 Long bones – assess for but do not be distracted by limb trauma.	Follow the management for haemorrhage control in Figures 4.1 and 4.2. Consider splinting: ● In the critical patient, **long bone fractures** should be splinted en-route to the trauma facility. ● **Pelvic fractures** should be stabilised at the earliest possible opportunity, preferably before the patient is moved – refer to **Major Pelvic Trauma**. **Fluid therapy** If fluid replacement is indicated refer to **Intravascular Fluid Therapy in Adults**. **TRANEXAMIC ACID** If a patient requires IV fluids and fulfils the criteria in steps 1 or 2 of the Pre-Hospital Major Trauma Triage Tool (Appendix) then they should receive a bolus of tranexamic acid (refer to **Tranexamic Acid**). In cases of internal or uncontrolled haemorrhage undertake a **TIME CRITICAL** transfer to appropriate hospital according to local procedures.

Trauma Emergencies in Adults – Overview

TABLE 4.3 – ASSESSMENT and MANAGEMENT of: Trauma Emergencies *(continued)*		
	Consider hypovolaemic shock but be aware that blood loss of 1000–1500 ml is required before classical signs start to appear. Signs of hypovolaemic shock include pallor, cool peripheries, anxiety and abnormal behaviour, increased respiratory rate and tachycardia. Signs of shock also appear much later in certain patient groups (e.g. pregnant women, patients on beta-blockers and the physically fit). There may well be little evidence of shock.	To minimise clot disruption avoid unnecessary movement in victims of blunt trauma: ● Log roll should be avoided wherever possible. ● Patients should be lifted from the ground using a scoop (bivalve) stretcher. ● Once on a scoop (bivalve) stretcher patients should be transported on it. ● A long spinal board is an extrication device and should not be used unless required – refer to **Spinal Injury and Spinal Cord Injury**. ● A patient with penetrating trauma who has no neurology and no possibility of direct trauma to the spinal column should NOT be immobilised.
D	**Disability** Obtain a full GCS (refer to Table 4.5) for the patient as this is required for the Pre-Hospital Major Trauma Triage Tool (Appendix).	
	Assess and note pupil size, equality and response to light.	
	Altered mental status.	Check blood glucose level to rule out hypo- or hyperglycaemia as the cause – refer to **Glycaemic Emergencies in Adults and Children**.
E	**EXPOSURE and ENVIRONMENT** At this stage further monitoring may be applied.	
	Exposure.	Ensure patient does not suffer from exposure to cold/wet conditions.
	Trapped patient.	Consider mobilising early senior clinical support.

TABLE 4.4 – Secondary Survey
ASSESSMENT
Head ● Re-assess airway. ● Check skin colour and temperature. ● Palpate for bruising/fractures. ● Check pupil size and reactivity. ● Examine for loss of cerebrospinal fluid. ● Establish Glasgow Coma Scale (refer to Table 4.5). ● Assess for other signs of basal skull fracture. **NB** For further information refer to **Head Injury**.
Neck ● The collar will need to be loosened for proper examination of the neck. ● Re-assess for signs of life-threatening injury using the mnemonic **TWELVE:** – **T**racheal deviation – **W**ounds, bruising or swelling – **E**mphysema (surgical)

(continued)

Trauma Emergencies in Adults – Overview

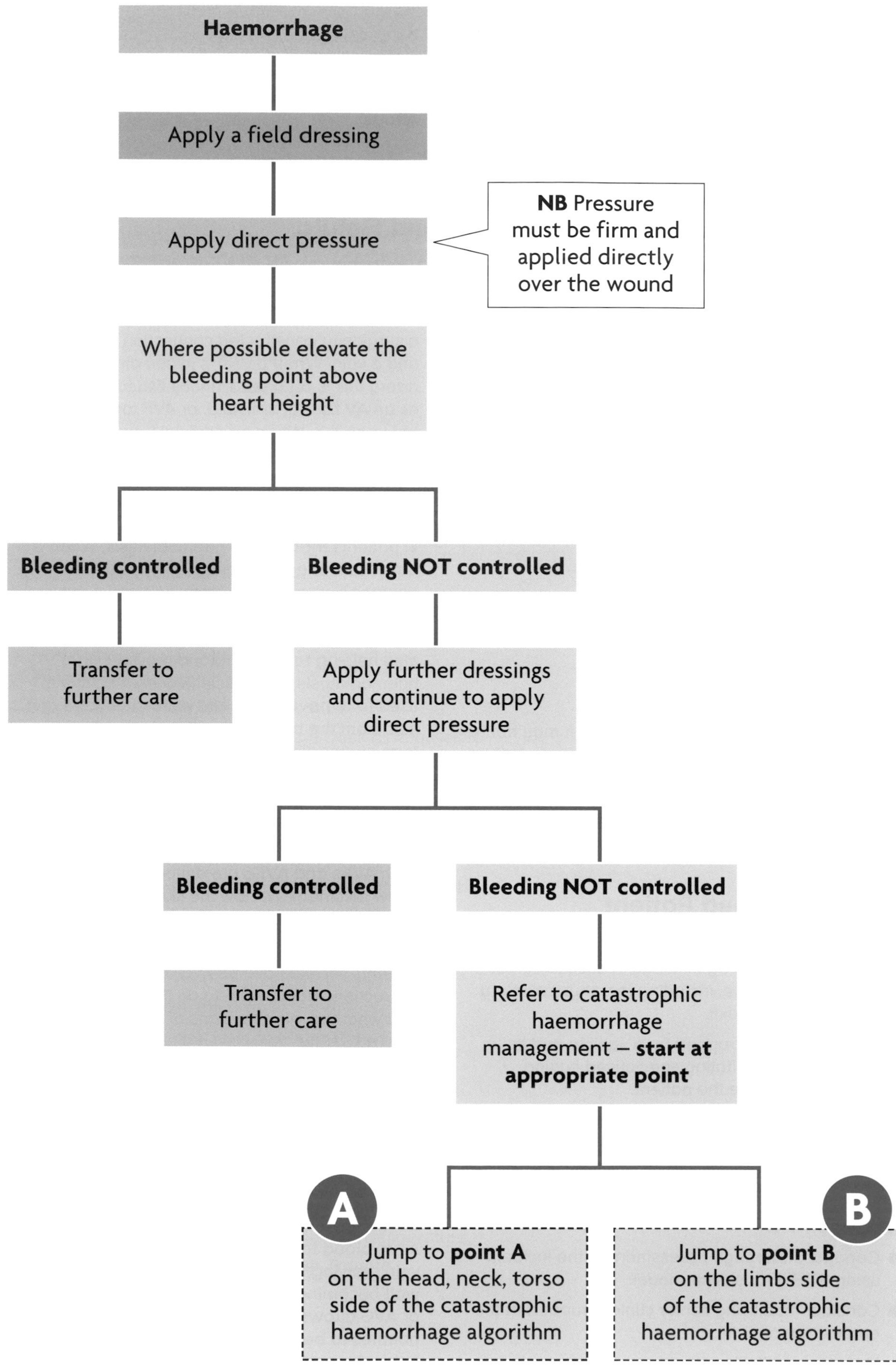
Haemorrhage
Apply a field dressing
Apply direct pressure
NB Pressure must be firm and applied directly over the wound
Where possible elevate the bleeding point above heart height
Bleeding controlled
Bleeding NOT controlled
Transfer to further care
Apply further dressings and continue to apply direct pressure
Bleeding controlled
Bleeding NOT controlled
Transfer to further care
Refer to catastrophic haemorrhage management – start at appropriate point
A
B
Jump to point A on the head, neck, torso side of the catastrophic haemorrhage algorithm
Jump to point B on the limbs side of the catastrophic haemorrhage algorithm

Figure 4.1 – The management of haemorrhage algorithm.

Trauma Emergencies in Adults – Overview

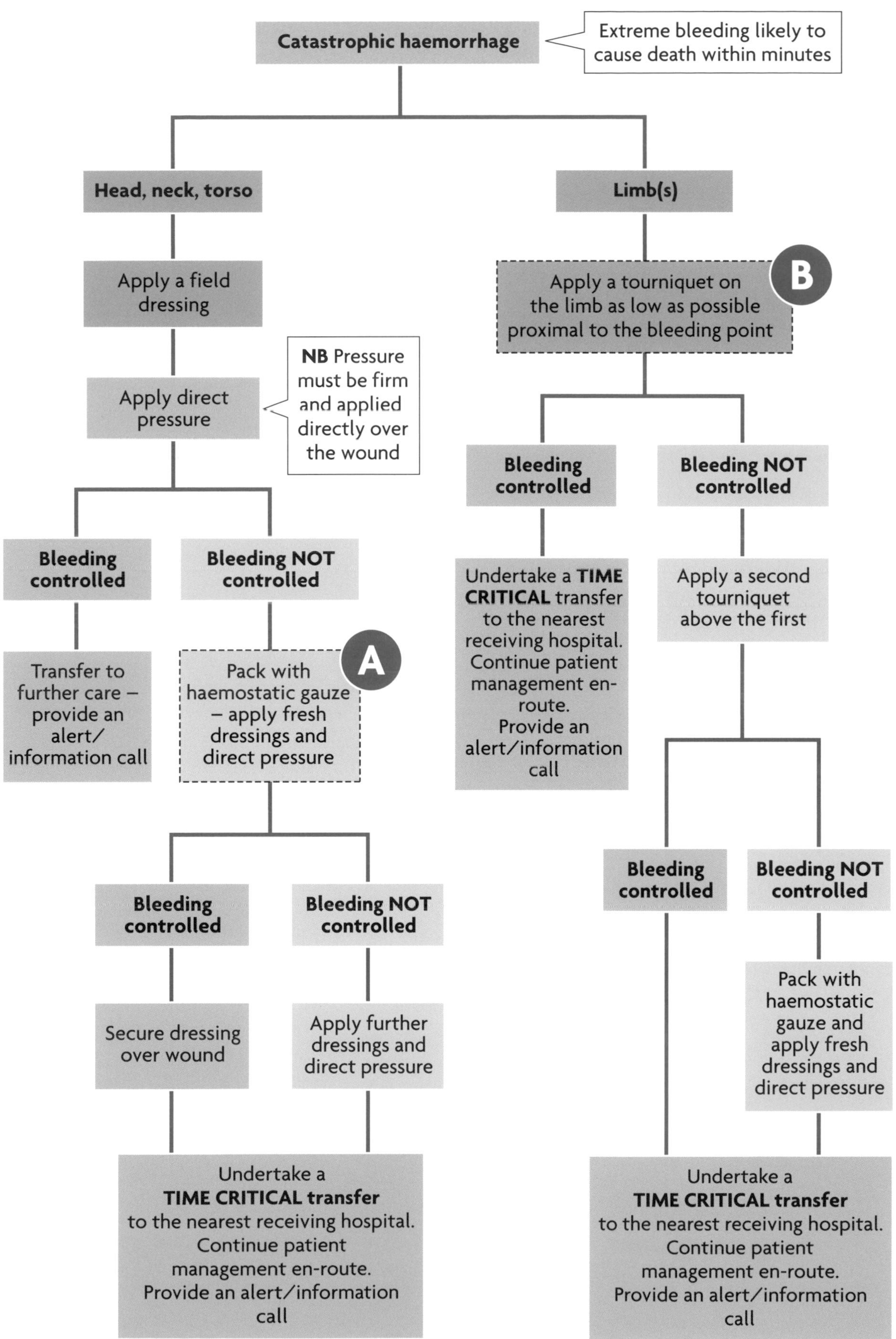

Catastrophic haemorrhage
Extreme bleeding likely to cause death within minutes
Head, neck, torso
Limb(s)
Apply a field dressing
Apply direct pressure
NB Pressure must be firm and applied directly over the wound
Bleeding controlled
Bleeding NOT controlled
Transfer to further care – provide an alert/information call
A
Pack with haemostatic gauze – apply fresh dressings and direct pressure
Bleeding controlled
Bleeding NOT controlled
Secure dressing over wound
Apply further dressings and direct pressure
Undertake a TIME CRITICAL transfer to the nearest receiving hospital. Continue patient management en-route. Provide an alert/information call
B
Apply a tourniquet on the limb as low as possible proximal to the bleeding point
Bleeding controlled
Bleeding NOT controlled
Undertake a TIME CRITICAL transfer to the nearest receiving hospital. Continue patient management en-route. Provide an alert/information call
Apply a second tourniquet above the first
Bleeding controlled
Bleeding NOT controlled
Pack with haemostatic gauze and apply fresh dressings and direct pressure
Undertake a TIME CRITICAL transfer to the nearest receiving hospital. Continue patient management en-route. Provide an alert/information call
SECTION 4 Trauma

Figure 4.2 – The management of catastrophic haemorrhage algorithm.

7.3 Why may an AV fistula haemorrhage?

- Over time, repeated needling of the AVF or AVG can result in weakening or thinning of the skin over them and/or the wall of the AVF or AVG itself. The AVF or AVG can also become infected as a result of the repeated needling. These can lead to scabs, ulcers and/or false aneurysms forming. Weakness of the fistula wall can lead to tear or rupture resulting in arterial blood at high pressure spurting from the opening. If no action is taken, the person can die from loss of blood very quickly.

7.4 Complications and increased risks of bleeding associated with AV fistulas and AV grafts

1. Infection of the AV fistula/graft site – indicated by redness or painful swelling, discharge or pus. This increases the risk of the fistula/graft rupturing and the patient bleeding catastrophically. An infected fistula/graft needs urgent treatment in hospital.
2. Damage or injury to the AV fistula/graft due to trauma or infection – anything which damages the fistula/graft (direct blow to the AV fistula/graft), increased pressure in the arm (e.g. lying on the arm when asleep or wearing a tight shirt above the fistula) or infection can cause serious damage. If the AV fistula/graft is punctured or cut it is likely to bleed very heavily.
3. Alteration in the fistula/graft, skin or arm – e.g. damaged skin, any abnormal lumps, a swollen or painful area, or altered sensation in the arm may indicate a serious problem with the AV fistula/graft.
4. Any non-healing scab/wound over the AV fistula/graft.
5. Prolonged bleeding – post haemodialysis or bleeding in between dialysis sessions.
6. Aneurysms that are increasing in size – either at cannulation sites or elsewhere.
7. Shiny, thin skin over the fistula/graft – particularly over aneurysms.
8. Other skin integrity issues in the vicinity of the AV fistula/graft.

7.5 Management of AV fistulas and AV grafts haemorrhage

- Management should be the same as for any external bleeding by applying direct pressure.
- The quickest and simplest first aid measure to control bleeding from an AVG or AVF is to use an inverted plastic bottle top (the concave/inside part of the bottle top applied to the skin) to seal it – sterility is not an issue in an emergency. Direct pressure can also be applied with the limb elevated directly over the artery feeding the fistula. The objective is to stop the bleeding, not to save the fistula/graft.
- Using tourniquets is not generally recommended as incorrect placement can exacerbate the bleeding significantly and therefore should only be used if other options have been unsuccessful. If used, a tourniquet should be positioned ‘above’ the bleeding site and as near to the axilla as possible i.e. between the heart and the bleeding site. The intention is to occlude the arterial blood flow which may be challenging due to the calcification of vessels. If applying a tourniquet, failure to occlude arterial flow can result in a venous tourniquet exacerbating haemorrhage.
- The high arterial pressure means that bleeding is profuse and therefore the length of time compression will be required will be longer than for other types of bleed.
- If available, an Olaes dressing is a suitable option, utilising the plastic cup component of the dressing (refer to Figure 4.4). The cup should be applied directly to the skin over the bleeding point and secured in place using the elasticated dressing to seal and tamponade the bleeding.

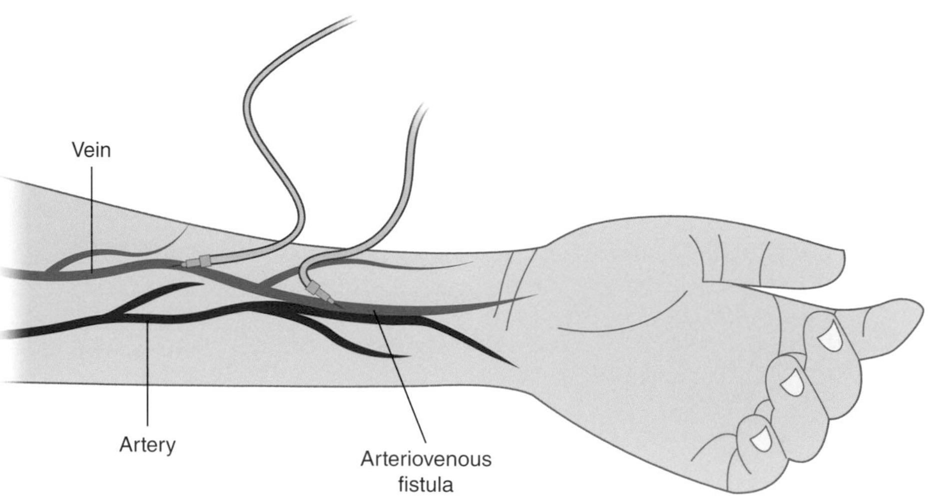

Figure 4.3 – AV fistula site.

Trauma Emergencies in Adults – Overview

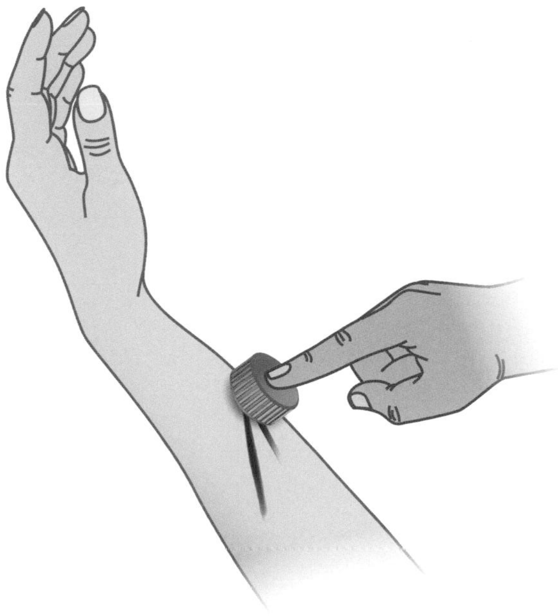

Figure 4.4 – AV fistula bleed.

It may be easiest to do this having removed the gauze from the dressing pocket of the dressing to debulk it.

- Do NOT use multiple ambulance absorbent dressings as these do not apply adequate pressure and therefore do not arrest the haemorrhage.
- Advice to first aiders or carers may have been given to control the bleeding using a plastic bottle top (concave/inside of bottle top in contact with the skin) and held in position with a secure dressing prior to the arrival of the ambulance service. If this is controlling the haemorrhage, do not take down the bottle top dressing as catastrophic bleeding may recur.
- All patients experiencing a spontaneous bleed from their AV fistula/graft (however minor) and/or felt to be at immediate risk of a bleed or further bleed MUST be conveyed to hospital for review.
- Consider direct admission to the regional renal transplant centre as per locally agreed care pathways.
- Most patients should be admitted for a period of observation.
- These patients should be discussed with and ideally seen by a surgeon who specialises in vascular access or, if unavailable, the renal team before they leave hospital.
- Those whose bleeding has been severe and uncontrolled will require surgical intervention as an emergency and lifesaving procedure.

7.6 Other considerations

- If you need to cannulate a patient with an AV fistula/graft never cannulate the fistula or the arm or limb it is sited on.
- Do not record a blood pressure on the arm with the fistula/graft.
- Patients with a fistula/graft may be prescribed anticoagulant medications during their dialysis treatment, which will increase the bleeding time.

KEY POINTS!

Trauma Emergencies Overview (Adults)

- **Overall assessment of safety is of prime importance: self, scene, casualties.**
- **The primary survey forms the basis of patient assessment, with due consideration for C-spine immobilisation.**
- **Arrest of external haemorrhage can be life saving.**
- **Consider seeking senior clinical advice/support at the earliest opportunity.**
- **All patients with a spontaneous bleed from their AV fistula/graft must be conveyed to hospital.**

Appendix – The NHS Clinical Advisory Group on Trauma

Pre-Hospital Major Trauma Triage Tool >12 years

The Major Trauma Triage Tool presented below is based on the American College of Surgeons Guidelines for Field Triage 2006 with minor modifications. In Step 2 'Flail chest' has been changed to 'Chest injury with altered physiology' and 'Paralysis' has been changed to 'Sensory or motor deficit (new onset following trauma)'. In Step 3 'feet' have been changed to 'metres' for distance fallen. 'Entrapment' has been added. In Step 4 Burns are considered special if they are facial, circumferential or 20% body surface area (BSA).

Entry criteria for use of triage is a judgement that the patient may have suffered significant trauma.

Step 1

Physiological:

- GCS < 14 (refer to Table 4.5)
- SBP < 90 mmHg.

SECTION 4 Trauma

Trauma Emergencies in Adults – Overview

If either of the above factors is present, activate a Major Trauma Alert and definitive care to be from Major Trauma Centre; otherwise proceed to Step 2.

Step 2

Anatomical:

- Penetrating to head/neck/torso/limbs proximal to elbow/knee.
- Chest injury with altered physiology.
- Two proximal long bone fractures.
- Crushed/degloved/mangled extremity.
- Amputation proximal to wrist/ankle.
- Pelvic fractures.
- Open or depressed skull fracture.
- Sensory or motor deficit (new onset following trauma).

If any of the above factors are present activate a Major Trauma Alert and definitive care to be from Major Trauma Centre; otherwise proceed to Step 3.

Step 3

Mechanism:

- Falls:
  - Fall > 6 m/2 storeys in adult
  - Fall > 3 m/2 times height in child.
- Motor vehicles:
  - Intrusion > 30 cm occupant site
  - Ejection partial/complete
  - Death in same passenger compartment
  - Vehicle telemetry data consistent with high risk of injury.
- Pedestrian/cyclist versus motor vehicle thrown/run over/with significant (> 20 mph) impact.
- Motorcycle crash > 20 mph.
- Entrapment.

If any of the above factors are present consider a Major Trauma Alert with further assessment by either Trauma Unit or Major Trauma Centre; otherwise proceed to Step 4.

Step 4

- Special considerations that should lower the threshold for a Trauma Alert:
  - Older adults (age > 55)
  - Children (to Paediatric Trauma Centre)
  - Anticoagulation/bleeding disorders
  - Burns: full thickness facial, circumferential or 20% body surface area (BSA)
  - Time-sensitive extremity injury
  - Dialysis-dependent renal disease
  - Pregnancy > 20 weeks
  - EMS provider judgement.

If any of the above factors are present consider a Major Trauma Alert with further assessment by either Trauma Unit or Major Trauma Centre.

Acknowledgements

We would like to gratefully acknowledge the contribution of John JM Black and Paul Gibbs to this JRCALC guideline.

Further Reading

British Renal Society. Vascular Access Special Interest Group – A multi professional initiative. Kidney Care. 2016, 1(3): 150–152.

Ellingson KD, Palekar RS, Lucero CA et al. Vascular hemorrhages contribute to deaths among hemodialysis patients. Kidney Int. 2012, 82(6): 686–692.

Inston N, Mistry H, Gilbert J, et al. Aneurysms in vascular access: State of the art and future developments. J Vasc Access. 2017, 18(6): 464–472.

Trauma Emergencies in Children – Overview

1. Introduction

- Paediatric trauma is managed following the standard **<C>ABCDE** approach to trauma, taking into account differences in the child's anatomy, relative size and physiological response to injury. These differences are addressed below.

2. Incidence

- 700 children die as a result of accidents in England and Wales each year.
- 50% of child trauma deaths occur in motor vehicle incidents. Children travelling by car should legally be restrained but this law is not always followed and many deaths and serious injuries occur following vehicular ejection. Additionally, child deaths from cycle and pedestrian incidents are also very common.
- 30% of child trauma deaths occur at home with burns and falls being the leading causes.
- Child death reviews often identify circumstances that could potentially have been avoided had injury prevention methods been rigorously applied.

3. Assessment: The Basic Trauma Approach

3.1 SCENE

Overall control of the incident allows paramedics to concentrate on patient assessment and management and it is recommended that a model, such as SCENE, is used to assess the initial trauma scene so that it can be managed effectively (see below).

3.2 Primary survey

- Catastrophic haemorrhage (refer to Figure 4.6).
- Airway with cervical spine control (refer to **Spinal Injury and Spinal Cord Injury**).
- Breathing.
- Circulation.
- Disability.
- Exposure.

The management of a child suffering a traumatic injury requires a careful approach, with an emphasis on explanation, reassurance and honesty. Trust of the carer by the child makes management much easier.

If possible, it is helpful to keep the child's parents/carers close by for reassurance, although their distress can exacerbate that of the child.

3.3 Stepwise primary survey assessment

As for all trauma care, a systematic approach, managing problems as they are encountered before moving on is required.

4. Catastrophic Haemorrhage

Catastrophic blood loss must be arrested immediately (refer to catastrophic haemorrhage control, Figure 4.6).

5. Airway

In small children, the relatively large occiput tends to flex the head forward. In order to return the head to the neutral position it may be necessary to insert a small amount of padding under the shoulders.

S	**Safety** Risk assessment. Perform a dynamic risk assessment. Are there any dangers now or will there be any that become apparent during the incident? This needs to be continually re-assessed throughout the incident. Appropriate personal protective equipment should be utilised according to local protocols.
C	**Cause including MOI** Establish the events leading up to the incident. Is this consistent with your findings? Read the scene/wreckage looking for evidence that children were involved (e.g. toys or child seats). These may provide a clue that a child has been ejected from the vehicle or wandered off from the scene but may still require medical attention or other care. Ask if children were involved.
E	**Environment** Are there any environmental factors that need to be taken into consideration? These can include problems with access or egress, weather conditions or time of day.
N	**Number of patients** Establish exactly how many patients there are during the initial assessment of the scene
E	**Extra resources needed** Additional resources should be mobilised now. These can include additional ambulances, helicopter or senior medical support. Liaise with the major trauma advisor according to local protocols.

Trauma Emergencies in Children – Overview

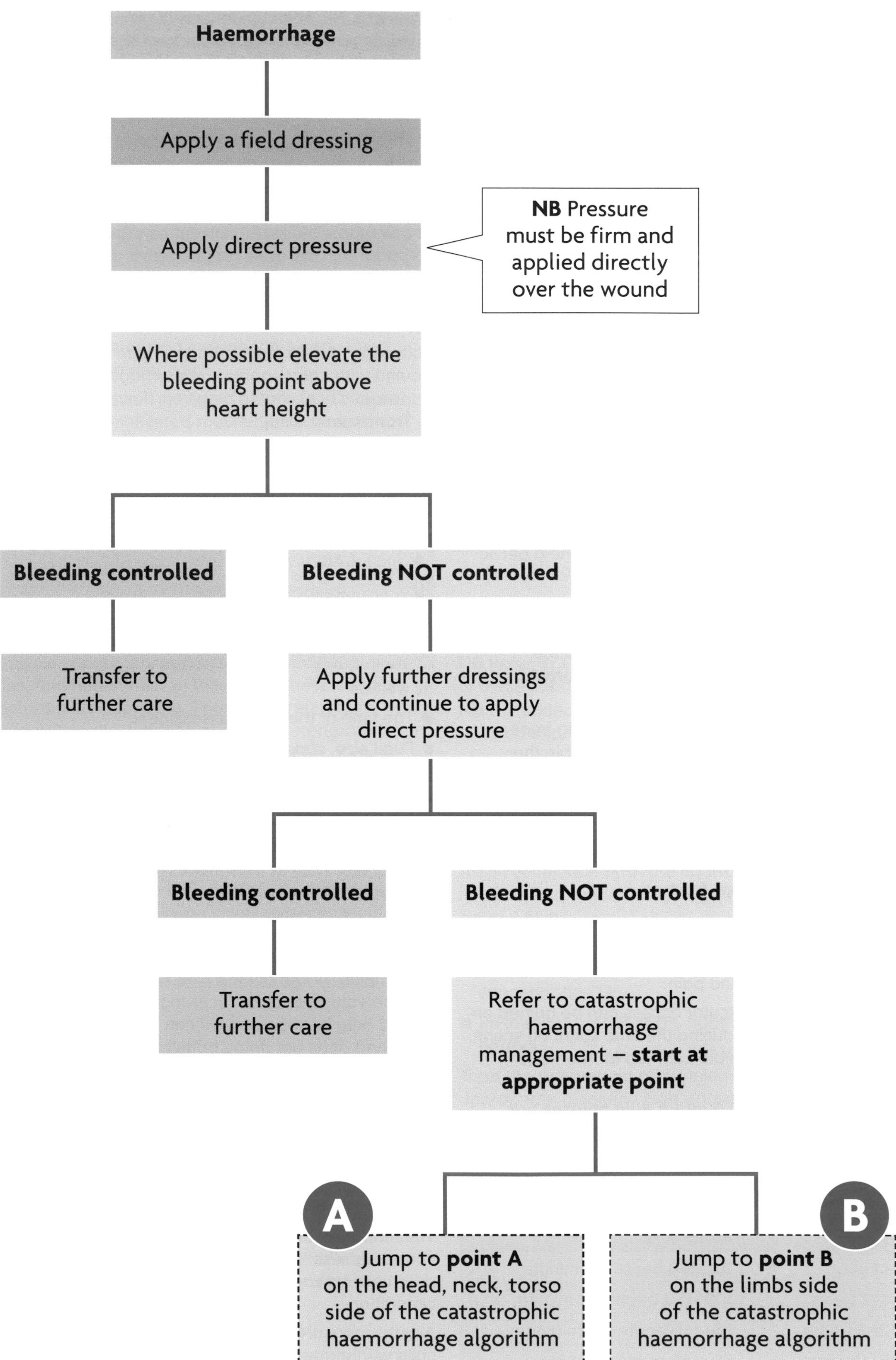

Haemorrhage
Apply a field dressing
Apply direct pressure
NB Pressure must be firm and applied directly over the wound
Where possible elevate the bleeding point above heart height
Bleeding controlled
Bleeding NOT controlled
Transfer to further care
Apply further dressings and continue to apply direct pressure
Bleeding controlled
Bleeding NOT controlled
Transfer to further care
Refer to catastrophic haemorrhage management – **start at appropriate point**
A
B
Jump to **point A** on the head, neck, torso side of the catastrophic haemorrhage algorithm
Jump to **point B** on the limbs side of the catastrophic haemorrhage algorithm

Figure 4.5 – The management of haemorrhage algorithm.

Trauma Emergencies in Children – Overview

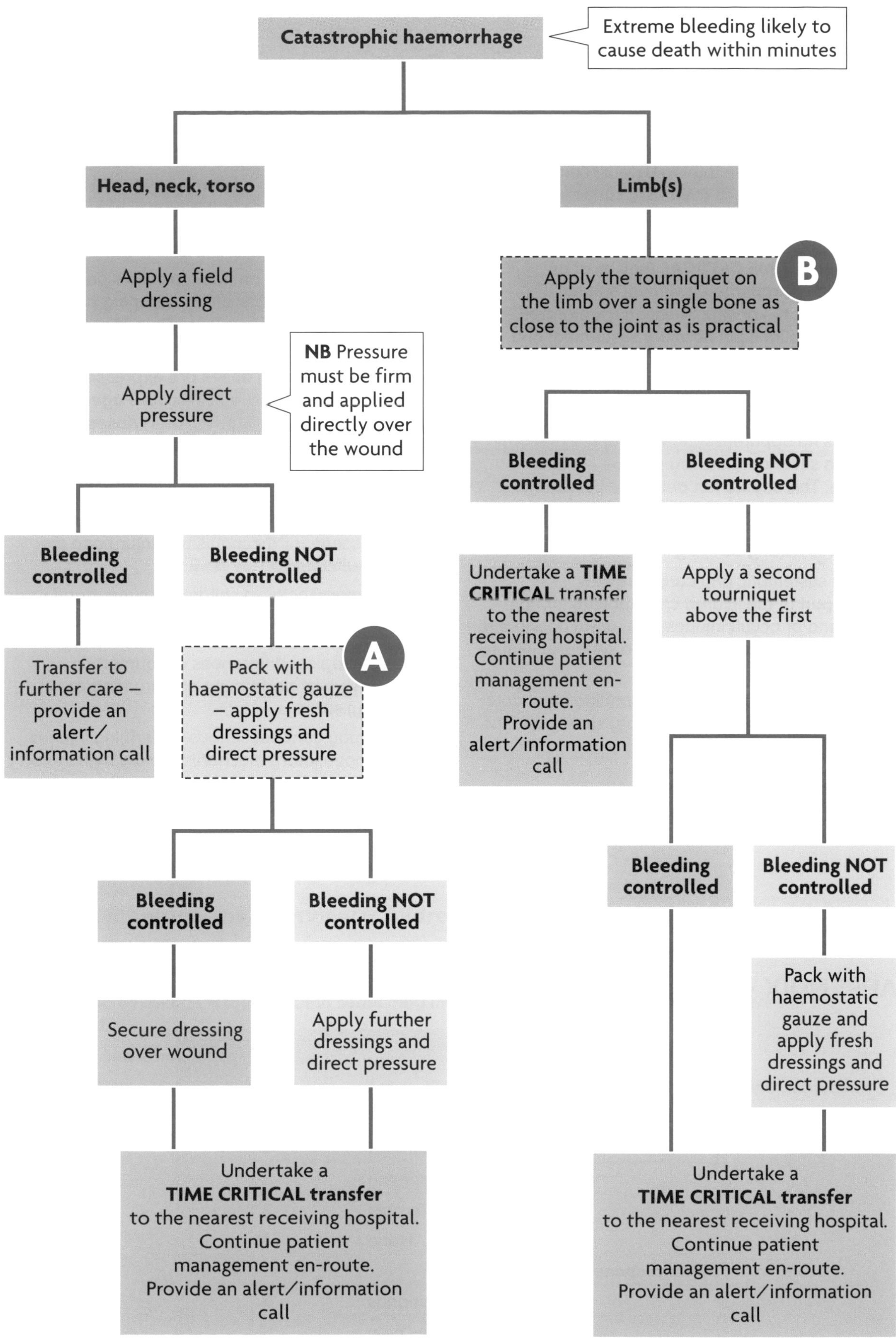
Catastrophic haemorrhage
Extreme bleeding likely to cause death within minutes
Head, neck, torso
Limb(s)
Apply a field dressing
Apply direct pressure
NB Pressure must be firm and applied directly over the wound
Bleeding controlled
Bleeding NOT controlled
Transfer to further care – provide an alert/ information call
Pack with haemostatic gauze – apply fresh dressings and direct pressure
A
Bleeding controlled
Bleeding NOT controlled
Secure dressing over wound
Apply further dressings and direct pressure
Undertake a TIME CRITICAL transfer to the nearest receiving hospital. Continue patient management en-route. Provide an alert/information call
Apply the tourniquet on the limb over a single bone as close to the joint as is practical
B
Bleeding controlled
Bleeding NOT controlled
Undertake a TIME CRITICAL transfer to the nearest receiving hospital. Continue patient management en-route. Provide an alert/information call
Apply a second tourniquet above the first
Bleeding controlled
Bleeding NOT controlled
Pack with haemostatic gauze and apply fresh dressings and direct pressure
Undertake a TIME CRITICAL transfer to the nearest receiving hospital. Continue patient management en-route. Provide an alert/information call

Figure 4.6 – The management of catastrophic haemorrhage algorithm.

Abdominal Trauma

1. Introduction

- Trauma to the abdomen can be extremely difficult to assess even in a hospital setting. In the field, identifying which abdominal structure(s) has been injured is less important than identifying that abdominal trauma itself has occurred.
- It is therefore, of major importance to note abnormal signs associated with blood loss and to establish that abdominal injury is the probable cause, rather than being concerned with, for example, whether the source of that abdominal bleeding originates from the spleen or liver.
- There may be significant intra-abdominal injury with very few, if any, initial indications of this at the time the abdomen is examined by the paramedic at the scene.

2. Severity and Outcome

The leading cause of morbidity and mortality is as a result of blunt trauma. Mortality from isolated abdominal stab wounds is approximately 1–2%.

3. Pathophysiology

The abdomen may be described as three anatomical areas:

a **Abdominal cavity**

b **Pelvis**

c **Retro-peritoneal area.**

a **Abdominal cavity** – extends from the diaphragm to the pelvis. It contains the stomach, small intestine, large intestine, liver, gall bladder and spleen.

The upper abdominal organs are partly in the lower thorax and lie under the lower ribs; therefore fractures of lower ribs may damage abdominal structures such as the liver and spleen.

b **Pelvis** – contains the bladder, the lower part of the large intestine and, in the female, the uterus and ovaries. The iliac artery and vein overlie the posterior part of the pelvic ring and may be torn in pelvic fractures, adding to already major bleeding.

c **Retro-peritoneal area** – lies against the posterior abdominal wall, and contains the kidneys and ureters, pancreas, abdominal aorta, vena cava and part of the duodenum. These structures are attached to the posterior abdominal wall, and are often injured by shearing due to rapid deceleration forces.

4. Abdominal Injuries

Blunt trauma – is the most common pattern of injury seen and results from direct blows to the abdomen or rapid deceleration. Blunt trauma may also result from all phases of a blast.

- The spleen, liver (hepatic tear) and 'tethered' structures such as the duodenum are the most commonly injured. The small bowel, mesentery and aorta may also sustain injury.

Penetrating trauma – stab wounds, gunshot wounds, blast injuries and other penetrating injuries.

- **Stab wounds** – stab injures should be assumed to have caused serious damage until proved otherwise. Damage to liver, spleen or major blood vessels may cause massive haemorrhage. **NB** Upper abdominal stab wounds may have caused major intra-thoracic damage if the weapon was directed upwards (refer to **Thoracic Trauma**). Similarly, chest stabbing injuries may also cause intra-abdominal injury.
- **Gunshot wounds** – tend to cause both direct and indirect injury, due to the forces involved and the chaotic paths that bullets may take. The same rules apply to associated intra-thoracic injuries.
- **Blast injuries** – can lead to both blunt and penetrating injuries. Where an explosion occurs in a confined space the blast wave can cause injuries to the bowel (perforation and haemorrhage) and penetrating ballistics can lead to organ damage.

5. Assessment and Management

For the assessment and management of abdominal trauma refer to Table 4.10.

TABLE 4.10 – Assessment and Management of: Abdominal Trauma

ASSESSMENT	MANAGEMENT
• **Assess <C>ABCD**	• Control any external catastrophic haemorrhage – refer to **Trauma Emergencies Overview.** • If any of the following **TIME CRITICAL** features are present: – major **<C>ABCD** problems – haemodynamic compromise – decreased level of consciousness – neck and back injuries – refer to **Spinal Injury and Spinal Cord Injury**, then:

Abdominal Trauma

TABLE 4.10 – Assessment and Management of: Abdominal Trauma *(continued)*	
	• Start correcting **A** and **B** problems. • Undertake a **TIME CRITICAL** transfer to nearest appropriate receiving hospital. This may be a major trauma centre, refer to local protocols. • Provide an alert/information call. • Continue patient management en-route.
• Assess	• Ascertain the mechanism of injury: • **Road traffic collision:** look for impact speed and severity of deceleration; seat belt and lap belt use are particularly associated with torn or perforated abdominal structures. • **Stabbing and gunshot wound(s):** consider the length of the weapon used or the type of gun and the range. • **Blast injuries:** blast wave injuries and penetrating ballistics. Assess the chest and abdomen – **NB** Some abdominal organs (e.g. liver and spleen) are covered by lower ribs/chest margins. **ABDOMEN:** • Examine for signs of tenderness. • Examine for external signs of injury (e.g. contusions, seat/lap belt abrasions). • Evisceration (protruding abdominal organs). **GENTLY** palpate the four quadrants of the abdomen for signs of tenderness, guarding and rigidity. Shoulder-tip pain should increase suspicion of injury or internal bleeding. **NB** Significant **INTRA-ABDOMINAL TRAUMA** may show little or no evidence in the early stages, therefore **DO NOT** rule out injury if initial examination is normal. **CHEST:** • Fractures of the lower ribs – if confirmed or suspected refer to **Thoracic Trauma**.
• Evisceration	• **DO NOT** push protruding abdominal organs back into the abdominal cavity. • Cover protruding abdominal organs with warm moist dressings.
• Impaling objects	• Leave impaling objects (e.g. a knife) **IN-SITU** • Secure the object prior to transfer to further care. If the object(s) is pulsating, **DO NOT** completely immobilise it, but allow it to pulsate.
• Haemorrhage	• In the case of external haemorrhage apply a field dressing and direct pressure – refer to **Trauma Emergencies Overview**.
• Oxygen	• Administer high levels of supplemental oxygen (aim for SpO_2 94–98%) – refer to **Oxygen**. • Apply pulse oximeter.
• Ventilation	Consider assisted ventilation at a rate of 12–20 respirations per minute if: • Oxygen saturation (SpO_2) is <90% on high levels of supplemental oxygen. • Respiratory rate is <10 or >30bpm. • Inadequate chest expansion. Refer to **Airway and Breathing Management**.
• Vital signs	• Monitor vital signs. • Monitor ECG.
• Pelvic injuries	• Consider pelvic injuries – if suspected refer to **Major Pelvic Trauma**.
• Thoracic injuries	• If the injury affects the chest refer to **Thoracic Trauma**.
• Pain management	• If pain relief is indicated refer to **Pain Management in Adults** and **Pain Management in Children**.

(continued)

- Blood glucose level must be checked as part of initial assessment as alteration in behaviour or conscious level may be attributed to this.
- History taking must include assessment of medications (i.e. anticoagulants) and other factors that place the patient either at higher risk of serious underlying injury or which may suggest that the patient cannot be safely discharged at the scene.

3.2 Focal Neurological Deficit

- Focal neurological deficit covers problems restricted to a particular part of the body or a particular activity, for example, difficulties with understanding, speaking, reading or writing; decreased sensation; loss of balance; general weakness; visual changes; abnormal reflexes; and problems walking.

3.3 Open or Depressed Base of Skull Fracture or Penetrating Head Injury

- Signs include clear fluid running from the ears or nose, black eye with no associated damage around the eyes ('panda eyes'), bleeding from one or both ears, bruising behind one or both ears, penetrating injury signs, visible trauma to the scalp or skull of concern to the clinician.

4. Management of Traumatic Brain Injury (TBI) in the Pre-Hospital Setting

4.1 Airway with Cervical Spine Control

- It is well recognised that airway obstruction or aspiration are significant and often preventable causes of death in patients with severe traumatic brain injury. Basic airway manoeuvres are essential to prevent primary airway obstruction and associated brain hypoxia. These should be instigated with consideration for protecting the cervical spine, as it is estimated that up to 10% of traumatic brain injuries are complicated by a cervical spine injury. However, there is also strong evidence to suggest that, probably due to compression of the jugular veins of the neck, tightly or poorly fitted rigid cervical spinal immobilisation collars create a detrimental rise in intracranial pressure (ICP). Such ICP rises should be avoided where possible in traumatic brain injury. Patients should be immobilised using the methods found elsewhere in these practice guidelines.
- Once standard immobilisation has been achieved, with the head and body secured, consideration should be given to loosening or removing the collar. This is to mitigate the effects of the collar on intracranial pressure and may help to reduce agitation. The decision to loosen or remove the collar is in no way a decision to clear the C-spine and the reasons for collar removal should be clearly documented and handed over to the receiving hospital team.
- In addition to maintaining C-spine immobilisation, evidence suggests that placing the patient in a 30° head-up position reduces the effects of a raised ICP in patients with TBI, and this is traditionally employed once the cervical collar is removed in the intensive care unit (ICU). The logistical challenges of elevating a patient to 30° while immobilised in the pre-hospital setting probably render this process all but redundant. However, clinicians should remain aware of the effect of positioning, and ensure the patient's head remains above, or at least level with the feet throughout extrication and transfer.
- For a patient with a severe head injury (GCS <8) and in patients unable to maintain their own airway; to prevent a worsening secondary brain injury the patient needs to have their airway secured and ventilation optimised, preferably at scene or while they are transferred to definitive care. Consideration should be given to whether an appropriately skilled and trained clinician is available to provide rapid sequence intubation (RSI) or whether immediate transfer should take place. The distance and journey time from an appropriate receiving unit should be considered in line with local procedures and pathways. Advice may be sought via senior advice systems within your employing service. The level of pre-hospital enhanced care available in any one area and at any time of the day is variable. Diverting to a trauma unit should only be for immediate airway compromise that cannot be managed in the pre-hospital setting.

4.2 Breathing and Ventilation

- Adequate ventilation is essential to the management of TBI through the avoidance of hypoxia and maintenance of 'normocapnia'. Numerous studies have demonstrated the correlation between arterial hypoxaemia and poor prognosis following TBI, with some even demonstrating increased mortality of up to 50% following only brief episodes of desaturation. Current evidence suggests that oxygen should initially be administered at 10–15 l/min via a non-rebreathing mask, with a target saturation of 94–98%.
- Evidence also demonstrates that those patients who remain normocapnic (4.6 and 6.0 kPa) following a TBI have significantly better outcomes. Hyperventilation reduces arterial carbon dioxide (CO_2) concentrations, and leads to a consequent vasoconstriction within the cerebral vasculature, worsening both cerebral hypoxia and oedema. Hypercapnia, associated with hypoventilation increases the vasodilatation of the cerebral blood vessels, which increases intracranial volumes and therefore ICP.

4.3 Circulation

- Estimates have previously suggested that between 8% and 13% of patients with severe traumatic head injuries are hypotensive either at the scene of the injury, or in the ED. In addition, a wealth of evidence demonstrates a strong correlation between hypotension and poor outcome in TBI, with some highlighting that a single episode of hypotension (SBP < 90 mmHg) is independently linked to a 100% increase in mortality rate.
- Mean arterial pressure (MAP) is considered to be a better guide to cerebral perfusion pressures (CCP) than the systolic blood pressure alone, but intracranial pressure measurement is required to established the optimum MAP. This leads to the obvious conclusion that effective management of hypotension in the pre-hospital setting improves the outcomes of patients with TBI.
- Haemorrhage control (especially from the highly vascular scalp) should be established early to avoid the unnecessary consumption of coagulation products, and where hypotension is identified intravenous fluid resuscitation should be commenced. Unfortunately, there still remains a lack of clear research evidence to demonstrate the most appropriate fluid for resuscitation in TBI when blood products are unavailable and in most cases it will be dictated by local service interpretations and current formulary restrictions.

4.4 Disability

- The patients GCS should be calculated, as this can be an important prognostic indicator and is useful for monitoring injury progression over time.
- Pupils should be examined for size, reaction and whether they are equal.

4.5 Exposure/Environment/Extricate

- There is a high incidence of associated injuries found in patients with TBI, and an attempt to identify these during the secondary survey should be made, while remaining aware of the severe impacts of prolonged scene delays.
- Over recent years there has been a growing interest in the potential benefits of therapeutic hypothermia in TBI, although to date, research has failed to demonstrate any statistical benefit in long-term outcome. The key message therefore is the patient should be maintained within a 'normothermic' range.
- Time on scene should be kept to a minimum.

4.6 Pain and Agitation

- Agitation in TBI has a number of potential causes. One commonly overlooked cause of agitation in patients with a TBI is pain, either from the head injury itself or associated injuries sustained at the time of the TBI. Managing pain in TBI poses a challenge for the pre-hospital clinician; a patient in pain will be agitated, more difficult to manage, and may place themselves at risk of further cerebral hypoxia.
- The administration of opiates in severe TBI can be considered but there is a need to be aware of the potential for exaggerated respiratory depression, hypoventilation, hypercapnia and increased ICP. The decision whether to use opiates in those with a TBI is therefore a clinical one, underpinned by careful assessment and close monitoring for adverse effects.
- Clinicians might consider requesting more senior assistance for patients whose TBI is complicated by agitation associated with acute pain. Midazolam can be considered as an adjunct to help settle an agitated patient (refer to Section 5 below).

4.7 Evacuation Considerations

- The underlying principles of effective pre-hospital management of TBI are rapid assessment; swift and appropriate management; and timely transportation to a receiving centre with sufficient expertise to manage the patient. This will be dependent upon local resources and operational plans for those sustaining significant trauma, but clinicians should consider the most appropriate mode of evacuation early in the incident, to reduce on-scene time as much as possible.
- Helicopter emergency medical services (HEMS) may be able to facilitate more rapid transfer and evacuation but the decision to wait for HEMS arrival should be a balanced decision based on journey time to receiving unit and the need for additional transfer to HEMS at both incident and hospital end.
- A pre-alert call and a detailed clinical hand-over using ATMIST to the receiving unit is imperative for all patients with a significant TBI.

4.8 Special Considerations

Head Injuries in the Older Person

- Although significant head injury is predominantly a condition seen in the younger generation, a second peak in incidence occurs in those > 65 years. A number of age-related structural changes in the cerebral architecture leaves older people with increased susceptibility to intracranial haemorrhage following what may be an apparently minor head injury. In addition, older people are at increased risk of intracranial bleeding following head injury due to co-morbidities such as clotting derangements or polypharmacy. Older patients may present to healthcare services in an atypical way following a head injury, due to altered intracranial anatomy or pre-existing cognitive decline. Clinicians should suspect TBI in all older patients identified to have sustained trauma of any significance, and ensure that they maintain a high index of suspicion when assessing and treating older patients with traumatic injuries.

5. Midazolam in Traumatic Brain Injury

- Patients with TBI can pose a challenge for management in the pre hospital setting, and any associated hypoxia, hypercapnia and intracranial hypertension can contribute significantly to a poorer prognosis. Although not robust, the evidence suggests that the therapeutic benefits of midazolam for these patients can include amnesia, anxiolysis and most critically, an ability to effectively provide oxygenation and ventilation, which may help reduce the detrimental secondary brain injury they incur. However, sedating agents will reduce systemic blood pressure leading to a decrease in cerebral perfusion pressure (CPP), in addition to further jeopardising the patient's airway. Therefore, the decision to use midazolam to facilitate safe patient management needs to be carefully considered. Such interventions should only be undertaken after additional training and confirmation of ability to deal with the complications of midazolam use. Remember – Midazolam is a sedating agent with an unpredictable dose response relationship in a head injured patient and may cause a patient to rapidly become deeply sedated requiring immediate enhanced care intervention. Any practitioner considering the use of midazolam in head injuries should be specifically trained in and capable of undertaking the additional interventions required.

6. Assessment and Management of Mild to Moderate Head Injury

- Ambulance clinicians need to consider early detection and treatment of life-threatening brain injury, where present, but also be able to safely discharge patients with negligible risk of brain injury. Ninety-five per cent of people who have sustained a head injury present with a normal or minimally impaired conscious level (GCS greater than 12).
- Additional care should be taken when assessing children, the older person and other patient

TABLE 4.11 – Conveyance Decision Tool

Red criteria

Refer to local major trauma triage tool and consider the need for immediate transfer to a major trauma centre and/or pre-alert call.

Immediately transport to hospital if any one of the following is found:

- Glasgow coma scale (GCS) score of less than 15 on initial assessment.
- Any loss of consciousness as a result of the injury.
- Any focal neurological deficit since the injury.
- Any suspicion of a skull fracture or penetrating head injury since the injury.
- Amnesia for events before or after the injury.
- Persistent headache since the injury.
- Any vomiting episodes since the injury (clinical judgement should be used regarding the cause of vomiting in those aged 12 years or younger and the need for referral).
- Any seizure since the injury.
- Any previous brain surgery.
- A high-energy head injury.
- Any history of bleeding or clotting disorders.
- Current anticoagulant therapy such as warfarin (see further detail below).
- Current drug or alcohol intoxication.
- Any safeguarding concerns (for example, possible non-accidental injury or a vulnerable person is affected).
- Continuing concern by the ambulance clinician about the diagnosis.
- Irritability or altered behaviour, particularly in infants and children aged under 5 years.
- No visible trauma to the head but still of concern to the clinician.
- No one is able to observe the injured person at home.
- Continuing concern by the injured person or their family or carer about the diagnosis.

TABLE 4.11 – Conveyance Decision Tool *(continued)*
Green criteria Consider discharge where all of the following can be met: • No Red criteria are identified. • Able to appropriately safety-net the patient in the community with suitable supervision arrangements. If the patient has no carer at home or lives alone only discharge them if suitable supervision arrangements have been organised, or when the risk of late complications is deemed negligible. For example, arranging for a relative, friend or neighbour to visit regularly. • Verbal and written advice can be given to the patient and those supervising. • Patient, carers and clinician have no ongoing concerns.
Additional considerations Patients currently undergoing anticoagulant therapy should be assessed in hospital. Common anticoagulants include: • Warfarin • Rivaroxaban • Apixaban • Dabigatran • Edoxaban • Heparin • Dalteparin • Enoxaparin • Tinzaparin Patients undergoing anti-platelet therapy do not automatically require assessment in hospital. Have a lower threshold for conveyance of patients on dual anti-platelets and refer to local procedures. Common anti-platelets include: • Aspirin • Clopidogrel • Ticagrelor

groups such as patients with dementia, underlying chronic neurological disorders or learning disabilities. These can be more difficult to accurately assess and have a higher rate of additional and non-accidental injuries. In some patients the pre-injury baseline GCS may be less than 15. Establish this where possible, and take it into account during assessment. History taking must include assessment of medications (e.g. anticoagulants) and other factors that place the patient either at higher risk of serious underlying injury or which may suggest that the patient cannot be safely discharged at the scene.

- The following guidance is written to highlight key features of head injuries that require hospital attendance and those patients who can be safely cared for in the community. The list is not exhaustive – a holistic assessment of the patient, mechanism of injury, symptoms, observations and the scene in general must be made. Where any doubt exists regarding the suitability of a patient for discharge they should be referred to the emergency department.

6.1 Discharge at the Scene

- Not all patients who have sustained a head injury will require further assessment in a hospital. Where no red features are present and where all green conditions can be met, patients may be discharged from the scene.
- Complications from head injuries can develop over a number of hours or days and as such any decision to discharge a patient from the scene needs to be supported by appropriate safety netting. At a minimum this should include a period of time, for example up to 24 hours, in which the patient can be supervised by a suitable adult who is able to call for help should there be any deterioration. Verbal and written advice that is age appropriate should be given in line with NICE Guideline CG176 (2014). Guidance should refer, at a minimum, to any potential for a developing head injury that would require further assessment, common symptoms that do not require further treatment, and guidance around what the patient can or cannot do while recovering from the injury.

Head Injury

Assessment	Management
C - Catastrophic haemorrhage manage catastrophic haemorrhage (see management of catastrophic haemorrhage algorithm)	• See guidelines for management of catastrophic haemorrhage
A – Airway and C spine Establish current or impending airway loss. Consider C spine status	• Establish and maintain a patent airway • Protect cervical spine to prevent secondary spinal cord injury
B – Breathing: Assess rate, pattern and effectiveness of respiration. Obtain oxygen saturations and CRT	• Maintain O_2 saturations with supplemental O_2 as required (See target values) • Instigate capnographic monitoring if available • Avoid hyper / hypoventilation of mechanically ventilated patients (See target values)
C – Circulation Assess pulse rate, rhythm and volume. Assess BP. Confirm control of significant haemorrhage	• Instigate and maintain haemorrhage control • Avoid any episodes of unmanaged hypotension (See target values) • Obtain IV access • Adult: use 250ml boluses of selected fluid to ensure BP remains above 90 mmHg • Children: avoid hypotension (see age specific systolic BP targets) • Avoid excessive dilution of clotting factors through excessive fluid therapy
D – Disability Assess GCS Measure temperature and blood glucose Identify associated injuries taking account of mechanism and injury patterns Check pupil reaction	• Cover patients to prevent heat loss during extrication and evacuation • Avoid using cool or cold infusions • Correct abnormalities of blood glucose • Manage pain in accordance with local or national guidelines • Monitor level of consciousness and be prepared for impending management challenges in those with a diminishing GCS • Treat seizures according to established JRCALC guidelines
Evacuation considerations	• Early referral to specialist neurosurgical centre* • Monitor for deterioration Consider 30° head up tilt • Early pre-alert call to receiving unit

Treatment Goals (Adults):
SPO_2 : >94%
Systolic Blood Pressure: >90 mmHg
$ETCO_2$: 35–40 mmHg

Treatment goals (children):
SPO_2: 95%
$ETCO_2$: 35–40 mmHg
Blood Pressure: see age-specific systolic BP targets

Age-specific systolic Blood Pressure targets (children)	
< 1 year	> 80 mmHg
1–5 years	> 90 mmHg
5–14 years	> 100 mmHg
> 14 years	> 110 mmHg

Figure 4.9 – Assessment and management of head injury

SECTION 4 Trauma

Head Injury

Bibliography

1. National Institute for Health and Clinical Excellence. *Head injury: assessment and early management.* London: NICE, 2017. Available from: https://www.nice.org.uk/guidance/cg176.
2. Bayless P, Ray VG. Incidence of cervical spine injuries in association with blunt head trauma. *Am J Emerg Med* 1989; 7:139–42.
3. Boer C, Franschman G, Loer S. Prehospital management of severe traumatic brain injury: conecpts and ongoing controversies. *Curr Opin Anesthesio*l 2012 25:556–562
4. Chestnut R, Marshall L, Klauber M et al. Early and late systemic hypotension as a frequent and fundamental source of cerebral ischaemia following severe brain injry in the Traumatic Coma Data Bank. *Acta Neurochir Suppl* 1993 59:121–1253.
5. Clifton G, Valadka A, Zygun D et al. Very early hypothermia induction in patients with severe brain injury (The National Acute Brain Injury Study: hypothermia II): a randomized trial. *Lancet Neurol* 2011; 10: 131–139.
6. Dubick MA, Shek P, Wade CE. ROC trials update on prehospital hypertonic saline resuscitation in the aftermath of the US-Canadian trials. *Clinics* 2013;68(6):883–886.
7. Dumont T, Visioni A, Rughani A et al. Inappropriate pre-hospital ventilation in severe traumatic injuries increases in-hospital mortality. *J Neurotrauma* 27:1223–1241
8. Ferguson J, Mardel SN, Beattie TF, Wytch R. Cervical collars: a potential risk to the head-injured patient. *Injury* 1993, 24(7): 454–6.
9. Flanagan S, Hibbard M, Riordan B. Traumatic Brain Injury in the Elderly: Diagnostic and Treatment Challenges. Clin Geriatr Med 2006 22:449–468.
10. Gu J, Yang T, Kuang Y et al. Comparison of the safety and efficacy of propofol with midazolam for sedation of patients with severe traumatic brain injury: A meta-analysis. *Journal of Critical Care* 2014; 29 287–290.
11. Ho AM, Fung KY, Joynt GM, Karmakar MK, Peng Z. Rigid cervical collar and intracranial pressure of patients with severe head injury. *J Trauma* 2002; 53:1185–8.
12. Holly LT, Kelly DF, Counelis GJ, Blinman T, McArthur DL, Cryer HG. Cervical spine trauma associated with moderate and severe head injury: Incidence, risk factors, and injury characteristics. *J Neurosurg* 2002; 96 (Suppl 3):285–91.
13. Hunt K, Hallworth S, Smith M. The effects of rigid collar placement on intracranial and cerebral perfusion pressures. *Anaesthesia* 2001; 56:511–3.
14. Langlois JA, Kegler SR, Butler JA, et al. Traumatic brain injury–related hospital dis- charges: results from a 14-state surveillance system, 1997. MMWR CDC Surveill Summ 2003;52:1–20.
15. Ng I, Lim J, Wong H. Effects of head posture on cerebral hemodynamics: its influences on intracranial pressure, cerebral perfusion pressure, and cerebral oxygenation. Neurosurgery 2004; 54(3):593–7.
16. O'Driscoll B, Howard L, Davison A (On behalf of the British Thoracic Society Emergency Oxygen Guideline Development Group). Guidelines for Emergency Oxygen Use in Adult Patients. Thorax. *Thorax* 63 (Suppl VI): 2008 doi:10.1136/thx.2008.102947.
17. Peterson K, Carson S, Carney N: Hypothermia treatment for traumatic brain injury: a systematic review and meta-analysis. *J Neurotrauma* 2008 25:62-71.
18. Piatt JI I., Jr Detected and overlooked cervical spine injury among comatose trauma patients: From the Pennsylvania trauma outcomes study. *Neurosurg Focus.* 2005; 19 :E6.
19. Piek J, Chesnut R, Marshall L et al. Extracranial complications of severe head injury. *J Neurosurg* 1992. 77:901–907.
20. Stiver S, Manley G. Prehospital management of traumatic brain injury. *Neurosurg Focus* 2008 25(4): E5
21. Stocchetti N, Furlan A Volta F: Hypoxemia and arterial hypotension at the accident scene in head injury. *J Trauma* 1996 40: 764–767.
22. Tian HL, Guo Y, Hu J, Rong BY, Wang G, Gao WW, et al. Clinical characterization of comatose patients with cervical spine injury and traumatic brain injury. *J Trauma.* 2009; 67 :1305–10.
23. Trunkey D. Towards Optimal Trauma Care. Arch Emerg Med. 1985 2: 181–195.
24. Urwin SC, Menon DK. Comparative tolerability of sedative agents in head-injured adults. *Drug Saf* 2004;27:107–33.

Limb Trauma

TABLE 4.15 – ASSESSMENT and MANAGEMENT of: Limb Trauma

ASSESSMENT	MANAGEMENT
● Assess **<C>ABCDE**	● Control any external catastrophic haemorrhage (refer to **Trauma Emergencies Overview**). ● If any of the following **TIME CRITICAL** features are present: – major **<C>ABC** complications – haemodynamic instability (refer to **Intravascular Fluid Therapy in Adults**) – altered level of consciousness (refer to **Altered Level of Consciousness**) – neck and back injuries (refer to **Spinal Injury and Spinal Cord Injury**) – threatened limb – loss of neurovascular function (e.g. resulting from a dislocation that requires prompt realignment), then: ● Correct **<C>ABC** complications. ● Mid shaft femoral fracture – apply a traction splint if this can be done quickly without delaying transfer, otherwise apply manual traction where sufficient personnel are available – once applied it should not be released. ● Undertake a **TIME CRITICAL** transfer to a major trauma centre, unless the patient needs an immediate lifesaving intervention, in which case transfer to nearest trauma unit. ● Provide a pre-alert using ATMIST. ● Continue patient management en-route.
● Specifically assess	● Ascertain the mechanism of injury and any factors indicating the forces involved (e.g. the pattern of fractures may indicate mechanism of injury): – fractures of the heel in a fall from a height may be accompanied by pelvic and spinal crush fractures (refer to **Major Pelvic Trauma** and **Spinal Injury and Spinal Cord Injury**) – 'dashboard' injury to the knee may be accompanied by a fracture or dislocation of the hip – humeral fractures from a side impact are associated with chest injuries (refer to **Thoracic Trauma**) – tibial fractures are rarely isolated injuries and are often associated with high energy trauma and other life-threatening injuries. ● Assess all four limbs for injury to long bones and joints – in suspected fracture, expose site(s) to assess swelling and deformity. ● Assess neurovascular function – MSC × 4: motor, sensation and circulation, distal to the fracture site. Assess foot pulses; palpate dorsalis pedis as capillary refill time can be misleading. ● Assess general skin colour. ● Assess age of patient – consider greenstick fractures in children, and fractures of wrist and hip in older people. ● For accompanying illnesses: – some cancers can involve bones (e.g. breast, lung and prostate) and result in fractures from minor injuries – osteoporosis in older females makes fractures more likely. **NB** Where possible avoid unnecessary pain stimulus.
● Oxygen	● Administer high levels of supplemental oxygen (aim for SpO_2 94–98%) (refer to **Oxygen**).
● Splintage	In pre-hospital care it is difficult to differentiate between ligament sprain and a fracture; therefore ASSUME a fracture and immobilise. ● Remove and document jewellery from the affected limbs before swelling occurs. ● Check and record the presence/absence of pulses, and muscle function distal to injury.

TABLE 4.15 – ASSESSMENT and MANAGEMENT of: Limb Trauma *(continued)*	
	• Consider realignment of grossly deformed limbs to a position as close to normal anatomic alignment as possible. Where deformity is minor and both distal sensation and circulation are intact, then realignment may not be necessary. • Apply splintage (refer to Table 4.14). • Guidance on alignment: Deformed fracture dislocation of the ankle is the most common deformity that may benefit from manipulation in the pre-hospital environment. Indications to attempt manipulation are: – Vascular impairment – Absent or very weak distal pulse – Significantly prolonged capillary refill – Critical skin over the fracture site (blanching or discolouration). • Manipulation into alignment as close to normal should be considered when any of these features are present and transfer to an appropriate ED cannot be managed in a suitable time frame.
• Compound fracture	• Gross contamination can be removed from wounds but do not irrigate open fractures of the long bones, hindfoot or midfoot in pre-hospital settings as it may force contamination deeper into the bone or tissue. • Apply a saline-soaked dressing and cover with an occlusive layer. • Any gross displacement from normal alignment must, where possible, be corrected, and splints applied (refer to Table 4.14). **NB** Document the nature of the contamination, as contaminates may be drawn inside following realignment.
• Amputations, partial amputations and degloving	• Do not irrigate grossly contaminated wounds with saline. • Immobilise a partially amputated limb in a position of normal anatomical alignment. • Where possible dress the injured limb to prevent further contamination. • Apply a saline-soaked dressing covered with an occlusive layer. **NB** Reimplantation following amputation or reconstruction following partial amputation may be possible. In order that the amputated parts are maintained and transported in the best condition possible: • remove any gross contamination • cover the part(s) with a moist field dressing • secure in a sealed plastic bag • place the bag on ice – do not place body parts in direct contact with ice as this can cause tissue damage; the aim is to keep the temperature low but not freezing.
• Neck of femur fractures	• Assess for shortening and external rotation of the leg on the injured side, with pain in the hip and referred pain in the knee. • Ascertain whether the patient has been on the floor for some time, assess for signs of hypothermia, dehydration, pressure ulcers and chest infection. • Monitor vital signs. • Immobilise by strapping the injured leg to the normal one with foam padding between the limbs – extra padding with blankets and strapping around the hips and pelvis can be used to provide additional support while moving the patient (refer to Table 4.14).
• Compartment syndrome	• Consider the need for rapid transfer to nearest appropriate hospital as per local trauma care pathway, as the patient may require immediate surgery; elevate limb and consider pain relief en-route.

(continued)

Spinal Injury and Spinal Cord Injury

1. Introduction

- In the major trauma patient, spinal injuries are common. The majority are stable; some are unstable, risking spinal cord damage, and a small number are associated with spinal cord injury at the outset. Differentiation between stable and unstable injuries requires specific imaging in the ED.
- Effective management from the time of injury is important to ensure optimal outcomes. This guideline provides guidance for the assessment and initial management of cervical spine and spinal trauma, including indicators to guidance for related conditions.

2. Pathophysiology

- The spinal cord runs in the spinal canal down to the level of the second lumbar vertebra in adults.
- The amount of space in the spinal canal in the upper neck is relatively large, and risk of secondary injury in this area can be reduced if adequate immobilisation is applied. In the thoracic area the cord is wide and the spinal canal relatively narrow; injury in this area is more likely to completely disrupt and damage the spinal cord.
- Spinal shock is a state of complete loss of motor function and often sensory function found sometimes after SCI. This immediate reaction may go on for some considerable time, but some recovery may well be possible. Complete and incomplete cord injury cannot be distinguished in the presence of spinal shock.
- Neurogenic shock is the state of poor tissue perfusion caused by sympathetic tone loss after spinal cord injury.

3. Incidence

- Falls are a frequent cause of SCI in the older person. Maintain a high index of suspicion in cases of older people who have had low energy falls.
- SCI affects young and fit people and will continue to affect them to a varying degree for the rest of their lives.
- Road traffic collisions, falls and sporting injuries are the most common causes of SCI – as a group, motorcyclists occupy more spinal injury unit beds than any other group involved in road traffic collisions. Rollover road traffic collisions where occupants are not wearing seatbelts, and the head comes into contact with the vehicle body, and pedestrians struck by vehicles are likely to suffer SCI. Ejection from a vehicle increases the risk of injury significantly.
- UK Trauma Audit Research Network (TARN) data has shown that, in the presence of a cervical bony injury, 13.4% of patients have associated injuries elsewhere in the thoracic and lumbar spine.

3.1 Risk Factors

- Road traffic collisions (RTC):
  - rollover RTC
  - non-wearing of seatbelts
  - ejection from vehicle
  - struck by a vehicle.
- Sporting injuries:
  - diving into shallow water
  - horse riding
  - rugby
  - gymnastics and trampolining.
- Falls:
  - older people.
  - rheumatoid arthritis.
- Violent attacks and domestic incidents
- Certain sporting accidents, especially diving into shallow water, horse riding; rugby, gymnastics and trampolining have a higher than average risk of SCI. Rapid deceleration injury such as gliding and light aircraft accidents also increase the risk of SCI.
- Older people and those with rheumatoid arthritis are prone to odontoid peg fractures that may be difficult to detect clinically. Such injuries can occur from relatively minor trauma (e.g. falls from a standing height).

3.2 Cauda Equina Syndrome (CES)

- Cauda equina syndrome is caused by compression of the nerves in the spinal canal below the end of the spinal cord (at L2 vertebra level). It can occur in patients with trauma, a herniated disc, chronic or acute low back pain, and patients with tumours or infection.
- Clinical diagnosis of CES is not easy. Most cases are of sudden onset and progress rapidly within hours or days. However, CES can evolve slowly and patients do not always complain of pain. Roughly 50–70% of patients have urinary retention on presentation.
- CES is an acute surgical emergency; early diagnosis is essential and the patient requires immediate conveyance to hospital for investigation if CES is suspected. Early surgical decompression is crucial to prevent permanent neurological damage.

Spinal Injury and Spinal Cord Injury

Red flag signs and symptoms of CES

⚑ Loss of bladder and/or bowel dysfunction control, causing incontinence.

⚑ Reduced sensation in the saddle (perineal) area.

⚑ New onset sexual dysfunction.

⚑ Neurological deficit in the lower limb (motor/sensory loss, reflex changes).

4. Severity and Outcome

- Injury most frequently occurs at the junctions of mobile and fixed sections of the spine. Hence fractures are more commonly seen in the lower cervical vertebrae, where the cervical and thoracic spine meets (C5, 6, 7/T1 area), and the thoracolumbar junction. Of patients with one identified spinal fracture, 10–15% will be found to have another.
- In the extreme, SCI may prove immediately fatal where the upper cervical cord is damaged, paralysing the diaphragm and respiratory muscles.
- Partial cord damage, however, may solely affect individual sensory or motor nerve tracts producing varying long-term disability. It is important to note that there is an increasing percentage of cases where the cord damage is only partial and quality recovery is possible, providing the condition is recognised and managed appropriately.

5. Immobilisation

- All patients with the possibility of spinal injury should have manual immobilisation commenced at the earliest time, while initial assessment is undertaken.
- If immobilisation is indicated then the whole spine must be immobilised. There are differences between the types of semi-rigid collar; acceptable methods of immobilisation are:
  - manual immobilisation while the spine is supported
  - collar, head blocks and spinal support.

The following techniques may be used:

- Patient lying supine:
  - Use a scoop stretcher and cervical spine immobilisation. To minimise movement of the spine, utilise a 10-degree tilt to the left and right.
  - Patients should be transported on the scoop stretcher unless there is a prolonged journey time, when a vacuum mattress should be utilised.
  - To utilise the vacuum mattress, lift the patient using the scoop stretcher, then insert the mattress underneath and remove the scoop stretcher.
- Patient lying prone:
  - Log roll the patient with manual immobilisation of the cervical spine to enable a scoop stretcher to be used.
  - Perform a 2-stage log roll onto a vacuum mattress.
- Patient requiring extrication:
  - Extrication devices should be used if there is any risk of rotational movement.
  - Rearward extrication on an extrication board.
  - Side extrication invariably involves some rotational component and therefore has higher risks in many circumstances.

NB The longboard should only be used as an extrication device. Do not transport patients to hospital on a longboard.

5.1 Extrication

- Consider asking a patient who is not physically trapped to self-extricate, providing they have none of the following:
  - significant distracting injuries
  - abnormal neurological symptoms (paraesthesia or weakness or numbness)
  - spinal pain or tenderness.
- Explain to a patient who is self-extricating that they should stop moving and wait to be moved if they develop any spinal pain, numbness, tingling or weakness.
- When a patient has self-extricated:
  - ask them to lay supine on a stretcher positioned adjacent to the vehicle or incident
  - assess them further for any signs of spinal injury, spinal tenderness or abnormal neurology in the ambulance.
- **Inviting a patient to self-extricate is not clearing the cervical spine.**
- Any patient who has not had a cervical spine clearance documented in the ambulance clinician's notes should be treated as an uncleared spine whether immobilised or not, and that information must be specifically relayed to staff on handover.

Emergency Extrication

- If there is an immediate threat to a patient's life and rapid extrication is needed, make all efforts to limit spinal movement without delaying treatment.

5.2 Cautions/Precautions

Vomiting

- Vomiting and consequent aspiration are serious consequences of immobilisation. Ambulance clinicians must always have a plan of action in case vomiting should occur.

Spinal Injury and Spinal Cord Injury

TABLE 4.16 – ASSESSMENT and MANAGEMENT of: Cervical Spine and Spinal Trauma *(continued)*

• Rapidly assess to determine the presence and estimate the level of spinal cord injury	• The following signs may indicate injury: – diaphragmatic or abdominal breathing – hypotension (BP often <80–90 mmHg) with bradycardia – warm peripheries or vasodilatation in the presence of low blood pressure – flaccid (floppy) muscles with absent reflexes – priapism – partial or full erection of the penis. • In a conscious patient – assess sensory and motor function: – use light touch and response to pain – examine upper limbs and hands – examine lower limbs and feet – examine both sides – undertake the examination in the MID-AXILLARY line, NOT the MID-CLAVICULAR line, as C2, C3 and C4 all supply sensation to the nipple line; use the forehead as the reference point to guide what is normal sensation. **NB** Always presume a SCI in the unconscious trauma patient.
• If the patient is non-time critical, perform a more thorough assessment with a brief secondary survey	
• Assess for neurogenic shock	• Diagnosis is difficult in pre-hospital care – the aim is to: – maintain blood pressure of approximately 90 mmHg systolic – obtain IV access – determine the need for fluid replacement but DO NOT delay on scene (refer to **Intravascular Fluid Therapy in Adults** and **Intravascular Fluid Therapy in Children**). • In neurogenic shock, a few degrees of head-down tilt may improve the circulation, but remember that in cases of abdominal breathing, this manoeuvre may further worsen respiration and ventilation. This position is also unsuitable for a patient who has, or may have, a head injury. • If bradycardia is present consider atropine (refer to **Atropine**) – but it is important to rule out other causes (e.g. hypoxia, severe hypovolaemia).
• Assess the need for assisted ventilation	• Refer to **Airway and Breathing Management**.
• Steroids	• Steroids have no part to play in the pre-hospital management of acute spinal cord injuries.
• At hospital	• The patient should be on a scoop stretcher. • Complete documentation and, if possible, record information whether the assessments show that the patient's condition is improving or deteriorating.
• Additional Information	• Transportation of spinal patients: – Driving should balance the advantages of smooth driving and time to arrival at hospital. No immobilisation technique eliminates movement from vehicle swaying and jarring. – There is no evidence to show advantage of direct transport to a spinal injury centre. – Patients should be transported on the scoop stretcher unless there is a prolonged journey time, when a vacuum mattress should be utilised. – As half of all cases of spinal injuries have other serious injuries, any unnecessary delay at the scene or in transit should be avoided.

SECTION 4 Trauma

Spinal Injury and Spinal Cord Injury

Patients with a history of trauma
Is there a potential for spinal injury in an adult >16 years old?

Yes ↓

- Under the influence of drugs or alcohol?
- Is confused or uncooperative?
- Has a reduced level of consciousness?
- Has any spinal pain (or pain elicited on coughing)?
- Any motor weakness in hands or feet?
- Any history of past spinal problems, including previous spinal surgery, severe osteoarthritis, ankylosing spondylitis?
- Any priapism?

Yes → IMMOBILISE

No ↓

High Risk?

- Dangerous mechanism of injury (fall from a height of >1 metre or five steps, axial load to the head - e.g. diving, high-speed motor vehicle collision, rollover motor accident, ejection from a motor vehicle, accident involving motorised recreational vehicles, bicycle collision, horse riding accidents)

Yes → IMMOBILISE

No ↓

Upon Examination:

- Any abnormal neurology (loss of sensation; numbness; 'pins and needles'; burning pain)?
- Any bony spinal pain anywhere along the spine (at rest or on coughing)?
- Any distracting injury?

Yes → IMMOBILISE

No ↓

Low Risk?

- Was involved in a minor rear-end motor vehicle collision
- Is comfortable in a sitting position
- Has been ambulatory at any time since the injury
- Has no midline cervical spine tenderness (answer 'no' if patient has pain)
- Delayed onset of neck pain

No → IMMOBILISE

Yes ↓

Is the patient able to actively rotate their head 45° to the left and right?
and
Is the patient able to mobilise without pain or abnormal neurology?

No → IMMOBILISE

Yes ↓

Spine Cleared

Use of spinal immobilisation devices may be difficult (e.g. in people with short/wide necks, or people with a pre-existing deformity) and could be counterproductive (i.e. increasing pain, worsening neurological signs and symptoms). In uncooperative, agitated or distressed people, think about letting them find a position where they are comfortable with manual in-line spinal immobilisation.

IMMOBILISE

Immobilise the entire spine.

If the patient is ambulatory or has been ambulatory at the scene, they can self-extricate if appropriate and may be guided to lie down onto the scoop stretcher to be immobilised.

The scoop should be placed on the trolley and located as close as practicable to the patient.

Patients MUST NOT be encouraged to walk up any steps (causes potential axial loading).

Patients with suspected spinal injury with abnormal neurology must be transferred to a Major Trauma Centre

Figure 4.10 – Immobilisation algorithm

Republished with permission of Yorkshire Ambulance Service.

Major Pelvic Trauma

The incidence of rectal injury ranges from 17% to 64% dependent upon type of fracture. Bowel entrapment is rare.

Pelvic injury is commonly associated with concomitant intra-thoracic and/or intra-abdominal injury.

TABLE 4.17 – ASSESSMENT and MANAGEMENT of: Major Pelvic Trauma	
ASSESSMENT ● Assess: **<C> ABCD; <C> catastrophic haemorrhage** – Airway – Breathing – Disability (mini neurological examination). ● Evaluate whether patient is **TIME CRITICAL** or **NON-TIME CRITICAL** following criteria as per trauma emergencies guideline. If patient is **TIME CRITICAL, correct A and B problems, stabilise the pelvis on scene and rapidly transport to nearest suitable receiving hospital. Provide an alert/information call.** En-route, continue patient management of pelvic trauma (see below). ● In **NON-TIME CRITICAL** patients perform a more thorough patient assessment with a brief secondary survey. **Specifically Consider** ● Pelvic fracture should be considered based upon the mechanism of injury. ● Clinical assessment of the pelvis includes observation for physical injury such as bruising, bleeding, deformity or swelling to the pelvis. Shortening of a lower limb may be present (see also **limb trauma guideline)** ● Assessment by compression or distraction (e.g. springing) of the pelvis is unreliable and may both dislodge clots and exacerbate any injury and should not be performed. Any patient with a relevant mechanism of injury and concomitant hypotension **MUST** be managed as having a **time critical pelvic injury** until proven otherwise.	**MANAGEMENT** ● Control any external catastrophic haemorrhage – **refer to trauma emergencies overview**. **Oxygen Therapy** ● Major pelvic injury falls into the category of critical illness and requires high levels of supplemental oxygen regardless of initial oxygen saturation reading (SpO_2). Maintain high flow oxygen (15 litres per minute) until vital signs are normal; thereafter reduce flow rate, titrating to maintain oxygen saturations (SpO_2) in the 94–98% range (**Oxygen**). **Pelvic Stabilisation** There is currently no evidence to suggest that any particular pelvic immobilisation device or approach is superior in terms of outcome in pelvic trauma and a number of methods have been reported. Effective stabilisation of the pelvic ring should be instigated at the earliest possible opportunity, preferably before moving the patient, and may be achieved by: ● Use of an appropriate pelvic splint. ● Apply the pelvic splint directly to skin, if this can be done easily with minimal handling. ● Expert consensus suggests the use of an appropriate pelvic splint is preferable to improvised immobilisation techniques. In all methods, circumferential pressure is applied over the greater trochanters and not the iliac crests. Care must be exercised so as to ensure that the pelvis is not reduced beyond its normal anatomical position. ● Pressure sores and soft tissue injuries may occur when immobilisation devices are incorrectly fitted. ● Reduction and stabilisation of the pelvic ring should occur as soon as is practicable whilst still on scene, as stabilisation helps to reduce blood loss by realigning fracture surfaces, thereby limiting active bleeding and additionally helping to stabilise clots. Reduction of the pelvis may have a tamponade effect, particularly for venous bleeding; however, there is little evidence to support this belief. ● Log rolling of the patient with possible pelvic fracture should be avoided as this may exacerbate any pelvic injury; where possible utilise an orthopaedic scoop stretcher to lift patients off the ground and limit movement to a 15° tilt. **Fluid therapy** ● There is little evidence to support the routine use of IV fluids in adult trauma patients; **refer to Intravascular Fluid Therapy in Adults** and **Intravascular Fluid Therapy in Children**. **Pain management** ● Patients' pain should be managed appropriately (refer to **Pain Management** guidelines); analgesia in the form of Entonox (refer to **Entonox** for administration and information) or morphine sulfate may be appropriate (refer to **Morphine Sulfate** for dosages and information).

Major Pelvic Trauma

5. Referral Pathway

5.1 The following cases should ALWAYS be transferred to further care:

- Any patient with hypotension and potential pelvic injury **MUST** be treated as a **TIME CRITICAL** pelvic injury until proven otherwise.
- Any patient with sufficient mechanism of injury to cause a pelvic injury.

5.2 The following cases MAY be considered suitable/safe to be left at home:

- None.

6. Special Considerations for Children

- Pelvic fractures represent 1–3% of all fractures in children, thus there is a lower incidence compared with adults.
- In children, pelvic injuries have a lower mortality accounting for 3.6–5.7% of trauma deaths, with fewer deaths occurring as a direct result of pelvic haemorrhage; blood loss is more likely to be from solid visceral injury than the pelvis.
- Different injury patterns – multi-system injuries in 60%; greater incidence of diaphragmatic injury.
- Principles of management are the same, with the exception of fluid and oxygen therapy (refer to **Intravascular Fluid Therapy in Adults**, **Intravascular Fluid Therapy in Children** and **Oxygen**).
- Clinical findings in small children can be unreliable.

7. Audit Information

- Incidence of suspected/actual pelvic fracture.
- Incidence of concomitant hypotension.
- Frequency of pelvic immobilisation when pelvic fracture suspected.
- Method of pelvic immobilisation.

KEY POINTS!

Major Pelvic Trauma

- **Pelvic fracture should be considered based upon mechanism of injury.**
- **The majority of pelvic fractures are stable pubic ramus or acetabular fractures.**
- **Any patient with hypotension and potentially relevant mechanism of injury MUST be considered to have a TIME CRITICAL pelvic injury.**
- **'Springing' or distraction of the pelvis must not be undertaken.**
- **Pelvic stabilisation should be implemented as soon as is practicable whilst still on scene.**
- **Consider appropriate pain management.**
- **The use of a scoop stretcher is recommended to avoid log rolling the patient unless extrication is required.**

SECTION 4 Trauma

Bibliography

1. Brown JK, Jing Y, Wang S, Ehrlich PF. Patterns of severe injury in pediatric car crash victims: Crash Injury Research Engineering Network database. *Journal of Pediatric Surgery* 2006, 41(2): 362–367.
2. O'Brien DP, Luchette FA, Pereira SJ, Lim E, Seeskin CS, James L, et al. Pelvic fracture in the elderly is associated with increased mortality. *Surgery* 2002, 132(4): 710–714.
3. Stein DM, O'Connor JV, Kufera JA, Ho SM, Dischinger PC, Copeland CE et al. Risk factors associated with pelvic fractures sustained in motor vehicle collisions involving newer vehicles. *Journal of Trauma* 2006, 61(1): 21–30.
4. Dalai SA, Burgess AR, Siegel JH, Young JW, Brumback RJ, Poka A, et al. Pelvic fracture in multiple trauma: classification by mechanism is key to pattern of organ injury, resuscitative requirements, and outcome. *Journal of Trauma* 1989, 29(7): 981–1000; discussion 1000–2.
5. Demetriades D, Karaiskakis M, Toutouzas K, Alo K, Velmahos G, Chan L. Pelvic fractures: epidemiology and predictors of associated abdominal injuries and outcomes. *Journal of the American College of Surgeons* 2002, 195(1): 1–10.
6. Demetriades D, Murray J, Brown C, Velmahos G, Salim A, Alo K et al. High-level falls: type and severity of injuries and survival outcome according to age. *Journal of Trauma* 2005, 58(2): 342–345.
7. Ferrera PC, Hill DA. Good outcomes of open pelvic fractures. *Injury* 1999, 30(3): 187–90.
8. Gustavo Parreira J, Coimbra R, Rasslan S, Oliveira A, Fregoneze M, Mercadante M. The role of associated injuries on outcome of blunt trauma patients sustaining pelvic fractures. *Injury* 2000, 31(9): 677–682.
9. Inaba K, Sharkey PW, Stephen DJG, Redelmeier DA, Brenneman FD. The increasing incidence of severe

83. Scurr JH, Cutting P. Tight jeans as a compression garment after major trauma. *British Medical Journal (Clinical Research Edition)* 1984, 288(6420): 828.

84. Simpson T, Krieg JC, Heuer F, Bottlang M. Stabilization of pelvic ring disruptions with a circumferential sheet. *Journal of Trauma, Injury, Infection, & Critical Care* 2002, 52(1): 158–161.

85. Vermeulen B, Peter R, Hoffmeyer P, Unger PF. Prehospital stabilization of pelvic dislocations: a new strap belt to provide temporary hemodynamic stabilization. *Swiss Surgery* 1999, 5(2): 43–6.

86. Nunn T, Cosker TDA, Bose D, Pallister I. Immediate application of improvised pelvic binder as first step in extended resuscitation from life-threatening hypovolaemic shock in conscious patients with unstable pelvic injuries. *Injury* 2007, 38(1): 125–128.

87. Krieg JC, Mohr M, Mirza AJ, Bottlang M. Pelvic circumferential compression in the presence of soft-tissue injuries: a case report. *Journal of Trauma, Injury, Infection, & Critical Care* 2005, 59(2): 470–472.

88. Ismail N, Bellemare JF, Mollitt DL, DiScala C, Koeppel B, Tepas IJJ. Death from pelvic fracture: children are different. *Journal of Pediatric Surgery* 1996, 31(1): 82–5.

89. Junkins EPJ, Nelson DS, Carroll KL, Hansen K, Furnival RA. A prospective evaluation of the clinical presentation of pediatric pelvic fractures. *Journal of Trauma* 2001, 51(1): 64–68.

90. Silber JS, Flynn JM, Koffler KM, Dormans JP, Drummond DS. Analysis of the cause, classification, and associated injuries of 166 consecutive pediatric pelvic fractures. *Journal of Pediatric Orthopaedics* 2001, 21(4): 446–450.

91. Junkins EP, Furnival RA, Bake RG. The clinical presentation of pediatric pelvic fractures. *Pediatric Emergency Care* 2001, 17(1): 15–18.

Thoracic Trauma

1. Introduction

- In pre-hospital care, the most common problem associated with severe thoracic injuries is hypoxia, either from impaired ventilation or secondary to hypovolaemia from massive bleeding into the chest (haemothorax) or major vessel disruption (e.g. ruptured thoracic aorta).

2. Incidence

- Severe thoracic injuries are one of the most common causes of death from trauma, accounting for approximately 25% of such deaths.

3. Severity and Outcome

- Despite the very high percentage of serious thoracic injuries, the vast majority of them can be managed in hospital with chest drainage and resuscitation, and only 10–15% require surgical intervention.

4. Pathophysiology

- The mechanism of injury is an important guide to the likelihood of significant thoracic injuries. Injuries to the chest wall usually arise from direct contact, for example, intrusion of wreckage in a road traffic collision or blunt trauma arising from direct blow. Seat belt injuries fall into this category and may cause fractures of the sternum, ribs and clavicle.
- If the force is sufficient, the deformity and the damage to the chest wall structures may induce tearing and contusion to the underlying lung and other structures. This may produce a combination of severe pain on breathing (pleuritic pain) and a damaged lung, both of which will significantly reduce the ability to ventilate adequately. This combination is a common cause of hypoxia.
- Blunt trauma to the sternum may cause myocardial contusion, which may result in cardiac rhythm disturbances.
- Penetrating trauma may well damage the heart, the lungs and great vessels both in isolation or combination. It must be remembered that penetrating wounds to the upper abdomen and neck may well have caused injuries within the chest remote from the entry wound. Conversely, penetrating wounds to the chest may well involve the liver, kidneys and spleen.
- The lung may be damaged with bleeding causing a haemothorax or an air-leak causing a pneumothorax. Penetrating or occasionally a blunt injury may result in cardiac injuries. Blood can leak into the non-elastic surrounding pericardial sac and build up pressure to an extent that the heart is incapable of refilling to pump blood into circulation. This is known as cardiac tamponade and can be fatal if not rapidly relieved at hospital (see additional information in Table 4.19).
- Rapid deceleration injuries may result in sheering forces sufficient to rupture great vessels such as the aorta, caused by compressing the vessels between the sternum and spine.
- The five major thoracic injuries encountered in the pre-hospital setting include:
  1. tension pneumothorax
  2. massive haemothorax (following uncontrolled haemorrhage into the chest cavity)
  3. open chest wounds
  4. flail chest
  5. cardiac tamponade.

5. Assessment and Management

For the assessment and management of thoracic trauma refer to Table 4.18 and Table 4.19.

TABLE 4.18 – ASSESSMENT and MANAGEMENT of: Thoracic Trauma

ASSESSMENT	MANAGEMENT
• Assess **<C>ABCDE**	• Control any external catastrophic haemorrhage (refer to **Trauma Emergencies Overview**). • If any of the following **TIME CRITICAL** features are present: – major **<C>ABCD** complications – penetrating chest injury – flail chest – tension pneumothorax – cardiac tamponade – surgical emphysema – blast injury to the lungs.

(continued)

a Patients should normally be transported in a semi-recumbent or upright posture; however, this may often not be possible due to other injuries present or suspected.

Thoracic Trauma

TABLE 4.18 – ASSESSMENT and MANAGEMENT of: Thoracic Trauma *(continued)*	
	• Correct **<C>ABC** problems. • Undertake a **TIME CRITICAL** transfer to a major trauma centre.[1] • Major unmanageable **A** and **B** problems should be transferred to nearest trauma unit. • Provide a pre-alert using ATMIST. • Continue patient management en-route.
• Specifically consider: – tension pneumothorax – open chest wounds – flail chest – surgical emphysema – cardiac tamponade – impaling objects	• Refer to Table 4.19 for the assessment and management of these conditions/situations.
• If the patient is **NON-TIME CRITICAL**, undertake a secondary survey	• A load and go approach is particularly important with penetrating injuries, unless enhanced care support is likely to arrive before the patient can reach an appropriate hospital.
• Monitor SpO_2 and assess for signs of hypoxia	• Administer high levels of supplemental oxygen until the vital signs are normal, then aim for a target saturation within the range of 94–98% (refer to **Oxygen**).
• Assess breathing adequacy, respiratory rate, effort and volume, and equality of air entry	• Consider assisted ventilation at a rate of 12–20 respirations per minute, if any of the following are present: – SpO_2 <90% on high levels of supplemental oxygen. – Respiratory rate is <10 or >30 breaths per minute. – Inadequate chest expansion. **NB** Exercise caution, as any positive pressure ventilation may increase the size of a pneumothorax.
• Monitor nasal $EtCO_2$	• $EtCO_2$ presents an immediate picture of the patient's condition.
• Monitor heart rate and rhythm	• Attach ECG monitor.
• Consider the need for IV fluids	• Obtain IV access. • Refer to **Intravascular Fluid Therapy in Adults** and **Intravascular Fluid Therapy in Children** – **DO NOT** delay on scene.
• Assess patient's level of pain	• Refer to **Pain Management in Adults** and **Pain Management in Children**. **NB** Avoid Entonox in a patient with a chest injury as there is a significant risk of enlarging a pneumothorax. **NB** Adequate morphine analgesia may improve ventilation by allowing better chest wall movement, but high doses may induce respiratory depression. Careful titration of doses is therefore required (refer to **Morphine Sulfate**).
• Assessment (children) • Assess as above	**Management (children)** Manage as above but consider: • Children can have severe internal chest injuries with minimal or no external evidence of chest injuries. • Children show signs of shock late due to good compensatory mechanisms. • Always consider multiple injuries in children with rib fractures, as this suggests a significant mechanism of injury and isolated chest injuries are rare in children. • Consider non-accidental injury.

Thoracic Trauma

TABLE 4.18 – ASSESSMENT and MANAGEMENT of: Thoracic Trauma *(continued)*	
• Additional Information	• Chest trauma is treated with difficulty in the field, and prolonged treatment before transportation is **NOT** indicated if significant chest injury is suspected. • Open chest wounds – seal the wound with a proprietary dressing with a valve, but if none are available use a three-sided dressing. • Specifically consider the need for thoracic surgery intervention. • Impaling objects – handle carefully, secure the object with a dressing and if the object is pulsating do not completely immobilise it but allow the object to pulsate. **NB** Be vigilant – the patient may try to remove the object and this could be used as a weapon. • Remember any stab or bullet wound to the chest, abdomen or back may penetrate the heart. • Patients with significant chest trauma may often insist on sitting upright and this is especially common in patients with diaphragmatic injury who may get extremely breathless when lying down. In this instance, the patient is best managed sitting upright or at 30–45 degrees, and it must be documented that the spine has not been cleared. • In the rare incident of gunshot/stab injury to personnel wearing protection vests (e.g. ballistic and stab), these may protect from penetrating injury. However, serious underlying blunt trauma (e.g. pulmonary contusion) may be caused to the thorax. • **NEVER UNDERESTIMATE THESE INJURIES.** There is a strong link between serious blunt chest wall injury and thoracic spine injury. Maintain a high index of suspicion.

TABLE 4.19 – ASSESSMENT and MANAGEMENT of: Specific Thoracic Trauma	
Flail Chest	
Flail chest is usually the result of a significant blunt chest injury, causing two or more rib fractures in two or more places. A sternal flail can also occur where the ribs or costal cartilages are fractured on both sides of the chest. This results in a flail segment that moves independently of the rest of the chest during respiration leading to inadequate ventilation. The ensuing pulmonary insufficiency is caused by three pathophysiological processes: 1 The negative pressure required for effective ventilation is disrupted due to the paradoxical motion of the flail segment. 2 The underlying pulmonary contusion, which causes haemorrhage and oedema of the lung. 3 The pain associated with the multiple rib fractures will result in a degree of hypoventilation. – Small flail segments may not be detectable. – Large flail segments may impair ventilation considerably as a result of pain.	
ASSESSMENT	**MANAGEMENT**
• Assess for signs of a flail chest	• Flail segments should not be immobilised and efforts to maintain ventilation are the priority. • Allow the patient to sit supported at 30–45 degrees rather than try to make them stay on a scoop stretcher. **NB** Traditionally, the patient has been turned onto the affected side for transportation, but this CANNOT be achieved on a scoop stretcher.

(continued)

SECTION 4 Trauma

Thoracic Trauma

TABLE 4.19 – ASSESSMENT and MANAGEMENT of: Specific Thoracic Trauma *(continued)*	
• Assess the patient's level of pain	• Consider the need for analgesia (if indicated refer to **Pain Management in Adults** and **Pain Management in Children**).
• Transfer	• Undertake a **TIME CRITICAL** transfer to a major trauma centre, unless the patient needs an immediate lifesaving intervention, in which case transfer to nearest trauma unit. • Provide a pre-alert using ATMIST. • Continue patient management en-route.
Tension Pneumothorax	
• This is a rare respiratory emergency, which may require immediate action at the scene or en-route to further care. A tension pneumothorax occurs when a damaged area of lung leaks air out into the pleural space on each inspiration, but does not permit the air to exit from the chest via the lung on expiration. • This progressively builds up air under tension on the affected side collapsing that lung and putting increasing pressure on the heart and great vessels and the opposite lung. Decreased venous return is significantly affected by the kinking of the vessels, especially the inferior vena cava, as the mediastinum is pushed towards the contralateral side. Coughing and shouting can make a situation worse. If this air is not released externally, the heart will be unable to fill and the other lung will no longer be able to ventilate, inducing cardiac arrest. • Tension pneumothorax is most often related to penetrating trauma, but can arise spontaneously from blunt or crushing injuries to the chest and as the result of a blast wave. This will present rapidly with an increase in breathlessness and extreme respiratory distress (respiratory rate often >30 breaths per minute). Subsequently the patient may deteriorate and the breathing rate may rapidly slow to <10 breaths per minute before the patient arrests. • Signs and symptoms: – The chest on the affected side may appear to be moving poorly or not at all. – At the same time, the affected chest wall may appear to be over-expanded (hyperexpansion). – Air entry will be greatly reduced or absent on the affected side. – In the absence of shock, the neck veins may become distended. – Later, the trachea and apex beat of the heart may become displaced away from the side of the pneumothorax, and cyanosis and breathlessness may appear. – Hyperresonance may be present. – Occasionally, the patient will only present with rapidly deteriorating respiratory distress. – The patient may appear shocked as a result of decreased cardiac output. – Patients are usually tachycardic and hypotensive. • Ventilation of a patient with a chest injury is a common cause of tension pneumothorax in the pre-hospital setting. Forcing oxygenated air down into the lung under positive pressure will progressively expand a small, undetected simple pneumothorax into a tension pneumothorax. This will take some minutes and may well be several minutes after ventilation has commenced. It is usually noticed by increasing back pressure during ventilation; either by the bag becoming harder to squeeze or the ventilator alarms sounding.	
ASSESSMENT	**MANAGEMENT**
• Assess breathing adequacy, respiratory rate, volume, and equality of air entry. FEEL, LOOK, AUSCULTATE and PERCUSS • View both sides of the chest and check they are moving; auscultate to ensure air entry is present and percuss on both sides	• **Only perform needle thoracocentesis in a patient if there is haemodynamic instability, hypotension, or increasing respiratory compromise.** • If a tension pneumothorax is likely, decompress rapidly by needle thoracocentesis. • If the patient requires positive pressure ventilation, an open thoracostomy should be performed if an appropriately skilled practitioner is available (**Caution** - performing a thoracostomy on a spontaneously breathing patient will leave a simple pneumothorax with a poorly ventilated lung. Bilateral thoracostomies on a spontaneously breathing patient should only be done one at a time, and appropriate chest seal dressings should be applied).

SECTION 4 Trauma

TABLE 4.19 – ASSESSMENT and MANAGEMENT of: Specific Thoracic Trauma *(continued)*	
• Observe the patient for signs of recurrence of the tension pneumothorax	• If the procedure was unsuccessful, repeat the thoracocentesis. • Consider the use of a thicker needle in patients with a thicker chest wall, following your organisation's guidelines.
• Transfer	• Undertake a **TIME CRITICAL** transfer to a major trauma centre, unless the patient needs an immediate lifesaving intervention, in which case transfer to nearest trauma unit. • Provide a pre-alert using ATMIST. **NB** Needle thoracocentesis may not always decompress pneumothoraces in large patients. In such cases, a thoracostomy with or without a chest drain may need to be performed. This needs to be done either in hospital or by appropriately skilled practitioners (e.g. BASICS or HEMS doctors on scene or in hospital).
Cardiac Tamponade	
The heart is enclosed in a tough, non-elastic membrane, called the pericardium. A potential space exists between the pericardium and the heart itself. If a penetrating wound injures the heart, the blood may flow under pressure into the pericardial space. As the pericardium cannot expand, a leak of as little as 20–30 ml of blood can cause compression of the heart. This decreases cardiac output and causes tachycardia and hypotension. Further compression reduces cardiac output and cardiac arrest may occur.	
ASSESSMENT	**MANAGEMENT**
• Assess for signs of cardiac tamponade • Signs of hypovolaemic shock, tachycardia and hypotension, accompanied by blunt or penetrating chest trauma may be an indication of cardiac tamponade • Note the presence of distended neck veins and muffled heart sounds when listening with a stethoscope	• Cardiac tamponade is a **TIME CRITICAL, LIFE-THREATENING** condition that requires rapid surgical intervention, resulting in an open chest operation to evacuate the compressing blood. • DO NOT delay on scene inserting cannulae or commencing fluid therapy.
• Transfer	• Undertake a **TIME CRITICAL** transfer to a major trauma centre, unless the patient needs an immediate lifesaving intervention, in which case transfer to nearest trauma unit. • Provide a pre-alert using ATMIST.
• Re-assess **ABC** en-route to hospital	**NB** Pericardiocentesis is not recommended in the pre-hospital setting, as it is rarely successful, has significant complications and delays definitive care.
Surgical Emphysema	
• Surgical emphysema produces swelling of the chest wall, neck and face with a cracking feeling under the fingers when the skin is pressed. This indicates an air leak from within the chest, either from a pneumothorax, a ruptured large airway or a fractured larynx. • Normally it requires no specific treatment, but it does indicate potentially SERIOUS underlying chest trauma. Sometimes the surgical emphysema might be extensive and cause the patient to swell up. Where the emphysema is progressively increasing, look for a possible underlying tension pneumothorax. • In some cases, surgical emphysema may become so severe as to tighten the overlying skin and restrict chest movement. A tension pneumothorax must be excluded as above. If there is no improvement, the patient must be transferred to hospital as soon as possible.	

(continued)

TABLE 4.19 – ASSESSMENT and MANAGEMENT of: Specific Thoracic Trauma *(continued)*	
ASSESSMENT	**MANAGEMENT**
• Assess for signs of surgical emphysema, swelling of the chest wall, neck and face with a cracking feeling under the fingers when the skin is pressed	
• Consider possible underlying tension pneumothorax	• Refer to tension pneumothorax guidance above.
Blast Injury	
Blast injury is caused by three mechanisms: 1 Rupture of air-filled organs. 2 Missiled debris. 3 Contact injury. Although rare in survivors, strongly suspect a blast lung injury if the patient is suffering from tympanic injury. However, the absence of a tympanic injury DOES NOT exclude lung injury. **NB** Being shielded from blast debris DOES NOT exclude lung injury.	
ASSESSMENT	**MANAGEMENT**
• Assess for blast injury	• Pre-hospital management is supportive.

KEY POINTS!

Thoracic Trauma

- **Thoracic injury is commonly associated with hypoxia, either from impaired ventilation or secondary to hypovolaemia from massive bleeding into the chest (haemathorax) or major vessel disruption.**
- **Count the respiratory rate and look for asymmetrical chest movement.**
- **Pulse oximetry must be used as this will assist in recognising hypoxia.**
- **The mechanism of injury is an important guide to the likelihood of significant thoracic injury.**
- **Blunt trauma to the sternum may induce myocardial contusion, which may result in ECG rhythm disturbances.**
- **ECG monitoring.**
- **Impaling objects should be adequately secured. If the object is pulsating do not completely immobilise, but allow the object to pulsate.**
- **Do not probe or explore penetrating injuries.**

Bibliography

1. National Institute for Health and Clinical Excellence. Fractures (Complex): Assessment and Management (NG37). London: NICE, 2016. Available from: https://www.nice.org.uk/guidance/ng37.
2. National Institute for Health and Clinical Excellence. Fractures (Non-complex): Assessment and Management (NG38). London: NICE, 2016. Available from: https://www.nice.org.uk/guidance/ng38.
3. National Institute for Health and Clinical Excellence. Major Trauma: Assessment and Initial Management (NG39). London: NICE, 2016. Available from: https://www.nice.org.uk/guidance/ng39.
4. National Institute for Health and Clinical Excellence. Major Trauma: Service Delivery (NG40). London: NICE, 2016. Available from: https://www.nice.org.uk/guidance/ng40.
5. National Institute for Health and Clinical Excellence. *Spinal Injury: Assessment and Initial Management* (NG41). London: NICE, 2016. Available from: https://www.nice.org.uk/guidance/ng41.
6. National Institute for Health and Clinical Excellence. *When to Suspect Child Maltreatment* (CG89). London: NICE, 2009. Available from: https://www.nice.org.uk/guidance/cg89.

7. Revell M, Porter K, Greaves I. Fluid resuscitation in pre-hospital trauma care: a consensus view. *Emergency Medicine Journal* 2002, 19(6): 494–498.

8. Lee C, Revell M, Porter K, Steyn R. The pre-hospital management of chest injuries: a consensus statement. Faculty of Pre-hospital Care, Royal College of Surgeons of Edinburgh. *Emergency Medicine Journal* 2007, 24(3): 220–224.

9. Warner KJ, Copass MK, Bulger EM. Paramedic use of needle thoracostomy in the pre-hospital environment. *Prehospital Emergency Care* 2008, 12(2): 162–168.

10. Waydhas C, Sauerland S. Pre-hospital pleural decompression and chest tube placement after blunt trauma: a systematic review. *Resuscitation* 2007, 72(1): 11–25.

11. Dretzke J, Sandercock J, Bayliss S, Burls A. Clinical effectiveness and cost effectiveness of pre-hospital intravenous fluids in trauma patients. *Health Technology Assessment* 2004, 8(23).

12. Turner J, Nicholl J, Webber L, Cox H, Dixon S, Yates D. A randomised controlled trial of prehospital intravenous fluid replacement therapy in serious trauma. *Health Technology Assessment* 2000, 4(31).

13. Stern SA. Low-volume fluid resuscitation for presumed hemorrhagic shock: helpful or harmful? *Current Opinion in Critical Care* 2001, 7(6): 422–430.

14. Pepe PE, Mosesso VNJ, Falk JL. Pre-hospital fluid resuscitation of the patient with major trauma. *Prehospital Emergency Care* 2002, 6(1): 81–91.

15. Borman JB, Aharonson-Daniel L, Savitsky B, Peleg K. Unilateral flail chest is seldom a lethal injury. *Emergency Medicine Journal* 2006, 23(12): 903–905.

16. BMJ Evidence Centre. Best Practice: Cardiac tamponade. Available from: http://bestpractice.bmj.com/best-practice/monograph/459.html, 2012.

17. Fitzgerald M, Spencer J, Johnson F, Marasco S, Atkin C, Kossmann T. Definitive management of acute cardiac tamponade secondary to blunt trauma. *Emergency Medicine Australasia* 2005, 17(5–6): 494–499.

18. Friend KD. Prehospital recognition of tension pneumothorax. *Prehospital Emergency Care* 2000, 4(1): 75–77.

19. Massarutti D, Trillo G, Berlot G, Tomasini A, Bacer B, D'Orlando L et al. Simple thoracostomy in pre-hospital trauma management is safe and effective: a 2-year experience by helicopter emergency medical crews. *European Journal of Emergency Medicine* 2006, 13(5): 276–280.

20. Wanek S, Mayberry JC. Blunt thoracic trauma: flail chest, pulmonary contusion, and blast injury. *Critical Care Clinics* 2004, 20(1): 71–81.

21. Blaivas M. Inadequate needle thoracostomy rate in the pre-hospital setting for presumed pneumothorax. *Journal of Ultrasound in Medicine* 2010, 29(9): 1285–1289.

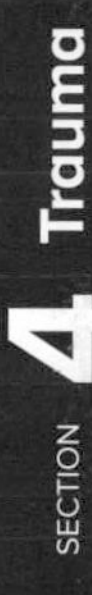

Falls in Older Adults

1. Introduction

- Falls are defined as an unintentional or unexpected loss of balance resulting in coming to rest on the floor, the ground or an object below knee level. The impact of a fall on the individual and their family is not to be underestimated, with falls often leading to a fear of falling and potentially having psychological, as well as physical effects. A fall is distinguished from a collapse, which occurs as a result of an acute medical problem such as an acute arrhythmia, a transient ischaemic attack or vertigo.[1] A fall can be precipitated by an acute medical condition, and the actual cause of the fall can be very difficult to establish on initial presentation. This guideline covers falls from a standing height. Falls from above standing height or 2 metres above the ground, are not covered in this guideline (refer to **Section 4 – Trauma**).
- The term 'mechanical fall' is **not** an appropriate term to use when describing a fall; it implies that a benign aetiology for an older person's fall exists and it is inaccurate, inconsistently used, is not associated with a discrete fall evaluation and does not predict outcomes.[2]
- Older people in contact with healthcare professionals for any reason should be asked routinely whether they have fallen in the past year, asked about the frequency, context and characteristics of the falls and referred to appropriate falls prevention pathways as per local arrangements. Recently the SAFER 2 study (a large multi-centre cluster randomised controlled trial) has shown that a paramedic protocol for assessment of older patients (aged ≥65) who have fallen, with an option to refer direct to a community-based falls service (in place of conveyance to the ED), is safe, inexpensive and reduced subsequent 999 calls in those patients. There was no overall difference in outcomes (whether taken to hospital or managed at home) between the trial arms.

2. Incidence

- Falls are the leading cause of emergency calls in the over 65s and account for 10–25% of emergency ambulance responses each year for adults aged over 65 years.[3] In the London Ambulance Service alone, there were 70,380 incidents of people aged 65 and over who were coded as presenting with a fall in the period for 2015–16.
- Falls represent the second leading cause of accidental injury death worldwide and the leading cause of injury-related mortality in the UK.[4] Every year 1 in 3 people aged over 65 and up to 1 in 2 aged over 80 will fall at least once.[5] By 2025 it is estimated that this will account for over 3.2 million falls in people over the age of 65 in England alone.[6] Up to 14,000 people will die each year as a result of a fall and a subsequent fractured neck of femur.[7]
- A fall of <2 metres is the commonest mechanism of injury in older patients.[8]

3. Severity and Outcome

- As part of the normal ageing process there is a loss of bone density, muscle tone, skin changes and often increased poly-pharmacy. A simple fall in an older person may result in a much more significant injury than would be seen in a younger person. Clinicians should have a higher index of suspicion of injury in older people. However, falls are not a part of normal ageing and are typically due to pathological changes described earlier.
- The Silver Book[9] recommends ways in which emergency admissions for older people can be reduced and emphasises that health and social care services must adapt to meet older people's urgent care needs, including ambulance services.
- Falls can be a marker of frailty, which is associated with common syndromes of ageing including immobility, incontinence, susceptibility to the side effects of medication, delirium and dementia, all of which increase the complexity of the presentation and may indicate a change in normal health status. Frail older people typically suffer falls indoors. For a person with frailty a relatively small event (e.g. a minor infection, a new medication or constipation) may trigger a sudden and dramatic functional decline. Frailty is a clinically recognised state of increased vulnerability. It results from ageing associated with a decline in the body's physical and psychological reserves. This can cause the person to fall and also to struggle to recover following a fall. It is important to recognise the presence of frailty in weighing the benefits and risks of any intervention or treatment plan. Even if no injury has been sustained, further assessment and support post-fall will enable the provision of the right care and support for the person.

4. Risk Factors for Falls

Refer to Table 4.20.

- Risk factors for falls can be broadly classified into three categories:
  - intrinsic factors – relating to the person
  - extrinsic factors – relating to the person's environment
  - exposure to risk.
- However, it is recognised that falls often result from the dynamic interactions of risks in all categories.
- Intrinsic risk factors include changes in the body caused by the normal ageing process, certain medical conditions, excessive alcohol, being physically inactive or a combination of these.

Falls in Older Adults

- It is important to consider dementia and cognitive impairment in the assessment of a patient who has fallen. As many as 11–26% of patients presenting with a fall will have cognitive impairment, some of which will be undiagnosed.[10,11] Patients with dementia are more likely to fall, have more falls and are more likely to sustain an injury (such as a hip fracture or head injury) from the fall. If sustaining an injury, the outcomes are worse for the patient, their family, the health service and society at large. It is therefore vital to recognise this as a high-risk group.
- It is important that the cause of the fall is considered so that the correct pathways are chosen or excluded; red flags should always be excluded and modifiable factors considered.

Many medicines cause postural hypotension and may contribute to over 20% of extrinsic falls. Common causes are:

- cardiac drugs:
  - antiarrhythmics (e.g. digoxin)
  - alpha-blockers (e.g. doxazosin)
  - beta-blockers (e.g. bisoprolol, atenolol)
  - ACE inhibitors (e.g. ramipril, lisinopril)
  - angiotensin 2 blockers (e.g. losartan, candesartan)
  - diuretics (e.g. furosemide, bumetanide, spironolactone, bendroflumethiazide)
  - calcium channel blockers (e.g. amlodipine, diltiazem)
- urological drugs (e.g. oxybutynin)
- neuropsychiatric drugs:
  - Parkinson's drugs (e.g. madopar, sinemet, ropinirole)
  - tricyclic antidepressants (e.g. amitriptyline)
  - antipsychotics (e.g. haloperidol, risperidone)
  - painkillers (e.g. opioids)
- In these patients a formal medicines optimisation review may be indicated by the GP practice or another clinical lead (following local guidance).

Certain activities can be 'high risk' because of the specific interaction of risk factors involved, for example, poor balance combined with standing on a stool to change a light bulb or reach a high shelf. To understand falls risk in the environment fully, it is important to observe a person moving around in their environment; referral for a falls assessment in line with local pathways/guidelines will facilitate this.

TABLE 4.20 – Intrinsic and Extrinsic Falls Risk Factors[12]

Common intrinsic risks of falls[13]	**Common extrinsic risk factors of falls**
• lower extremity weakness • previous falls • gait and balance disorders • visual impairment • depression • functional and cognitive impairment • dizziness • low body mass index • urinary incontinence • postural hypotension • female sex • being over age 80. **Other intrinsic causes of falls** • sensory deficit (poor vision, peripheral neuropathy) • musculoskeletal disease (osteoarthritis, proximal muscle weakness, previous joint replacement) • other neurodegenerative conditions • central nervous system disease (cognitive dysfunction, vestibular hypofunction, cerebrovascular disease, cerebral hypoperfusion) • Parkinson's disease and Parkinsonism.	• polypharmacy (use of multiple medications) • psychotropic medications • poor lighting (especially on stairs), glare and shadows • low ambient temperature • wet, slippery or uneven floor surfaces • thresholds at room entrances • obstacles and tripping hazards, including clutter • chairs, toilets or beds being too high, low or unstable • inappropriate or unsafe walking aids • inadequately maintained wheelchairs, for example, brakes not locking • improper use of wheelchairs, for example, failing to clear foot plates • unsafe or absent equipment, such as handrails • pets, such as cats and dogs • loose fitting footwear and clothing, such as trailing dressing gowns • access to the property, wheelie bins, the garden, uneven ground.

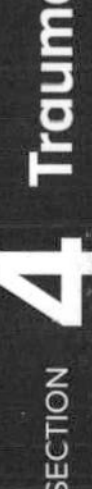

Falls in Older Adults

Early warning sign - blanching erythema

Areas of discoloured tissue that blanch when fingertip pressure is applied and the colour recovers when pressure is released, indicating damage is starting to occur but can be reversed.

On darkly pigmented skin, blanching does not occur and changes to colour, temperature and texture of skin are the main indicators.

Grade 1	Grade 2	Grade 3	Grade 4
Non-blanchable erythema	**Partial thickness skin loss**	**Full thickness skin loss**	**Full thickness tissue loss**
Intact skin with non-blanchable redness, usually over a bony prominence. Darker skin tones may not have visible blanching but the colour may differ from the surrounding area. The affected area may be painful, firmer, softer, warmer or cooler than the surrounding tissue.	Loss of the epidermis/dermis presenting as a shallow open ulcer with a red/pink wound bed without slough or bruising.[1] May also present as an intact or open/ruptured blister.	Subcutaneous fat may be visible but bone, tendon or muscle is not visible or palpable. Slough may be present but does not obscure the depth of tissue loss. May include undermining or tunnelling.[2]	Extensive destruction with exposed or palpable bone, tendon or muscle. Slough may be present but does not obscure the depth of tissue loss. Often includes undermining or tunnelling.[2]

Moisture lesions

Moisture lesions are skin damage due to exposure to urine, faeces or other body fluids.

a) Location:
Located in peri-anal, gluteal, cleft, groin or buttock area. Not usually over a bony prominence.

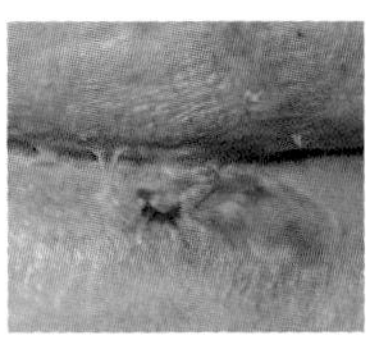

b) Shape:
Diffuse often multiple lesions. May be 'copy', 'mirror' or 'kissing' lesion on adjacent buttock or anal cleft. Linear.

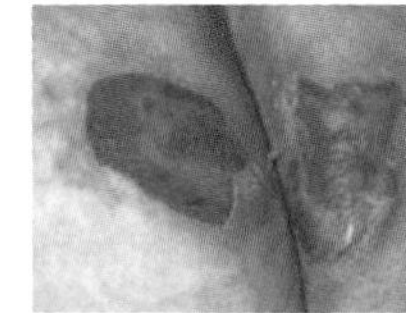

c) Edges:
Diffuse irregular edges.

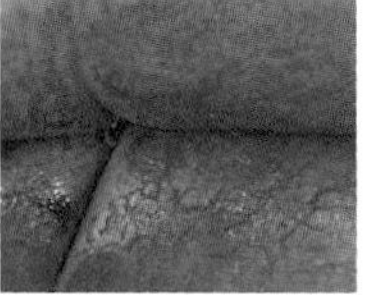

d) Necrosis:
No necrosis or slough. May develop slough if infection present.

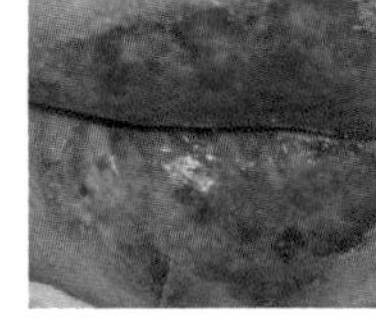

e) Depth:
Superficial partial thickness skin loss. Can enlarge or deepen if infection present.

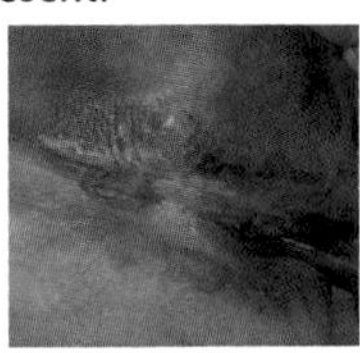

f) Colour:
Colour of redness may not be uniform. May have pink or white surrounding skin (maceration). Peri-anal redness may be present.

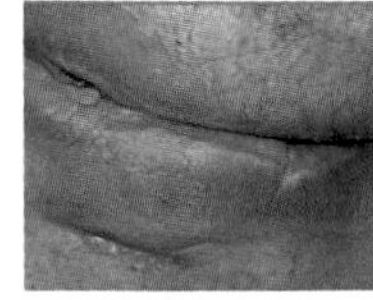

Where pressure ulcers commonly occur

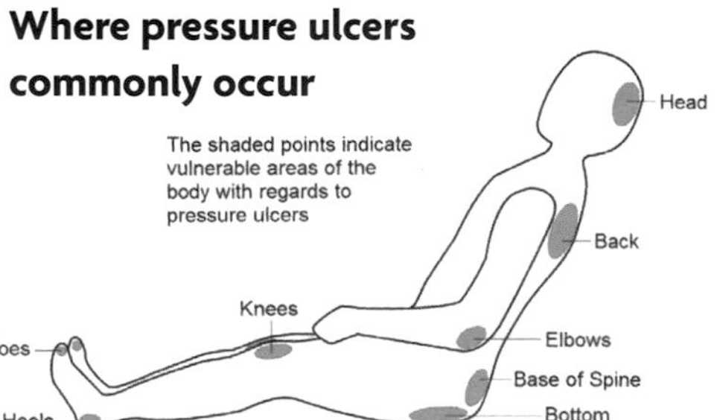

[1] Bruising can indicate deep tissue injury

[2] The depth of a Grade 3 or 4 pressure ulcer varies by anatomical location. Areas such as the bridge of the nose, ears, occiput and malleolus do not have fatty tissue so the depth of these ulcers may be shallow. In contrast areas which have excess fatty tissue can develop deep Grade 3 pressure ulcers where bone, tendon, muscle is not directly visible or palpable.

Figure 4.11 – Grading tool for assessing skin breakdown. Reproduced with kind permission of Healthcare Improvement Scotland.

6.7 Continence

- Confirm the patient's usual toileting/continence regime. Consider new symptoms, including dysuria, increased frequency of urination, suprapubic tenderness, urgency and polyuria, but do not carry out a urine dipstick in the absence of symptoms of UTI.[15]
- If continent/partially continent; consider if they are likely to be able to locate and physically get to the toilet/commode, rearrange clothes and clean the genital area and hands.
- If incontinent/partially continent; consider if the patient/carer is able to manage pads/catheter care, rearrange clothes, clean the genital area and hands and dispose of waste safety. Community nursing services may be available to provide rapid continence assessment including recatheterisation.

6.8 How to Decide If the Patient Could Be Managed in the Community?

- Decisions on whether to manage a patient at home/in the community can be challenging and should be made following a comprehensive history, clinical assessment and examination. Decisions on the best management of an older person who has fallen are made on a risk/benefit basis and may benefit from discussion with locally agreed clinical contacts. These could include ambulance service clinical advice lines, or other healthcare professionals clinical advice lines using a shared decision making approach, and should always consider the views of the patient and relatives/carers. The final referral decision will also depend on the availability and responsiveness of local community health and social care services. Well-structured advice on how to assess and make decisions related to choosing an appropriate clinical pathway, improves patient safety and outcomes.[16]
- There are also risks in taking an older person to hospital, including institutionalisation and/or deconditioning (the consequence of prolonged bed-rest, leading to loss of functional status through reduced muscle mass and strength). The decline in muscle mass and strength has been linked to falls, functional decline, increased frailty, immobility and healthcare-associated infection.[17]
- Some older people who fall may prefer to be managed in the community or at home, and where possible this should be supported, particularly where family/carers can also provide support. Following a comprehensive patient assessment and wider review of the circumstances of the fall (having excluded injuries/acute illness), ambulance clinicians should provide the referral for this to occur in line with local pathways and guidance.

6.9 Ongoing Referral

- All older people who have fallen resulting in an ambulance call/attendance, but are then managed at home, should be offered referral pathways as per local guidelines. The purpose of referral/re-referral is to prevent further falls and injury.
- Referrals should take into account current care plans and other health and social care organisations already involved in the patient's care.
- Decision making should be a shared process, including the patient and their family/carers/other health and social care professionals/any person holding their lasting power of attorney for health and welfare.
- Referral to services via locally agreed pathways may result in:
  - multifactorial falls risk assessment
  - frailty assessment
  - assessment of care needs, including telecare.

6.10 Falls Prevention[4]

- Ambulance clinicians have a role to play in having conversations with people who are at risk of falling, or who have fallen, to try and prevent further falls. The evidence-based Making Every Contact Count (MECC) approach[18] can be applied or other locally agreed methods of ensuring health prevention messages can be given. A MECC interaction takes a matter of minutes and is not intended to add to busy workloads, but should be part of the conversations after a fall or with patients who have been identified as at risk of falling. Evidence suggests that the broad adoption of the MECC approach could potentially have a significant impact on the health of the population.
- Support can be given to older people at risk of falling by routinely asking them about falls and encouraging them to stay active, connected, eat well and reduce alcohol intake, to reduce the risk of falling and to improve outcomes if a fall happens. Consider discussing the measures a person can take to reduce their risk factors for falling, doing exercises recommended by falls teams or other health care professionals, the preventable nature of some falls and where they can seek further advice and assistance.
- Consider leaving the patient with an information leaflet about falls prevention and suggesting telecare options, such as a pendant type alarm so help can be summoned for any further falls, or simple solutions to providing a safer physical environment. Conversations can take place with carers/family members if the person has cognitive impairment.

Falls in Older Adults

TABLE 4.21 – ASSESSMENT and MANAGEMENT of: Falls in Older People *(continued)*	
ASSESSMENT	**MANAGEMENT**
– **Time** of day the fall occurred (falls in the morning could be due to postural hypotension and later in the day could be due to fatigue)	– Can the history of the fall be corroborated by a reliable third party? – Is there a history of previous falls? When did these occur, with what frequency, were any injurious? – Is this fall consistent with previous falls or different? – Is there a new onset of confusion? – Are alcohol/drugs/medication involved?
FUNCTIONAL ASSESSMENT – MOBILITY	
• Mobility must be considered to: – help exclude injury – determine if mobility is a factor contributing to falls risk – ascertain a person's ability to function safely at home following the fall • Observe the person getting up from their chair, balancing on standing, walking round their home (including turning) and sitting down again – using their usual walking aid if applicable) • A formal test may be used as per local guidance, such as the 'get up and go' test or the 'turn 180 degrees' test[28,29,30] • A mobility assessment should also take into account the use and the state of repair of walking aids • While the person is moving around, check they can weight-bear and consider how steady, safe and confident they are • Where possible, find out the person's normal mobility status; it may be that a person has limited mobility normally but is managing well with regular visits from family or carers and/or with equipment such as a commode	• Consider whether the person is able to: – get to the toilet/commode and transfer on and off it safely – access a drink or simple snack – manage on the stairs if this is essential to get to the toilet/bed or other rooms – take essential medications as prescribed – summon help. • If the person receives care, consider the timing of the next visit. Contact the agency if possible. Information may be found in a care plan. • Consider local services that may be available to respond to support the person in remaining at home and avoiding hospital admission.
OTHER CONSIDERATIONS	
• General	• Look/ask for other information about the patient, such as anticipatory care plans that may detail preferences for place of care, clinical management, home care input, nursing/therapy input, including access to electronic care records. • Ask about lasting power of attorney/end of life and DNACPR/ReSPECT decisions. • In cases of worsening chronic confusion, consider referral back to GP/local pathway. • Consider frailty in line with local guidance. • Consider the need for senior clinical advice/support.

Falls in Older Adults

TABLE 4.21 – ASSESSMENT and MANAGEMENT of: Falls in Older People *(continued)*	
ASSESSMENT	**MANAGEMENT**
• Extrinsic factors	• Walking aids (consider correct use, state of repair, suitability for the patient). • Footwear (good fit, not worn out, adequate grip and support). • Floor surfaces (clear of obstructions, carpets and rugs not frayed or lifted, not slippery or wet/ greasy). • Lighting. • Temperature. • Spectacles and hearing aids, telecare alarm (worn, clean and working, regular check-ups). • Home safety, smoke alarms, clutter and other trip hazards, exit routes, crime risks, ability to self-evacuate, home adaptations. • Shared decision making with patients and families/carers/other health and social care professionals. • Respect the autonomy of the individual.
• Safeguarding	• Ask the patient if they feel safe. • Consider the need for additional support, protection or referral for safeguarding. • Refer to **Safeguarding Adults at Risk**.
• Social context	• Housing type. • Living alone or with spouse/family/partner. – What is the level of support offered by the above? – Does the patient have caring responsibilities? What are they and are they affected by the fall? – What are the existing support/care packages in place? When is the next planned visit of carers? – Are the patient/relatives and carers coping or in denial? • Is support/care assessment required? • Does the family and carer burden/need require assessment? • Does the patient suffer social isolation/ loneliness?
• Referral and safety-netting	• Follow local policies or guidelines. • Patients who have fallen should be offered referral to a community-based falls service to enable secondary prevention as per local policies.[16]
• Prevention	• Self-care and links to the voluntary sector. • Signposting. • Local leaflets, contacts and information. • Written advice for non-injury falls. • Advice for the patient, their relatives and carers. • Make every contact count (MECC) opportunities.

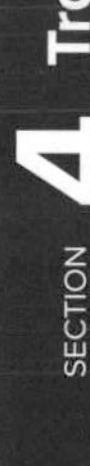

Burns and Scalds

1. Introduction

- Burns arise in a number of accident situations, and may have a variety of presentations (refer to Table 4.22), accompanying injuries or pre-existing medical problems associated with the burn injury. Scalds, flame or thermal burns, chemical and electrical burns will all produce a different burn pattern, and inhalation of smoke or toxic chemicals from the fire may cause serious accompanying complications.
- A number of burn patients will also be seriously injured following falls from a height in fires, or injuries sustained as a result of road traffic collision where a vehicle ignites after a collision or crash.
- Explosions will often induce flash burns, and other serious injuries due to the effect of the blast wave or flying debris.
- Inhalation of superheated smoke, steam or gases in a fire, will induce major airway swelling and respiratory obstruction – refer to Table 4.23 for signs of airway burns. The likelihood of an airway injury increases with the presence of multiple risk factors or signs.
- Non-accidental injury should always be considered when burns have occurred in children and vulnerable adults including older people, in particular where the mechanism of injury described does not match the injury sustained, or there is inconsistency in the history (refer to **Safeguarding Children** and **Safeguarding Adults at Risk**).
- Preceding long-term illness, especially chronic bronchitis and emphysema, will seriously worsen the outcome from airway burns.
- Remember that a burn injury may be preceded by a medical condition causing a collapse (e.g. elderly patient with a stroke collapsing against a radiator).
- Burns can be very painful (refer to **Pain Management in Adults** and **Pain Management in Children**).

TABLE 4.22 – Burns/Scalds
Electrical
Search for entry and exit sites. Assess ECG rhythm. The extent of burn damage in electrical burns is often impossible to assess fully at the time of injury (refer to **Electrical Injuries**).
Thermal
The skin contact time and temperature of the source determines the depth of the burn. Scalds with boiling water are frequently of short duration as the water flows off the skin rapidly. Record the type of clothing (e.g. wool retains the hot water). Those resulting from hot fat and other liquids that remain on the skin may cause significantly deeper and more serious burns. Also the time to cold water and removal of clothing is of significant impact.
Chemical
It is vital to note the nature of the chemical. Alkalis in particular may cause deep, penetrating burns, sometimes with little initial discomfort. Certain chemicals such as phenol or hydrofluoric acid can cause poisoning by absorption through the skin and therefore must be irrigated with COPIOUS amounts of water for a minimum of 15 minutes (this should be continued until definitive care is available if patient condition and water supply allows) (refer to **Major, Complex and High Risk Incidents**).

2. Burn Severity

- Refer to Wallace's Rule of Nines or the Lund and Browder chart to assess total body surface area (TBSA).
- For small or large burns (<15% or > 85%) it is acceptable to use the patient's palmar surface including the fingers as a size estimate. This equates to approximately 1% TBSA.
- Be aware of the risk of underestimating the size of burns with patients with large breasts or the obese patient. These factors can significantly affect the proportion of total body surface area using standardised charts.
- Use all of the burn area, but do not consider areas of erythema as this is often transient in the initial phases of a burn. Do not try to differentiate between levels of burn (superficial, partial thickness, full thickness etc.) as it is impractical to estimate the depth of burns in the initial hours following injury.
- Only a rough estimate is required; an accurate measure is not possible in the early stages; however, the size of a burn may well influence referral and management pathways.

TABLE 4.23 – Signs/Increased Risk of Airway Burns
Signs
• Facial or neck burns.
• Soot in the nasal and oral cavities.
• Coughing up blackened sputum.
• Cough and hoarseness.
• Difficulty with breathing and swallowing.
• Blistering around the mouth and tongue.
• Scorched hair, eyebrows or facial hair.
• Stridor or altered breath sounds such as wheezing.
• Loss of consciousness.
• Fires/blasts in enclosed spaces.

SECTION 4 Trauma

Burns and Scalds

3. Assessment and Management

- For the assessment and management of burns and scalds in adults refer to Table 4.24.

TABLE 4.24 – ASSESSMENT and MANAGEMENT of: Burns and Scalds

ASSESSMENT	MANAGEMENT
• Ensure scene safety for rescuer and patient	**If safe to do so, stop the burning process:** • Remove from the burn source. • Brush off dry chemical.
• Assess **<C>ABCD**	• If any of the following **TIME CRITICAL** features present: – major **<C>ABCD** problems – airway burns (soot or oedema around the mouth and nose) – history of hot air or gas inhalation; these patients may initially appear well but can deteriorate very rapidly and need complex airway intervention – respiratory distress – evidence of circumferential (completely encircling) burns of the chest, neck, limb – significant facial burns – burns >15% in adults and >10% in children TBSA – presence of other major injuries, then: • Start correcting A and B and undertake a **TIME CRITICAL** transfer to nearest appropriate hospital according to local care pathways. • Continue patient management en-route. • Provide an alert/information call.
• Specifically assess	• Airway patency as early intervention may be required with inhalational burns; if intubation is impossible, needle cricothyroidotomy is the management of choice. • Waveform capnography should be used whenever intubation is performed. • Breathing for rate, depth and any breathing difficulty – refer to **Airway and Breathing Management**. • Evidence of trauma – for neck and back trauma refer to **Spinal Injury and Spinal Cord Injury**. • Co-existing or precipitating medical conditions.
• Oxygen	• Administer supplemental **oxygen** via a non-rebreathing mask – SpO_2 readings may be false due to carboxyhaemoglobin.
• Cool/irrigate the burn	• Irrigate with copious amounts of water as soon as is practicable, this can still be effective up to three hours after the injury. For chemical burns, irrigate for a minimum of 15 minutes up to a maximum of one hour. For all other burns, irrigate for a maximum of 20 minutes for avoid hypothermia. • Cut off burning, or smouldering clothing, providing it is not adhering to the skin. • Remove any constricting jewellery including rings. • **DO NOT** use ice or ice water as this can worsen the burn injury and exaggerate hypothermia. • Use saline if no other irrigant available. • Gel based dressings may be used but water treatment is preferred. • Alkali burns require prolonged irrigation – continue until definitive care.

(continued)

TABLE 4.24 – ASSESSMENT and MANAGEMENT of: Burns and Scalds *(continued)*	
	– If possible, get the patient to do as much as possible with directions; this may not always be possible but will greatly reduce the exposure to the first responders. – Do not apply any form of dressing or gel until the burn has been adequately irrigated. – Minimise on scene duration for patients with large burns or burns on the face, eyes or hands.

KEY POINTS!

Burns and Scalds

- **Airway status can deteriorate rapidly and may need complex interventions available at the emergency departments.**
- **Stopping the burning process is essential.**
- **The time from burning is an essential piece of information.**
- **Pain relief is important.**
- **Consider non-accidental injury in children and vulnerable adults including older people.**
- **When irrigating the eyes ensure that the fluid runs away from the contralateral eye to avoid contamination.**

Bibliography

1. The Royal Children's Hospital Melbourne. *Burns/management of burn wounds* Available from: https://www.rch.org.au/clinicalguide/guideline_index/Burns/, 2018.
2. National Institute for Health and Care Excellence. *Burns and Scalds* Clinical Knowledge Summaries. Available from: https://cks.nice.org.uk/burns-and-scalds#!scenario, 2017.
3. Porter A, Snooks H, Youren A, Gaze S, Whitfield R, Rapport F et al. 'Covering our backs': ambulance crews' attitudes towards clinical documentation when emergency (999) patients are not conveyed to hospital. *Emergency Medicine Journal* 2008, 25(5): 292–295.
4. Ayers DE, Kay AR. Management of burns in the wilderness. *Travel Medicine and Infectious Disease* 2005, 3(4): 239–48.
5. Boots RJ, Dulhunty JM, Paratz J, Lipman J. Respiratory complications in burns: an evolving spectrum of injury. *Clinical Pulmonary Medicine* 2009, 16(3): 132–8.
6. Cancio LC. Airway management and smoke inhalation injury in the burn patient. *Clinics in Plastic Surgery* 2009, 36(4): 555–67.
7. Enoch S, Roshan A, Shah M. Emergency and early management of burns and scalds. *British Medical Journal* 2009, 338(7700): 937–41.
8. Hassan Z, Wong JK, Bush J, Bayat A, Dunn KW. Assessing the severity of inhalation injuries in adults. *Burns: Journal of the International Society for Burn Injuries* 2010, 36(2): 212–16.
9. Hermans MHE. A general overview of burn care. *International Wound Journal* 2005, 2(3): 206–20, 222–3.
10. Karpelowsky JS, Rode H. Basic principles in the management of thermal injuries. *South African Family Practice* 2008, 50(3): 24–31.
11. Karpelowsky JS, Wallis L, Madaree A, Rode H. South African Burn Society burn stabilisation protocol. *South African Medical Journal* 2007, 97(8): 574–7.
12. Marek K, Piotr W, Stanislaw S, Stefan G, Justyna G, Mariusz N, et al. Fibreoptic bronchoscopy in routine clinical practice in confirming the diagnosis and treatment of inhalation burns. *Burns: Journal of the International Society for Burn Injuries* 2007, 33(5): 554–60.
13. Mlcak RP, Suman OE, Herndon DN. Respiratory management of inhalation injury. *Burns: Journal of the International Society for Burn Injuries* 2007, 33(1): 2–13.
14. Muehlberger T, Ottomann C, Toman N, Daigeler A, Lehnhardt M. Emergency pre-hospital care of burn patients. *The Surgeon: Journal of the Royal Colleges of Surgeons of Edinburgh & Ireland* 2010, 8(2): 101–4.
15. New Zealand Guidelines Group. *Management of Burns and Scalds in Primary Care.* Wellington: Accident Compensation Corporation, 2007. Available from: http://www.moh.govt.nz/notebook/nbbooks.nsf/0/BD251444C120DC0FCC2573210070271D/$file/burns_full.pdf.
16. Palmieri TL. Inhalation injury: research progress and needs. *Journal of Burn Care and Research* 2007, 28(4): 549–54.
17. Pham TN, Gibran NS. Thermal and electrical injuries. *Surgical Clinics of North America* 2007, 87(1): 185–206.
18. Singh S, Handy J. The respiratory insult in burns injury. *Current Anaesthesia and Critical Care* 2008, 19(5–6): 264–8.
19. Spanholtz TA, Theodorou P, Amini P, Spilker G. Severe burn injuries: acute and long-term treatment. *Deutsches Arzteblatt* 2009, 106(38): 607–13.

20. Suzuki M, Aikawa N, Kobayashi K, Higuchi R. Prognostic implications of inhalation injury in burn patients in Tokyo. *Burns: Journal of the International Society for Burn Injuries* 2005, 31(3): 331–6.

21. Walton JJ, Manara AR. Burns and smoke inhalation. *Anaesthesia & Intensive Care Medicine* 2005, 6(9): 317–21.

22. Wasiak J, Cleland H, Campbell F. Dressings for superficial and partial thickness burns. *Cochrane Database of Systematic Reviews* 2007, 3: CD002106.

23. Durrant CAT, Simpson AR, Williams G. Thermal injury: the first 24 h. *Current Anaesthesia and Critical Care* 2008, 19(5–6): 256–63.

24. Freiburg C, Igneri P, Sartorelli K, Rogers F. Effects of differences in percent total body surface area estimation on fluid resuscitation of transferred burn patients. *Journal of Burn Care and Research* 2007, 28(1): 42–8.

25. Hackenschmidt A. Burn trauma priorities for a patient with 80% total body surface area burns. *Journal of Emergency Nursing* 2007, 33(4): 405–8.

26. Hussain S, Ferguson C. Assessing the size of burns: which method works best? *Emergency Medicine Journal* 2009, 26(9): 664–6.

27. Singer AJ, Dagum AB. Current management of acute cutaneous wounds. *New England Journal of Medicine* 2008, 359(10): 1037–46.

28. Williams C. Successful assessment and management of burn injuries. *Nursing Standard* 2009, 23(32): 53–4.

29. Allison K, Porter K. Consensus on the pre-hospital approach to burns patient management. *Emergency Medicine Journal* 2004, 21(1): 112–14.

30. Williams G, Dziewulski P. Intravascular fluid therapy in burns injury. In Group. TJRCALGD, editor, 2011.

31. Blackhurst H. Estimation of burn surface area using the hand. *BestBets* 2007. Available from: http://www.bestbets.org/bets/bet.php?id=01516.

32. Jose RM, Roy DK, Vidyadharan R, Erdmann M. Burns area estimation: an error perpetuated. *Burns: Journal of the International Society for Burn Injuries* 2004, 30(5): 481–2.

33. Jose RM, Roy DK, Wright PK, Erdmann M. Hand surface area: do racial differences exist? *Burns: Journal of the International Society for Burn Injuries* 2006, 32(2): 216–17.

34. Lee J-Y, Choi J-W, Kim H. Determination of hand surface area by sex and body shape using alginate. *Journal of Physiological Anthropology* 2007, 26(4): 475–83.

35. Liao C-Y, Chen S-L, Chou T-D, Lee T-P, Dai N-T, Chen T-M. Use of two-dimensional projection for estimating hand surface area of Chinese adults. *Burns: Journal of the International Society for Burn Injuries* 2008, 34(4): 556–9.

36. Yu C-Y, Hsu Y-W, Chen C-Y. Determination of hand surface area as a percentage of body surface area by 3D anthropometry. *Burns: Journal of the International Society for Burn Injuries* 2008, 34(8): 1183–9.

37. Hidvegi N, Nduka C, Myers S, Dziewulski P. Estimation of breast burn size. *Plastic and Reconstructive Surgery* 2004, 113(6): 1591–7.

38. Ichiki Y, Kato Y, Kitajima Y. Assessment of burn area: most objective method. *Burns: Journal of the International Society for Burn Injuries* 2008, 34(3): 425–6.

39. Singer AJ, Brebbia J, Soroff HH. Management of local burn wounds in the ED. *American Journal of Emergency Medicine* 2007, 25(6): 666–71.

40. Cuttle L, Kravchuk O, Wallis B, Kimble RM. An audit of first-aid treatment of pediatric burns patients and their clinical outcome. *Journal of Burn Care & Research: Official publication of the American Burn Association* 2009, 30(6): 1028–34.

41. Health Protection Agency. *HPA Compendium of Chemical Hazards*. London: HPA, 2007. Available from: http://www.hpa.org.uk/Topics/ChemicalsAndPoisons/CompendiumOfChemicalHazards.

Electrical Injuries

1. Introduction

- Electrical injury is potentially life-threatening.
- Incidents which occur in the workplace are likely to involve high voltage electricity (415 volts), whereas incidents which occur in the home are likely to involve lower voltage electricity (240 volts).
- Electrical injury may also result from a lightning strike which may deliver up to 300kV.

2. Incidence

- In the UK, approximately 1,000 people at work are injured following contact with an electrical supply; of these 25 will die from their injuries.[1]
- Approximately five fatalities from lightning strike are recorded in Britain each year.[2]

3. Severity and Outcome

- Electrical injury can cause serious multi-system damage leading to morbidity and mortality. This is caused by electric shock and tissue damage from the thermal effects along the current pathway.

The nature and extent of injury depends on:

- The voltage and whether it is alternating (AC) or direct (DC).
- The magnitude of the current.
- Resistance to current flow.
- Duration of exposure to the current.
- The pathway of the current – current traversing the myocardium is more likely to be fatal and hand-to-hand travel is more dangerous than hand-to-foot or foot-to-foot.

4. Pathophysiology

Injury occurs when electricity passes through the body causing:

- **Cardiac** arrhythmias (e.g. ventricular fibrillation); cardiorespiratory arrest can arise from the direct effects of the current on cell membranes and smooth muscle as it traverses the myocardium. Myocardial ischaemia can occur due to spasm of the coronary artery.
- **Burns** to the skin at the point of contact (entry and exit) and in deeper tissues, including viscera, muscles and nerves as thermal energy traverses the body and tends to follow neurovascular bundles. Unusual burn patterns may be left on the body following a lightning strike.
- **Trauma** including joint dislocation, fractures and compartment syndrome can arise from sustained tetanic muscle contraction, falling or being thrown.
- **Muscular paralysis** may occur from contact with high voltage electricity affecting the central respiratory control system or respiratory muscles.
- **Pregnancy** can be affected depending on the magnitude and duration of contact with the current.

5. Assessment and Management

For the assessment and management of electrical injuries refer to Table 4.25 and Figure 4.12.

Electrical Injuries

TABLE 4.25 – ASSESSMENT and MANAGEMENT of: Electrical Injuries	
ASSESSMENT ⚠ Ensure scene safety for rescuer and patient	**MANAGEMENT** ⚠ **DO NOT** approach the patient until the electricity supply is cut off and you are certain it is safe to approach.
	NOTE: Attach defibrillator pad at the earliest opportunity and keep defibrillator with the patient until hand-over to hospital staff.
• Assess **<C>ABCD**	• If any of the following **TIME CRITICAL** features present: – major **<C>ABCD** problems – cardiorespiratory arrest – refer to **Advanced Life Support**. – facial/airway burns – refer to **Airway and Breathing Management**. – cardiac arrhythmia – refer to **Cardiac Rhythm Disturbance**. – significant trauma – refer to **appropriate trauma guideline.** – extensive burns – refer to **Burns and Scalds**, then: • Start correcting <C>ABCD and undertake a **TIME CRITICAL** transfer to nearest receiving hospital or specialist burns unit if appropriate. • Continue patient management en-route. • Provide an alert/information call.
• Burn process	• Remove smouldering clothing and shoes to prevent further thermal injury – refer to **Burns and Scalds**.
• Specifically assess:	• Airway patency as early intervention may be required. • Breathing for rate, depth and any breathing difficulty – refer to **Airway and Breathing Management**. • Heart rate/rhythm – undertake a 12-lead ECG: – arrhythmias are unlikely to develop in cases of contact with domestic low voltage sources once the patient is isolated from the current – in cases of contact with high voltage sources arrhythmias may develop later. • Evidence of trauma (e.g. neck and back, burns) refer to **appropriate trauma guideline.** • Magnitude of the current, that is domestic low voltage (≤240 volts)/industrial high voltage (>480 volts).
• Oxygen	• Monitor the patient's SpO_2, administer oxygen to achieve saturations of >94% if the patient presents as hypoxaemic on air, refer to **Oxygen**.
• Fluid	• If fluid resuscitation indicated – refer to **Intravascular Fluid Therapy in Adults** and **Intravascular Fluid Therapy in Children**.
• Assess the need for pain relief	• If pain relief indicated – refer to **Pain Management in Adults** and **Pain Management in Children**
• Transfer to further care	• **ALL** patients exposed to high voltage current. • Patients exposed to a domestic or low voltage electrical source, who are asymptomatic, with no injuries and have normal initial 12-lead ECG may not require hospital assessment.

Electrical Injuries

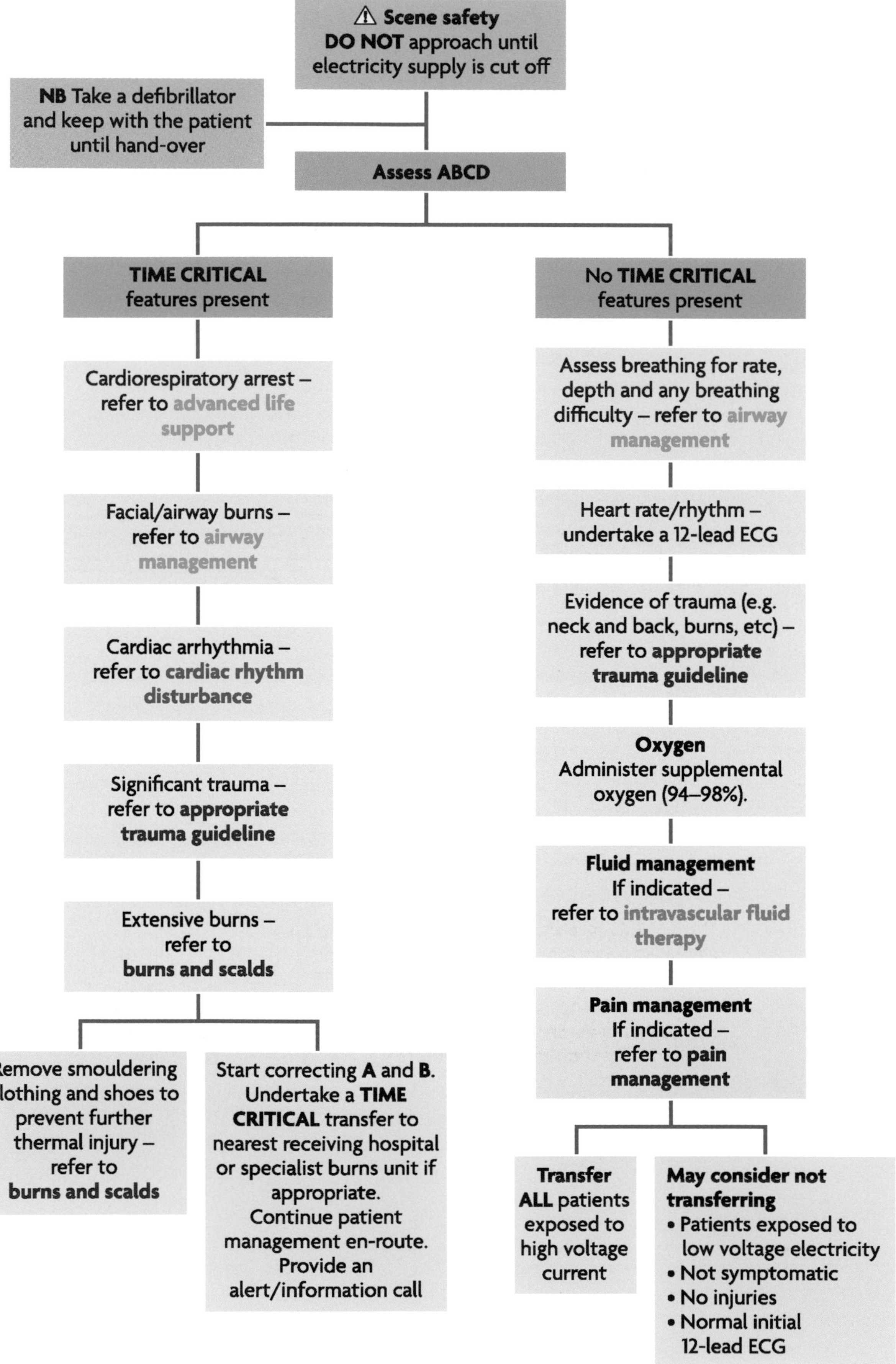

⚠ Scene safety
DO NOT approach until electricity supply is cut off
NB Take a defibrillator and keep with the patient until hand-over
Assess ABCD
TIME CRITICAL features present
Cardiorespiratory arrest – refer to advanced life support
Facial/airway burns – refer to airway management
Cardiac arrhythmia – refer to cardiac rhythm disturbance
Significant trauma – refer to appropriate trauma guideline
Extensive burns – refer to burns and scalds
Remove smouldering clothing and shoes to prevent further thermal injury – refer to burns and scalds
Start correcting A and B. Undertake a TIME CRITICAL transfer to nearest receiving hospital or specialist burns unit if appropriate. Continue patient management en-route. Provide an alert/information call
No TIME CRITICAL features present
Assess breathing for rate, depth and any breathing difficulty – refer to airway management
Heart rate/rhythm – undertake a 12-lead ECG
Evidence of trauma (e.g. neck and back, burns, etc) – refer to appropriate trauma guideline
Oxygen
Administer supplemental oxygen (94–98%).
Fluid management
If indicated – refer to intravascular fluid therapy
Pain management
If indicated – refer to pain management
Transfer ALL patients exposed to high voltage current
May consider not transferring
• Patients exposed to low voltage electricity
• Not symptomatic
• No injuries
• Normal initial 12-lead ECG

Figure 4.12 – Assessment and management of electrical injuries algorithm.

SECTION 4 Trauma

Electrical Injuries

KEY POINTS!

Electrical Injuries

- **Scene safety.**
- **Manage cardiac/respiratory arrest.**
- **Consider trauma.**
- **Severe tissue damage may be present despite apparently minor injury.**
- **Exposure to domestic voltage may not require hospitalisation.**

Further Reading

Further important information and evidence in support of this guideline can be found in the Bibliography.[3,4,5,6,7,8,9,10,11,1]

Bibliography

1. Health and Safety Executive. *Electrical injuries*. Available from: http://www.hse.gov.uk/electricity/injuries.htm, 2010.
2. Royal College of Emergency Medicine. *Electrical Injuries – Lightning* Clinical Knowledge Summaries. Available from: https://www.rcemlearning.co.uk/references/electrical-injuries-lightning/, 2017.
3. Soar J, Perkins GD, Abbas G, Alfonzo A, Barelli A, Bierens JJLM, et al. European Resuscitation Council Guidelines for Resuscitation 2010 Section 8: Cardiac arrest in special circumstances: electrolyte abnormalities, poisoning, drowning, accidental hypothermia, hyperthermia, asthma, anaphylaxis, cardiac surgery, trauma, pregnancy, electrocution. *Resuscitation* 2010, 81(10): 1400–1433.
4. Gauglitz GG, Herndon DN, Jeschke MG. Emergency treatment of severely burned pediatric patients: current therapeutic strategies. *Pediatric Health* 2008, 2(6): 761–75.
5. Yarrow J, Moiemen N, Gulhane S. Early management of burns in children. *Paediatrics and Child Health* 2009, 19(11): 509–16.
6. Ritenour AE, Morton MJ, McManus JG, Barillo DJ, Cancio LC. Lightning injury: a review. *Burns: Journal of the International Society for Burn Injuries* 2008, 34(5): 585–94.
7. Dollery W. Cardiac monitoring not needed in household electrical injury if the patient is asymptomatic and has a normal ECG. *BestBets*, 2003. Available from: http://www.bestbets.org/bets/bet.php?id=9.
8. Bailey B, Gaudreault P, Thivierge RL. Cardiac monitoring of high-risk patients after an electrical injury: a prospective multicentre study. *Emergency Medicine Journal* 2007, 24(5): 348–52.
9. Adukauskiene D, Vizgirdaite V, Mazeikiene S. Electrical injuries. [In Lithuanian]. *Medicina (Kaunas)* 2007, 43(3): 259–66. Abstract in English available from: http://www.ncbi.nlm.nih.gov/pubmed/17413256.
10. Spies C, Trohman RG. Narrative review: electrocution and life-threatening electrical injuries. *Annals of Internal Medicine* 2006, 145(7): 531–7.
11. Vierhapper MF, Lumenta DB, Beck H, Keck M, Kamolz LP, Frey M. Electrical injury: a long-term analysis with review of regional differences. *Annals of Plastic Surgery* 2011, 66(1): 43–6: doi 10.1097/SAP.0b013e3181f3e60f.

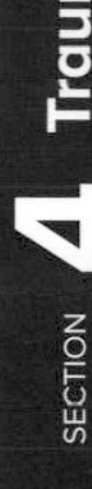

Immersion and Drowning

1. Introduction

- Drowning is a common cause of accidental death.
- **Drowning** refers to the 'process resulting in primary respiratory impairment from submersion/ immersion in a liquid medium'. Thus the person is prevented from breathing air due to liquid medium at the entrance of the airway. **NB** Drowning does not infer that the patient has died.
- **Immersion** refers to being covered in a liquid medium and the main problems will be hypothermia and cardiovascular collapse from the removal of hydrostatic pressure of the surrounding water on the lower limbs.
- **Submersion** refers to the entire body, including the airway being under the liquid medium and the main problems are asphyxia and hypoxia.
- **Exacerbating factors** – intoxication from alcohol or drugs may often accompany incidents. Occasionally, an immersion incident may be precipitated by a medical cause such as a convulsion.

2. Incidence

- Worldwide there are approximately 450,000 deaths per year with 205 deaths from accidental drowning occurring in England and Wales in 2009; with many more near-drownings. A high percentage of deaths will involve young males and children.

3. Severity and Outcome

- The extent of hypoxia and hypothermia, resulting from duration of immersion and/or submersion and/or the temperature of the liquid medium will determine severity and outcome.
- Concomitant trauma may result; for example, <0.5% of patients may suffer neck and/or head injury; diving into shallow water is a common cause.

4. Pathophysiology

- Following submersion, the patient will initially try to hold their breath. They may develop laryngospasm as water irritates the vocal cords or may aspirate large quantities of water. Both processes result in rapid hypoxia and hypercapnia.
- If rescue is not made, the patient will aspirate water into their lungs, exacerbating hypoxia. The patient will become bradycardic and sustain a cardiac arrest; thus correction of hypoxaemia is critical to obtaining a return of spontaneous circulation. In 10–15% of cases, the laryngeal spasm is so intense, none of the liquid medium enters the lungs.
- Changes in haemodynamics after immersion (the 'hydrostatic squeeze effect') make positional hypotension likely. If the patient is raised vertically from the water their blood pressure will fall – 'after-drop' – which may lead to cardiovascular collapse. Therefore it is recommended that rescuers must always attempt to maintain the patient flat and avoid vertical removal from water.

5. Rescue and Resuscitation

⚠ Safety first – **DO NOT** put yourself in danger. Carry out a dynamic risk assessment and undertake measures to preserve your own safety and that of other rescuers.

- Establish the number of patients involved.
- History is often incomplete at the scene, both relating to the incident and the patient.

5.1 Aquatic rescue

- When the patient is rescued, attempt to maintain the patient flat and avoid vertical removal from water.
- If neck and back trauma is suspected, wait until the patient has been rescued before attempting to apply spinal immobilisation, but limit neck flexion and extension.

5.2 Airway and breathing

- Alleviate hypoxaemia as soon as possible, as adequate ventilation and oxygenation may restore cardiac activity.
- In patients in cardiac arrest clear airway, provide ventilations and commence CPR as soon as the patient is rescued. Refer to **Advanced Life Support**.
- Administer supplemental oxygen, preferably via bag-valve-mask. Apply pulse oximeter. If the patient does not respond to oxygen therapy consider assisted ventilation.
- Mechanical drainage of water from the lungs should not be carried out. The lungs can be ventilated even with large volumes of water inside them, although ventilation may be difficult due to reduced lung compliance.
- Approximately 80% of patients will aspirate water into their stomach. There is a high risk of regurgitation of the stomach contents, especially if the patient has ingested alcohol/drugs – have suction at hand. Tilting to drain aspirated water simply empties water from the stomach into the pharynx, risking further airway contamination.

5.3 For the management of cardiac arrest following drowning

- Refer to **Advanced Life Support: Drowning**.

5.4 For the management of hypothermia

- Refer to **Hypothermia** and **Advanced Life Support: Hypothermia**.

Immersion and Drowning

- If the patient is hypothermic, the heart rate may be extremely slow and external cardiac compression may be required – refer to **Cardiac Rhythm Disturbance**. **NB** Bradycardia often responds to improved ventilation.

5.5 Intravascular fluid therapy

- Following prolonged immersion patients may become hypovolaemic – if fluid resuscitation indicated refer to **Intravascular Fluid Therapy in Adults** and **Intravascular Fluid Therapy in Children**.

5.6 Survival and submersion

Research has shown that there is little accurate data on which factors predict survival, following submersion. Submersion time is a significant factor but there is little accurate data. In order to obtain more accurate data on the factors associated with good outcomes following submersion, data will be collected on a number of parameters, such as:

- Time of the incident.
- Time the patient was rescued.
- Time of first effective CPR.
- Duration of submersion.
- Water temperature.
- Type (salt, fresh, contaminated).
- Precipitating factors (e.g. intoxication from alcohol or drugs, convulsion etc).

As it is often difficult to obtain accurate time information from witnesses, for the purpose of deciding whether to commence resuscitation the submersion time is measured from the time of initial call to ambulance control centre.

6. Assessment and Management

For the assessment and management of the immersion incident refer to Table 4.26.

TABLE 4.26 – ASSESSMENT and MANAGEMENT of: Immersion Incident

⚠ **Safety First – DO NOT put yourself in danger – carry out a dynamic risk assessment and undertake measures to preserve your own safety, and where possible that of the patient, bystanders and other rescuers.** • **Take a defibrillator at the earliest opportunity.** • **Ascertain how many patients are involved.** • **NB Information may be incomplete at the scene.** • **Note the environment – in certain circumstances hair may become entangled in a drain/filter (e.g. pools/hot tubs).**	**NB The duration of hypoxia is the most important factor in determining outcome. Oxygenate and restore circulation at the earliest opportunity.**
ASSESSMENT	**MANAGEMENT**
• Assess **<C>ABCDE**	• If any of the following **TIME CRITICAL** features present: – major **<C>ABCDE** problems – refer to **Trauma Emergencies in Adults – Overview Trauma Emergencies in Children – Overview**. – pulseless and apnoeic – refer to relevant **Resuscitation** guidelines. – major life-threatening trauma – refer to relevant **Trauma** guidelines. – neck and back injuries – refer to **Spinal Injury and Spinal Cord Injury**, then: • Start correcting any <C>ABCD problems. • Undertake a TIME CRITICAL transfer to nearest appropriate receiving hospital. • Continue patient management en route. • Provide an ATMIST information call. • Administer high levels of supplemental oxygen – refer to **Oxygen**. • Prevent further heat loss/consider warming the patient – refer to **Hypothermia**.

(continued)

Immersion and Drowning

TABLE 4.26 – ASSESSMENT and MANAGEMENT of: Immersion Incident *(continued)*	
• Airway	• Clear airway. • There is a high risk of regurgitation of the stomach contents, especially if the patient has ingested alcohol/drugs – have suction at hand.
• Respiratory rate	• Measure and record respiratory rate.
• Ventilation	• Adequate ventilation and oxygenation may restore cardiac activity. Consider assisted ventilation if: – SpO_2 is <90% with oxygen therapy – respiratory rate <10 or >30 breaths per minute – expansion is inadequate. **NB** Ventilation may be difficult due to reduced lung compliance if water has been inhaled – refer to **Airway and Breathing Management**.
• Oxygen	• Administer supplemental oxygen – refer to **Oxygen**. • Apply pulse oximeter – **NB** the measurement may be unreliable in patients with cold peripheries. – **children** – administer high levels of supplemental oxygen – **adults** – aim for a target saturation within the range of 94–98%.
• Pulse	• Measure and record pulse.
• Heart rate	• In the presence of hypothermia the heart rate may be extremely slow and external cardiac compression may be required – refer to **Cardiac Rhythm Disturbance**. **NB** Bradycardia often responds to improved ventilation and oxygenation.
• Concomitant injuries	• Consider concomitant injuries. • Consider neck and back injuries – refer to **Spinal Injury and Spinal Cord Injury**. • Treat associated injuries – refer to specific guideline(s).
• ECG	• Monitor and record 12-Lead ECG. Assess for abnormality, refer to **Cardiac Rhythm Disturbance**.
• Blood pressure and fluids	• Measure and record blood pressure. • In cases of prolonged immersion patients may become hypovolaemic – if fluid resuscitation indicated refer to **Intravascular Fluid Therapy in Adults** and **Intravascular Fluid Therapy in Children**.
• Blood glucose	• If appropriate, measure and record blood glucose for hypo/hyperglycaemia, refer to **Glycaemic Emergencies in Adults and Children**.
• Temperature	• Measure and record temperature.
• Position	• If possible, the patient should be removed from the water and managed in a horizontal position, especially in rescue involving a helicopter or large vessel, where the patient is lifted more than a few metres – however, in **TIME CRITICAL** conditions speed of removal from the water takes precedence over method of removal.
• Assess the patient's pain	• Where present, assess the **SOCRATES** of pain and record initial and subsequent pain scores. • Consider analgesia if appropriate, refer to **Pain Management in Adults** and **Pain Management in Children**.

Immersion and Drowning

TABLE 4.26 – ASSESSMENT and MANAGEMENT of: Immersion Incident *(continued)*	
• Transfer to further care	• Transfer all patients to further care. • If neck and back injury not suspected transfer in the recovery position. • If the patient is immobilised prepare for side-tilt. • Prevent further heat loss/consider warming the patient – refer to **Hypothermia**. • Provide an ATMIST information call. • Continue patient management en-route.
• Discontinuation of resuscitative efforts	• Refer to **Advanced Life Support**.
• Documentation	• Complete documentation to include all clinical findings, advice from other clinicians, onward referral and worsening advice given.

KEY POINTS!

Immersion and Drowning

- **Ensure own personal safety.**
- **Successful resuscitations have occurred after prolonged submersion/immersion.**
- **Hypothermia is a condition often associated with the immersion incident.**
- **There are special considerations in cardiac arrest treatment in the presence of hypothermia.**
- **Severe complications may develop several hours after submersion/immersion.**

Bibliography

1. Soar J, Perkins GD, Abbas G, Alfonzo A, Barelli A, Bierens JJLM, et al. European Resuscitation Council Guidelines for Resuscitation 2010 Section 8: Cardiac arrest in special circumstances: electrolyte abnormalities, poisoning, drowning, accidental hypothermia, hyperthermia, asthma, anaphylaxis, cardiac surgery, trauma, pregnancy, electrocution. *Resuscitation* 2010, 81(10): 1400–1433.
2. Brenner RA, Taneja GS, Haynie DL, Trumble AC, Qian C, Klinger RM, et al. Association between swimming lessons and drowning in childhood: a case-control study. *Archives of Pediatrics & Adolescent Medicine* 2009, 163(3): 203–10.
3. Durchholz C, Peters J, Staudt F, Pontz B. Childhood drowning: a retrospective analysis. *Notarzt* 2004, 20(5): 168–72.
4. Ross FI, Elliott EJ, Lam LT, Cass DT. Children under 5 years presenting to paediatricians with near-drowning. *Journal of Paediatrics and Child Health* 2003, 39(6): 446–50.
5. Bierens JJLM, Knape JTA, Gelissen HPMM. Drowning. *Current Opinion in Critical Care* 2002, 8(6): 578–86.
6. Kemp A, Sibert JR. Drowning and near drowning in children in the United Kingdom: lessons for prevention. *British Medical Journal* 1992, 304(6835): 1143–6.
7. Cummings P, Quan L. Trends in unintentional drowning: the role of alcohol and medical care. *Journal of the American Medical Association* 1999, 281(23): 2198–202.
8. Franklin RC, Scarr JP, Pearn JH. Reducing drowning deaths: the continued challenge of immersion fatalities in Australia. *Medical Journal of Australia* 2010, 192(3): 123–6.
9. Youn CS, Choi SP, Yim HW, Park KN. Out-of-hospital cardiac arrest due to drowning: an Utstein Style report of 10 years of experience from St Mary's Hospital. *Resuscitation* 2009, 80(7): 778–83.
10. Barbieri S, Feltracco P, Delantone M, Spagna A, Michieletto E, Bortolato A, et al. Helicopter rescue and pre-hospital care for drowning children: two summer season case studies. *Minerva Anestesiologica* 2008, 74(12): 703–7.
11. Hyder AA, Borse NN, Blum L, Khan R, El Arifeen S, Baqui AH. Childhood drowning in low- and middle-income countries: urgent need for intervention trials. *Journal of Paediatrics and Child Health* 2008, 44(4): 221–7.
12. Salomez F, Vincent J-L. Drowning: a review of epidemiology, pathophysiology, treatment and prevention. *Resuscitation* 2004, 63(3): 261–8.
13. Peden MM, McGee K. The epidemiology of drowning worldwide. *International Journal of Injury Control and Safety Promotion* 2003, 10(4): 195–9.
14. Franklin RC, Scarr JP, Pearn JH. Reducing drowning deaths: the continued challenge of immersion fatalities in Australia. *Medical Journal of Australia* 2011, 192(3): 123–6.
15. al-Talafieh A, al-Majali R, al-Dehayat G. Clinical, laboratory and X-ray findings of drowning and near-drowning in the Gulf of Aqaba. *Eastern Mediterranean Health Journal* 1999, 5(4): 706–9.
16. Papa L, Hoelle R, Idris A. Systematic review of definitions for drowning incidents. *Resuscitation* 2005, 65(3): 255–64.

Immersion and Drowning

17. Diplock S, Jamrozik K. Legislative and regulatory measures for preventing alcohol-related drownings and near-drownings. *Australian & New Zealand Journal of Public Health* 2006, 30(4): 314–17.
18. Driscoll TR, Harrison JA, Steenkamp M. Review of the role of alcohol in drowning associated with recreational aquatic activity. *Injury Prevention* 2004, 10(2): 107–13.
19. Eksborg S, Rajs J. Causes and manners of death among users of heroin, methadone, amphetamine, and cannabis in relation to postmortem chemical tests for illegal drugs. *Substance Use and Misuse* 2008, 43(10): 1326–39.
20. Lossius R, Nakken KO. Epilepsy and sudden death. *Tidsskrift for Den norske legeforening* 2002, 122(11): 1114–17.
21. Office for National Statistics. *Deaths Registered in England and Wales in 2010, By Cause.* Available from: http://www.ons.gov.uk, 2010.
22. Watson RS, Cummings P, Quan L, Bratton S, Weiss NS. Cervical spine injuries among submersion victims. *Journal of Trauma* 2001, 51(4): 658–62.
23. Hwang V, Shofer FS, Durbin DR, Baren M. Prevalence of traumatic injuries in drowning and near drowning in children and adolescents. *Archives of Pediatrics & Adolescent Medicine* 2003, 157(1): 50–3.
24. Faddy S. Drowning and near-drowning: the physiology and pathology. *Australian Journal of Medical Science* 2001, 22(1): 4–13.
25. Layon AJ, Modell JH. Drowning: update 2009. *Anaesthesiology* 2009, 110(6): 1390–401.
26. Ouanes-Besbes L, Dachraoui F, Ouanes I, Abroug F. Drowning: pathophysiology and treatment. *Reanimation* 2009, 18(8): 702–7.
27. Claesson A, Svensson L, Silfverstolpe J, Herlitz J. Characteristics and outcome among patients suffering out-of-hospital cardiac arrest due to drowning. *Resuscitation* 2008, 76(3): 381–7.
28. Edwards ND, Timmins AC, Randalls B, Morgan GA, Simcock AD. Survival in adults after cardiac arrest due to drowning. *Intensive Care Medicine* 1990, 16(5): 336–7.
29. Lee LK, Mao C, Thompson KM. Demographic factors and their association with outcomes in pediatric submersion injury. *Academic Emergency Medicine* 2006, 13(3): 308–13.
30. Modell JH, Graves SA, Ketover A. Clinical course of 91 consecutive neardrowning victims. *Chest* 1976, 70(2): 231–8.
31. Modell JH, Idris AH, Pineda JA, Silverstein JH. Survival after prolonged submersion in freshwater in Florida. *Chest* 2004, 125(5): 1948–51.
32. Nussbaum E, Maggi JC. Pentobarbital therapy does not improve neurologic outcome in nearly drowned, flaccid-comatose children. *Pediatrics* 1988, 81(5): 630–4.
33. Suominen P, Baillie C, Korpela R, Rautanen S, Ranta S, Olkkola KT. Impact of age, submersion time and water temperature on outcome in near-drowning. *Resuscitation* 2002, 52(3): 247–54.
34. Wollenek G, Honarwar N, Golej J, Marx M. Cold water submersion and cardiac arrest in treatment of severe hypothermia with cardiopulmonary bypass. *Resuscitation* 2002, 52(3): 255–63.
35. Wyatt JP, Tomlinson GS, Busuttil A. Resuscitation of drowning victims in south-east Scotland. *Resuscitation* 1999, 41(2): 101–4.

5

Maternity Care

Maternity Care (including Obstetric Emergencies Overview)

1. Introduction

- Any woman of childbearing age may be pregnant and, unless there is a history of hysterectomy, there must be a high index of suspicion that any abdominal pain or vaginal bleeding may be pregnancy related.
- There are three fundamental rules which must be followed at all times when dealing with a pregnant woman:
  - a Resuscitation of the mother must always be the priority.
  - b Manual uterine displacement must be employed to support resuscitation measures beyond 20 weeks gestation, refer to Figure 5.1.
  - c Hypotension is a late sign of shock. Any signs of hypovolaemia during pregnancy are likely to indicate a 35% (class III) blood loss and must be treated aggressively.
- In cases of maternal cardiac arrest requiring ongoing cardiopulmonary resuscitation, pre-alert the nearest emergency department with an obstetric unit when transferring a pregnant woman in order to ensure preparedness for an emergency perimortem caesarean section (resuscitative hysterotomy), as delivering the fetus may be required to help facilitate maternal resuscitation. **NB Effective resuscitation of the mother will provide effective resuscitation of the fetus.**
- When ambulance clinicians attend an obstetric emergency, they should work as a team, with the paramedics responsible and accountable for the care of the woman or newborn baby and delegating tasks accordingly.
- When a midwife is present, paramedics and midwife must work together to act in the best interests of the woman and the newborn baby.

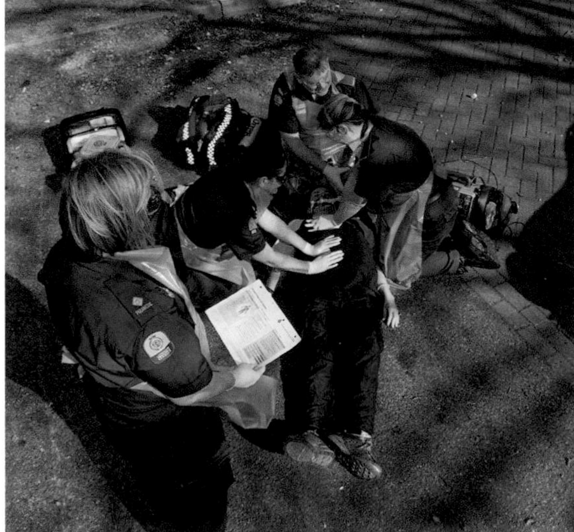

Figure 5.1 – Manual uterine displacement.

If both mother and newborn baby are clinically well, the midwife is the responsible and accountable clinician. The midwife can either discharge the ambulance clinicians, and arrange for ongoing community midwifery care, or arrange conveyance of the mother and baby together to the most appropriate facility.

- In the event of a newborn requiring conveyance to hospital ahead of the mother, it may be preferable that the midwife remains on scene with the mother to manage the third stage of labour, assess for perineal trauma, and manage any ongoing post-partum bleeding. Ambulance clinicians can manage ongoing care of the newborn, utilise the established communication channels, and pre-alert the nearest ED where the baby can be assessed. The mother should be repatriated with the baby as soon as reasonably possible at the same location.
- The MBRRACE-UK annual report, Saving Lives, Improving Mothers' Care, reviews maternal deaths in the UK and produces recommendations relating to care provision. The report continues to show an overall decrease in the maternal death rate, which is currently 8.5 women per 100,000 maternities.
  - Maternal deaths from direct causes – complication from the pregnancy itself such as bleeding, blood clots, pre-eclampsia or infection – continue to decrease.
  - Maternal deaths from indirect causes – pre-existing conditions that are not direct pregnancy complications such as heart disease, epilepsy, mental health problems or cancer – remain high.
  - Deaths from mental health problems contribute to around a quarter of maternal deaths occurring between six weeks and one year after the end of pregnancy.
  - The focus of care must be upon establishing appropriate resuscitative measures, placing a pre-alert to the nearest emergency department with an obstetric unit attached, conveying the woman, with manual uterine displacement in place, and preparation for further assessment and treatment, including a perimortem caesarean section if necessary.
  - Effective communication is therefore essential to ensure clinical information being passed on is complete and relevant, utilising a structured communication tool.

2. Communication, Information Sharing and Consent

All women who are booked for maternity care should have access to their handheld maternity records. These will provide key information regarding medical history, previous and current pregnancies, obstetric problems as well as emergency contact details for care providers, including next of kin. Information within these notes may aid assessment during the primary and/or secondary survey. Maternity units may also have their own unique set of handheld records or, in some cases, these may be electronic.

2.1 Human Factors and 'SBAR'

- Clinical performance and safe practice can be enhanced through an understanding of the effects of teamwork, tasks, equipment, workspace, culture and organisation on human behaviour and abilities, and application of that knowledge within a clinical setting.
- Increasing situational awareness and the utilisation of communication tools (such as SBAR) help to promote a safer environment and enhance clinical outcome. Awareness of what is happening around us can be reduced during emergency situations, and this can lead to near misses and/or adverse outcomes. It is therefore essential that enhanced communication skills, and an environment in which open and honest lines of communication is encouraged, are maintained.
- The use of the Situation, Background, Assessment, Recommendation (SBAR) communication tool is recommended in order to optimise transfer of information between members of the multi-disciplinary team. The purpose of SBAR is to promote the accurate and unambiguous handover of clinically relevant information regarding care of the mother from one healthcare professional to another. The use of SBAR has the potential to improve the speed at which care is delivered and the quality of care that is ultimately provided.

2.2 Consent

- Consent to treatment is the principle that a person must give permission before they receive any type of medical treatment, investigation or examination. Consent from a woman is needed regardless of the procedure. For consent to be valid it must be voluntary and informed, and the person consenting must have the capacity to make the decision. If an adult has the capacity to make a voluntary and informed decision to consent to or refuse a particular treatment, their decision must be respected. This is still the case even if refusing treatment would result in their death, or the death of their unborn child.
- The provision of adequate information should include the benefits and risks of the proposed treatments, and alternative treatments. If the woman is not offered as much information as they reasonably need to make their decision, and in a format that they can understand, their consent will not be valid.
- Consent can be given verbally or in writing and should be given to the health care professional directly responsible for the person's current treatment.
- Consent may not be necessary if a person requires emergency treatment that is believed to be in their best interests or to save their life and they are unable to give consent due to a lack of capacity caused by either mental or physical complications.
- During obstetrics emergencies, it may be necessary to perform intimate examination in order to perform lifesaving treatment. Practitioners must, where possible, obtain informed consent and offer the woman a chaperone. All examinations must be carried out sensitively, with respect for the woman's dignity, cultural beliefs and confidentiality.

3. Physiological Changes in Pregnancy

Pregnancy is timed from the FIRST day of the last period and may last up to or in excess of 42 weeks. The pregnancy is divided into three trimesters (1–12 weeks +6 days, 13–25 weeks +6 days and 26 weeks+). These terms are used with the maternity handheld records, they will also detail the lead clinician, i.e. the midwife or the obstetrician who is responsible for the provision of maternity care with the woman.

There are a multitude of physiological and anatomical changes during pregnancy that may influence the management of the pregnant woman. These changes include:

- Cardiovascular system:
  - An increase in cardiac output by 20–30% in the first 10 weeks of pregnancy.
  - An increase in average maternal heart rate by 10–15 beats per minute.
  - A decrease in systolic and diastolic blood pressure by an average of 10–15 mmHg due to a reduction in peripheral resistance caused by an increase in the release of the progesterone hormone.
  - The weight of the gravid uterus, from 20 weeks gestation onwards, may cause compression of the inferior vena cava (IVC), reducing venous return, and lowering cardiac output, by up to 40%, for women in the supine position; this in turn can reduce blood pressure. The combined effects of the gravid uterus on the IVC and a reduction in peripheral vascular resistance can result in the woman feeling faint or having an episode of syncope, resolved by repositioning her onto her side or into the lateral position.
  - An increase in blood volume through haemodilution (increasing by 45%) occurs together with a small increase in the numbers of red blood cells. The disproportionate

increase of plasma volume relative to the increase in red cell mass can lead to a 'physiological' anaemia in the mother from around 27 weeks gestation. Due to the increase in blood volume, a pregnant woman is able to tolerate greater blood loss before showing signs of hypovolaemia. This compensation is at the expense of shunting blood away from the uterus and placenta, and therefore fetus.

- Respiratory system:
  - An increase in breathing rate and effort and a decrease in vital capacity, as the gravid uterus enlarges and the diaphragm becomes splinted. Some shortness of breath is common during pregnancy but early consideration should be given to the need for increased oxygen requirements.
  - Oedema of the larynx may compromise airway management and a collapsed pregnant woman requires the airway to be secured as soon as possible.
  - Placement of an advanced airway (supraglottic airway or endotracheal intubation) should be secured in all maternal cardiac arrests (refer to **Maternal Resuscitation**).
- Gastrointestinal system:
  - An increase in the acidity of the stomach contents, due to a delay in gastric emptying, caused by progesterone-like effects of the placental hormones.
  - Relaxation of the cardiac sphincter makes regurgitation of the stomach contents more likely (refer to **Maternal Resuscitation**).
  - Nausea and vomiting can occur around 4–8 weeks gestation and continue until around 14–16 weeks. Some severe cases may continue for a longer period of time and can result in rapid dehydration (hyperemesis gravidarum) requiring hospital assessment/admission.

4. Appropriate Destination for Conveyance

- The choice of destination to convey mother and baby should be carefully considered and in line with local procedures. Ideally mother and baby should be conveyed to the same destination. There are units, commonly called birth/birthing centres (or 'standalone' maternity units), that are solely midwifery-led. Be aware that there are no resident obstetricians, anaesthetists or neonatologists with the capability of performing advanced obstetric or neonatal interventions at these sites. There are no specialist neonatal facilities.
- The mother may choose to book for delivery at a particular unit and request to be conveyed there; however, in an emergency situation this may have to be overridden:
  - The nearest ED will be the appropriate destination when there is cardiac arrest, major airway problems, ongoing eclamptic convulsions and severe uncontrollable bleeding.
  - In other obstetric emergencies (e.g. shoulder dystocia, mild to moderate bleeding etc.) transfer to the nearest full obstetric unit (i.e. not a birthing centre or 'standalone' midwifery unit) will be appropriate. Remember, that in many cases, a full obstetric unit will be co-located with an ED but this may not always be the case.
- Careful consideration should always be given to the most appropriate destination in each case. Also consider carefully the accessibility of a unit (e.g. out-of-hours, locked doors, corridors and lifts). In line with local procedures, pre-alert arrangements and telephone numbers should be agreed and readily available to clinicians.

5. Assessment

- Critical assessment of the mother is vital in all situations, while fetal assessment may be indirect based on reported movements etc. Refer to Table 5.1
- Neonatal assessment is also important, with particular reference to respiratory effort and maintaining body temperature. Refer to Table 5.5.

6. Special Cases

6.1 Concealment, Denial and Unknown Pregnancy

Occasionally pregnancy may be concealed or denied until labour commences. In both situations there may have been no antenatal care. There may be mental health, drug and alcohol abuse issues and safeguarding concerns (refer to **Safeguarding Adults at Risk** and **Safeguarding Children**). Some concealed pregnancies may result in the birth occurring in secret. Ambulance clinicians must be aware that the consequences of concealment and denial can have a fatal outcome for both mother and baby.

- Always consider the possibility of pregnancy in any woman of reproductive age. Ask the woman if she could be pregnant. Be aware that a young teenage girl may not want to answer such a question in the presence of a parent or carer.
- It may be necessary to visually inspect and palpate the abdomen for evidence of a pregnant uterus.
- If labour is confirmed and birth is not imminent, determine if there is any relevant medical history. Transfer the woman to the nearest obstetric unit.
- Determine how many weeks pregnant the woman is if known, or by visual inspection of the

Maternity Care (including Obstetric Emergencies Overview)

TABLE 5.1 – ASSESSMENT

• Quickly assess the woman and scene as you approach	
• Primary survey	• It is important to remember that a woman and, if born, a newborn baby will require assessment. • The aim of the primary survey is to identify any life-threatening problems, to enable management to be commenced as rapidly as possible, and to reach an early determination of the priority for transportation. The primary survey should be modified in the presence of actual or suspected trauma (refer to **Trauma in Pregnancy**).
• Massive external haemorrhage	• Is there a significant volume of blood visible without the need to disturb the woman's clothing? – Is the woman's clothing soaked? – Is there blood on the floor? – Are there a number of blood-soaked sanitary pads visible?
• Airway	• Is the woman able to talk? (Yes = airway open.) If the woman is unresponsive, refer to **Maternal Resuscitation**. • Is the woman making unusual sounds? (Gurgling = fluid in the airway.) • Is suction required? (Snoring = tongue/swelling/foreign body obstruction.) • If the woman is unresponsive, open the airway and look in – suction for fluids, manually remove solid obstructions.
• Breathing	• Document respiratory rate and effort. (Are accessory muscles being used?) • Obtain oxygen saturations as soon as possible. • Auscultate for added sounds. (Wheeze = bronchospasm; coarse sounds = pulmonary oedema.) • Assess for the presence of cyanosis. • Give oxygen based on clinical findings (not routinely).
• Circulation	• Document radial pulse rate and volume. (Capillary refill time (CRT) may be used if neither the radial nor carotid pulses can be palpated.) • Assess skin colour and temperature (to touch). (Pallor, or cold or damp skin = an adrenergic reaction to shock.) • Record blood pressure – the systolic is most valuable if you suspect shock. • Visually inspect the abdominal area and gently palpate for evidence of internal bleeding (indicated by tenderness, guarding, firm woody uterus).
• Disability	• Perform an AVPU assessment of consciousness level (is the woman Alert, responding only to Voice, responding only to Pain or Unresponsive?). • Document the woman's posture (normal, convulsing (state whether focal or generalised), abnormal flexion, abnormal extension). • Document pupil size and reaction (PEaRL – pupils equal and reacting to light).
• Expose/ environment/ evaluate	• Ensuring consent is obtained, expose and visually inspect the vaginal opening: – Is there any evidence of bleeding? – Can you see a presenting part of the baby? – Is there a prolapsed loop of cord? – Have the waters broken (and if so, is the amniotic fluid clear, blood stained or meconium stained)? – Does the perineum bulge with each contraction? – If the baby has been born, is there a significant perineal tear? Can you see any part of the uterus?

(continued)

TABLE 5.1 – ASSESSMENT *(continued)*	
	● Assess the environment: – Is the woman or baby at risk of hypothermia? – Are the surroundings as clean as you can make them if the birth is imminent? – Are there other children present (this may indicate a previous pregnancy with live birth)? ● Evaluate how time critical the woman's condition is. – If it is time critical, decide immediately whether you need to transport the woman urgently to the nearest hospital with an obstetric unit, placing a pre-alert as early as reasonably possible. (The nearest hospital with an obstetric unit may not be the booked unit; however, it is critical the woman has rapid obstetric or appropriate assessment at the nearest facility.) – If the birth is imminent, remember to call for additional clinical resource. This may include midwifery assistance, which may be deployed from the nearest maternity unit to the location of the woman (follow local guidelines).
● Fundus	● Make a quick assessment of fundal height: a fundus at the level of the umbilicus equates to a gestation of approximately 22 weeks. By definition, if fundal height is below the umbilicus, this suggests that if the fetus is delivered, it is unlikely to survive.
● Fetal activity	● Ask the mother when she last felt her baby move.
● Secondary survey	● If any critical problems are identified during the primary survey, the secondary survey should only be undertaken when any **ABCDE** problems have been addressed and transportation to definitive care has commenced (if this is possible). In many cases where critical problems are identified, it will not be possible or appropriate to undertake a secondary survey in the pre-hospital phase of care.

abdomen; where the uterine fundus is at the level of the umbilicus the pregnancy may be more than 22 weeks.

- If birth is in progress or occurs en-route, request a midwife from the nearest maternity unit, if this service is available, and additional resources and prepare for birth (see Table 5.1).
- Once the baby has been born and assessed, transfer mother and baby to the nearest obstetric unit.
- If the woman is unaware of pregnancy, consider birth/miscarriage in any significant PV bleed that cannot be explained.
- Pre-alert the nearest obstetric unit or nearest ED with an obstetric unit, dependent upon considered gestation.
- Discuss at handover any safeguarding concerns identified when attending the home environment (refer to **Safeguarding Adults at Risk** and **Safeguarding Children**).

6.2 Female Genital Mutilation (FGM)

These women should have had their delivery planned with a consultant obstetrician and a midwife who have received special training in the management of FGM. If de-infibulation (reversal of FGM) is required, it may have been undertaken antenatally or may have been planned to be undertaken in labour or after a planned caesarean section.

- Some women with previous pregnancies may have had an illegal re-infibulation operation after childbirth.
- Unless the mother has had a previous normal vaginal delivery and has not had a de-infibulation, she must be regarded as having a high risk of perineal trauma and haemorrhage.
- If de-infibulation is planned, when in labour, the woman must be transferred immediately to her booked obstetric unit. However, if this is likely to incur a delay, the woman must be conveyed to the nearest obstetric unit.
- If a woman has not received antenatal care and evidence of FGM is noted upon arrival of ambulance clinicians at a birth, further resources should be requested and an early attempt at conveying the woman to the nearest obstetric unit made.
- An information call should be placed to the identified obstetric unit informing them of the additional indications of transfer.

7. Glossary of Terms

Table 5.2 provides a glossary of abbreviations specific to maternity and commonly used in handheld maternity records.

Maternity Care (including Obstetric Emergencies Overview)

UNDERTAKE PRIMARY SURVEY
Establish gestation and frequency of contractions

BIRTH IMMINENT

↓

Request midwife if available
Prepare for newborn life support
Reassure the woman and support her in a comfortable position, avoiding the supine position
Provide Entonox for pain relief

↓

Support the birth of the baby's head by applying gentle pressure as head advances

↓

Support the baby during the birth and place on the maternal abdomen

↓

Thoroughly dry the baby with a warm towel and wrap with a dry towel

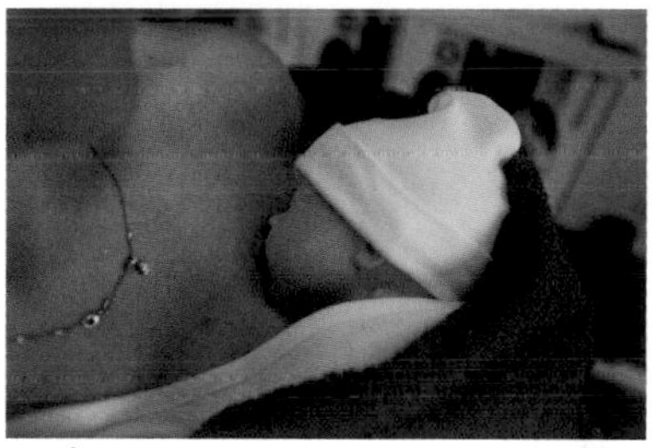

↓

If the baby is crying provide 'skin-to-skin' contact with the mother

→ If the baby is not crying refer to **Newborn Life Support**

↓

Allow the umbilical cord to stop pulsating prior to clamping and cutting

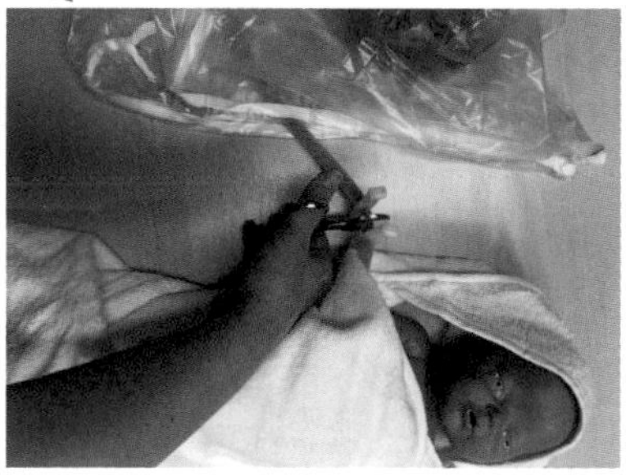

↓

The placenta may take 15–20 mins to birth – **DO NOT** pull on the cord – encourage the mother to pass urine

Deliver the placenta into a plastic bag for the midwife to inspect and check for completeness

Assess and record estimated blood loss

If the placenta remains undelivered with minimal bleeding, plan to transfer to the nearest appropriate destination as agreed locally

Maternal safety is the prime consideration

Consider the specific clinical situation **and which interventions may be required for the woman and baby on arrival**

Refer to 'Appropriate Destination for Conveyance' in **Maternity Care**

If the placenta remains undelivered and bleeding refer to Figure 5.5

BIRTH NOT IMMINENT

↓

Contact booked unit for advice if no time critical features present
(The woman may travel by car or taxi to booked unit if ambulance is not required)

Figure 5.2 – Pre-hospital maternity emergency management – normal birth.

Maternity Care (including Obstetric Emergencies Overview)

TABLE 5.2 – Glossary	
Abbreviation	**Term**
LMP	Last menstrual period.
EDD	Estimated date of delivery – the timing of the pregnancy is written in the notes in the format 12/40, i.e. 12 weeks have elapsed out of the 40-week pregnancy.
T or D	Term or expected date of delivery/pregnancy, therefore T+3 or D+3 in the notes is 3 days over the EDD.
CEPH	Cephalic (head).
BR	Breech.
G	Gravida, the number of times a woman has been pregnant (including the present pregnancy), e.g. G3.
P	Parity, the number of times a woman has given birth to a liveborn or stillborn baby, e.g. P3. A second figure implies previous miscarriages or terminations, e.g. P3+2.

KEY POINTS!

Maternity Care (including Obstetric Emergencies Overview)

- **Any woman of childbearing age MAY be pregnant.**
- **Due to the increase in blood volume, the pregnant woman is able to tolerate greater blood or plasma loss before showing signs of hypovolaemia, establish large bore (16G) IV cannulation early.**
- **A pregnant woman in cardiac arrest must ideally be conveyed with left manual uterine displacement after 20 weeks gestation. (Maintaining left lateral tilt is an alternative but may be more difficult to use effectively in the pre-hospital care environment.)**
- **The use of SBAR to communicate between ambulance clinicians and maternity clinicians can optimise transfer of information.**

Further Reading

Further important information and evidence in support of this guideline can be found in the Bibliography.

Bibliography

1. Knight M, Tuffnell D, Kenyon S, Shakespeare J, Gray R, Kurinczuk JJ (eds) on behalf of MBRRACE-UK. *Saving Lives, Improving Mothers' Care – Surveillance of maternal deaths in the UK 2011–13 and lessons learned to inform maternity care from the UK and Ireland Confidential Enquiries into Maternal Deaths and Morbidity 2009–13*. Oxford: National Perinatal Epidemiology Unit, University of Oxford, 2015.
2. Catchpole (2010), cited in Department of Health. *Human Factors Reference Group Interim Report, 1 March 2012*. National Quality Board. Available from: http://www.england.nhs.uk/ourwork/part-rel/nqb/ag-min/, 2012.
3. Woollard M, Hinshaw K, Simpson H, Wieteska S, (eds). *Pre-hospital Obstetric Emergency Training*. Oxford: Wiley-Blackwell, 2009.
4. Centre for Maternal and Child Enquiries. Saving mothers' lives: reviewing maternal deaths to make motherhood safer: 2006–2008. *BJOG: An International Journal of Obstetrics & Gynaecology* 2011, 118 (suppl. 1).
5. Bourjeily G, Paidas M, Khalil H, Rosene-Montella K, Rodger M. Pulmonary embolism in pregnancy. *The Lancet* 2010, 375(9713): 500–12.

Birth Imminent: Normal Birth and Birth Complications

1. Introduction

The best clinical management for a woman who is experiencing an abnormal labour or complications with the birth is to be transferred to the NEAREST appropriate unit without delay. This will usually be the nearest obstetric unit but in certain circumstances may involve transfer to the nearest ED (refer to 'Appropriate Destination for Conveyance' in Maternity Care).

When there is a midwife on scene it is their responsibility to manage the labour and birth, and ambulance clinicians should work under their direction, while working together as a team. If the midwife is not present, the decision on whether to convey the woman should be based on the principle that any situation that deviates from a normal uncomplicated labour should result in the woman being transported immediately to the nearest hospital with an obstetric unit once the appropriate number of conveying resources are available.

In this situation the ambulance clinicians must alert the hospital either directly or via the emergency operations centre (EOC). An early assessment of the need for additional resources may be necessary, including the request for a second ambulance where a newborn baby is required to be conveyed separately from the woman. Ensure that the request is made as soon as possible.

The most important feature of attending a pregnant woman is to complete a rapid assessment, to ascertain whether there is anything abnormal taking place.

The maternal assessment process outlined in Table 5.3 MUST be followed in order to decide whether to:

- STAY ON SCENE AND REQUEST A MIDWIFE (if not already present and available within the locality).
- TRANSFER TO FURTHER CARE IMMEDIATELY.

In maternity cases where birth is not imminent and there are no complications, it may be appropriate to contact the midwife in the booked maternity unit for advice regarding the transport arrangements. This may involve the woman making her own way to her planned place of birth if there are no immediately time critical features, or conveying her to the nearest maternity unit for assessment.

The assessment should be repeated en-route and, if any complications occur, the condition should be treated appropriately and destination changed if a nearer facility is available. If the woman is booked into a unit that is not within a reasonable distance or travelling time, ambulance clinicians should base their judgements on the maternal assessment, and take her to the nearest appropriate unit.

TABLE 5.3 – Assessment and Management of: Normal Birth

ASSESSMENT	MANAGEMENT
• Quickly assess the woman and scene as you approach • Undertake a primary survey **<C>ABCDE**	• If any time critical features are present, correct **<C>ABC** problems and transport to the nearest ED with an obstetric unit (refer to **Medical Emergencies in Adults – Overview** and **Medical Emergencies in Children – Overview**). • Provide a pre-alert.
• Ascertain the period of gestation • Ask the woman, and also review the woman's maternity records. Refer to antenatal pages for assessment of any obstetric risk factors or complications	
Assess for: • operculum (show) • ruptured amniotic fluid sac (waters broken) • contractions • and/or bleeding (See Figure 5.2 . For additional information, refer to **Maternity Care**)	If **NONE** of these indications is present **AND** there is no other medical/traumatic condition, discuss the woman's management with the **BOOKED OBSTETRIC UNIT**, informing of: • woman's name • woman's age and date of birth • woman's hospital registration number • name of lead clinician (midwifery or obstetric led care) • history of this pregnancy • estimated date of delivery (EDD) • period of gestation (number of weeks pregnant) • previous obstetric history.

(continued)

SECTION 5 Maternity Care

TABLE 5.3 – Assessment and Management of: Normal Birth *(continued)*	
If ANY of the above indications are present, assess: • contraction interval • the urge to push or bear down • crowning/top of the baby's head/ breech presentation visible at the vulva	• Undertake a visual inspection of the vaginal entrance if there are regular contractions (1–2 minute intervals) and an urge to push or bear down.
• If birth is imminent, that is regular contractions (1–2 minute intervals) and an urge to push or bear down and or crowning/top of the baby's head/breech presentation visible at the vulva	• Remain on scene, request a midwife if available in the locality and an additional ambulance with a paramedic if not already present, and prepare for the birth of the baby (see below).
• Second stage of labour (from full dilatation of the cervix until complete birth of the baby) • Continue assessing the woman's level of pain	• Reassure the woman, tell her what you are doing and include her birth partner if present. • Ensure the environment is safe and secure for the birth of the baby with particular attention to the temperature of the room: – incontinence pads – cover the ambulance stretcher or birthing area – maternity pack – open and set out – towels (warm towels if possible) – enough to dry and wrap the baby – blanket(s) – cover the mother for warmth and modesty – heat – turn the heat up in the birth area (aim for 25°C). 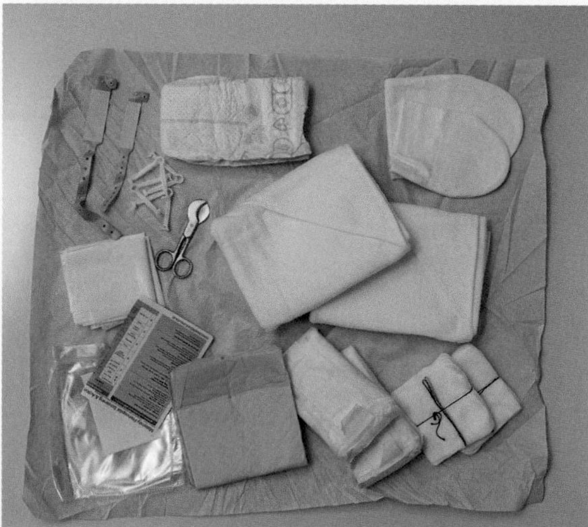 Contents of the maternity pack. • Support the woman in any position she finds comfortable – discourage her from lying flat on her back because of the risk of supine hypotension. • Encourage the woman to continue taking Entonox to relieve pain/discomfort if necessary. • **CAUTION** – at this stage, morphine should only be administered in exceptional circumstances due to the risk of neonatal respiratory depression. • To allow for the baby's head to be born slowly, encourage the woman to concentrate on panting or breathing out during the birth. The use of Entonox can assist here.

TABLE 5.3 – Assessment and Management of: Normal Birth *(continued)*	
	● Consider applying gentle pressure to the top of the baby's head as it advances through the vaginal entrance to prevent very rapid birth of the head. Pressure may also assist in keeping the head flexed to allow the smallest diameter of the fetal skull to be born. This may reduce perineal trauma. ● The umbilical cord may be around the baby's neck and does not require removal, as the baby can be born with the cord left in place. ● Hold the baby as it is born and lift it towards the woman's abdomen. ● Wipe any obvious large collections of mucous from the baby's mouth and nose.
● Undertake an initial **ABCD** assessment of the baby – include head, trunk, axilla and groin	● Newborns are at risk of hypothermia. ● **CAUTION** – premature babies lose heat faster than full term babies (refer to **Care of the Newborn**). ● Quickly and thoroughly dry the baby using a warm towel while you make your initial assessment. ● Remove the now wet towel and wrap the baby in a dry towel to minimise heat losses.
● Assess the baby's airway	● If the baby is crying, it has a clear airway. ● If the baby is not breathing, confirm that the airway is open – the head is ideally placed in the 'neutral' position, i.e. not the extended 'sniffing position'. Figure reproduced with the kind permission of the Resuscitation Council (UK). ● **SUCTION IS NOT USUALLY NECESSARY** – if required, use the suction unit on low power (around 75 mmHg) with a CH 12–14 catheter and then only within the oral cavity. **ONLY** use suction to remove **VISIBLE** thick particulate lumps of meconium. During suctioning, the tip of the catheter should be visible to the operator. **DO NOT** probe blindly with the catheter as this can cause a vagal response and depress respiration. ● If the baby is not breathing refer to **Newborn Life Support**. ● Once the baby is breathing adequately, cyanosis will gradually improve over several minutes – if the cyanosis is not clearing, enrich the atmosphere near the baby's face with a low flow of oxygen at 2 litres. ● Where available, oxygen saturation probes should be used. Refer to **Care of the Newborn**.

(continued)

Birth Imminent: Normal Birth and Birth Complications

TABLE 5.4 – Assessment and Management of: Birth Complications *(continued)*

● Re-assess the mother constantly en-route	● Should birth take place en-route assess both the mother and the baby and take appropriate action. ● Keeping the baby warm is a priority in the preterm newborn (refer to **Newborn Life Support**). ● Convey mother and baby to the **NEAREST** obstetric unit or ED with an obstetric unit dependent on local policy. ● Provide a pre-alert to enable a midwifery and neonatal team to receive the mother and newborn baby upon your arrival. ● In some circumstances, it may be necessary to convey the baby separately from the mother, dependent upon the clinical condition of either newborn or mother. In this instance, mother and baby should be conveyed to the same ED with an ID bracelet placed on each of them. ● If transfer to further care is not possible because the birth is imminent, request a midwife plus an additional ambulance and inform the EOC. ● Once the baby is born, utilise the additional ambulance to transport the baby **IMMEDIATELY** to the **NEAREST** appropriate destination as agreed locally. ● The baby should be transported once appropriate resource is available even if the midwife has not yet arrived. ● Provide a pre-alert to the hospital (it will be necessary to identify the nearest, most appropriate ED with an obstetric unit, with the necessary neonatal facilities). ● The mother should be transferred to the same location as the baby; where no complications are identified, a courtesy call should be placed ahead of her arrival.
2. Maternal convulsions (eclampsia) (see Figure 5.3)	
ASSESSMENT ● Quickly assess the woman and scene as you approach	**MANAGEMENT** ● Refer to **Pregnancy-induced Hypertension (including Eclampsia)**. ● **ALL** generalised tonic/clonic type convulsions after 24th week of pregnancy should be regarded as eclampsia until proved otherwise, **EVEN IF THERE IS A HISTORY OF EPILEPSY**. ● If the woman is convulsing, refer to **Convulsions in Adults** and **Convulsions in Children**.
Undertake a primary survey **<C>ABCDEF** Assess for **TIME CRITICAL** features	● Correct A and B problems and transfer to the nearest ED with an obstetric unit.
3. Prolapsed umbilical cord (see Figure 5.4)	
ASSESSMENT The descent of the umbilical cord into the lower uterine segment. This is a **TIME CRITICAL EMERGENCY** requiring immediate intervention, rapid removal and transfer to the nearest obstetric unit	**MANAGEMENT** Avoid handling the umbilical cord. Using a dry pad, replace the cord GENTLY within the opening of the vulva to keep it warm and prevent spasm, and use the pad to prevent further prolapse. (Do not use moist/wet pads as this will make the cord cold). If available, use underwear to hold the pad in position. If attending as a solo responding clinician, position the woman in the knee/chest position while awaiting an ambulance.

TABLE 5.4 – Assessment and Management of: Birth Complications *(continued)*

	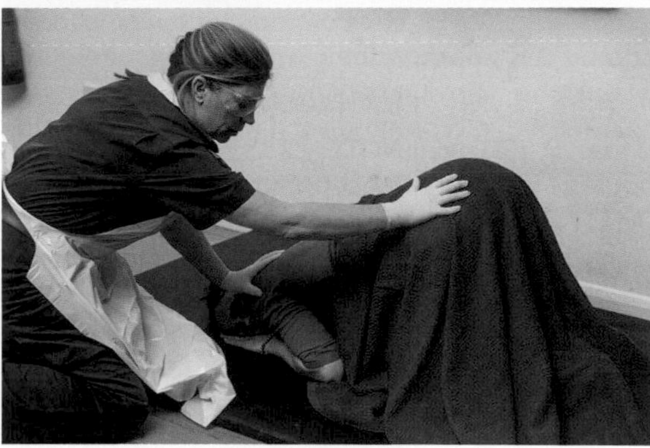 To enable rapid transfer to the ambulance, the woman can be walked, avoiding the use of the carry chair where possible. Once in the ambulance, position the mother on her side with padding placed under her hips to raise the pelvis and reduce pressure on the cord. 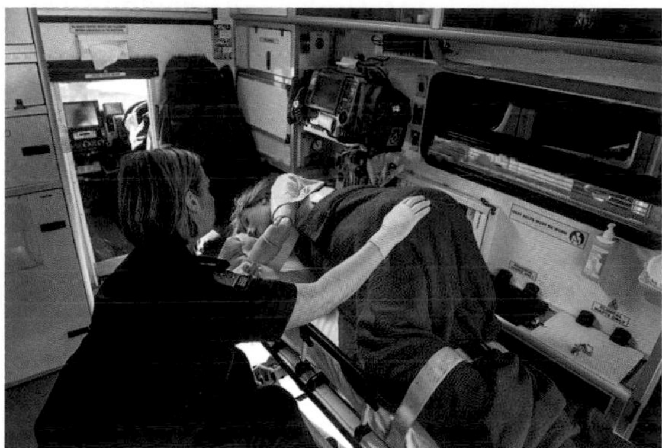 Administer Entonox if the mother experiences pain or the urge to push. Provide ongoing assessment of the woman to ensure that birth is not imminent (if birth is imminent, refer to the normal birth section of this guideline.) It is not safe to convey the woman in the all fours position in the ambulance. • Transfer to the nearest obstetric unit. • Place an early pre-alert stating the obstetric emergency of cord prolapse. • It may be necessary to request maternity staff to meet the ambulance clinicians at a suitable entrance to avoid any delays due to accessing lifts or entry to buildings.

(continued)

<table>
<tr><th colspan="2">TABLE 5.4 – Assessment and Management of: Birth Complications (continued)</th></tr>
<tr><td>● Assess if any/either baby requires resuscitation</td><td>● Refer to Newborn Life Support.</td></tr>
<tr><td colspan="2">6. Malpresentation – including vaginal breech birth (see Figure 5.6)</td></tr>
<tr><td>ASSESSMENT
● Vaginal breech birth is where the feet or buttocks of the baby present first rather than the baby's head
● NB Cord prolapse is more common with a breech presentation (refer to 3 above); follow local guidelines</td><td>MANAGEMENT
Vaginal breech birth – if birth is NOT in progress:
● Recognise breech presentation (may be documented in the woman's antenatal notes, thick meconium may be seen at vaginal opening, fetal buttocks or feet visible at vaginal opening).
● Transfer mother to the nearest obstetric unit without delay.
● Constantly re-assess en-route and take appropriate action if the circumstances change.
Vaginal breech birth – if birth IS in progress:
● Request a midwife (if available locally) and additional resources.
● Prepare for newborn resuscitation (refer to Newborn Life Support).
● Encourage the woman to adopt a position to enable gravity to help the birth of the baby, for example the edge of the bed, the edge of a sofa or the 'all fours' position.
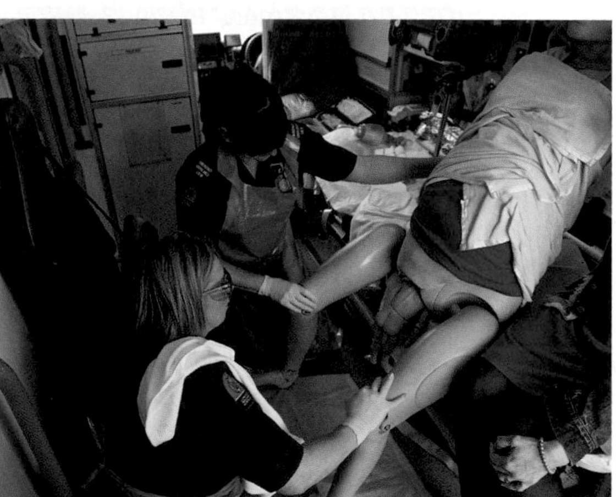
Breech delivery with mother semi-recumbent. Note – the fetal back should be upwards.
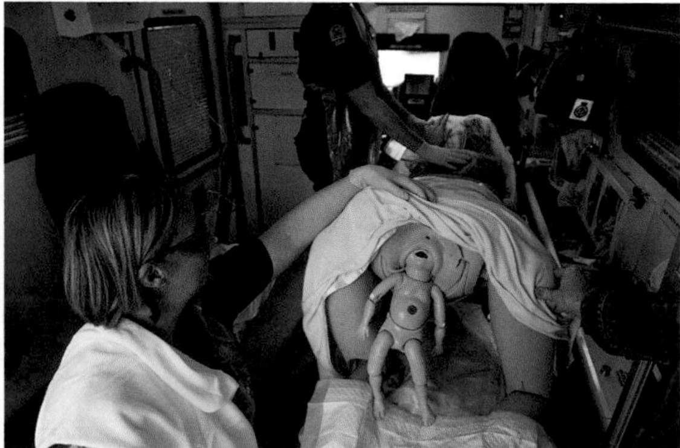
Breech delivery in 'all fours' position. Note – the fetal abdomen should face upwards (i.e. the fetal back faces the maternal abdomen).</td></tr>
</table>

TABLE 5.4 – Assessment and Management of: Birth Complications *(continued)*

	• Allow breech to descend spontaneously with maternal pushing, and maintain a 'hands off' position. It is not necessary to touch the baby or handle the umbilical cord during the birth. • The baby's legs and arms will spontaneously birth and do not require any assistance. • Only assist to ensure the baby's back remains facing towards the woman's abdomen. • If the baby's back rotates away from the woman's abdomen, handle the baby over the hips (the bony pelvis) and gently rotate the baby's back to face towards the woman's abdomen. • In the semi-recumbent position, once the baby's body is born to the nape of the neck, allow slow spontaneous birth of the head by supporting the baby's body on your forearm and gently lift the baby to facilitate birth of the baby's head. In the all fours position, as the head delivers the baby's body will deliver onto the bed/trolley. • Once the birth is complete, if the baby does not require any resuscitation, management of the umbilical cord should be as per normal birth guidelines, and should be left to stop pulsating. • Breech babies are more likely to be covered in meconium and may require resuscitation (refer to **Newborn Life Support**). • If delays occur during the birth: – **Legs.** If the legs delay birth of the body, apply gentle pressure to the back of the baby's knee (popliteal fossa) enabling birth of each individual leg. – **Arms.** If the arms are extended, gently rotate baby's pelvis 180 degrees to bring the posterior arm anterior (i.e. uppermost) and deliver that arm first, then rotate the baby in the opposite direction 180 degrees and release the other arm. – **Head.** If the head does not deliver in the semi-recumbent position (with the baby's body supported on your forearm), *apply pressure to the back of the baby's head with the fingers of your other hand*, to aid flexion while the head delivers. • Where ambulance clinicians have received appropriate training in management of breech birth, additional manoeuvres can be undertaken as detailed above for management of the legs, arms and head where delays in birth are identified. • Where the ambulance clinician has not received appropriate training, the nearest obstetric unit can be contacted to provide guidance on the ongoing management of the birth. Any presenting body part other than the head, buttocks or feet (e.g. one foot or a hand/arm). • Transfer the mother immediately to the nearest obstetric unit. • Provide a pre-alert. It may be necessary to request maternity staff meet the ambulance clinicians at a suitable entrance to avoid any delays due to accessing lifts.

(continued)

TABLE 5.4 – Assessment and Management of: Birth Complications *(continued)*

	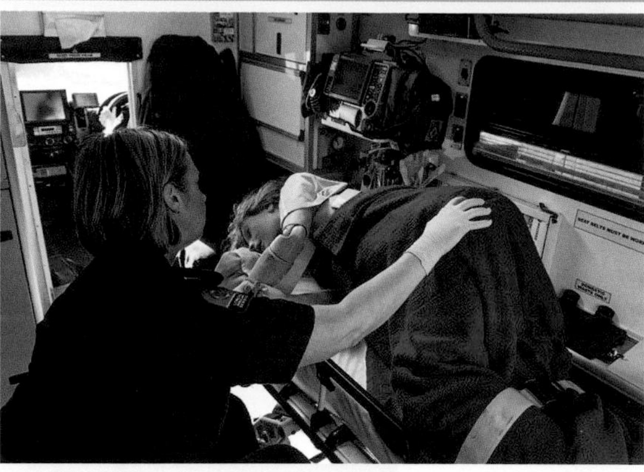 ● Convey the woman to the nearest obstetric unit positioned in a lateral position using a pillow to seperate the woman's legs and avoid pressure on the baby's head. Offer Entonox to provide analgesia if required. Do not delay to await arrival of the midwife. ● Place a pre-alert stating the obstetric emergency of shoulder dystocia. It may be necessary to request maternity staff meet the ambulance clinicians at a suitable entrance to avoid any delays due to accessing lifts or access to buildings. **The use of internal manoeuvres by ambulance clinicians** ● Where McRoberts manoeuvre, suprapubic pressure and all fours position have been attempted to expedite the birth, the use of specific internal manoeuvres may be appropriate where a registered paramedic has received additional training to undertake them. ● In a pre-hospital setting where a lone attending clinician is first on scene, the use of all fours position may facilitate the removal of the posterior arm, notably when awaiting an ambulance to the scene.

KEY POINTS!

Birth Imminent: Normal Birth and Birth Complications

- **For a woman experiencing an abnormal labour or birth, transfer immediately to the nearest obstetric unit. This includes:**
  - **severe vaginal bleeding**
  - **preterm or multiple births**
  - **prolapsed umbilical cord**
  - **continuous severe abdominal/epigastric pain**
  - **maternal convulsions (eclampsia)**
  - **presentation of the baby other than the head (e.g. arm or leg or buttocks)**
  - **shoulder dystocia.**
- **If the woman presents with an obvious medical or traumatic condition that puts her life in imminent danger, transfer to the nearest ED with an obstetric unit.**
- **The period of gestation is important in informing the appropriate course of action, including the most appropriate location for conveyance, namely an ED, an early pregnancy unit or an obstetric unit.**
- **In the event of an obstetric emergency, detailing the exact emergency via a pre-alert call will assist the ED or maternity unit to summon the appropriate staff.**
- **Maintaining normothermia in the newborn is critical while on scene and during conveyance. The optimum body temperature of the baby should be between 36.5 and 37.5 degrees.**

Birth Imminent: Normal Birth and Birth Complications

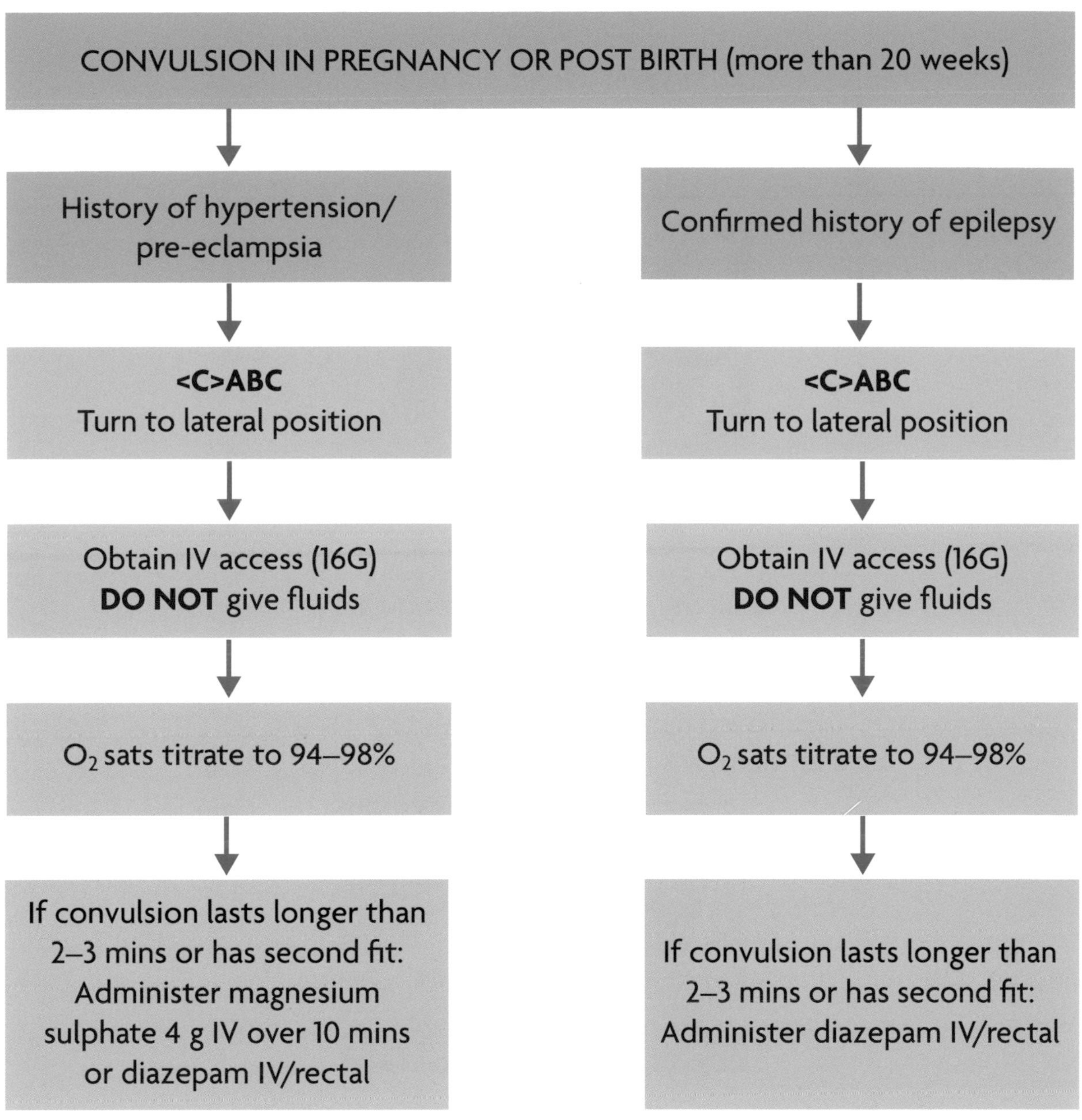
CONVULSION IN PREGNANCY OR POST BIRTH (more than 20 weeks)
History of hypertension/ pre-eclampsia
<C>ABC
Turn to lateral position
Obtain IV access (16G)
DO NOT give fluids
O_2 sats titrate to 94–98%
If convulsion lasts longer than 2–3 mins or has second fit: Administer magnesium sulphate 4 g IV over 10 mins or diazepam IV/rectal
Confirmed history of epilepsy
<C>ABC
Turn to lateral position
Obtain IV access (16G)
DO NOT give fluids
O_2 sats titrate to 94–98%
If convulsion lasts longer than 2–3 mins or has second fit: Administer diazepam IV/rectal

Transfer to nearest appropriate destination as agreed locally
Maternal safety is the prime consideration
Consider the specific clinical situation **and which interventions may be required for the woman and baby on arrival**
Refer to 'Appropriate Destination for Conveyance' in **Maternity Care**
Pre-alert stating obstetric emergency eclampsia
Take maternity notes if available

Figure 5.3 – Pre-hospital maternity emergency – management of eclampsia.

Birth Imminent: Normal Birth and Birth Complications

Breech position noted in maternal notes or thick meconium seen at vaginal opening

↓ BREECH BIRTH IMMINENT

Request midwife if available
Prepare for newborn life support

↓

Position on edge of bed/trolley
or on all fours

↓

HANDS OFF
Allow breech to descend spontaneously with maternal pushing
DO NOT touch baby or handle umbilical cord

↓

In either position, ensure the baby's back is always facing towards the maternal abdomen

↓

Support baby as head births

↓

Treat as normal birth or
refer to Newborn Life Support

↓ BREECH BIRTH NOT IMMINENT OR ANY OTHER PRESENTING PART (i.e. hand/arm)

Transfer to nearest appropriate destination as agreed locally
Maternal safety is the prime consideration
Consider the specific clinical situation **and which interventions may be required for the woman and baby on arrival**
Refer to 'Appropriate Destination for Conveyance' in **Maternity Care**
Continuously assess for birth imminent en-route

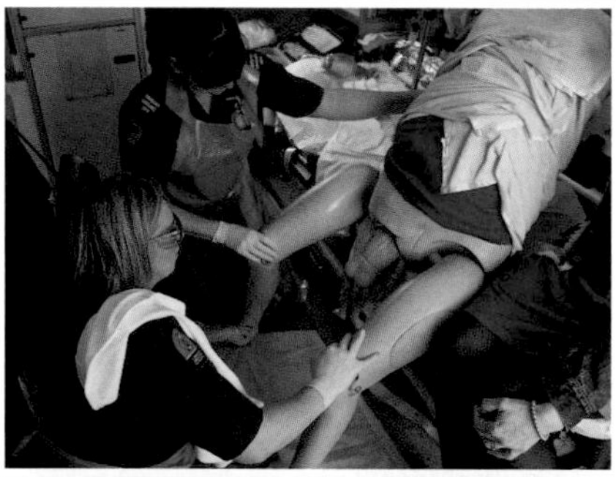

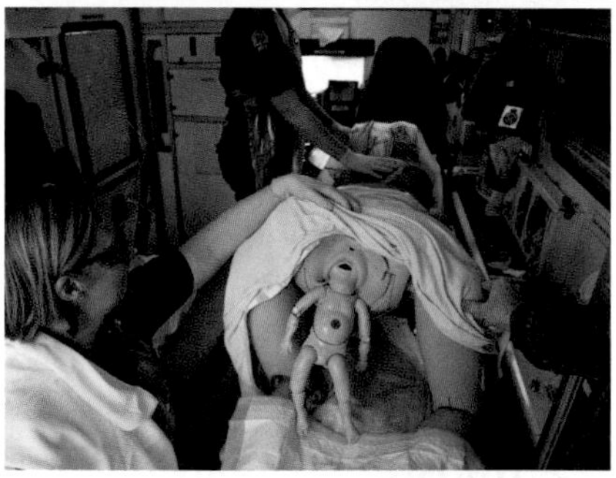

IF DELAY OCCURS DURING THE BIRTH:

LEGS: apply gentle pressure behind the baby's knee
ARMS: gently rotate the baby's pelvis 90 degrees to aid birth of the first arm – rotate the baby's body in the opposite direction if required to birth the second arm – allow the baby's body to hang unassisted
HEAD: support the baby with one arm and use the other hand to aid flexion of the back of the baby's head while delivering baby

DO NOT PULL ON THE BABY
DO NOT CLAMP AND CUT THE UMBILICAL CORD DURING THE BIRTH

Figure 5.6 – Pre-hospital maternity emergency – management of breech birth.

Birth Imminent: Normal Birth and Birth Complications

REQUEST A MIDWIFE IF AVAILABLE AND PREPARE FOR NEWBORN LIFE SUPPORT
Position the woman in the McRoberts position
For a solo clinician – ask the woman to hold her legs and push with her next contraction

If shoulders do not release:
Attempt to deliver the baby
- With your hands on the baby's head apply gentle 'axial' traction, keeping the baby's head in line with its spine for up to 30 seconds

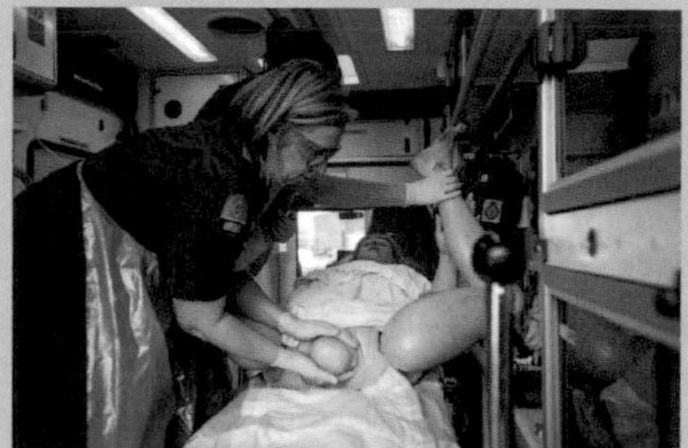

Undelivered?

Apply suprapubic pressure with the woman in the McRoberts position
- Identify the position of the fetal back and place assistant on that maternal side
- Using a CPR grip, apply continuous pressure downwards and lateral for 30 seconds (2 fingers above symphysis pubis)
- Encourage the woman to push **OR** attempt gentle 'axial' traction to deliver baby

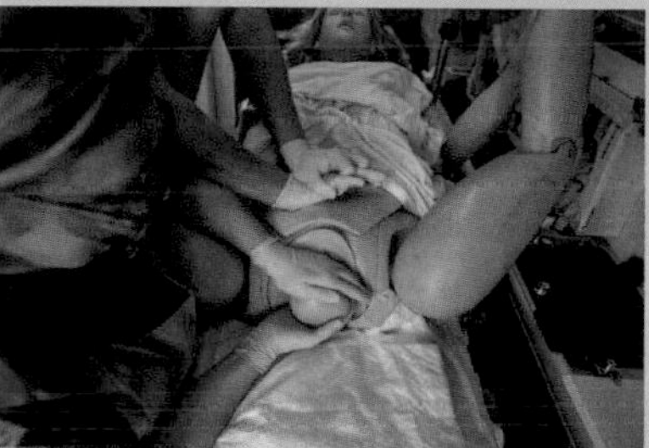

Undelivered?

- Attempt intermittent 'rocking' suprapubic pressure for 30 seconds and encourage woman to push
- Or attempt gentle 'axial' traction to deliver baby

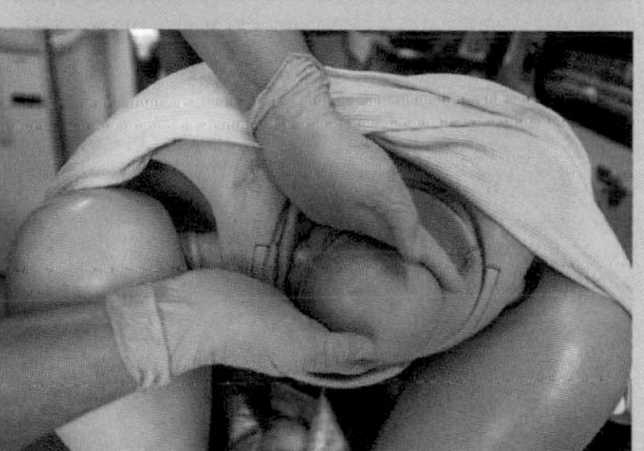

Undelivered?

- Change the woman's position to 'all fours' and encourage her to push
- Or attempt gentle 'axial' traction to deliver baby

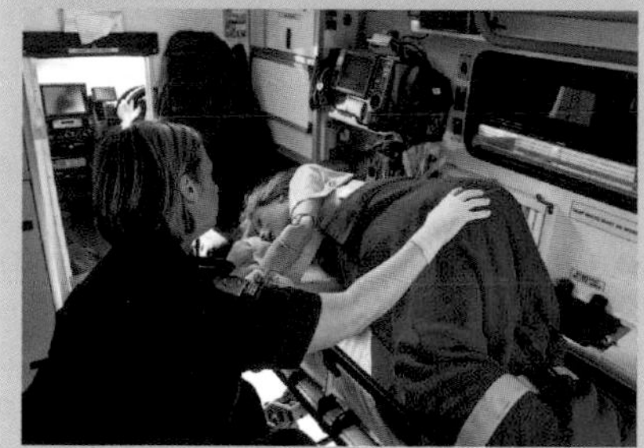

Undelivered?

- Walk the woman to the ambulance and anticipate the birth during transfer
- Convey in a lateral position with legs separated by a blanket to protect the baby's head
- Reassure the woman and provide Entonox as required.

Baby born
Refer to **Care of the Newborn**

Transfer to the nearest appropriate destination as agreed locally
Maternal safety is the prime consideration
Consider the specific clinical situation **and which interventions may be required for the woman and baby on arrival**
Refer to 'Appropriate Destination for Conveyance' in **Maternity Care**
Pre-alert stating the obstetric emergency shoulder dystocia
Keep a log of the time each intervention is attempted

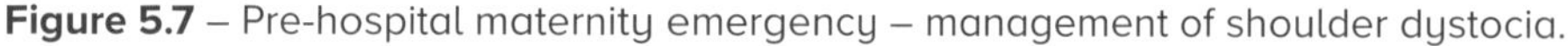

Figure 5.7 – Pre-hospital maternity emergency – management of shoulder dystocia.

cooling during the transfer to hospital. Accidental hypothermia in all babies, but especially in the premature baby, can be harmful.For each degree below 36.5°C, the risk of mortality increases by 28%. A cold baby has increased oxygen consumption, and is at risk of hypoglycaemia and acidosis, and is associated with an increased mortality. It is therefore important that the baby is kept warm during the transfer in the ambulance, to prevent hypoglycaemia and these complications.

2.3 Hypoglycaemia

- The newborn baby has a relatively immature liver with limited glycogen stores and so low blood sugars are not an uncommon problem. It is therefore important to encourage and support early breastfeeding where possible.
- In a baby without any abnormal signs and symptoms (see list below), and no risk factors (see list below), hypoglycaemia is defined as any single blood glucose (BG) reading with a value of <1.0 mmol/l, even if a subsequent reading is normal. In a baby who is at-risk (see list below), hypoglycaemia is defined as two consecutive blood glucose readings of <2.0 mmol/l. In a baby with abnormal signs and symptoms, a single reading of <2.5 mmol/l can be used to diagnose hypoglycaemia. If the BG is <1.1 mmol/L, remains <2.6 mmol/L or if the baby is symptomatic, they must be reviewed urgently by a paediatrician and the baby requires admission to the neonatal unit.
- Glucose is the main energy source for the fetus and neonate, and the newborn brain depends almost exclusively on glucose for energy metabolism.
- Hypoglycaemia can therefore lead to convulsions and brain injury. Severe and prolonged hypoglycaemia may result in long-term neurological damage. It is therefore important to prevent and treat a low blood sugar level as soon as it is detected.
- Signs and symptoms of hypoglycaemia include:
  - jitteriness
  - irritability
  - lethargy
  - apnoeic episodes
  - convulsions
  - BG <1.5 mmol/L.

NB Many hypoglycaemic babies are asymptomatic, hence the importance of routine blood glucose checks in babies at risk. Those at risk of hypoglycaemia include babies who are:

- premature
- small for gestational age
- <2.5kg at birth
- in need of resuscitation at birth
- born to diabetic mothers, due to high circulating maternal insulin levels
- born to mothers using beta blockers (labetalol)
- suffering from perinatal hypoxia
- suffering from hypothermia
- suffering from sepsis.

After birth, encourage the mother to feed her baby as soon as possible (or at least within the first hour). Failing this, intravenous glucose may be needed, depending on (i) the baby's condition and (ii) the blood glucose level. The newborn baby's liver has very limited glycogen stores, so hypoglycaemia must not be treated using intramuscular glucagon (glucagon works by stimulating the liver to convert glycogen into glucose). A baby found to have hypoglycaemia (as previously defined) must be transported to hospital for further investigation and management.

2.4 Neonatal Jaundice

- Jaundice refers to the yellow colouration of the skin and sclera caused by a raised bilirubin level. About 60% of term and 80% of pre-term babies develop jaundice in the first week of life. Physiological jaundice occurs around day 2–7, although 10% of breast fed babies are still jaundiced at 1 month of age. Physiological jaundice is due to increased breakdown of haemoglobin in red blood cells to bilirubin, and the immature liver is unable to handle the conversion of bilirubin to a form that can be excreted in the gut. Jaundice is harmless unless the bilirubin level is very high, when this can cross the blood–brain barrier.
- Unconjugated bilirubin is potentially toxic to brain tissue causing kernicterus and brain damage. Different treatment thresholds are recommended for different gestations and ages (see graphs published by National Institute for Health and Care Excellence). Jaundice is treated with phototherapy or exchange transfusion, depending on the level of bilirubin and the cause. Early jaundice (occurring before day 2) or prolonged jaundice (after day 14) may be due to other pathological causes or underlying diseases and requires investigation. Babies with early jaundice occurring <2 days of age must be referred for an urgent medical review.

2.5 Preterm Delivery

- Prematurity is defined as <37 weeks gestation. Premature infants are more likely to need assistance with ventilation.
- At <32 weeks gestation spontaneous breathing will be inadequate and this group of babies are likely to be deficient in surfactant (surfactant reduces alveolar surface tension and keeps the lung alveoli open during expiration), necessitating surfactant replacement and/

or ventilatory support, and immediate transfer to the nearest ED with an obstetric unit will be necessary.

- At <32 weeks gestation the risk of intracranial bleeds is increased.
- Other complications of prematurity include hypothermia, hypoglycaemia and a higher risk of infection.
- Improving neonatal intensive care has seen better outcomes for babies born pre-term (especially in babies born after 28 weeks gestation). However, the EPICure study following up babies born in the UK at the limits of viability before 26 weeks gestation showed a high mortality and morbidity. Overall survival was only 39% and survivors commonly have severe disabilities. Hypothermia was one of the factors associated with death.

Birth at Less Than 24 Weeks Gestation

Ambulance clinicians may attend births at extremes of prematurity and viability. The guidance regarding newborn resuscitation in the pre-hospital phase of care is less well defined than in a maternity unit, where access to neonatal expertise can enable a plan to be discussed with the woman based upon the clinical assessment of the pregnancy to date. The following guidance acts to enable clinicians working in the pre-hospital setting to be supported when faced with a baby born prematurely between 20 and 24 weeks gestation:

- When attending a birth at 20–24 weeks **OR** the gestation is unknown, and there are signs of life, the recommendations are:
  - Maintain ventilation using the smallest paediatric mask – size 00.
  - Provide effective ventilations with the baby lying flat, assess heart rate and do not expect the chest to move at this gestation. If ventilations are effective the heart rate will remain stable or improve.
  - Where neonatal wraps or cribs are available these should be used to minimise heat loss.
  - Ensure the head is covered with the small baby hat.
  - Place a pre-alert stating whether the mother is travelling with the baby.
  - Convey to the nearest ED with an obstetric unit, requesting the neonatal team.
- Where there are signs of life, ventilations should be continued until the neonatal team can assess the gestation and weight of the baby. The team will then consider the ongoing management in the best interests of the baby and the family.
- Neither a midwife nor an ambulance clinician should discontinue resuscitative attempts; this decision sits within the expertise of the neonatologist.

2.6 Congenital Abnormalities

- The outcome of babies born with congenital abnormalities varies but is improving with advancement in medical therapies and interventions. The abnormality may have been detected on previous antenatal scans or may have been undiagnosed until birth. Hence all babies who are known to have a congenital abnormality should be transferred to hospital where the abnormality can be assessed and treated, even when the baby appears to be normal at birth.
- Cling film the defect to reduce fluid and heat losses.

NB Do not wrap the cling film circumferentially around the newborn's body as this will inhibit breathing.

2.7 Early Onset Neonatal Sepsis

Early onset neonatal sepsis can be life-threatening and it is important that it is recognised and treated early. The following **red flags** ⚑ suggest a high risk of early onset neonatal sepsis:

- Maternal risk factors:
  - ⚑ systemic antibiotic treatment given to the mother for confirmed or suspected invasive bacteria
  - ⚑ group B streptococcus (GBS)
  - ⚑ E.coli
  - ⚑ listeria
  - ⚑ other organisms, such as anaerobes (rare)
  - ⚑ GBS colonisation, bacteriuria or infection in CURRENT pregnancy
  - ⚑ a previous baby with invasive GBS infection
  - ⚑ preterm, pre-labour rupture of membranes of any duration
  - ⚑ suspected or confirmed intrapartum rupture of membranes >18 hours.
- Neonatal risk factors
  - ⚑ convulsions in the baby
  - ⚑ signs for shock in the baby
  - ⚑ need for mechanical ventilation in a term baby
  - ⚑ suspected or confirmed infection in a co-twin.

3. Assessment and Management

The baby's condition can be assessed quickly just from their colour, heart rate and breathing effort. For the initial clinical assessment of the newborn baby the following should be undertaken (refer to Table 5.5):

- Colour – useful for assessing the initial condition of the baby at birth.

4. Wyllie J, Perlman JM, Kattwinkel J, et al. Part 7: Neonatal resuscitation: 2015 International Consensus on Cardiopulmonary Resuscitation and Emergency Cardiovascular Care Science with Treatment Recommendations. *Resuscitation* 2015; 95: e169–201.

5. Hawdon JM. Investigation, prevention and management of neonatal hypoglycaemia (impaired postnatal metabolic adaptation). *Paediatrics and Child Health* 2012, 22(4): 131–135.

6. Cornblath M, Hawdon JM, Williams AF, Aynsley-Green A, Ward-Platt MP, Schwartz R, et al. Controversies regarding definition of neonatal hypoglycemia: suggested operational thresholds. *Pediatrics* 2000, 105 (5): 1141–1145.

7. Woollard M, Hinshaw K, Simpson H, Wieteska S. Care of the baby at birth. In *Pre-hospital Obstetric Emergency Training*. Oxford: Wiley-Blackwell, 2009: 125–135.

8. National Collaborating Centre for Women's and Children's Health. *Diabetes in Pregnancy* (CG63). London: National Institute for Health and Clinical Excellence, 2008.

9. Beard L, Lax P, Tindall M. Physiological effects of transfer for critically ill patients. *Anaesthesia Tutorial of the Week* 2016, 330. Available from: http://anaesthesiology.gr/media/File/pdf/330-Physiological-effects-of-transfer-for-critically-ill-patients.pdf.

10. National Institute for Health and Clinical Excellence. Neonatal Jaundice: Treatment Threshold Graphs. London: NICE, 2010. Available from: https://www.nice.org.uk/guidance/cg98/evidence/full-guideline-pdf-245411821.

Haemorrhage During Pregnancy (including Miscarriage and Ectopic Pregnancy)

1. Introduction

- This guidance is for the assessment and management of women with bleeding during early and late pregnancy (including miscarriage and ectopic pregnancy). For postpartum haemorrhage refer to **Birth Imminent: Normal Birth** and **Birth Complications**. For complications associated with therapeutic termination ('abortion') refer to **Vaginal Bleeding: Gynaecological Causes**.
- Any bleeding from the genital tract during pregnancy is of concern and in early pregnancy may indicate miscarriage or an ectopic pregnancy. This more commonly occurs in the first three months (weeks 1–12) but can also occur in the second trimester. Haemorrhage may:
  - present with evident vaginal loss of blood (e.g. miscarriage in early pregnancy and placenta praevia in late pregnancy)
  - occur mainly (or completely) within the abdomen (e.g. ruptured ectopic pregnancy) or uterus (e.g. concealed placental abruption). This presents with little or no external loss, but pain and signs of hypovolaemic shock. Pregnant women may appear well even with a large amount of concealed blood loss. Tachycardia may not appear until 30% or more of the circulating volume has been depleted.
- Bleeding in pregnancy is broadly divided into two timeframes: bleeding that occurs in the early part of pregnancy, such as miscarriage or ectopic pregnancy (less than 24 weeks), and that occurring in the late second and third trimesters of pregnancy, such as placenta praevia or placental abruption (i.e. after 24 weeks).

2. Haemorrhage in Early Pregnancy (≤24 weeks)

Haemorrhage in early pregnancy may indicate miscarriage or ectopic pregnancy

2.1 Incidence

Miscarriage is most common in the first 12 weeks of gestation. The mother will often be anxious as to what is happening and can be very concerned as to the health and wellbeing of her unborn baby.

2.2 Pathophysiology

- Miscarriage is the loss of pregnancy before 24 completed weeks. It is most commonly seen at 6–14 weeks of gestation but can occur after 14 weeks.
- Miscarriage occurs when some of the early fetal or placental tissue (known as 'products of conception') are partly passed through the cervix and may become trapped, leading to continuing blood loss. If shock ensues, it is may be out of proportion to the amount of blood loss (i.e. when there is an added vagal component due to tissues trapped in the cervix).

Risk factors – miscarriage
• Previous history of miscarriage. • Previously identified potential miscarriage at scan. • Smoker. • Obesity.

Symptoms:

- Bleeding – light or heavy, often with clots and or jelly-like tissue.
- Pain – central, crampy, suprapubic or backache.
- Signs of pregnancy may be subsiding, e.g. nausea or breast tenderness.
- Significant symptoms (including hypotension) without significant external blood loss may indicate 'cervical shock' due to retained miscarriage tissue stuck in the cervix. Symptomatic bradycardia may arise due to vagal stimulation.

Symptoms characteristic of a ruptured ectopic pregnancy:

- Usually presents at around 6–8 weeks gestation, so usually only one period has been missed.
- Acute lower abdominal pain.
- Slight bleeding or brownish vaginal discharge.
- Tachycardia and skin coolness can indicate significant hidden bleeding within the abdomen.

Other suspicious symptoms:

- Unexplained fainting.
- Shoulder-tip pain.
- Unusual bowel symptoms.
- Intra-uterine contraceptive device fitted.
- Previous ectopic pregnancy.
- Tubal surgery.
- Sterilisation or reversal of sterilisation.
- Endometriosis.
- Pelvic inflammatory disease.
- Subfertility (delay in conceiving).

2.3 Management of Pregnancy Loss and Fetal Tissue in Early Pregnancy (<22 weeks)

Ambulance clinicians are often called to attend women who may have miscarried before the clinicians' arrival, or during the episode of care. This can be a very distressing time for the woman, her family and the ambulance clinicians involved.

Fetal tissue, including the baby, may be passed by the mother during the miscarriage. It may resemble blood-stained tissue, or demonstrate a discernible baby with placenta still attached. The management of fetal tissue must follow the principles below to ensure that all staff comply with the Human Tissue Act (March 2015).

Haemorrhage During Pregnancy (including Miscarriage and Ectopic Pregnancy)

TABLE 5.7 – Assessment and Management of: Haemorrhage During Pregnancy *(continued)*

• Assess woman's level of pain	• Titrate pain relief against pain (refer to **Pain Management in Adults** and **Pain Management in Children**): – **Paracetamol.** – **Entonox.** – **Morphine**: **NOTE** administer cautiously if the woman is hypotensive. • Nil by mouth. • Symptomatic bradycardia due to vagal stimulation can be treated with atropine (refer to **Atropine** and **Cardiac Rhythm Disturbance**). • Adjust woman's position as required. • If **TIME CRITICAL** features present, transfer to the nearest appropriate destination with a pre-alert stating the emergency. • Dependent upon locally agreed pathways and the gestational age of the pregnancy, it may be necessary to take the woman directly to the nearest maternity unit.

KEY POINTS!

Haemorrhage During Pregnancy (including Miscarriage and Ectopic Pregnancy)

- **Haemorrhage during pregnancy is broadly divided into two categories, occurring in early and late pregnancy.**
- **Haemorrhage may be revealed (evident vaginal blood loss) or concealed (little or no obvious loss).**
- **Pregnant women may appear well even when a large amount of blood has been lost (tachycardia may not appear until 30% of circulating volume as symptoms of hypovolaemic shock occur very late, by which stage the woman is critically ill).**
- **Obtain venous access with large bore cannulae (16G).**
- **In the presence of a confirmed miscarriage, intramuscular Syntometrine administration should be considered.**

Bibliography

1. Soar J, Perkins GD, Abbas G, Alfonzo A, Barelli A, Bierens JJLM, et al. European Resuscitation Council Guidelines for Resuscitation 2010 Section 8: Cardiac arrest in special circumstances: electrolyte abnormalities, poisoning, drowning, accidental hypothermia, hyperthermia, asthma, anaphylaxis, cardiac surgery, trauma, pregnancy, electrocution. *Resuscitation* 2010, 81(10): 1400–1433.
2. Woollard M, Simpson H, Hinshaw K, Wieteska S. Obstetric services. In *Pre-hospital Obstetric Emergency Training.* Oxford: Wiley-Blackwell, 2009: 1–6.
3. Woollard M, Hinshaw K, Simpson H, Wieteska S. Anatomical and physiological changes in pregnancy. In *Pre-hospital Obstetric Emergency Training.* Oxford: Wiley-Blackwell, 2009: 18–27.
4. Woollard M, Hinshaw K, Simpson H, Wieteska S. Structured approach to the obstetric patient. In *Pre-hospital Obstetric Emergency Training.* Oxford: Wiley-Blackwell, 2009: 38–52.
5. Woollard M, Hinshaw K, Simpson H, Wieteska S. Emergencies in early pregnancy and complications following gynaecological surgery. In *Pre-hospital Obstetric Emergency Training.* Oxford: Wiley-Blackwell, 2009: 53–61.
6. Woollard M, Hinshaw K, Simpson H, Wieteska S. Emergencies in late pregnancy. In *Pre-Hospital Obstetric Emergency Training.* Oxford: Wiley-Blackwell, 2009: 62–110.
7. Human Tissue Authority (2015) *Guidance on the Disposal of Pregnancy Remains Following Pregnancy Loss or Termination.* Available from: https://www.hta.gov.uk/sites/default/files/Guidance_on_the_disposal_of_pregnancy_remains.pdf, 2015.
8. Royal College of Nursing. *Managing the Disposal of Pregnancy Remains. RCN Guidance for Nursing and Midwifery Practice.* Available from: https://www2.rcn.org.uk/__data/assets/pdf_file/0008/645884/RCNguide_disposal_pregnancy_remains_WEB.pdf, 2015.

Haemorrhage During Pregnancy (including Miscarriage and Ectopic Pregnancy)

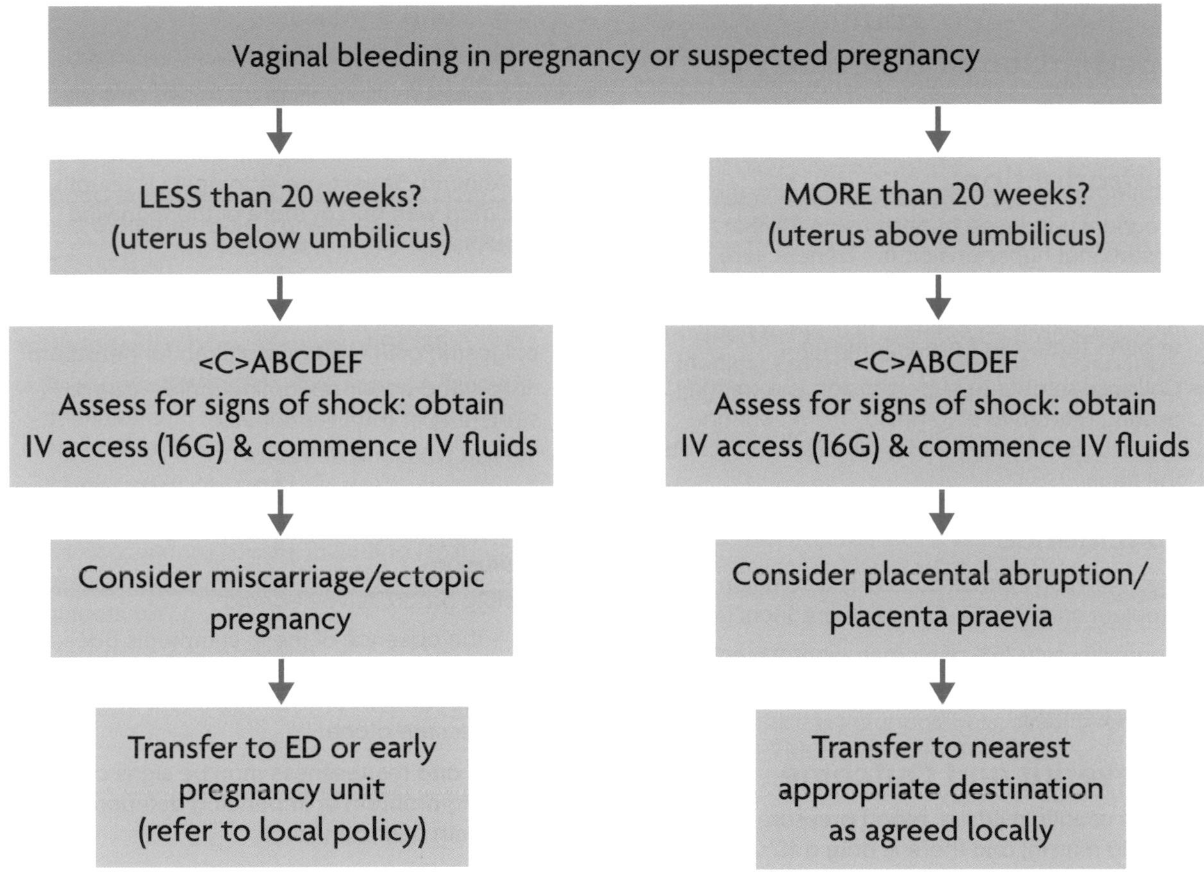

Maternal safety is the prime consideration

Consider the specific clinical situation **and which interventions may be required for the woman and baby on arrival**

Refer to 'Appropriate Destination for Conveyance' in **Maternity Care**

- If significant shock or compromise, consider ED in the first instance
- Take maternity notes if available

Figure 5.9 – Pre-hospital maternity emergency management – haemorrhage during pregnancy.

Pregnancy-induced Hypertension (including Eclampsia)

SECTION 2 – Eclampsia

1. Introduction

- Eclampsia is generalised tonic/clonic convulsion and identical to an epileptic convulsion.
- Many patients will have had pre-existing pre-eclampsia (of a mild, moderate or severe degree), but cases of eclampsia can present acutely with no prior warning – ONE THIRD of cases present for the FIRST TIME post-delivery (usually in the first 48 hours). **THE BP MAY ONLY BE MILDLY ELEVATED AT PRESENTATION** (i.e. 140/80–90 mmHg).
- Refer to **Convulsions (Adults)** and **Convulsions (Children)**.

2. Incidence

- Eclampsia occurs in approximately 2.7:10,000 deliveries, usually beyond 24 weeks.

3. Severity and Outcome

- Eclampsia is one of the most dangerous complications of pregnancy, and is a significant cause of maternal mortality, with a mortality rate of 2% in the UK.
- Convulsions are usually self-limiting, but may be severe and repeated.
- Other complications associated with eclampsia include renal failure, hepatic failure and DIC.

4. Pathophysiology

- The hypoxia caused during a tonic/clonic convulsion may lead to significant fetal compromise and death.

Risk factors – eclampsia
• Known pre-eclampsia. • Primiparity or first child with a new partner. • Previous severe pre-eclampsia. • Essential hypertension. • Diabetes. • Obesity. • Twins or higher multiples. • Renal disease. • Advanced maternal age (over 35 years). • Young maternal age (less than 16 years).

5. Assessment and Management

- For the assessment and management of eclampsia and eclamptic convulsion, refer to Table 5.10.

TABLE 5.10 – Assessment and Management of: Eclampsia

Definition – generalised tonic/clonic convulsion and identical to an epileptic convulsion.

ASSESSMENT	MANAGEMENT
• Undertake a primary survey **ABCDEF** • Assess for **TIME CRITICAL** features such as recurrent convulsions	• Correct **A** and **B** and transport to a consultant-led obstetric unit (refer to **Medical Emergencies in Adults – Overview** and **Medical Emergencies in Children – Overview**). • Obtain IV (LARGE BORE cannulae) or IO access. DO NOT administer fluid boluses because of the risk of provoking pulmonary oedema. • Provide a pre-alert stating the obstetric emergency of eclampsia.
• If **NON-TIME CRITICAL**, perform a more thorough assessment of the woman with secondary survey, including fetal assessment (refer to **Maternity Care** for guidance)	**NOTE:** epileptic patients may suffer tonic/clonic convulsions. • If >20 weeks gestation with a history of hypertension or pre-eclampsia, treat as for eclampsia – refer to Table 5.8 and Table 5.9. • If there is no history of hypertension or pre-eclampsia and blood pressure is normal, treat as for epilepsy (refer to **Convulsions (Adults)** and **Convulsions (Children)**). • Protect the airway. Place the woman in a full lateral ('recovery') position – do not use the supine position with left lateral tilt. If formal resuscitation is required, use the supine position with manual uterine displacement (refer to **Maternal Resuscitation**).
• Monitor SpO_2 (94–98%)	• Attach pulse oximeter; if SpO_2 <94%, administer O_2 to aim for a target saturation within the range of 94–98%.
• Continuous or recurrent convulsion	• If the patient convulses for longer than 2–3 minutes or has a second or subsequent convulsion, administer diazepam IV/PR (refer to **Diazepam** for dosages and information). **NOTE:** IV magnesium sulphate (4 g slow IV over 10 minutes) can be given if available and avoids the use of multiple drugs.

Pregnancy-induced Hypertension (including Eclampsia)

KEY POINTS!

Pregnancy-induced Hypertension (including Eclampsia)

- **Pregnancy-induced hypertension and pre-eclampsia commonly occur beyond 24–28 weeks gestation but can occur as early as 22 weeks.**
- **Pre-eclampsia can present up to 6 weeks post-delivery.**
- **Diagnosis of pre-eclampsia includes an increase in blood pressure above 140/90 mmHg, oedema and detection of protein in the woman's urine.**
- **Eclampsia is one of the most dangerous complications of pregnancy.**
- **Only administer diazepam or magnesium sulphate if the convulsions are prolonged or recurrent.**
- **Severe pre-eclampsia and eclampsia are TIME CRITICAL EMERGENCIES for both mother and fetus.**

Bibliography

1. Soar J, Perkins GD, Abbas G, Alfonzo A, Barelli A, Bierens JJLM, et al. European Resuscitation Council Guidelines for Resuscitation 2010 Section 8: Cardiac arrest in special circumstances: electrolyte abnormalities, poisoning, drowning, accidental hypothermia, hyperthermia, asthma, anaphylaxis, cardiac surgery, trauma, pregnancy, electrocution. *Resuscitation* 2010, 81(10): 1400–1433.
2. Centre for Maternal and Child Enquiries. Saving mothers' lives: reviewing maternal deaths to make motherhood safer: 2006–2008. *BJOG: An International Journal of Obstetrics & Gynaecology* 2011, 118 (suppl. 1).
3. Woollard M, Simpson H, Hinshaw K, Wieteska S. Obstetric services. In *Pre-hospital Obstetric Emergency Training.* Oxford: Wiley-Blackwell, 2009: 1–6.
4. Woollard M, Hinshaw K, Simpson H, Wieteska S. Anatomical and physiological changes in pregnancy. In *Pre-hospital Obstetric Emergency Training.* Oxford: Wiley-Blackwell, 2009: 18–27.
5. Woollard M, Hinshaw K, Simpson H, Wieteska S. Structured approach to the obstetric patient. In *Pre-hospital Obstetric Emergency Training.* Oxford: Wiley-Blackwell, 2009: 38–52.
6. Woollard M, Hinshaw K, Simpson H, Wieteska S. Emergencies in late pregnancy. In *Pre-Hospital Obstetric Emergency Training.* Oxford: Wiley-Blackwell, 2009: 62–110.

Vaginal Bleeding: Gynaecological Causes

1. Introduction

- A number of conditions can cause vaginal bleeding that is different from normal menstruation. Such conditions may result in a call to the ambulance service, including:
  - excessive menstrual period
  - normal or excessive menstrual period associated with severe abdominal pain
  - following surgical or medical therapeutic termination ('abortion') (**NB** – bleeding often continues for up to 10 days after treatment)
  - following gynaecological surgery (e.g. hysterectomy) (**NB** – heavy, ongoing bleeding commencing 7-14 days after surgery can indicate pelvic infection requiring antibiotics and may require hospital assessment)
  - colposcopy (**NB** – slight bleeding may occur up to 10 days after a colposcopy). A colposcopy is an outpatient test where the cervix is inspected following an abnormal cervical smear. Treatment such as cone biopsy for the abnormal smear may have been undertaken. Heavy bleeding post-colposcopy affects very few women in this situation. Heavy, ongoing bleeding at 7–14 days post-procedure can indicate infection requiring antibiotics and may require hospital assessment
  - gynaecological cancers, either before diagnosis or after treatment (i.e. cervix, uterus or vagina) may present with heavy vaginal bleeding
  - trauma; this can include post-coital tears and may be caused by sexual assault/rape.
- This guideline provides guidance for the assessment and management of gynaecological vaginal bleeding. For causes of bleeding in early or late pregnancy, refer to **Haemorrhage During Pregnancy**.

2. Incidence

- Women over 50 years are more at risk of cancers of the uterus and cervix.

3. Severity and Outcome

- The majority of causes of vaginal bleeding do not compromise the circulation, but blood loss can be alarming.

Sexual assault

- In sexual assault cases, there may be other injuries.
- When sexual assault is suspected (especially in a child or vulnerable adult), there are clear safeguarding issues (refer to **Safeguarding Children** and **Safeguarding Adults at Risk**).
- It is not the role of the ambulance service to investigate. This is a police matter.
- Remember that the victim of sexual assault has physical forensic evidence on their body and clothing, and represents a 'crime scene' (refer to **Sexual Assault**).

4. Assessment and Management

For the assessment and management of vaginal bleeding, refer to Table 5.11.

TABLE 5.11 – Assessment and Management of: Vaginal Bleeding

ASSESSMENT	MANAGEMENT
• Quickly assess the woman and scene as you approach • Undertake a primary survey <C>ABCDEF • Evaluate whether the woman has any **TIME CRITICAL** features or any signs of hypovolaemic shock	• If any **TIME CRITICAL** features are present, correct **A** and **B** and transport to nearest suitable receiving hospital (refer to **Medical Emergencies in Adults – Overview** and **Medical Emergencies in Children – Overview**). • Provide an alert/information call.

SECTION 5 Maternity Care

Vaginal Bleeding: Gynaecological Causes

TABLE 5.11 – Assessment and Management of: Vaginal Bleeding *(continued)*	
• Assess blood loss – ask about clots, blood-soaked clothes, bed sheets, number of soaked tampons/towels/pads, and where necessary, visibly inspect **NB** Blood under the feet or between toes indicates significant bleeding • If **NON-TIME CRITICAL**, perform a more thorough assessment of the woman with brief secondary survey for lower abdominal tenderness or guarding • Measure temperature and consider sepsis (refer to **Sepsis**) • Check the woman's age: – >50 years – more at risk of cancers of the uterus/cervix – <50 years – may be pregnant	• Obtain IV access – insert a **LARGE BORE (16G)** cannula. • If there is visible external blood loss >500 ml, refer to **Intravascular Fluid Therapy (Adults)** and **Intravascular Fluid Therapy (Children)**. 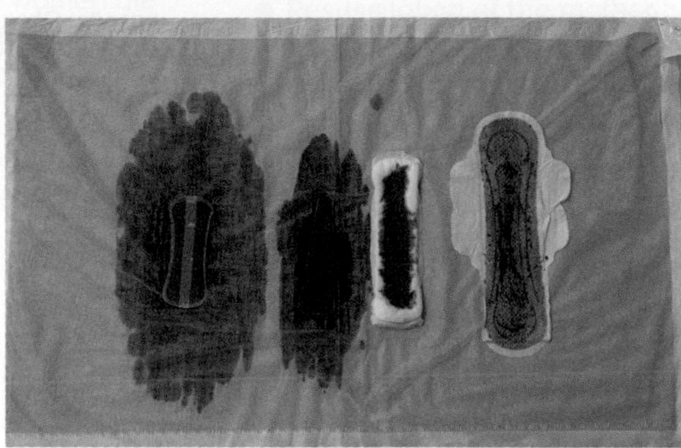 50 ml blood loss on various sanitary towels. 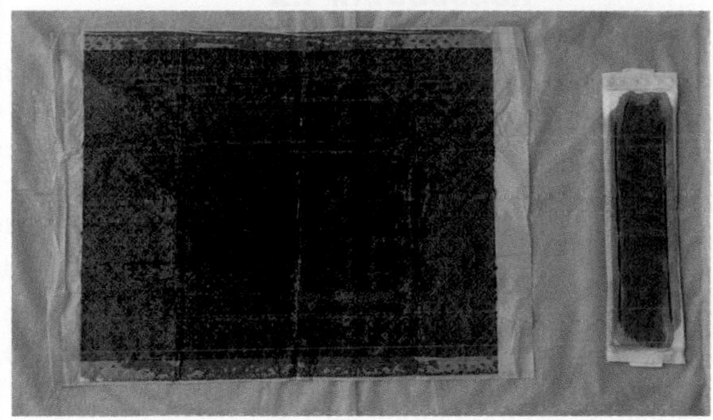 500 ml blood loss on maternity pad and 50 ml on maternity towel.
• Monitor SpO_2 (94–98%)	• If oxygen (SpO_2) <94%, administer O_2 to aim for a target saturation within the range of 94–98%.
• Assess the woman's level of pain	• Titrate analgesia against pain (refer to **Pain Management in Adults** and **Pain Management in Children**): – Paracetamol – Entonox – Morphine – **NB** administer cautiously if the patient is hypotensive.
• Assess the woman's comfort	• Nil by mouth. • Adjust the woman's position as required. • Transfer to further care.

KEY POINTS!

Vaginal Bleeding: Gynaecological Causes

- **The majority of vaginal bleeding episodes do not compromise circulation, but blood loss can be alarming.**
- **Following gynaecological surgical interventions, heavy, ongoing vaginal bleeding commencing 7–14 days post-procedure may indicate underlying infection.**
- **Assess blood loss; ask about number of soaked tampons/towels/pads and visually inspect.**
- **Provide analgesia where indicated.**
- **If you suspect a miscarriage or ectopic pregnancy refer to Haemorrhage During Pregnancy.**

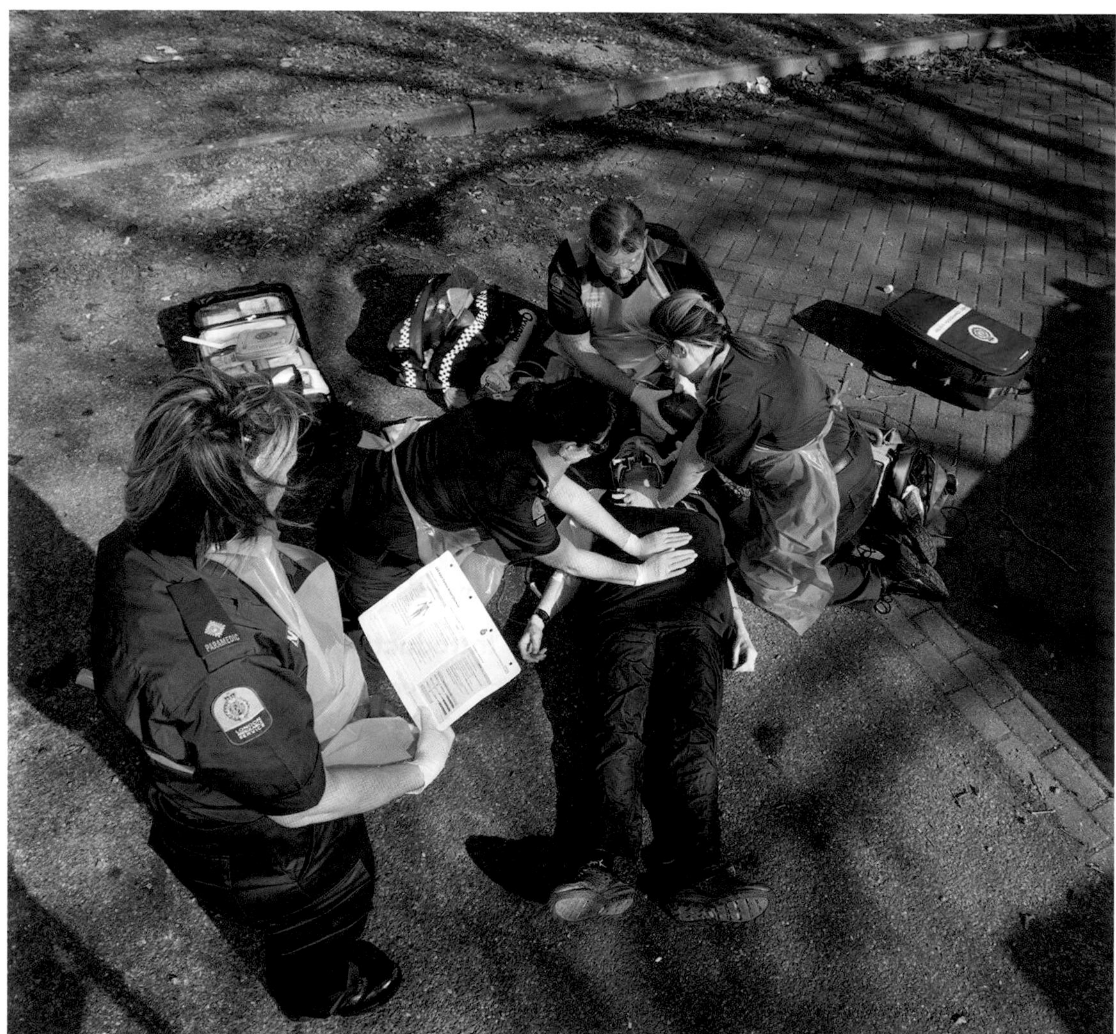

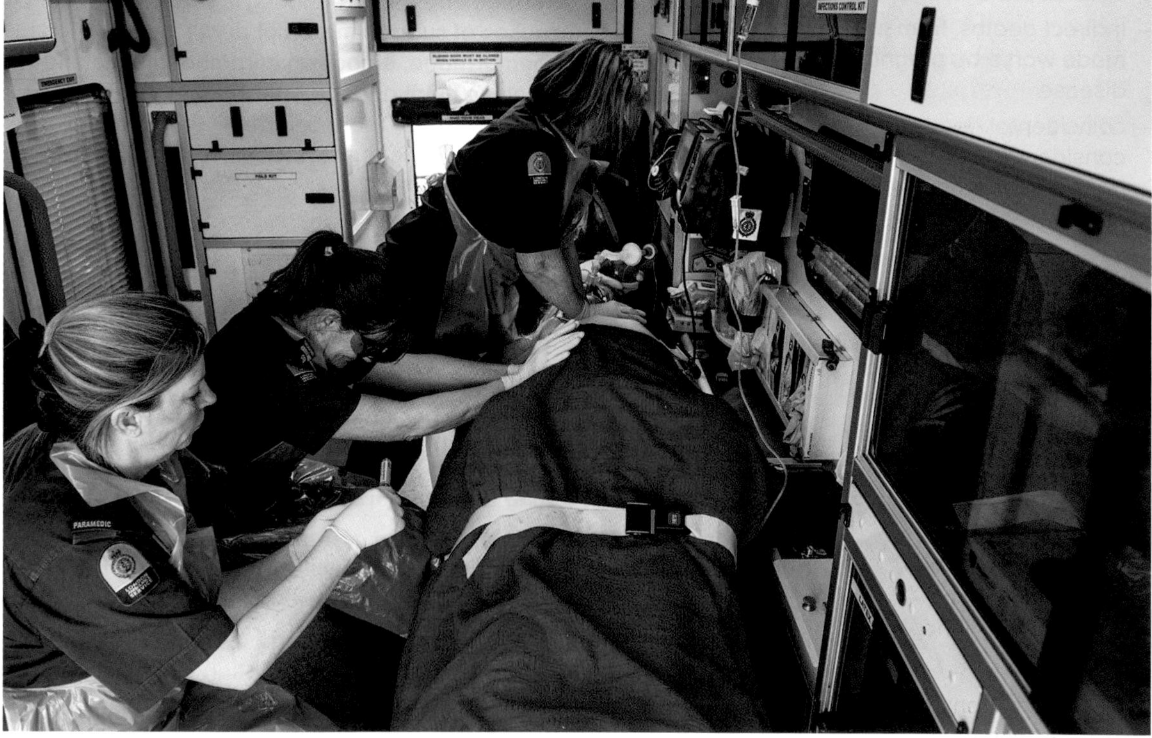

Figure 5.10 – Manual uterine displacement during resuscitation.

Maternal Resuscitation

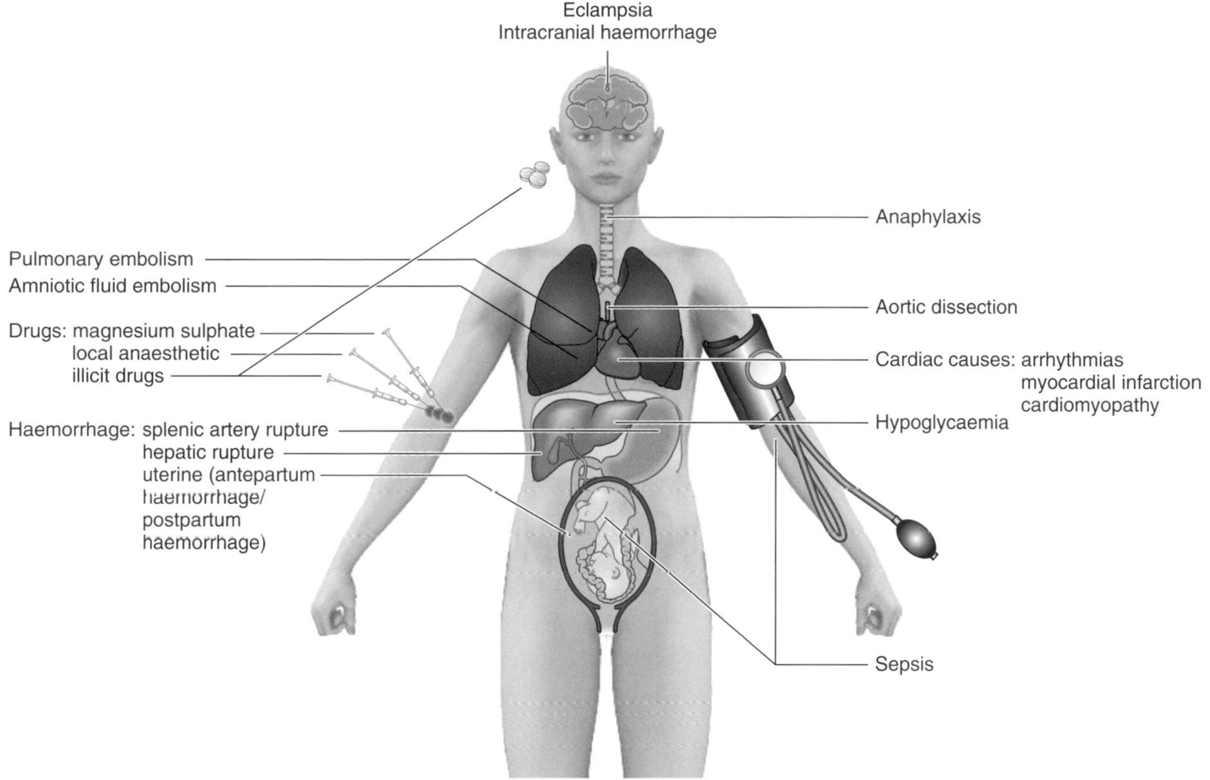

Figure 5.11 – Causes of maternal collapse.

Republished with kind permission of the Royal College of Obstetricians and Gynaecologists.

TABLE 5.13 – Reversible Causes of Maternal Collapse[3]

Reversible Cause		**Cause in Pregnancy**
4Hs	• Hypovolaemia • Hypoxia • Hypo/hyperkalaemia and other electrolyte disturbances • Hypothermia	• Bleeding (may be concealed) (obstetric/other) or relative hypovolaemia of dense spinal block; septic or neurogenic shock. • Pregnant women become hypoxic rapidly. • Cardiac events: peripartum cardiomyopathy, myocardial infarction, aortic dissection, large-vessel aneurysms. • No more likely.
4Ts	• Thromboembolism • Toxicity • Tension pneumothorax • Tamponade (cardiac) • Eclampsia and pre-eclampsia	• Amniotic fluid embolus, pulmonary embolus, air embolus, myocardial infarction. • Local anaesthetic, magnesium, other. • Following trauma/suicide attempt • Includes intracranial haemorrhage.

2.3 Modifications for Cardiac Arrest in Pregnancy

For the assessment and management of cardiac arrest during pregnancy refer to Table 5.14.

Key points are listed below:

- Start resuscitation according to standard ALS guidelines with manual displacement of the uterus to the maternal left to minimise inferior vena caval compression (spinal board will not achieve the required left lateral tilt).
- The hand position for chest compressions may need to be slightly higher (2–3 cm) on the sternum for patients with advanced pregnancy (e.g. >28 weeks).
- Consider using a tracheal tube 0.5–1.0 mm smaller than usual as the trachea can be narrowed by oedema and swelling. Supraglottic

Maternal Resuscitation

TABLE 5.14 – ASSESSMENT and MANAGEMENT of: Cardiac Arrest During Pregnancy

ASSESSMENT	MANAGEMENT
• Undertake a primary survey **ABCDE** • At 20 weeks, the uterine fundus will be below the umbilicus	• Manage as per standard advanced life support (refer to **Advanced Life Support in Adults**). • Assess and exclude reversible causes (see Table 5.13). • Caution – ventilation with a bag-valve-mask may lead to regurgitation and aspiration. A supraglottic airway device may reduce the risk of gastric aspiration and make ventilation of the lungs easier (refer to **Airway and Breathing Management**). • If there is no response to CPR after 5 minutes, undertake a **TIME CRITICAL** transfer to the nearest ED with an obstetric unit attached. Place a pre-alert as soon as possible to enable the ED team to organise a maternity team, as an immediate peri-mortem caesarean section (resuscitative hysterotomy) may be performed. • For pregnant women at 20 weeks gestation or more, use manual uterine displacement (to the maternal left side) to avoid compression of the inferior vena cava. • Manual displacement can be applied from either the maternal left or right side with the assistant ensuring the uterus is displaced toward the maternal left. (Resuscitation Council, 2015) • Within the ambulance saloon, manual uterine displacement must be maintained. • Establish IV or IO access as soon as possible, preferably at a level above the diaphragm.

airway devices are a suitable alternative in the pre-hospital setting and may provide a more rapid means of oxygenation than potentially prolonged intubation attempts.[4]

- Defibrillation energy levels are as recommended for standard defibrillation. If large breasts make it difficult to place an apical defibrillator electrode, use an antero-posterior or bi-axillary electrode position.
- Establish IV or IO access as soon as possible, preferably at a level above the diaphragm.
- Identify and correct the cause of the arrest using 4Hs and 4Ts as appropriate.
- Administer 100% supplemental oxygen (refer to **Oxygen**).
- Undertake a **TIME CRITICAL** transfer to the nearest ED with an obstetric unit attached. Place a pre-alert as soon as possible to enable the ED team to organise a maternity team, as an immediate peri-mortem caesarean section (resuscitative hysterotomy) may be performed.

2.4 The Team Approach to Pre-hospital Resuscitation (Resuscitation Council 2015)

- Resuscitation requires a system to be in place to achieve the best possible chance of survival. The system requires technical and non-technical skills (teamwork, situational awareness, leadership, decision making) in the pregnant woman, this will also involve consideration for manual uterine displacement.

Allocation of Roles

- Appoint a team leader as early as possible; ideally they should be a paramedic or clinician experienced in pre-hospital resuscitation.
- The team leader should assign team members specific roles, which they clearly understand and are capable of undertaking. This will promote teamwork, reduce confusion and ensure organised and effective management of resuscitation.
- Minimum of four trained staff is required to deliver high quality resuscitation. This will necessitate dispatch of more than one ambulance resource.
- Ensure there is 360° access to the patient ('Circle of Life'):
  - Position 1: Airway (at head of patient) – the person must be trained and equipped to provide the full range of airway skills.
  - Position 2: High quality chest compressions and defibrillation if needed – at patient's left side. Be prepared to alternate with the operator at position 3 to avoid fatigue.

- Position 3: High quality chest compressions and access to the circulation (intravenous, intraosseous) – at patient's right side.
- Position 4: Team leader – stand back and oversee the resuscitation attempt, only becoming involved if required. The team leader should have an awareness of the whole incident and ensure high quality resuscitation is maintained and appropriate decisions made.

The team leader will need to allocate the role of manual uterine displacement and may necessitate the involvement of additional resources where available.

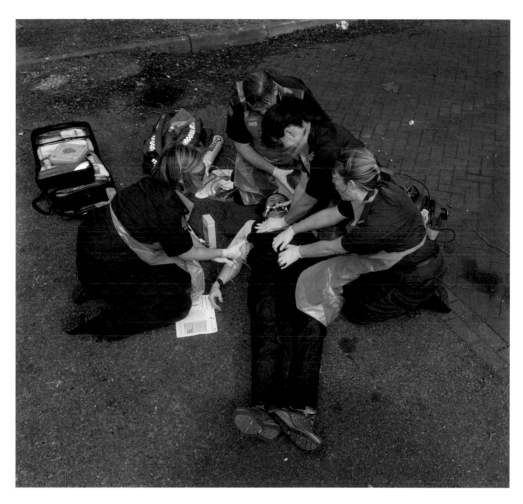

Figure 5.12 – Working as a team.

KEY POINTS!

Maternal Resuscitation

- **DO NOT withhold or terminate maternal resuscitation.**
- **ALWAYS manage pregnant women in cardiac arrest at greater than 20 weeks' gestation with manual displacement of the uterus to the maternal left.**
- **If resuscitation attempts fail to achieve ROSC within 5 minutes of the cardiac arrest, undertake a TIME CRITICAL transfer to the nearest ED with an obstetric unit attached.**
- **Provide an early pre-alert to enable the ED team to summon the maternity team, as an immediate peri-mortem caesarean section (resuscitative hysterotomy) may be performed.**

Further Reading

Further important information and evidence in support of this guideline can be found in the Bibliography.[5,6,7,8]

Newborn Life Support

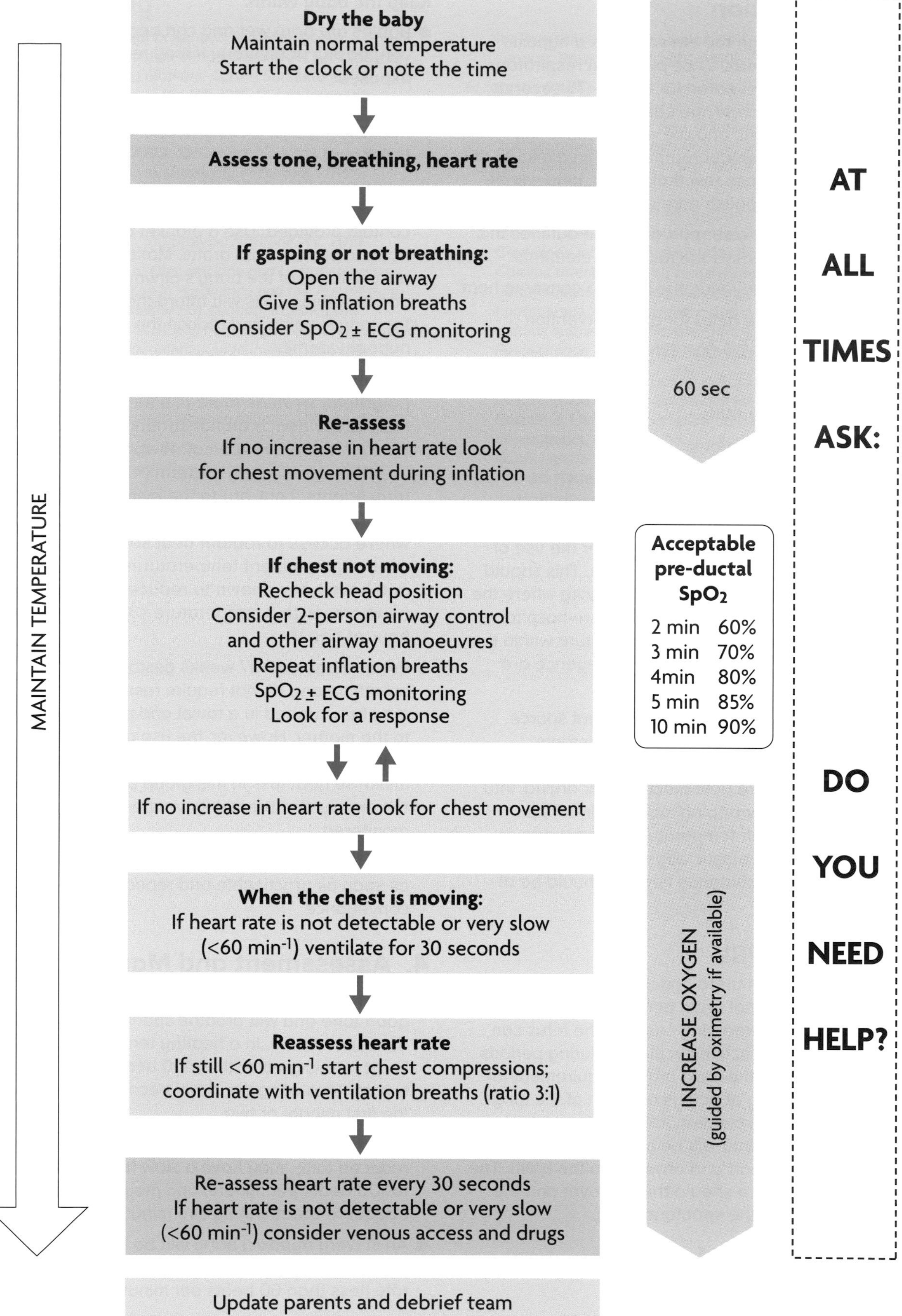

Dry the baby
Maintain normal temperature
Start the clock or note the time
Assess tone, breathing, heart rate
If gasping or not breathing:
Open the airway
Give 5 inflation breaths
Consider SpO2 ± ECG monitoring
Re-assess
If no increase in heart rate look for chest movement during inflation
If chest not moving:
Recheck head position
Consider 2-person airway control and other airway manoeuvres
Repeat inflation breaths
SpO2 ± ECG monitoring
Look for a response
If no increase in heart rate look for chest movement
When the chest is moving:
If heart rate is not detectable or very slow (<60 min-1) ventilate for 30 seconds
Reassess heart rate
If still <60 min-1 start chest compressions; coordinate with ventilation breaths (ratio 3:1)
Re-assess heart rate every 30 seconds
If heart rate is not detectable or very slow (<60 min-1) consider venous access and drugs
Update parents and debrief team
MAINTAIN TEMPERATURE
60 sec
Acceptable pre-ductal SpO2
2 min 60%
3 min 70%
4min 80%
5 min 85%
10 min 90%
INCREASE OXYGEN
(guided by oximetry if available)
AT ALL TIMES ASK:
DO YOU NEED HELP?

Figure 5.13 – Newborn life support algorithm – modified from the Resuscitation Council (UK) Guidelines 2015 algorithm (www.resus.org.uk).

Newborn Life Support

TABLE 5.15 – Assessment and Management of: Newborn Life Support	
ASSESSMENT	**MANAGEMENT**
• In all cases	• Ensure the ambient temperature is as high as possible. • Close windows and doors to reduce cold draughts. • Position the baby where there is 360-degree access to enable management of the airway and chest in case further intervention is required. • Dry the baby from head to toe while completing **ABC** assessment. • Apply appropriately sized newborn hat and wrap in a warm dry towel. • Delay clamping and cutting of the umbilical cord unless resuscitation is required.
• Assess	• Colour. • Tone. • Breathing rate. • Heart rate: – Assess heart rate by listening with a stethoscope (feeling for a peripheral pulse is not reliable). – In noisy or very cold environments, palpating the pulse at the umbilical cord may be an alternative and may save unwrapping the baby (this is only reliable when the pulse is >100 bpm). – Attach a pulse oximeter. **NB** Attaching to the right wrist using an infant probe can give an accurate heart rate in approximately 90 seconds, and provides an accurate oxygen saturation.
• Re-assess breathing and heart rate, every 30 seconds	• An increase in heart rate is usually the first clinical sign of improvement.
• Decide whether help is required (and likely to be available) and whether rapid evacuation to hospital is indicated. If transferring to hospital, follow pre-alert procedure	• Ensure the heater in the ambulance is set to maximum. • Once the baby is in the ambulance, continue to monitor its condition and repeat the temperature en-route.
Airway	• Place the baby on its back with the head in a neutral position, neither flexed nor extended. • If the baby is very floppy, a chin lift or jaw thrust may be required. • A small pad (2 cm) can be placed under the shoulders to assist in maintaining the neutral position.

(continued)

Newborn Life Support

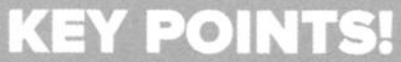

Newborn Life Support

- **Passage through the birth canal is a hypoxic event and some babies may require help to establish normal breathing after birth.**
- **Babies become cold very easily; dry the baby, remove any wet towels and wrap with dry ones. Once in the ambulance keep the compartment as warm as possible.**
- **Ensure the airway is open by placing the baby on its back with the head in a neutral position.**
- **If the baby is very floppy, it may be necessary to apply a chin lift or jaw thrust.**
- **If the baby is not breathing adequately within 60 seconds, give 5 inflation breaths.**
- **If chest compressions are necessary, compress the chest quickly and firmly at a ratio of 3:1 compressions to inflations using a two-thumbs encircling technique.**

Further Reading

Further important information and evidence in support of this guideline can be found in the Bibliography.[3,4]

Bibliography

1. Belsches TC, Tilly AE, Miller TR, Kambeyanda RH, Leadford A, Manasyan A, Chomba E et al. Randomised trial of plastic bags to prevent term neonatal hypothermia in a resource-poor setting. Pediatrics 2013, 132(3). Available from: http://pediatrics.aappublications.org/content/132/3/e656.
2. Leadford AE, Warren JB, Manasyan A, Chomba E, Salas AA, Schelonka R, Carlo WA. Plastic bags for prevention of hypothermia in preterm and low birth weight infants. Pediatrics 2013, 132(1). Available from: http://pediatrics.aappublications.org/content/132/1/e128.
3. Wyllie J, Bruinenberg J, Roehr CC, Rüdiger M, Trevisanuto D, Urlesberger B. European Resuscitation Council Guidelines for Resuscitation 2015: Section 7. Resuscitation and support of transition of babies at birth. *Resuscitation* 2015, 95: 249–263.
4. Wyllie J, Perlman JM, Kattwinkel J, et al. Part 7: Neonatal resuscitation: 2015 International Consensus on Cardiopulmonary Resuscitation and Emergency Cardiovascular Care Science with Treatment Recommendations. *Resuscitation* 2015, 95:e169–201.

Trauma in Pregnancy

1. Introduction

- The management of pregnant women with traumatic injuries requires a special approach.
- Mechanism of injury may indicate possible trauma to enlarged internal organs and structures, especially trauma occurring in the third trimester. For example, trauma to the gravid uterus during domestic violence can be linked to placental abruption (refer to **Birth Imminent: Normal Birth and Birth Complications**).
- It is important to remember that resuscitation of the mother may facilitate resuscitation of the fetus.

2. Incidence

- In the UK, 5% of maternal deaths are as a result of trauma, with a high proportion related to domestic violence and road traffic collisions.

Mechanism of injury

- Domestic violence.
- High energy transfer (especially road traffic accidents).
- Fall from height.

3. Severity and Outcome

- Managing a pregnant woman with major trauma is rare; however, both blunt and penetrating trauma can cause catastrophic haemorrhage.
- Trauma can lead to major placental abruption (separation) with significant hidden blood loss within the uterus and no visible vaginal bleeding abruption (refer to **Birth Imminent: Normal Birth and Birth Complications**).

4. Pathophysiology

- There are a number of physiological and anatomical changes during pregnancy that may influence the management of the pregnant woman with trauma (refer to **Maternity Care (including Obstetric Emergencies Overview)**).

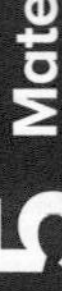

TABLE 5.16 – ASSESSMENT and MANAGEMENT of: Trauma in Pregnancy

ASSESSMENT	MANAGEMENT
• Quickly assess the scene and the woman as you approach • Undertake a primary survey **<C>ABCDEF** – specifically assess for: – abdominal pain – should be presumed to be significant and may be associated with internal concealed blood loss – vaginal blood loss – abruption may occur 3–4 days after the initial incident – stage of the pregnancy and impact on resuscitation if >20 weeks gestation – any medical problems with the pregnancy or relevant previous medical history – twins or multiple pregnancy – fetal movements (refer to **Maternity Care**) • Review the maternity handheld record if available • If domestic violence is suspected, consider any other children/adults present who may be at risk (refer to **Safeguarding Adults at Risk** and **Safeguarding Children**)	• Control external catastrophic haemorrhage using direct and indirect pressure or tourniquets where indicated (refer to **Trauma Emergencies Overview**). • Refer to **Maternal Resuscitation** where cardiac/ respiratory arrest is identified. • Open, maintain and protect the airway in accordance with the woman's clinical need. • Administer high levels of supplemental oxygen and aim for a target saturation within the range of 94–98% (refer to **Oxygen**). Provide assisted ventilation as indicated (refer to **Airway Management**). • If the woman is unable to position herself (e.g. if she is unconscious), she should be positioned on the left (right side up) by using a spinal board and monitor the airway. Where resources allow, the uterus can be manually displaced to the maternal left side (and this must be recorded on the patient record form) as illustrated in Figure 5.1. • Provide cervical spine protection as necessary (refer to **Spinal Injury and Spinal Cord Injury**). • Manage thoracic injuries (refer to **Thoracic Trauma**). **NB** The management of thoracic injuries is the same as for the non-pregnant woman. • Insert a minimum of one large bore IV cannula (16G) – do not delay transfer. • Administer intravascular fluids as indicated to maintain a systolic blood pressure above 90 mmHg (refer to **Intravascular Fluid Therapy in Adults**).

(continued)

Trauma in Pregnancy

TABLE 5.16 – ASSESSMENT and MANAGEMENT of: Trauma in Pregnancy *(continued)*	
• Undertake a secondary survey **<C>ABCDEF**	
• Assess the woman's level of pain	• Pain management (refer to **Pain Management in Adults**). **NB** Administer morphine cautiously if the patient is hypotensive. • Apply splints as appropriate, for example to pelvis (refer to **Pelvic Trauma**) or long bone fractures (refer to **Limb Trauma**).
• Assess blood glucose	• Measure blood glucose en-route to the appropriate facility. • Nil by mouth.
• Assess for burns and scalds	• For the management of burns, treat as non-pregnant woman (refer to **Burns and Scalds** and **Intravascular Fluid Therapy**).

SECTION **5** Maternity Care

KEY POINTS!

Trauma in Pregnancy

- **All trauma is significant.**
- **If the pregnant woman is found in cardiac arrest or develops cardiac/respiratory arrest en-route, commence advanced life support and pre-alert the nearest ED with an obstetric unit.**
- **Resuscitation of the woman may facilitate resuscitation of the fetus.**
- **Compression of the inferior vena cava by the gravid uterus (>20 weeks) is a serious potential complication; manually displace the uterus to the maternal left. Maintain during transfer.**
- **Due to the physiological changes in pregnancy, signs of shock may be slow to appear following trauma, hypotension being an extremely late indication of volume loss. Signs of hypovolaemia during pregnancy are likely to indicate a 35% (class III) blood loss and must be treated aggressively.**
- **Abruption may occur 3–4 days after the initial incident.**
- **If sexual assault or domestic violence is suspected, consideration must be given to potential safeguarding issues and provision made to ensure safety is maintained (refer to Safeguarding Adults at Risk).**

Bibliography

1. Centre for Maternal and Child Enquiries. Saving mothers' lives: reviewing maternal deaths to make motherhood safer: 2006–2008. *BJOG: An International Journal of Obstetrics & Gynaecology* 2011, 118 (suppl. 1).
2. Woollard M, Simpson H, Hinshaw K, Wieteska S. Obstetric services. In *Pre-hospital Obstetric Emergency Training.* Oxford: Wiley-Blackwell, 2009: 1–6.
3. Woollard M, Hinshaw K, Simpson H, Wieteska S. Anatomical and physiological changes in pregnancy. In *Pre-hospital Obstetric Emergency Training.* Oxford: Wiley-Blackwell, 2009: 18–27.
4. Woollard M, Hinshaw K, Simpson H, Wieteska S. Structured approach to the obstetric patient. In *Pre-hospital Obstetric Emergency Training.* Oxford: Wiley-Blackwell, 2009: 38–52.
5. Woollard M, Hinshaw K, Simpson H, Wieteska S. Emergencies in late pregnancy. In *Pre-Hospital Obstetric Emergency Training.* Oxford: Wiley-Blackwell, 2009: 62–110.
6. Woollard M, Hinshaw K, Simpson H, Wieteska S. Emergencies after delivery. In *Pre-hospital Obstetric Emergency Training.* Oxford: Wiley-Blackwell, 2009: 111–124.
7. Woollard M, Hinshaw K, Simpson H, Wieteska S. Management of non-obstetric emergencies. In *Pre-hospital Obstetric Emergency Training.* Oxford: Wiley-Blackwell, 2009: 136–165.

6

Special Situations

Major, Complex and High Risk Incidents

1. Specialist Capabilities

- Ambulance services maintain a range of specialist capabilities to support the response to complex incidents. These capabilities are interoperable, which means they can be used locally or combined to provide a national response.
- When responding to a complex or high-risk incident, it is essential for ambulance staff to request these specialist services early. They can be easily stood down if not required.
- The specialist capabilities are summarised in Table 6.1.

TABLE 6.1 – Ambulance Service Specialist Capabilities

Core Capability	Tactical Options	
Hazardous Area Response Teams (HART)	Hazardous materials	• Working inside the inner cordon • Industrial accidents • High risk infectious diseases • Complex transportation accidents
	Chemical, biological, radiological, nuclear explosives (CBRNe)	• Specialist operational response (SOR) • Component part of wider CBRNe capability
	Marauding terrorist attack (MTA)	• Specialist support to warm zone operations • Component part of wider MTA capability
	Safe working at height (SWaH)	• Manmade structures • Natural environments
	Confined space	• Substantially enclosed spaces • Building collapse • Compromised atmospheres • Entrapments
	Unstable terrain	• Active rubble pile • Rural access/difficult terrain
	Water operations	• Swift water rescue • Urban and rural flooding • Boat operations
	Support to security operations (SSO)	• Support to security operations • Support to Police operations • Illicit drug laboratories • VIP close protection support
Marauding terrorist attack (MTA)	• Working inside a ballistically unsafe area (warm zone) • Siege/stronghold	
Chemical, biological, radiological, nuclear explosives (CBRNe)	• Initial operational response (IOR) • Specialist operational response (SOR)/provided by HART • Interim decontamination of casualties • Full wet decontamination of casualties	
Command and control (C2)	• Strategic command of major and critical incidents • Tactical command of major and critical incidents • Operational command of major and critical incidents • National Interagency Liaison Officers (NILOs) • Strategic and tactical advisors • Medical advisors	

TABLE 6.1 – Ambulance Service Specialist Capabilities *(continued)*	
Core Capability	**Tactical Options**
Mass casualties	• Capabilities to treat large numbers of casualties • Casualty clearing stations (CCS) • National coordination of patient transfers

2. Security

2.1 UK Threat Levels

- The UK threat level is by set the Joint Terrorism Analysis Centre (JTAC) and is advised by intelligence or probability relating to international or Northern Island terrorism activities.
- Threat levels are designed to give a broad indication of the likelihood of terrorist attack.
  - **LOW** means an attack is unlikely.
  - **MODERATE** means an attack is possible but not likely.
  - **SUBSTANTIAL** means an attack is a strong possibility.
  - **SEVERE** means an attack is highly likely.
  - **CRITICAL** means an attack Is expected imminently.
- When the threat level is changed, particularly to **SEVERE** or **CRITICAL**, ambulance staff should seek specific advice from their own organisations. In general, staff should consider the following safety guidance:
  - For urgent information regarding suspicious activities, contact the police in the first instance.
  - For information regarding less imminent terrorist activities, contact the Anti-Terrorist Hotline: 0800 789 321.
  - For more information on UK threat levels visit: https://www.mi5.gov.uk/threat-levels.

2.2 Personal Safety

If there is an increase in threat level or there is a heightened state of security, the following steps will help to ensure personal safety. However, these are sensible precautions for clinicians to apply at all times:

- Challenge anyone on site who is not visibly displaying ID.
- Know the exits on all sites that are regularly visited or worked at.
- Consider means and routes for leaving the building or site.
- Beware of the surroundings. Look out for any suspicious or unusual behaviour, including unattended bags or packages.
- Vary routines, such as route to work or parking spot.
- Ensure your line manager knows where you are.
- Avoid travelling in uniform.
- Remove ID cards and vehicle car passes when leaving the workplace.
- Avoid drawing unnecessary attention to your occupation outside work.
- Update privacy settings on personal social media accounts so that information is only shared with known people. Never include operational or work information.

For more information regarding the Stay Safe campaign and other safety advice visit:

- https://www.gov.uk/government/publications/stay-safe-film
- https://www.gov.uk/government/publications/recognising-the-terrorist-threat

2.3 Protectively Marked Documents

- All information that the government needs to collect, store, process, generate or share to deliver services and conduct its business has intrinsic value and may require a degree of protection.
- Ambulance staff may come across protectively marked documents as part of routine work, especially work that may be associated with emergency preparedness. Failure to appropriately handle these documents (or associated materials) and the information contained within them can have serious consequences including dismissal and potential criminal liability.
- Security classifications indicate the sensitivity of information and the need to protect it. There are three levels of classification:
  - **OFFICIAL**: The majority of information that is created or processed by the public sector. This includes routine business operations and services, some of which could have damaging consequences if lost, stolen or published in the media, but are not subject to a heightened threat profile. 'Official classifications may be accompanied by a descriptor which will mandate special handling requirements. This includes 'Official - Sensitive'. If you receive material with an 'Official - Sensitive' descriptor, you must ensure you handle that material in accordance with the Government Protective Marking Scheme requirements.
  - **SECRET**: Very sensitive information that justifies heightened protective measures to defend against determined and highly capable threat actors. For example, where compromise could seriously damage military capabilities,

international relations or the investigation of serious organised crime.
- **TOP SECRET**: The government's most sensitive information requiring the highest levels of protection from the most serious threats. For example, where compromise could cause widespread loss of life or else threaten the security or economic wellbeing of the country or friendly nations.

2.4 Suspect Packages

- On discovery of a suspect package or if one is reported, follow these basic steps:
  1. Report the matter to the police via the ambulance control room (ACR).
  2. If possible, take a photograph of the package before withdrawing without touching or interfering with the package. If it is not possible to take a photograph, make a mental note of the size, location and any distinguishing features.
  3. If the police or fire and rescue service are not yet on scene, attempt to establish the following recommended minimum cordons:
     - small item (i.e. briefcase/rucksack) – 100 m
     - medium item (i.e. car) – 200 m
     - large item (i.e. van/lorry) – 400 m.
  4. Be mindful of the risk of secondary devices or other devices.
- The police will be able to assess the device with known intelligence and risk factors to decide how best to manage the situation. If the device is deemed to be credible, it will require a specialist multi-agency response. From an ambulance service perspective, request HART support via the ACR.

2.5 Initial Actions for a Major Incident

- Each NHS ambulance trust has a major incident plan, which will define key actions that ambulance staff must take if they are faced with a major incident. First and foremost, follow the plan of your service.
- The *Civil Contingencies Act 2004* defines an emergency of this magnitude in the following terms:
  a. An event or situation which threatens serious damage to human welfare in a place in the United Kingdom.
  b. An event or situation which threatens serious damage to the environment in a place in the United Kingdom.
  c. War, or terrorism which threatens serious damage to the security of the United Kingdom.
- An incident which requires a highly technical response, or the utilisation of specialist capabilities could also be termed a **CRITICAL** incident.
- The first clinician on scene at incidents such as these should provide an initial report back to the ACR using the METHANE model, which has been approved for use by each of the emergency services under the Joint Emergency Services Interoperability Programme (JESIP).
- The major incident standard messages are:
  - **Major incident alert/standby** – The term used by any member of staff to prefix messages indicating than an incident with the potential to generate a large number of casualties has or may have occurred.
  - **Major incident confirmed/declared** – The term used by any member of staff to prefix a message to confirm that a major incident has occurred, indicating that the plan should be implemented and a full pre-determined attendance/response is required.
  - **Major incident cancel** – The term used by a commander to cancel a major incident alert.
  - **Ambulance major incident stop** – The term used by a commander to indicate that sufficient ambulance and/or medical resources are available at the scene and that no further assistance is required.
  - **Ambulance major incident scene evacuation complete** – The term used by a Commander to indicate that the treatment and removal of casualties from the scene is complete.
  - **Ambulance major incident stand down** – The term used by a commander to indicate the conclusion of all ambulance service activity in connection with a declared major incident and a return to normal modes of operation.
- The early declaration of a major incident ensures that the appropriate resources are activated at the earliest opportunity. These messages should be part of a METHANE report, as outlined in Table 6.2.
- Now follow the Major Incident Action Cards of your ambulance trust.

2.6 Command and Control

- During a larger scale incident, a multi-agency command structure will form. The following information provides an overview of how the

TABLE 6.2 – METHANE Report Format

M	Major incident standby or declared
E	Exact location of incident
T	Type of incident
H	Hazards (present and potential)
A	Access and egress routes
N	Number, severity and type of casualties
E	Emergency services present on scene and further resources required

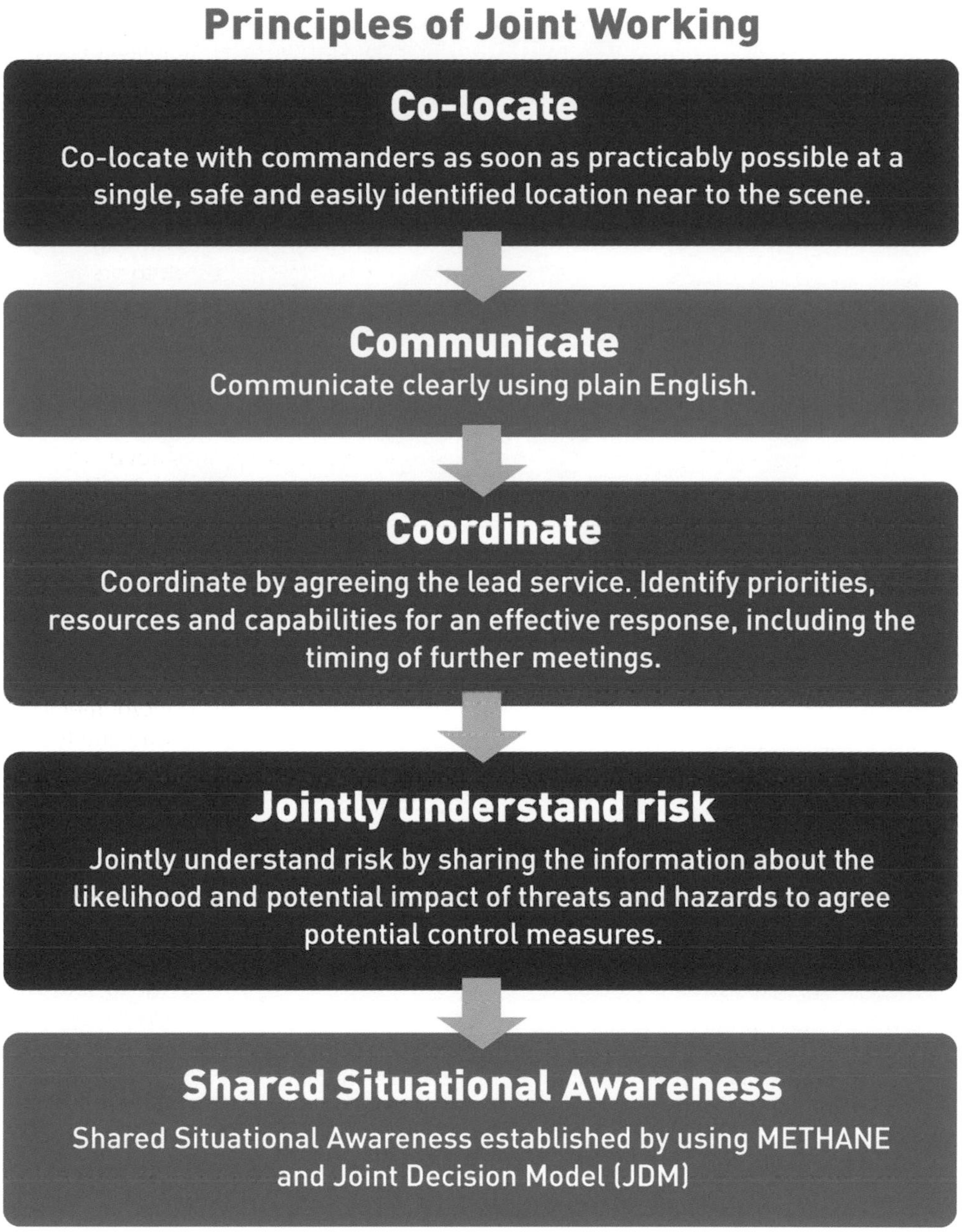

Principles of Joint Working

Co-locate

Co-locate with commanders as soon as practicably possible at a single, safe and easily identified location near to the scene.

Communicate

Communicate clearly using plain English.

Coordinate

Coordinate by agreeing the lead service. Identify priorities, resources and capabilities for an effective response, including the timing of further meetings.

Jointly understand risk

Jointly understand risk by sharing the information about the likelihood and potential impact of threats and hazards to agree potential control measures.

Shared Situational Awareness

Shared Situational Awareness established by using METHANE and Joint Decision Model (JDM)

Figure 6.1 – Joint working principles for the emergency services.

ambulance service will integrate in the wider command and control framework.

- There are NHS Standards for ambulance service command, to which local ambulance service plans are aligned. The ambulance service will work closely with other responding agencies using the joint working principles outlined in Figure 6.1.
- Important command decisions will be taken in the multi-agency setting using the joint decision model shown in Figure 6.2.
- Ambulance clinicians may be given a briefing by commanders. They may use the following 'IIMARCH' model, outlined in Table 6.3.
- All ambulance clinicians attending a major or complex incident have a responsibility to support risk management at the scene. Clinicians must ensure that a dynamic risk assessment is undertaken. The situation must be regularly reviewed and any hazards that need to be considered by commanders should be reported, i.e. those hazards that present a risk to patients and responders.
- Figure 6.3 provides an overview of how commanders and responders will approach assessing and then controlling the hazards and risks present at the scene.
- During a complex or major incident, ambulance responders may be assigned specific roles. This will include command roles and operational functions. Key roles are denoted by the nationally specified tabards shown in Figure 6.4.

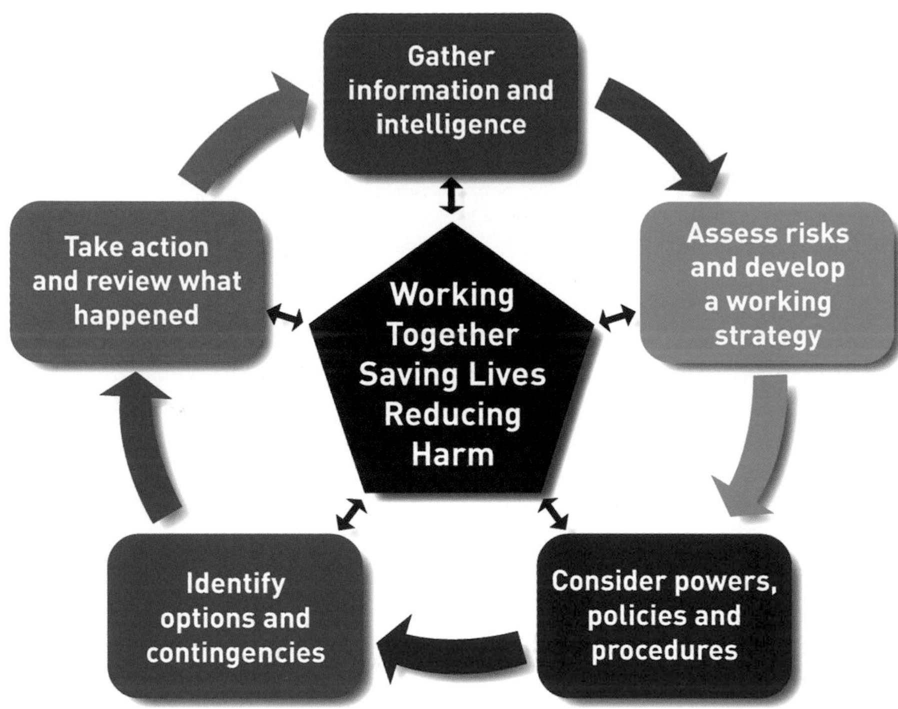
Gather information and intelligence
Assess risks and develop a working strategy
Consider powers, policies and procedures
Identify options and contingencies
Take action and review what happened
Working Together Saving Lives Reducing Harm

Figure 6.2 – Joint decision model.

TABLE 6.3 – IIMARCH

Initial	Item
I	Information: ● Where/what/how many? ● History (if applicable) use METHANE.
I	Intent: ● Why are we here? ● Strategy, tactical and operational plan.
M	Method: ● How are we going to do it? ● Tactical plan, policy, plans.
A	Administration: ● Command/media/dress code/decision logs/welfare/food/individual tasking/timing.
R	Risk assessment: ● Specific threat areas/PPE/filter changes.
C	Communications: ● Confirm radio callsigns. ● Indicate other means of communication if required. ● Ensure staff understand interagency communications.
H	Human rights: ● Disclosure details.

- National guidance on command and control can be found on the NARU website: www.naru.org.uk.
- Refer to local trust plans and procedures.

2.7 Triage

- During the initial stages of an incident with large numbers of casualties, there are unlikely to be enough clinical responders to stay with each casualty and provide treatment. Therefore, the triage sieve tool shown in Figure 6.5 should be applied to ensure the best for everyone is achieved until such time that resources are sufficient to provide further care.

3. Incidents Involving Firearms and Weapons

- The prevalence of criminal or terrorism-related incidents is a significant risk to the public and emergency services personnel. In recent times, Europe, the UK and indeed many other countries have seen numerous actual or attempted attacks on their sovereign soil by non-State actors.
- In the UK, violent criminal attacks, using bladed and other types of weapons are on the increase. Acts of terror have been conducted with varying degrees of sophistication ranging from attacks using easily accessible items, such as knives and vehicles, to more complex incidents involving firearms, home-made explosives (HME) and improvised explosive devices (IEDs).
- It may not be obvious to responders (especially those first on scene) that an incident involving

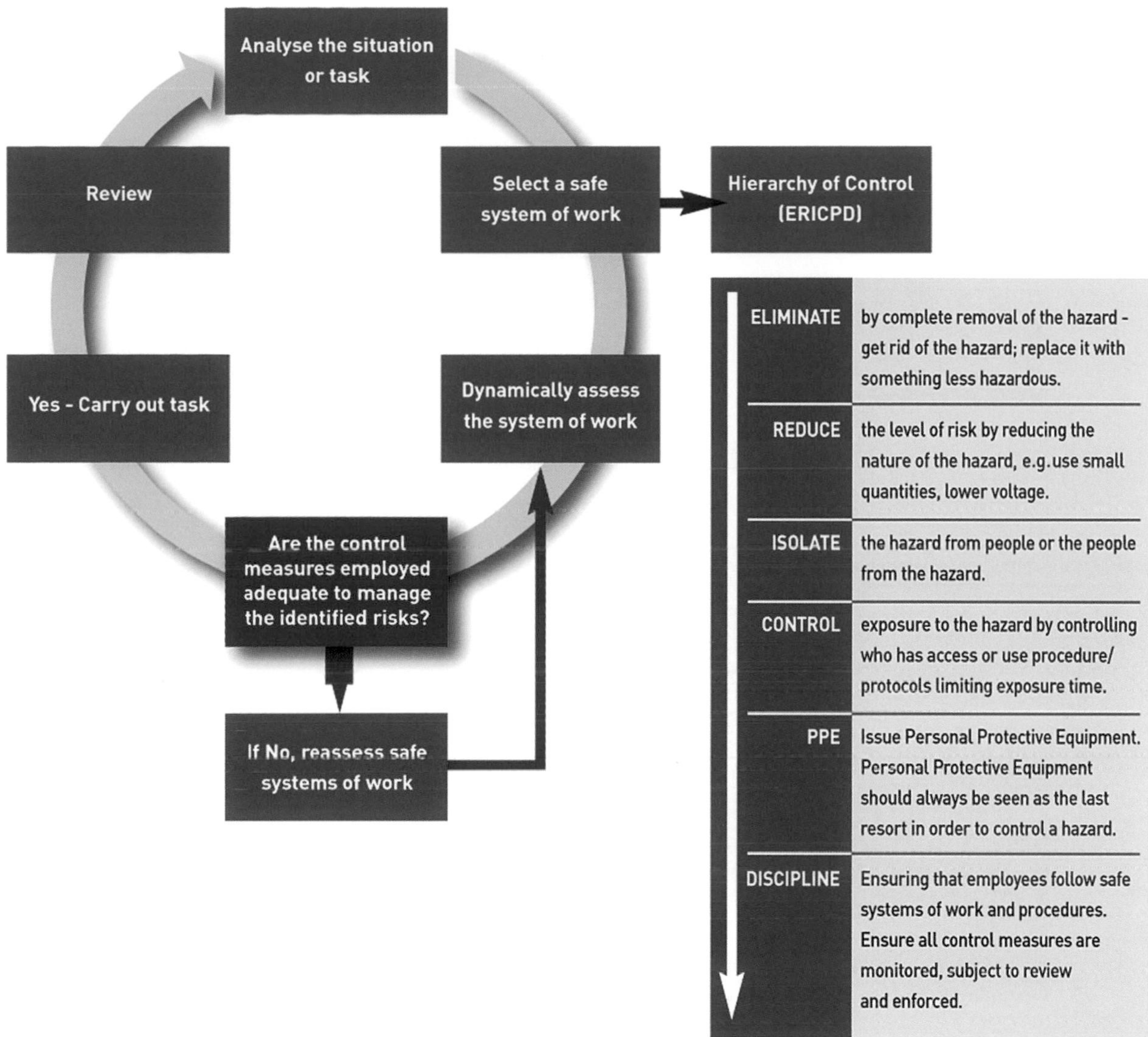

Figure 6.3 – Dynamic risk assessment model.

weapons has occurred and subsequently that there may still be a potential risk to the public and responders alike.

- Once on scene, incidents with mechanisms of injury (MoI) of penetrating and/or blast injury, particularly those with no apparent explanation, should be attended with caution. If either a criminal or terror-related act has occurred, then the safety of the responder(s) is paramount and unprotected responders should consider withdrawing from the area if they feel that their safety is compromised.
- The Home Office has issued specific advice to the public if they become caught up in a marauding terrorist attack (MTA) or an active shooter event in the form of the Run, Hide, Tell campaign (Figure 6.6).
- While aspects of the Home Office campaign are applicable to the ambulance service, ambulance responders also owe a duty of care to reported casualties (refer to **Duty of Care**).

The following guidance should be considered by ambulance personnel involved in an actual or suspected violent or terrorist attack:

- Withdraw from the scene as quickly as possible. If possible, take casualties and mission critical medical equipment.
- Move in a direction away from the actual or perceived threat and avoid running in straight lines.
- Move from point to point using hard cover as necessary and if available.
- The distance to withdraw to is situationally dependent and individual judgement should be used.
- If police and/or security services are present they may give a specific distance to move to.
- Safe distances in incidents involving firearms will vary depending on the type of weapon(s) being used. Some firearms have an effective range of as little as 50 m, while other types of weapon

Major, Complex and High Risk Incidents

COMMAND TABARDS

Tactical Commander (Ambulance Incident Commander)
White lower half with green & white checked shoulders.

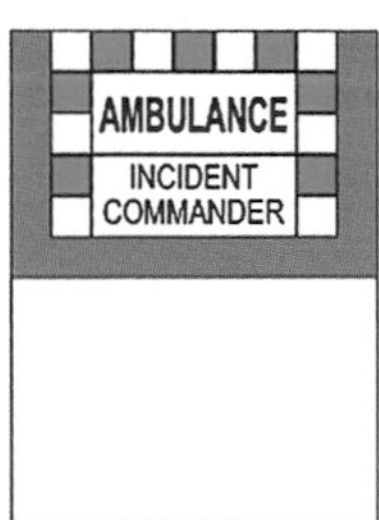

Ambulance Operational Commander and any functional role not individually listed
Saturn yellow lower half and green & white checked shoulders. Insert as per role.

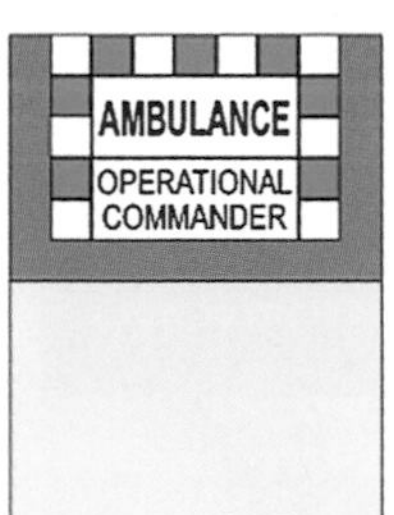

Airwave Tactical Advisor
Green & white check.

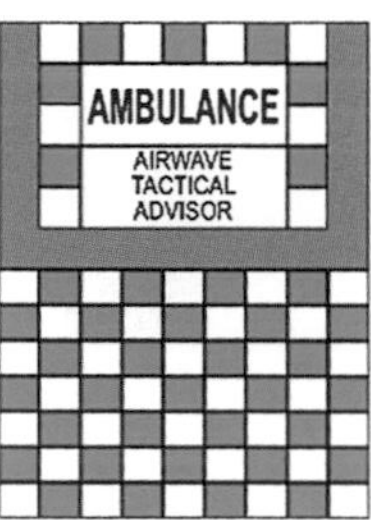

Ambulance Safety Officer (ASO)
Blue lower half with green & white checked shoulders.

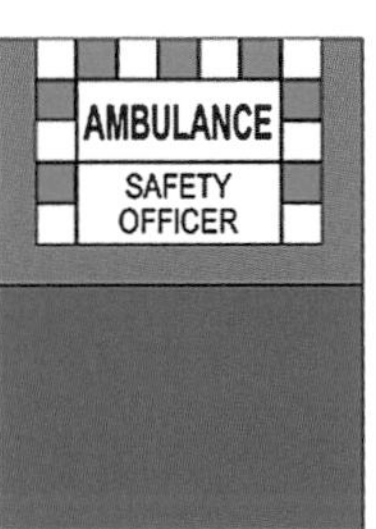

Decontamination Officer
Purple lower half with green & white checked shoulders.

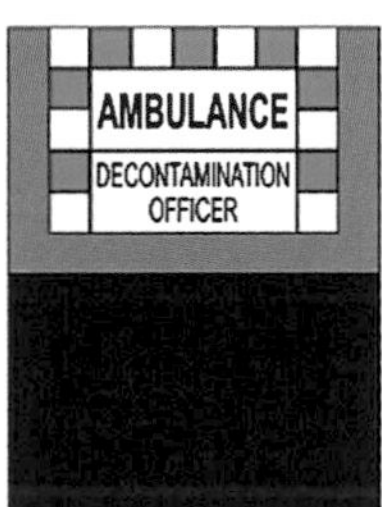

Doctor
Red lower half with green & white checked shoulders.

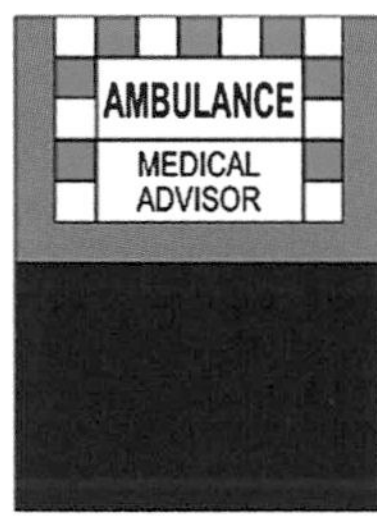

Strategic Advisor, Tactical Advisor or National Inter-Agency Liaison Officer (NILO)
Green lower half with green & white checked shoulders. Insert as per role.

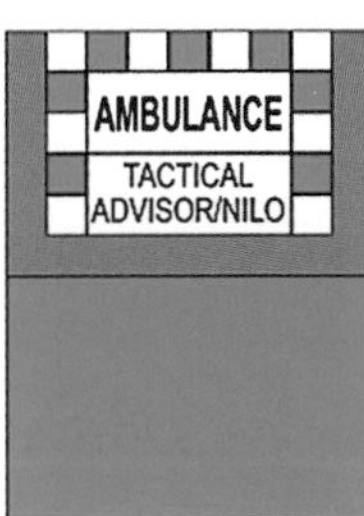

Ambulance Entry Control Officer (ECO)
Green & yellow all over check.

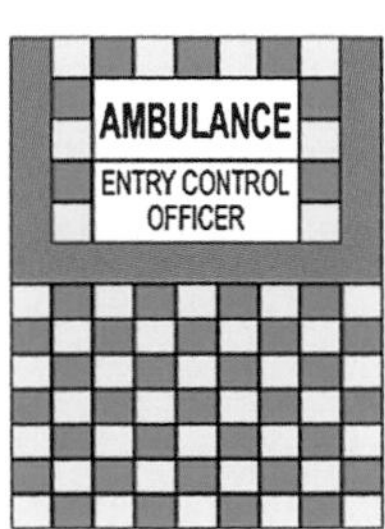

Loggist
Orange lower half and green & white checked shoulders. All orange is any support function.

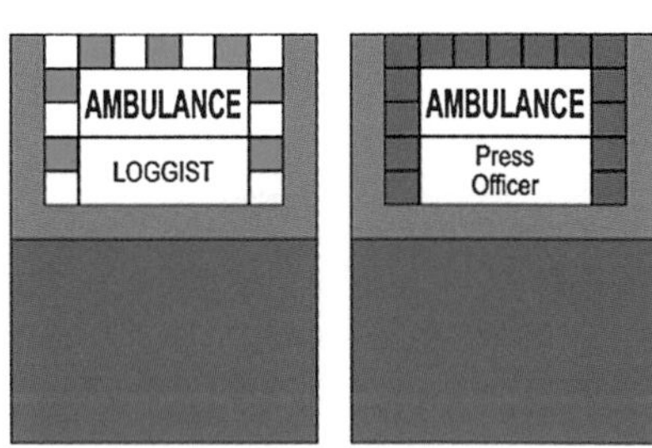

Figure 6.4 – National tabards for major incidents.

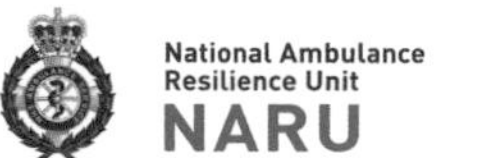
National Ambulance Resilience Unit
NARU

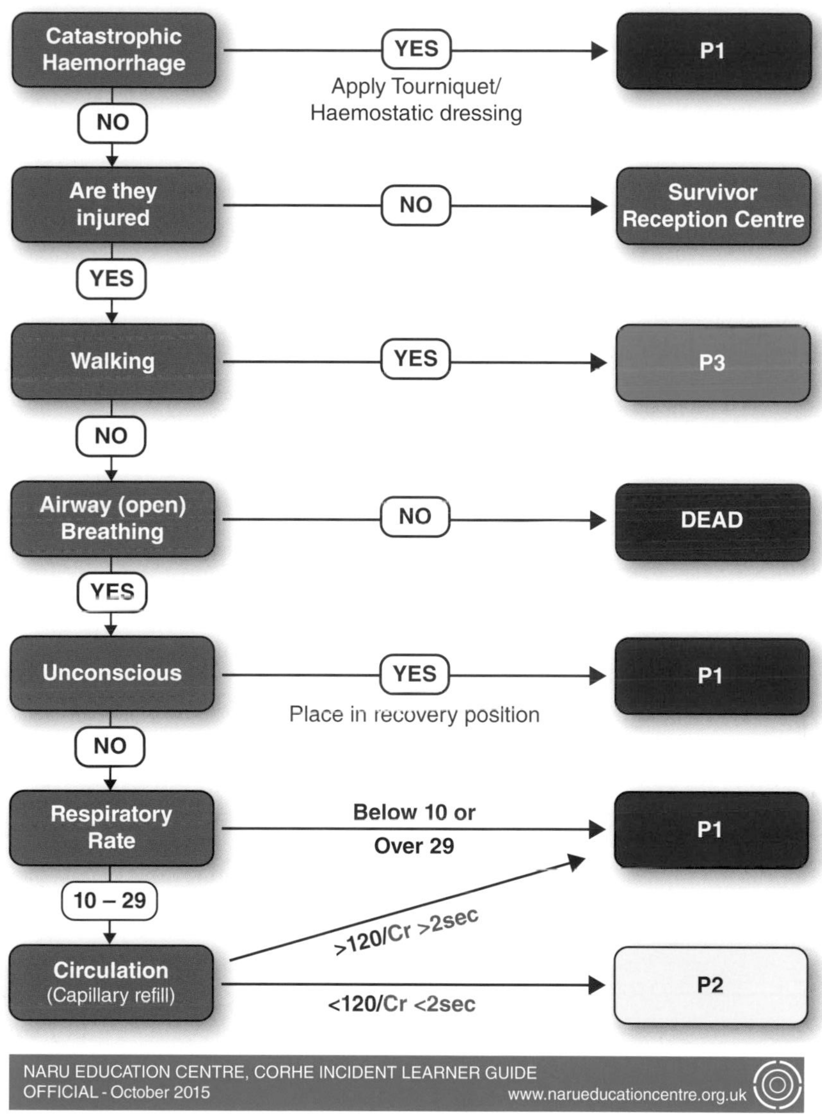

Figure 6.5 – Triage sieve tool.

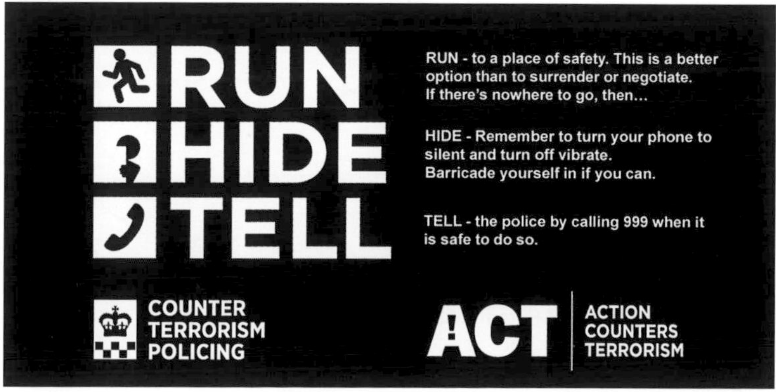
RUN
HIDE
TELL
RUN - to a place of safety. This is a better option than to surrender or negotiate. If there's nowhere to go, then...
HIDE - Remember to turn your phone to silent and turn off vibrate. Barricade yourself in if you can.
TELL - the police by calling 999 when it is safe to do so.
COUNTER TERRORISM POLICING
ACT
ACTION COUNTERS TERRORISM

Figure 6.6 – Run, Hide, Tell.

Source: Home Office, 2015.

systems may have an effective range of up to 400 m.

- When explosive devices are suspected to have been used or will be used, the minimum distance will again depend on the type and size of the device.
- Once at a safe distance, responders should seek cover that gives physical protection and protection from view. Cover from ballistic or explosive threats could be a solid structure like a building, for example.
- If physical cover is not achievable, then the responder should look for areas that will provide cover from view, for example a depression in the terrain.
- Once in cover, plan an escape route.
- Avoid isolated or obvious forms of cover, such as lone objects.
- Try to select cover that while providing protection also gives maximum fields of view.
- When in cover, scan the area for secondary threats and be prepared to move again if not satisfied with the area selected for cover.
- Stay calm and control breathing. Remain focused.
- Once it is safe to do so, it is imperative that the responders update the situation as soon as practicable using the METHANE reporting method.
- Ask for assistance from the police and the Hazardous Area Response Team (HART) if they are not already present or been dispatched.
- Continue to provide situational updates if practicable and safe to do so.
- Turn the volume down on the communication system and speak quietly. Where possible use an earpiece.
- Turn other mobile devices to silent (turn OFF any vibrating alert) while still in danger.
- HART units and ambulance intervention teams (AIT) are specifically trained and equipped with ballistic personal protective equipment (PPE) to operate within a ballistic warm zone while responding to marauding terrorist attacks (MTA). HART also provide support to security operations (SSO). For any incidents of criminal attack involving weapons or terrorism, HART should be deployed as a matter of reflex. The deployment of AIT will normally be a strategic decision based on the merits of the presenting situation.
- Incidents involving weapons carry with them their own injuries depending on the type of weapon(s) used. The MoI of incidents involving weapons do share some commonalities, and injury types may coexist (refer to Figure 6.7). For specific guidance on treatment algorithms, refer to **Trauma Emergencies Overview**, **Head Injury** and **Thoracic Trauma**.

4. Water Rescue

- Ambulance responders are frequently called to incidents involving water. Non-specialists should not enter fast moving water.
- Where patient(s) require life-saving interventions, there are steps that can be taken by all ambulance staff prior to specialist teams arriving. Consider the following:
  - Carry out a dynamic risk assessment.
  - Inform the ACR of the situation.

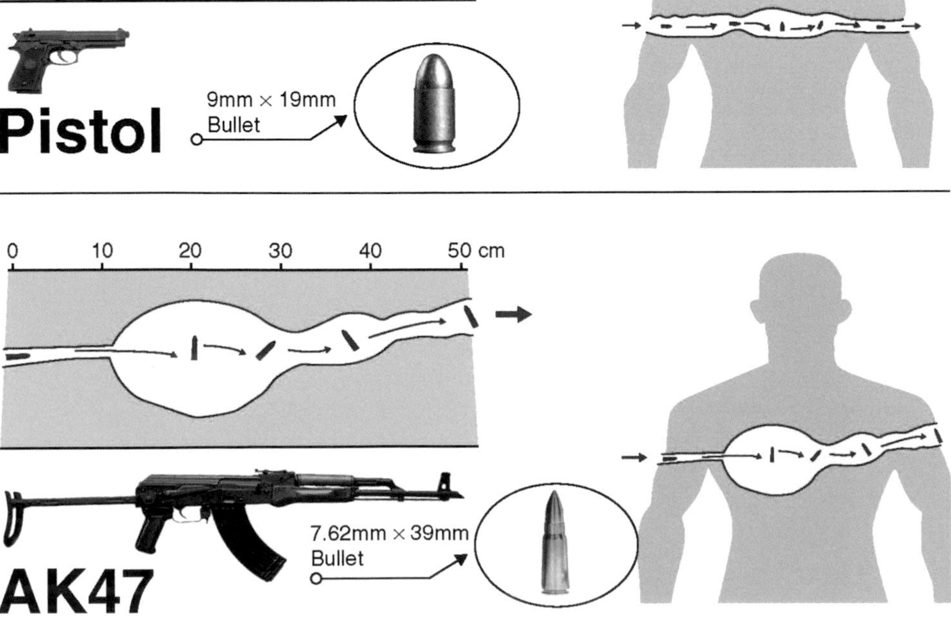

Figure 6.7 – Gunshot entry and exit wounds.

- Request specialist assistance, including HART assets, as soon as possible.
- Wear a life-jacket if working within the warm zone (3 m from water's edge).
- Shout at the patient to swim towards you.
- If they are unable to do so, throw a safety buoy (or similar) for them to hold on to and pull them to safety.
- Do not carry out a task that is likely to cause you to enter the water unintentionally and become a casualty yourself.
- Only enter the water if it is shallow enough and, based on the risk assessment, you are competent to do so (i.e. a shallow pool in a recreational park as opposed to a canal, lake or fast flowing river).
- Do not enter flood water without the support of specialist water responders.

- Ideally non-specialists should not be working within the warm zone without appropriate training, equipment or PPE but it is recognised that in some low risk incidents it is unacceptable to delay life-saving interventions awaiting specialist help. This must be managed appropriately within each trust.

5. High-consequence Infectious Disease

- Examples of high consequence infectious diseases are:
  - Ebola
  - Lassa fever
  - Marburg virus
  - pandemic influenza
  - other 'category 4' pathogens.
- It is crucial that the correct response to patient(s) with suspected/confirmed infectious disease is achieved to protect all those involved. The need for such a response will usually be pre-planned. Where this is not the case and an infectious disease is suspected, several precautions are needed.
- The patient should be isolated and further advice sought from a Tactical Advisor/NILO and trust protocols followed. Normally, universal precautions will be sufficient to protect ambulance responders. A more thorough history than normal will need to be obtained from the patient. Transfers of high-risk patients are usually completed by specialist HART staff who have access to additional protective equipment. If ambulance responders suspect they may have been exposed (i.e. needle stick injury), report and present for medical treatment immediately.

5.1 Pandemic Flu

- This is the highest-grade risk in the National Risk Register of Civil Emergencies. All ambulance responders should be familiar with their local trust's plans to respond to such patients. Universal precautions are normally appropriate. All ambulance responders should have access to FFP3 masks, or equivalent, and be appropriately fit tested. All ambulance responders are encouraged to receive an annual flu vaccination in order to protect themselves, their families and the public.

6. Transport Incidents

6.1 Rail Incidents

Table 6.4 outlines how to manage rail incidents.

TABLE 6.4 – Management of Rail Incidents

Non-specialists	Specialists (HART/CBRN)
Do not approach the track without authorisation from the Ambulance Operational Commander (if on scene or via EOC if they are en-route) that the power is off and trains stopped as confirmed by Network Rail Route Control.	
Request HART support and provide a METHANE report to control.	Have appropriate PPE and specialist equipment to deal with such an incident.
	Will provide medical support to partner agencies responding to the incident.
Use the mnemonic POWER: • **P**ower off and trains stopped confirmed by authorised person. When in doubt, contact EOC. • **O**ff the tracks unless the patient appears visible. • **W**ear PPE (minimum hi-vis jacket and helmet). • **E**nsure EOC and ambulance commander knows clinicians are entering or leaving trackside. • **R**apidly remove a viable patient and treat in the safest agreed area off the tracks.	
Identify your location at track to Network Rail Control via Ambulance Control (EOC) (Use signal; bridge or overhead line support number plates; quarter mile posts at track side; station or level crossing nearby; electrical substation name plate).	

6.2 Industrial Docks

- Report to the rendezvous point (RVP) to meet dock staff and be taken to the incident. If the activity is close to the water's edge, ensure HART attendance is requested early.
- Many docks contain structures that require staff to work at height or in confined spaces, i.e. ships, ISO container and cranes. An early request for specialist resources who are equipped, trained and authorised to work in such environments is imperative. Request HART early.
- Local ambulance services may have site-specific plans and arrangements for large dockland areas. For further information, contact the EPRR Department.

6.3 Airports

- Each airport will have a site-specific plan for incidents and emergencies on their site. This will have been developed in conjunction with the emergency services including ambulance services. When responding to an airport emergency, clinicians will usually be asked to report to a designed rendezvous point (RVP) where they will be met and taken airside by airport staff. Identify relevant RVPs in advance. These will be contained in your local plans.
- Each ambulance service will also have a pre-determined attendance (PDA) for such incidents. For further information on airport incidents, contact the EPRR Department.

6.4 Carriageways and Motorways

General guidelines:

- Blue lights and hazard warning lights should be left ON, unless the scene has been secured and a major incident has been declared.
- Ensure hi-vis PPE is worn, and consider a helmet to provide protection from debris and during any extrication.
- Approach from the rear of the incident, if possible, at low speed.
- Identify hazards, consider parking position and identify a safe area of work.
- Request police/Highways England if not already present.
- Follow the flow of traffic unless directed otherwise by police or Highways England.
- Do not stop on the non-incident carriageway to gain access to an incident on the opposite side, irrespective of how urgent the situation appears on the affected carriageway nor the distance to the next junction or crossing point.
- In multiple vehicle collisions, it may be necessary to sectorise the scene to promote understanding and aid communication.

Actions on arrival:

- Ensure the road is closed or restricted.
- The first vehicle should park before the incident and additional vehicles should park beyond it creating a boundary for a safe working area (except on motorways, where all vehicles should park beyond the incident in the obstructed lane).
- Exit the vehicle on the side away from moving traffic.
- Liaise with police, Highways England and the fire and rescue service (FRS).
- Ascertain the number and location of casualties trapped or injured and report to the control room.
- Ensure an operational commander is appointed to coordinate ambulance resources and stand back to liaise with other agencies.
- Prioritise extrication and request further resources if required (i.e. HART for additional equipment and capabilities).
- Establish an inner and outer cordon around the scene of operations, if appropriate.
- Keep the working area clear by creating an equipment dump.
- Treat all non-activated SRS devices as live; high voltage electrical systems should all be treated as live even when the engine is not running.
- Fires in an LPG-powered car will be treated by the FRS as a cylinder incident.

Agencies use Table 6.5 as a guide to help inform lane closures.

Leaving the incident:

- Do not move any vehicles, especially those providing the fend-off protection, before consulting with other emergency services.

TABLE 6.5 – Lane Closures for Road Incidents

Incident Location	Lane Closures Required
Two-way local roadway	Both lanes
Hard shoulder of the motorway or similar	Hard shoulder and lane 1
Lane 1 of a 3-lane roadway	Hard shoulder, lane 1 and lane 2
Lane 2 of a 3-lane roadway	Lanes 1, 2 and 3
Lane 3 of a 3-lane roadway	Lanes 2 and 3
Across the central reservation	Lanes 2 and 3 of both carriageways

- Maintain high visibility when moving away from the incident and re-joining traffic flows. Use warning lights until clear of the incident.

'All lane running':

- Some sections of the motorway may be utilised for 'all lane running' (Figure 6.8). On these sections the hard shoulder area may be used for live traffic at certain times. Lanes are then described as 1–4.

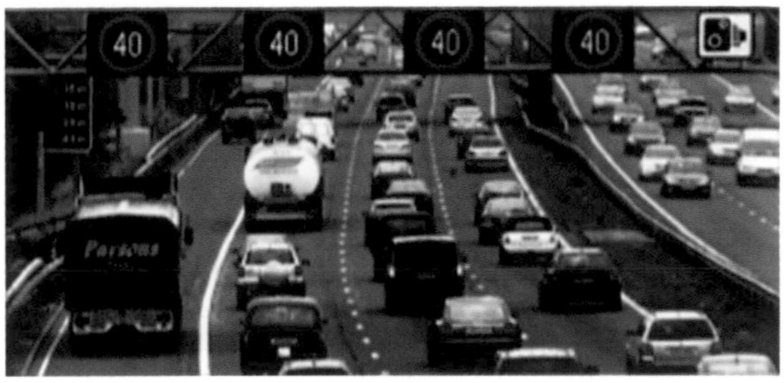

Incidents in tunnels:

- Attending resources should consider entering from both directions.
- Utilise both bores of the tunnel if possible and confirm that traffic has stopped.
- Utilise the non-incident bore for casualty treatment and loading if appropriate.

Figure 6.8 – All lane running.

- Ensure that all responders are aware when operations are utilised in the non-incident bore.
- Consider fume build up in a protracted incident.

Bibliography

1. Public Health England. *Chemical, biological, radiological and nuclear incidents: recognise and respond*. Available from: https://www.gov.uk/government/publications/chemical-biological-radiological-and-nuclear-incidents-recognise-and-respond, 2018.
2. NHS England. *Clinical guidelines for major incidents and mass casualty events*. Available from: https://www.england.nhs.uk/publication/clinical-guidelines-for-major-incidents-and-mass-casualty-events/, 2018.
3. National Ambulance Resilience Unit. *Compliance & Quality Assurance: National Provisions for Interoperable Capabilities*. Available from: https://naru.org.uk, 2018.

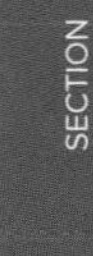

Police Incapacitants

1. Introduction

- The deployment of police incapacitants on individuals and/or groups can lead to conditions requiring pre-hospital care.
- The aim of this guideline is to support clinical decision making for the management of patients following the deployment of:
  - conducted electrical weapons (CEW), for example TASER® and stun guns
  - incapacitant sprays, i.e. CS/PAVA
  - projectiles
  - batons
- Not all patients exposed to police incapacitants will require hospital assessment; however, all patients should undergo a primary survey.
- Carry out a dynamic risk assessment; continually re-assess throughout the incident.

2. Conducted Electrical Weapons

CEWs are battery operated hand-held devices which deliver up to 50,000 volts of electricity, in rapid pulses, via two barbed electrodes (refer to Figure 6.9).

- The barbs are designed to stick into skin or clothes and connect to the device by fine long copper wires, or via two probes directly applied to the skin or clothes.
- Firing the device results in pain and a loss of voluntary control of muscles. These devices are currently in use by all police forces in the United Kingdom.
- Before touching the patient ensure the wires are disconnected from the device; the wires break easily by cutting with scissors.

There is an increased risk of combustion if a CEW is deployed after the deployment of incapacitant sprays or following contact with flammable liquids such as petrol.

Assessment and Management

- Most people incapacitated with a CEW do not require hospital assessment; however, patients should undergo a primary survey especially assessing for the presence of:
  - neck and back injuries
  - secondary injuries
  - cardiac symptoms
  - Acute Behavioural Disturbance (ABD)
  - attached electrodes.
- For the assessment and management of symptoms, conditions and injuries following deployment of CEW refer to Table 6.6.

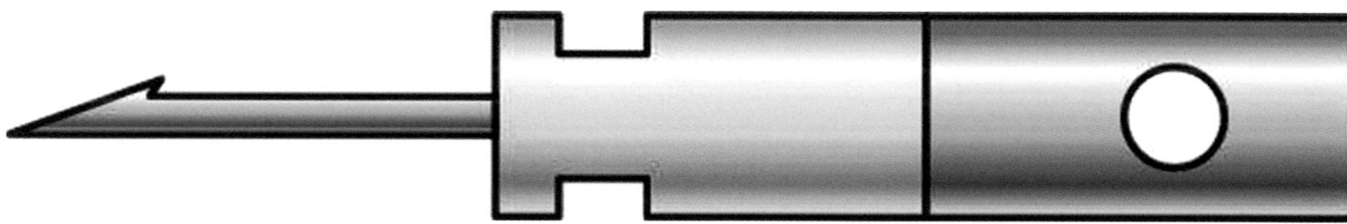

Figure 6.9 – CEW barb.

TABLE 6.6 – ASSESSMENT and MANAGEMENT following the Deployment of a CEW	
PRIMARY EFFECTS	
Effect	**Assessment/Management**
Pain	Refer to **Pain Management in Adults** and **Pain Management in Children**.
Electrode attachment The electrodes vary in length and have a 'fish hook' type end which is designed to stick to clothes and into the skin. **NB** Although the lengths of the barbs may vary, the management principles remain the same.	Electrode removal • Slightly stretch the skin around the electrode and pull sharply on the electrode. • Dispose of the electrode as clinical waste. • Clean the area. • Cover the site with an adhesive dressing. • Advise tetanus booster within 72 hours if not covered for tetanus.

TABLE 6.6 – ASSESSMENT and MANAGEMENT following the Deployment of a CEW *(continued)*

PRIMARY EFFECTS	
Effect	**Assessment/Management**
	NB If the electrode cannot be removed at the first attempt or breaks during attempted removal, leave in situ and transfer to definitive care. **DO NOT** attempt to remove the electrodes if they are: ● Attached to skin where blood vessels are close to the skin surface (e.g. neck and groin). ● Attached to one or both eye(s). ● Attached to the face. ● Attached to the genitalia. ● Attached to the mouth, throat or if the electrode has been swallowed. ● Firmly embedded in the scalp. ● Embedded in a joint (e.g. finger). ● Broken. In these circumstances, cut the wire close to the electrode leaving approximately 4 cm attached to the electrode and transfer to definitive care
Burns ● Superficial burns are likely around the area where the electrode attached to the skin and electricity was delivered. ● Burns may also occur if a CEW is deployed after the deployment of incapacitant sprays or following contact with flammable liquids such as petrol.	Refer to **Pain Management in Adults**, **Pain Management in Children** and **Burns and Scalds**.
Cardiac conditions/symptoms: ● Cardiac conditions have been reported following the deployment of a CEW, including increases in heart rate, cardiac rhythm disturbance and cardiac arrest.	ECGs are not needed for all patients. However, always undertake a 12-lead ECG and monitor blood pressure and oxygen saturation for patients: ● Complaining of chest pain. ● With cardiac symptoms (e.g. tachycardia, bradycardia). ● With significant cardiac history (e.g. angina, arrhythmias or a myocardial infarction). ● Fitted with pacemakers or cardioverter defibrillator. ● Cardiac arrhythmia: Refer to **Cardiac Rhythm Disturbance** for specific guidance. ● Cardiac arrest: Refer to the appropriate resuscitation guidelines.
Convulsions The deployment of a CEW may elicit a convulsion or epileptic fit.	For specific guidance refer to **Convulsions in Adults** and **Convulsions in Children**.
Obstetric and gynaecological conditions Spontaneous miscarriage has been reported following the deployment of CEW.	Refer to the appropriate **Maternity Care** guidelines.

(continued)

TABLE 6.6 – ASSESSMENT and MANAGEMENT following the Deployment of a Cew *(continued)*	
PRIMARY EFFECTS	
Effect	**Assessment/Management**
Soft tissue injury/injuries: ● Contusions ● Tendon damage ● Abrasions ● Lacerations ● Puncture wounds	Abrasions, lacerations and puncture wounds: ● Clean the area with an alcohol/antiseptic wipe. ● Cover the site with an adhesive dressing. ● Advise tetanus booster within 72 hours if not covered for tetanus. Contusions, damage to ligament and tendons: These injuries should be managed accordingly and transferred to definitive care.
Head injury Head injuries and loss of consciousness may also result from intracranial penetration of an electrode.	For specific guidance, refer to **Head Injury** and **Altered Level of Consciousness**.
SECONDARY EFFECTS	
Effect	**Assessment/Management**
Head, neck and back injuries, contusions, abrasions and lacerations: ● The powerful muscular contractions caused by the deployment of a CEW may result in thoracolumbar fractures. ● The loss of voluntary control of the muscles caused by the deployment of a CEW may result in falls, leading to injuries of the head, neck and back, contusions, abrasions, lacerations, ligament and tendon injury, etc.	For specific guidance refer to **Head Injury**, **Spinal Injury and Spinal Cord Injury**. Contusions, abrasions, lacerations, ligament and tendon injury: Manage as per soft tissue injuries above.
COINCIDENTAL EFFECTS	
Injuries and conditions unrelated to CEW deployment: ● Injuries and or conditions may be sustained or develop that are unrelated to the deployment of a CEW, for example, as the result of a physical struggle, the consumption of drugs and of physical exhaustion.	Assess and manage coincidental injuries as per condition, cognisant of the effects of drugs, dehydration or exhaustion.
Acute behavioural disturbance (ABD)	A CEW may be deployed on people in an aroused state which is sometimes described as 'excited delirium', ABD. People in this state may be at a greater risk of collapse, arrhythmias and sudden death following deployment of a CEW – undertake a **TIME CRITICAL** transfer and provide an alert/information call. The signs of excited delirium include: bizarre behaviour, physical aggression against people and objects, ripping off clothing, being under the influence of drugs or alcohol, abnormal physical strength and reduced perception of pain. **NB** A doctor may be required to administer rapid tranquilisation; assistance from the police may also be required.

3. Incapacitant Sprays

- Incapacitant sprays/peripheral chemosensory irritants (PCSIs) such as pepper spray (oleoresin, capsicum, pelargonic acid, vanillylamide), CS spray 2-chlorobenzalmalononitrile (O-chlorobenzylidene malononitrile) and PAVA are prepared with methyl isobutyl ketone (MIBK).
- The sprays cause irritation (burning sensation) when in contact with exposed skin and mucus membranes including eye, nose, and mouth and respiratory tract causing lacrimation, rhinorrhoea, sialorrhoea, disorientation, dizziness, breathing difficulties, coughing, vomiting.
- Avoid entering a contaminated or closed environment.

Assessment and Management

- Most people exposed to incapacitant sprays do not require hospital assessment.
- For the assessment and management of symptoms, and conditions following deployment of incapacitant sprays refer to Table 6.7.

TABLE 6.7 – ASSESSMENT and MANAGEMENT Following the Deployment of Incapacitant Sprays

Effect	Assessment/ Management
Lacrimation, rhinorrhoea, sialorrhoea, dizziness, coughing and vomiting	• Move the patient away from the source of the contamination. • Expose to fresh air. • For patients with heavy contamination of the skin and eyes irrigate with tap water. • If symptoms persist for longer than 15 minutes transfer to further care.
Breathing difficulties	For specific guidance refer to **Dyspnoea**.

4. Projectiles

Projectiles

- Projectiles such as plastic bullets, rubber bullets or bean bags can cause sudden death (after strikes to the head, chest and abdomen), dislocations, fractures, joint damage, ligaments and tendons, haemorrhage and haematoma, compartment syndrome, splenic rupture, subcapsular liver/haematoma, pneumothorax/ haemothorax, penetrating injuries to thorax, abdomen, eye, arm, leg, blood vessels.
- A sudden, single-blow blunt trauma to the front of the chest may on rare occasions lead to cardiac arrest due to the rhythm disturbance; this is the opposite of a pre-cordial thump for witnessed cardiac arrest. Refer to **resuscitation** guidelines.

Batons

- Baton strikes can cause:
  - Dislocations
  - Fractures
  - Joint, ligament and tendon damage
  - Haemorrhage and haematoma
  - Compartment syndrome
  - Death.
- Baton strikes to limbs will typically cause 'tramline bruising'; this is of no significant concern unless there is evidence of underlying fracture or neuromuscular condition.

KEY POINTS!

- **Ensure the wires are disconnected from the CEW before touching the patient.**
- **DO NOT remove electrodes in any of the instances listed in Table 6.6.**
- **Patients may also sustain secondary injuries (e.g. head injuries and fractures following a fall).**
- **Transfer to definitive care any patient with one or more of the following: cardiac symptoms, neck and back injuries and ABD.**
- **The symptoms of patients exposed to incapacitant sprays should settle after exposure to air. If symptoms do not persist after 15 minutes transfer to definitive care.**

Atropine for CBRNE

Presentation

- Pre-filled syringe containing 1 milligram atropine in 5 ml.
- Pre-filled syringe containing 1 milligram atropine in 10 ml.
- Pre-filled syringe containing 3 milligrams atropine in 10 ml.
- An ampoule containing 600 micrograms in 1 ml.
- Duodote® containing 2.1 milligrams of atropine sulphate.

Indications

Organophosphate (OP) poisoning.

Adults and children with a clinical diagnosis of poisoning by OP nerve agents, as an adjunct to maintenance of oxygenation.

Atropine should be administered for confirmed OP poisoning, or where features of OP poisoning develop. Clinical diagnosis of nerve agent poisoning (see below) is suggested by the characteristic features of nerve agent poisoning, associated with a history of possible exposure. Clinical features must include one or more of the following: bronchorrhoea, bronchospasm, severe bradycardia (<40 bpm).

Contra-Indications

Hypersensitivity to atropine sulphate or excipients in nerve agent poisoning.

Cautions

There are no other absolute criteria for the exclusion from administration of atropine in the treatment of OP poisoning, as the consequences of not instituting prompt treatment in poisoned patients will usually outweigh the risks associated with treatment. However, caution needs to be administered in the following:

- Patients with ulcerative colitis.
- Patients with risk of urinary retention.
- Patients with glaucoma.
- Patients with conditions characterised by tachycardia (e.g. thyrotoxicosis, heart failure).
- Patients with myasthenia gravis.

Side Effects

Reactions are mostly dose related and usually reversible and include:

- Loss of visual accommodation.
- Photophobia.
- Arrhythmias, transient bradycardia followed by tachycardia.
- Palpitations.
- Difficulty in micturition.

Additional Information

Toxic doses may cause CNS stimulation manifesting as restlessness, confusion, ataxia, lack of coordination, hallucinations and delirium. In severe intoxication CNS stimulation may give way to CNS depression, coma, circulatory and respiratory failure and death.

Characteristic features of nerve agent poisoning:

- Miosis, excess secretions (e.g. lacrimation and bronchorrhoea).
- Respiratory difficulty (e.g. bronchospasm or respiratory depression).
- Altered consciousness, convulsions, together with a history of possible exposure.

Nerve agent poisoning

- Atropine must only be administered after the patient is adequately oxygenated.
- In organophosphate poisoning there is no maximum dose and large doses (e.g. 20 milligrams) may be required to achieve atropinisation. Signs of atropinisation include: dry skin and mouth and an absence of bradycardia (e.g. heart rate adult ≥80; heart rate child HR ≥100 bpm). **NB** DO NOT rely on reversal of pinpoint pupils as a guide to atropinisation.
- Administering large volumes intramuscularly could lead to poor absorption and/or tissue damage; therefore administer the smallest volume possible and divide where necessary and practicable. Vary the site of injection for repeated doses; appropriate sites include: buttock (gluteus maximus), thigh (vastus lateralis), lateral hip (gluteus medius) and upper arm (deltoid).

Atropine for CBRNE

Dosage and Administration

Intravenous 1 milligram in 5 ml

Route: Intravenous/intraosseous/intramuscular (as appropriate).

AGE	INITIAL DOSE	REPEAT DOSE	DOSE INTERVAL	CONCENTRATION	VOLUME	MAX DOSE
≥8 years	2 milligrams	2 milligrams	5 minutes	1 milligram in 5 ml	10 ml	No limit
12 months – 7 years	600 micrograms	600 micrograms	5 minutes	1 milligram in 5 ml	3 ml	No limit
Birth – 9 months	200 micrograms	200 micrograms	5 minutes	1 milligram in 5 ml	1 ml	No limit

Intravenous 1 milligram in 10 ml

Route: Intravenous/intraosseous/intramuscular (administer the smallest volume possible and divide where necessary and practicable).

AGE	INITIAL DOSE	REPEAT DOSE	DOSE INTERVAL	CONCENTRATION	VOLUME	MAX DOSE
≥8 years	2 milligrams	2 milligrams	5 minutes	1 milligram in 10 ml	20 ml	No limit
12 months – 7 years	600 micrograms	600 micrograms	5 minutes	1 milligram in 10 ml	6 ml	No limit
Birth – 9 months	200 micrograms	200 micrograms	5 minutes	1 milligram in 10 ml	2 ml	No limit

Intravenous 3 milligrams in 10 ml

Route: Intravenous/intraosseous/intramuscular (as appropriate).

AGE	INITIAL DOSE	REPEAT DOSE	DOSE INTERVAL	CONCENTRATION	VOLUME	MAX DOSE
≥8 years	2 milligrams	2 milligrams	5 minutes	3 milligrams in 10 ml	6.7 ml	No limit
12 months – 7 years	600 micrograms	600 micrograms	5 minutes	3 milligrams in 10 ml	2 ml	No limit
Birth – 9 months	200 micrograms	200 micrograms	5 minutes	3 milligrams in 10 ml	0.6 ml	No limit

Intravenous 600 micrograms in 1 ml

Route: Intravenous/intraosseous/intramuscular.

AGE	INITIAL DOSE	REPEAT DOSE	DOSE INTERVAL	CONCENTRATION	VOLUME	MAX DOSE
≥8 years	2 milligrams	2 milligrams	5 minutes	600 micrograms in 1 ml	3.3 ml	No limit
12 months – 7 years	600 micrograms	600 micrograms	5 minutes	600 micrograms in 1 ml	1 ml	No limit
Birth – 9 months	200 micrograms	200 micrograms	5 minutes	600 micrograms in 1 ml	0.3 ml	No limit

DuoDote® auto-injector (atropine combined with Pralidoxime)

Presentation

Prefilled DuoDote® auto-injector providing a single intramuscular dose of atropine and pralidoxime chloride in a self-contained unit, specifically designed for administration by emergency medical services personnel.

When activated, each DuoDote® auto-injector delivers the following:

- 2.1 mg of atropine in 0.7ml of sterile, pyrogen-free solution
- 600 mg of pralidoxime chloride in 2 ml of sterile, pyrogen-free solution.

Indications

Adults and children ≥ 1 years with a clinical diagnosis of nerve agent or organophosphate poisoning suggested by the characteristic features associated with a history of possible exposure. Clinical features must include one or more of the following:

- bronchorrhoea (production of excess watery sputum)
- bronchospasm
- severe bradycardia (<40bpm).

Other signs may include:

- excess secretions e.g. lacrimation (tears)
- respiratory depression
- altered level of consciousness, convulsions.

Toxic doses of a nerve agent may cause CNS stimulation manifesting as restlessness, confusion, ataxia, lack of co-ordination, hallucinations, delirium. In severe intoxication CNS stimulation may give way to CNS depression, coma, circulatory and respiratory failure, and death.

DuoDote® should be used during pregnancy only if the potential benefit justifies the potential risk to the foetus.

The DuoDote® Auto-Injector is intended as an initial treatment of the symptoms of organophosphorus insecticide or nerve agent poisonings; definitive medical care should be sought immediately.

Actions

- Reduces secretions in the mouth and respiratory passages.
- Relieves airway constriction and respiratory muscle paralysis.

Contra-Indications

Children <1 year.

In the presence of life-threatening poisoning by organophosphorous nerve agents or insecticides, there are no absolute contra-indications to the use of DuoDote® in adults and children ≥ 1 year.

Cautions

When symptoms of poisoning are not severe, DuoDote® should be used with extreme caution in people with heart disease, arrhythmias, recent myocardial infarction, severe narrow angle glaucoma, pyloric stenosis, prostatic hypertrophy, significant renal insufficiency, chronic pulmonary disease, or hypersensitivity to any component of the product.

Myasthenia gravis.

Side Effects

- Loss of visual accommodation.
- Photophobia.
- Arrhythmias (transient bradycardia followed by tachycardia).
- Palpitations.
- Difficulty in micturition.

Additional Information

- Individuals should not rely solely upon DuoDote® to provide complete protection from chemical nerve agents and insecticide poisoning. Primary protection against exposure to chemical nerve agents and insecticide poisoning is the wearing of protective garments including masks designed specifically for this use. Evacuation and decontamination procedures should be undertaken as soon as possible. Staff assisting evacuated victims of nerve agent poisoning should avoid contaminating themselves by exposure to the victim's clothing.
- Organophosphorous nerve agent poisoning often causes bradycardia but can be associated with a heart rate in the low, high or normal range. Atropine increases heart rate and alleviates the bradycardia. In patients with a recent myocardial infarction and/or severe coronary artery disease, there is a possibility that atropine-induced tachycardia may cause ischaemia, extend or initiate myocardial infarcts, and stimulate ventricular ectopy and fibrillation.
- Explain treatment and associated side effects.
- All patients who receive Duodote® must be conveyed to hospital.

DuoDote® auto-injector (atropine combined with Pralidoxime)

Dosage and Administration

Route: Intramuscular (using built in needle) into the mid-lateral thigh. This is the initial treatment, all patients may require further ongoing countermeasures; seek senior clinical advice and evacuate to hospital.

In children under 1 DuoDote® should not be administered but atropine can be given. Refer to **Atropine**.

AGE	INITIAL DOSE	REPEAT DOSE	DOSE INTERVAL	MAX DOSE
≥12years	1 auto-injectors	1 auto-injectors	Every 15 mins if symptoms persist	3
Age 8-11	1 auto-injectors	1 auto-injectors	Every 15 mins if symptoms persist	2
Age 1-7	1 auto-injectors	NONE	N/A	1

Bibliography

South Western Ambulance Service Trust. *Medicines Protocol: DuoDote®*, 2017.

SECTION 6 Special Situations

7

Medicines

Medicines Overview

1. Introduction

- The guidelines contained in this section are the current medicines that are usually administered by registered paramedics, provided that they have the necessary legal authority. In the case of parenteral medicines this will be a prescription from an appropriate practitioner (including a Patient Specific Direction), an exemption from the Human Medicines Regulations 2012 (Schedule 17 for registered paramedics, Schedule 19 for anyone for the purpose of saving a life in an emergency) or a Patient Group Direction (See Schedule 16).[1]
- The Human Medicines Regulations 2012 and the Misuse of Drugs Regulations 2001 provide the underpinning legislation that governs what paramedics can administer.
- A Patient Group Direction (PGD) is required when an exemption, prescription or Patient Specific Direction (PSD) does not exist. A PGD is a legal document which defines the treatment that can be administered or supplied to a pre-defined population of patients and any administration outside of the scope of the PGD has no legal authority. JRCALC may include a monograph for medicines that are not covered by the paramedic exemption, but the monograph is not a legal authority to administer. A PGD must be supplied by the employing organisation. PGDs are not transferrable. You cannot use a PGD which is specific to one trust if you work for any other provider. The paramedic cannot delegate administration under a PGD, for example, to a colleague or a student.
- Medicines are classified as follows:
  - **General sales list (GSL).** These may be purchased by the public from retail outlets etc. without a prescription.
  - **Pharmacy medicines (P).** These can be sold from a registered pharmacy without a prescription but under the supervision of a pharmacist or a person under the supervision of a pharmacist.
  - **Prescription only medicines (POMs).** These require a prescription from an appropriate practitioner to authorise their administration or supply. All controlled drugs are POM. In addition to the paramedic exemption (Schedule 17, HMR 2012) there are other exemptions including an exemption for administration by anyone in an emergency to save a life (Schedule 19, HMR 2012). It is important to recognise that there is a difference between parenteral and non-parenteral medicines in legislation. The legislation is silent on who may administer a non-parenteral medicine but very specific about who may administer a parenteral medicine.

1.1 Safety aspects

- Anyone administering a medicine must check before administration:
  - That they have the right medication, for the right patient, with the right dose, for the right route, for the right reason, with the right documentation. They must witness any preparation by a third party and not administer anything for which they are not prepared to take responsibility. Controlled drugs must be administered in line with relevant legislation, organisational policies and procedures.
  - The right medication: correct expiry date, legible label, no discolouration or other signs of deterioration, no allergies. The drug name, strength and form.
  - Right dose for your patient: include previous doses administered.
  - Right route: consider oral dosing if not time critical as parenteral doses introduce the risk of infection.
  - Whether the packaging is intact, and the labelling is legible.

TABLE 7.1 – Documentation

Note the following:	✓	✗
Avoid unnecessary use of decimal points	3 mg	3.0 mg
Quantities of 1 gram or more should be written as	1 g	
Quantities less than 1 gram should be written in milligrams	500 mg	0.5 g
Quantities less than 1 mg should be written in micrograms	100 micrograms	0.1 mg
When decimals are unavoidable a zero should be written in front of the decimal point where there is no other figure	0.5 ml	.5 ml
Use of the decimal point is acceptable to express a range	0.5 to 1 g	
'Micrograms' and 'nanograms' should not be abbreviated nor should 'units'		
The term 'millilitre' is used	ml or mL	cubic centimetre, c.c., or cm^3

a Paramedic is defined as being on the register of paramedics maintained by the Health and Care Professions Council pursuant to HMR 2012.

SECTION 7 Medicines

– Check ampoules for particulate contamination, discolouration or physical changes, e.g. separation of oil and water phase of diazepam emulsion.
– Low fluid volume which may indicate evaporation of fluid through a hairline crack.

- Whenever possible a second check must be obtained prior to administration to reduce the risk of error. Further guidance on administration is included in the individual medicine monographs.

1.2 Prescribing terms

In the case of prescription medicines, a variety of abbreviations are used, some of which are described – refer to Table 7.2.

NB Internationally recognised units and symbols should be used where possible.

1.3 Drug routes

- Drug routes are classified as **parenteral** and **non-parenteral**:
  – **Parenteral routes** are those where a physical breach of the skin or mucous membrane is made, for example, by injection.
  – **Non-parenteral routes** are those where the drug is absorbed passively, for example, via the gastrointestinal tract, mucous membranes or skin.
- Drugs can be administered via a number of routes – refer to Table 7.3. It is important that the most appropriate route is selected, taking into account the patient's condition and the urgency of the situation, refer to Table 7.4.
- Drugs and their possible routes of administration and the risk of introducing infection: all parenteral routes have a risk introducing infection. In the emergency setting, the IV route is commonly used to give direct access to the systemic circulation without the need for an absorption phase. It allows the medicine to act rapidly but carries the highest risk of introducing infection so good aseptic technique is important. In most cases intravenous cannulation should be attempted, except for children in cardiac arrest where intraosseous cannulation is the preferred method. **NB** If a vein cannot be found it is not necessary to attempt IV cannulation. With intramuscular and subcutaneous routes, absorption may be erratic or incomplete if the patient is hypovolaemic or clinically unstable.

1.4 Paediatric doses

- Paediatric drug doses are based on a child's **weight**, on a milligram per kilogram basis.
- When a child's weight **is** known, it is better to administer according to their **weight** rather than their **age**.
- Often the child's weight is **not** known; in these situations **Page For Age** can provide an estimated drug dose, calculated according to 'average' growth chart weights for child of a given age.
- When a child is clearly larger or smaller than would be expected for their age (their parents/carers will often be aware of this), an 'older' or 'younger' **Page For Age** chart should be selected for that child, dependent on the chart that most closely reflects their actual weight.

TABLE 7.2 – Common Abbreviations

Abbreviation	Translation
ac	ante cibum (before food)
approx	approximately
bd	twice daily
CD	controlled drug subject to the Misuse of Drugs Regulations 2001
ec	enteric-coated (termed gastro-resistant in British Pharmacopoeia)
f/c	film-coated
IM	intramuscular
IO	intraosseous
IV	intravenous
m/r	modified-release
MAOI	monoamine-oxidase inhibitors
NSAID	non-steroidal anti-inflammatory drug
o.d	omni die (every day)
o.m	omni mane (every morning)
o.n	omni nocte (every night)
p.c	post cibum (after food)
p.o	oral
PGD	patient group direction
POM	prescription only medicine
pr	per rectum (rectally)
prn	when required
q.d.s	quater die sumendus (to be taken four times daily)
q.q.h	quarta quaque hora (every four hours)
s/c	subcutaneous
SSRI	selective serotonin re-uptake inhibitor
SR	slow release
stat	immediately
t.d.s	ter die sumendus (to be taken three times daily)
top	topical

Medicines Overview

TABLE 7.3 – Drug Routes
Parenteral routes
Intramuscular – Injection of the drug into muscle, which is then absorbed into the blood. Absorption may be decreased in poor perfusion states, e.g. hypothermia.
Intraosseous – A rigid needle inserted directly into the bone marrow. Resuscitation drugs and fluid replacement may be administered by this route. Absorption is as quick as by the intravenous route.
Intravenous – Direct introduction of the drug into the cardiovascular system without an absorption phase. Delivers the drug to the target organs very quickly.
Subcutaneous – Injection of the drug into subcutaneous tissue. This usually has a slower rate of absorption than from intramuscular injection and may be decreased in poor perfusion states. Useful in palliative care.
Non-parenteral routes
Inhaled – Gaseous drugs that are absorbed via the lungs.
Nebulisation – Liquid drugs agitated in a stream of gas such as oxygen to create fine droplets that are absorbed rapidly from the lungs.
Oral – The drug is swallowed and is absorbed into the blood from the gut. Absorption dependent. In serious trauma or illness, absorption may be delayed.
Rectal – The drug is absorbed from the wall of the rectum. This route is used for patients who are having seizures and who cannot be cannulated without risk to themselves or ambulance personnel. Effects usually occur 5–15 minutes after administration.
Sub-lingual – Tablet or aerosol spray is absorbed from the mucous membrane beneath the tongue. Effects usually occur within 2–3 minutes. Avoids first pass metabolism for GTN.
Transdermal – Absorption of a drug through the skin.
Buccal – Absorption via the mucous membrane.
Intranasal – Aerosol spray absorbed from the mucous membrane

TABLE 7.4 – Suggested Drug Routes

Drug/Route	**IV**	**IO**	**IM**	**SC**	**Oral**	**Sub-lingual**	**Buccal**	**Intranasal**	**Rectal**	**Inhaled**	**Nebulised**	**Transdermal**	**Flush**
Activated charcoal	N/A	N/A	N/A	N/A	✓	N/A	N/A	N/A	N/A	N/A	N/A	N/A	N/A
Adrenaline 1 in 10,000	✓	✓	N/A	N/A	N/A	N/A	N/A	N/A	N/A	N/A	N/A	N/A	N/A
Adrenaline 1 in 1,000	N/A	N/A	✓	✓	N/A	N/A	N/A	N/A	N/A	N/A	N/A	N/A	N/A
Amiodarone	✓	✓	N/A	N/A	N/A	N/A	N/A	N/A	N/A	N/A	N/A	N/A	N/A
Aspirin	N/A	N/A	N/A	N/A	✓	N/A	N/A	N/A	N/A	N/A	N/A	N/A	N/A
Atropine	✓	✓	N/A	N/A	N/A	N/A	N/A	N/A	N/A	N/A	N/A	N/A	N/A
Atropine (CBRNE)	N/A	N/A	✓	N/A	N/A	N/A	N/A	N/A	N/A	N/A	N/A	N/A	N/A
Benzylpenicillin	✓	✓	✓	N/A	N/A	N/A	N/A	N/A	N/A	N/A	N/A	N/A	N/A
Chlorphenamine	✓	✓	✓	N/A	✓	N/A	N/A	N/A	N/A	N/A	N/A	N/A	N/A
Clopidogrel	N/A	N/A	N/A	N/A	✓	N/A	N/A	N/A	N/A	N/A	N/A	N/A	N/A
Dexamethasone	N/A	N/A	N/A	N/A	✓	N/A	N/A	N/A	N/A	N/A	N/A	N/A	N/A
Diazepam*	✓	✓	N/A	N/A	N/A	N/A	N/A	N/A	✓	N/A	N/A	N/A	N/A
Entonox	N/A	N/A	N/A	N/A	N/A	N/A	N/A	N/A	N/A	✓	N/A	N/A	N/A
Furosemide	✓	N/A	N/A	N/A	N/A	N/A	N/A	N/A	N/A	N/A	N/A	N/A	N/A
Glucagon	N/A	N/A	✓	N/A	N/A	N/A	N/A	N/A	N/A	N/A	N/A	N/A	N/A
Glucose 10%	✓	✓	N/A	N/A	N/A	N/A	N/A	N/A	N/A	N/A	N/A	N/A	N/A
Glucose 40% gel	N/A	N/A	N/A	N/A	N/A	N/A	✓	N/A	N/A	N/A	N/A	N/A	N/A
Glyceryl trinitrate	N/A	N/A	N/A	N/A	N/A	✓	✓	N/A	N/A	N/A	N/A	N/A	N/A
Heparin*	✓	✓	N/A	N/A	N/A	N/A	N/A	N/A	N/A	N/A	N/A	N/A	N/A

Medicines Overview

TABLE 7.4 – Suggested Drug Routes *(continued)*													
Drug/Route	**IV**	**IO**	**IM**	**SC**	**Oral**	**Sub-lingual**	**Buccal**	**Intranasal**	**Rectal**	**Inhaled**	**Nebulised**	**Transdermal**	**Flush**
Hydrocortisone	✓	✓	✓	N/A	N/A	N/A	N/A	N/A	N/A	N/A	N/A	N/A	N/A
Ibuprofen	N/A	N/A	N/A	N/A	✓	N/A	N/A	N/A	N/A	N/A	N/A	N/A	N/A
Ipratropium bromide	N/A	N/A	N/A	N/A	N/A	N/A	N/A	N/A	N/A	N/A	✓	N/A	N/A
Ketamine	✓	✓	✓	N/A	N/A	N/A	N/A	N/A	N/A	N/A	N/A	N/A	N/A
Metoclopramide	✓	✓	✓	N/A	N/A	N/A	N/A	N/A	N/A	N/A	N/A	N/A	N/A
Midazolam*	✓	✓	N/A	N/A	N/A	N/A	✓	✓	N/A	N/A	N/A	N/A	N/A
Misoprostol	N/A	N/A	N/A	N/A	✓	✓	N/A	N/A	✓	N/A	N/A	N/A	N/A
Morphine sulfate	✓	✓	✓	✓	✓	N/A	N/A	N/A	N/A	N/A	N/A	N/A	N/A
Naloxone hydrochloride	✓	✓	✓	✓	N/A	N/A	N/A	✓	N/A	N/A	N/A	N/A	N/A
Ondansetron	✓	✓	✓	N/A	N/A	N/A	N/A	N/A	N/A	N/A	N/A	N/A	N/A
Oxygen	N/A	N/A	N/A	N/A	N/A	N/A	N/A	N/A	N/A	✓	N/A	N/A	N/A
Paracetamol	✓	✓	N/A	N/A	✓	N/A	N/A	N/A	N/A	N/A	N/A	N/A	N/A
Salbutamol	N/A	N/A	N/A	N/A	N/A	N/A	N/A	N/A	N/A	✓	✓	N/A	N/A
0.9% Sodium chloride	✓	✓	N/A	N/A	N/A	N/A	N/A	N/A	N/A	N/A	N/A	N/A	✓
Sodium lactate	✓	✓	N/A	N/A	N/A	N/A	N/A	N/A	N/A	N/A	N/A	N/A	N/A
Syntometrine	N/A	N/A	✓	N/A	N/A	N/A	N/A	N/A	N/A	N/A	N/A	N/A	N/A
Tenecteplase*	✓	N/A	N/A	N/A	N/A	N/A	N/A	N/A	N/A	N/A	N/A	N/A	N/A
Tranexamic acid*	✓	✓	N/A	N/A	N/A	N/A	N/A	N/A	N/A	N/A	N/A	N/A	N/A

*These medicines require a PGD.

KEY POINTS!

Medicines Overview

- **Before administration, always check the drug type, strength, that the label is legible, there is no damage to packaging that could have allowed deterioration, i.e. exposure to light or moisture, the clarity of fluid and the expiry date.**
- **Select the most appropriate route taking into account the patient's condition and the urgency of the situation.**
- **Whenever possible a second check by another member of staff must be obtained prior to administration. Do not administer anything unless you have seen the container from which the medicine originated. The person who administers is responsible for administration, regardless of whether or not they actually prepared the drug.**
- **Only administer drugs via the routes you have been trained to use.**
- **The drug codes are provided for INFORMATION ONLY.**
- **All medicine administration records must be complete, accurate and timely.**

Bibliography

1. The British National Formulary, British National Formulary for Children. Available from: http://www.bnf.org/bnf/index.htm, 2019.
2. UK Government. *The Human Medicines Regulations 2012*. London: The National Archives, 2012.
3. Royal Pharmaceutical Society. *Professional Guidance on the Administration of Medicines in Healthcare Settings*. London: RPS, 2019.
4. Royal Pharmaceutical Society. *Professional guidance on the safe and secure handling of medicines*. London: RPS, 2018.
5. National Institute for Health and Clinical Excellence. *Patient Group Directions. London: NICE, 2017.* Available from: https://www.nice.org.uk/guidance/mpg2

Adrenaline 1 milligram in 10 ml (1 in 10,000) ADX

Presentation

Pre-filled syringe containing 1 milligram of adrenaline (epinephrine) in 10 ml (1:10,000) ADX.

Indications

Cardiac arrest.

Actions

Adrenaline is a sympathomimetic that stimulates both alpha- and beta-adrenergic receptors.
As a result myocardial and cerebral blood flow is enhanced during CPR and CPR becomes more effective due to increased peripheral resistance which improves perfusion pressures.

Reverses allergic manifestations of acute anaphylaxis.

Relieves bronchospasm in acute severe asthma.

Cautions

Severe hypertension may occur in patients on non-cardioselective beta-blockers (e.g. propranolol).

Do **NOT** give repeated doses of adrenaline in hypothermic patients.

Dosage and Administration

Cardiac arrest:

- **Shockable rhythms:** administer adrenaline after the 3rd shock and then after alternate shocks (i.e. 5th, 7th etc).
- **Non-shockable rhythms:** administer adrenaline immediately IV access is achieved then alternate loops.

Route: Intravenous/intraosseous – **administer as a rapid bolus.**

AGE	INITIAL DOSE	REPEAT DOSE	DOSE INTERVAL	CONCENTRATION	VOLUME	MAX DOSE
≥12 years and adult	1 milligram	1 milligram	3–5 minutes	1 milligram in 10 ml (1:10,000)	10 ml	No limit
11 years	350 micrograms	350 micrograms	3–5 minutes	1 milligram in 10 ml (1:10,000)	3.5 ml	No limit
10 years	320 micrograms	320 micrograms	3–5 minutes	1 milligram in 10 ml (1:10,000)	3.2 ml	No limit
9 years	300 micrograms	300 micrograms	3–5 minutes	1 milligram in 10 ml (1:10,000)	3 ml	No limit
8 years	260 micrograms	260 micrograms	3–5 minutes	1 milligram in 10 ml (1:10,000)	2.6 ml	No limit
7 years	230 micrograms	230 micrograms	3–5 minutes	1 milligram in 10 ml (1:10,000)	2.3 ml	No limit
6 years	210 micrograms	210 micrograms	3–5 minutes	1 milligram in 10 ml (1:10,000)	2.1 ml	No limit
5 years	190 micrograms	190 micrograms	3–5 minutes	1 milligram in 10 ml (1:10,000)	1.9 ml	No limit
4 years	160 micrograms	160 micrograms	3–5 minutes	1 milligram in 10 ml (1:10,000)	1.6 ml	No limit
3 years	140 micrograms	140 micrograms	3–5 minutes	1 milligram in 10 ml (1:10,000)	1.4 ml	No limit
2 years	120 micrograms	120 micrograms	3–5 minutes	1 milligram in 10 ml (1:10,000)	1.2 ml	No limit
18 months	110 micrograms	110 micrograms	3–5 minutes	1 milligram in 10 ml (1:10,000)	1.1 ml	No limit
12 months	100 micrograms	100 micrograms	3–5 minutes	1 milligram in 10 ml (1:10,000)	1 ml	No limit

Adrenaline 1 milligram in 10 ml (1 in 10,000) ADX

AGE	INITIAL DOSE	REPEAT DOSE	DOSE INTERVAL	CONCENTRATION	VOLUME	MAX DOSE
9 months	90 micrograms	90 micrograms	3–5 minutes	1 milligram in 10 ml (1:10,000)	0.9 ml	No limit
6 months	80 micrograms	80 micrograms	3–5 minutes	1 milligram in 10 ml (1:10,000)	0.8 ml	No limit
3 months	60 micrograms	60 micrograms	3–5 minutes	1 milligram in 10 ml (1:10,000)	0.6 ml	No limit
1 month	50 micrograms	50 micrograms	3–5 minutes	1 milligram in 10 ml (1:10,000)	0.5 ml	No limit
Birth	35 micrograms	35 micrograms	3–5 minutes	1 milligram in 10 ml (1:10,000)	0.35 ml	No limit

Bibliography

National Institute for Health and Care Excellence. Adrenaline/Epinephrine. Available from: https://bnf.nice.org.uk/drug/adrenalineepinephrine.html, 2018.

Amiodarone Hydrochloride

AMO

Presentation

Pre-filled syringe containing 300 milligrams amiodarone in 10 ml.

Indications

Cardiac arrest

- **Shockable rhythms:** if unresponsive to defibrillation administer amiodarone after the 3rd shock and an additional bolus depending on age to unresponsive VF or pulseless VT following the 5th shock.

Actions

Antiarrhythmic; lengthens cardiac action potential and therefore effective refractory period. Prolongs QT interval on ECG.

Blocks sodium and potassium channels in cardiac muscle.

Acts to stabilise and reduce electrical irritability of cardiac muscle.

Contra-indications

No contra-indications in the context of the treatment of cardiac arrest.

Side Effects

Bradycardia.

Vasodilatation causing hypotension, flushing.

Bronchospasm.

Arrhythmias – Torsades de pointes.

Dosage and Administration

- Administer into large vein as extravasation can cause burns.
- Follow administration with a 0.9% sodium chloride flush – refer to **0.9% Sodium Chloride**.
- Cardiac arrest – Shockable rhythms: if unresponsive to defibrillation administer amiodarone after the 3rd shock.

Route: intravenous/intraosseous – **administer as a rapid bolus.**

AGE	INITIAL DOSE	REPEAT DOSE	DOSE INTERVAL	CONCEN-TRATION	VOLUME	MAX DOSE
Adult	300 milligrams (After 3rd shock)	150 milligrams	After 5th shock	300 milligrams in 10 ml	10 ml	450 milligrams
11 years	180 milligrams (After 3rd shock)	180 milligrams	After 5th shock	300 milligrams in 10 ml	6 ml	360 milligrams
10 years	160 milligrams (After 3rd shock)	160 milligrams	After 5th shock	300 milligrams in 10 ml	5.3 ml	320 milligrams
9 years	150 milligrams (After 3rd shock)	150 milligrams	After 5th shock	300 milligrams in 10 ml	5 ml	300 milligrams
8 years	130 milligrams (After 3rd shock)	130 milligrams	After 5th shock	300 milligrams in 10 ml	4.3 ml	260 milligrams
7 years	120 milligrams (After 3rd shock)	120 milligrams	After 5th shock	300 milligrams in 10 ml	4 ml	240 milligrams
6 years	100 milligrams (After 3rd shock)	100 milligrams	After 5th shock	300 milligrams in 10 ml	3.3 ml	200 milligrams
5 years	100 milligrams (After 3rd shock)	100 milligrams	After 5th shock	300 milligrams in 10 ml	3.3 ml	200 milligrams
4 years	80 milligrams (After 3rd shock)	80 milligrams	After 5th shock	300 milligrams in 10 ml	2.7 ml	160 milligrams

AGE	INITIAL DOSE	REPEAT DOSE	DOSE INTERVAL	CONCEN-TRATION	VOLUME	MAX DOSE
3 years	70 milligrams (After 3rd shock)	70 milligrams	After 5th shock	300 milligrams in 10 ml	2.3 ml	140 milligrams
2 years	60 milligrams (After 3rd shock)	60 milligrams	After 5th shock	300 milligrams in 10 ml	2 ml	120 milligrams
18 months	55 milligrams (After 3rd shock)	55 milligrams	After 5th shock	300 milligrams in 10 ml	1.8 ml	110 milligrams
12 months	50 milligrams (After 3rd shock)	50 milligrams	After 5th shock	300 milligrams in 10 ml	1.7 ml	100 milligrams
9 months	45 milligrams (After 3rd shock)	45 milligrams	After 5th shock	300 milligrams in 10 ml	1.5 ml	90 milligrams
6 months	40 milligrams (After 3rd shock)	40 milligrams	After 5th shock	300 milligrams in 10 ml	1.3 ml	80 milligrams
3 months	30 milligrams (After 3rd shock)	30 milligrams	After 5th shock	300 milligrams in 10 ml	1 ml	60 milligrams
1 month	25 milligrams (After 3rd shock)	25 milligrams	After 5th shock	300 milligrams in 10 ml	0.8 ml	50 milligrams
Birth	N/A	N/A	N/A	N/A	N/A	N/A

Bibliography

British National Formulary. Amiodarone Hydrochloride. Available from: https://bnf.nice.org.uk/drug/amiodarone-hydrochloride.html, 2018.

Route: Intravenous/intraosseous **administer as a rapid bolus**.

600 micrograms per ml

AGE	INITIAL DOSE	REPEAT DOSE	DOSE INTERVAL	CONCENTRATION	VOLUME	MAX DOSE	NOTE
≥12 years	600 micrograms	600 micrograms	3–5 minutes	600 micrograms per ml	1 ml	3 milligrams	The adult dosage can be given as 500 or 600 micrograms to a maximum of 3 milligrams depending on presentation available.
11 years	500 micrograms	NONE	N/A	600 micrograms per ml	0.8 ml	500 micrograms	
10 years	500 micrograms	NONE	N/A	600 micrograms per ml	0.8 ml	500 micrograms	
9 years	500 micrograms	NONE	N/A	600 micrograms per ml	0.8 ml	500 micrograms	
8 years	500 micrograms	NONE	N/A	600 micrograms per ml	0.8 ml	500 micrograms	
7 years	400 micrograms	NONE	N/A	600 micrograms per ml	0.7 ml	400 micrograms	
6 years	400 micrograms	NONE	N/A	600 micrograms per ml	0.7 ml	400 micrograms	
5 years	300 micrograms	NONE	N/A	600 micrograms per ml	0.5 ml	300 micrograms	
4 years	300 micrograms	NONE	N/A	600 micrograms per ml	0.5 ml	300 micrograms	
3 years	240 micrograms	NONE	N/A	600 micrograms per ml	0.4 ml	240 micrograms	
2 years	240 micrograms	NONE	N/A	600 micrograms per ml	0.4 ml	240 micrograms	
18 months	200 micrograms	NONE	N/A	600 micrograms per ml	0.3 ml	200 micrograms	
12 months	200 micrograms	NONE	N/A	600 micrograms per ml	0.3 ml	200 micrograms	
9 months	120 micrograms	NONE	N/A	600 micrograms per ml	0.2 ml	120 micrograms	
6 months	120 micrograms	NONE	N/A	600 micrograms per ml	0.2 ml	120 micrograms	
3 months	120 micrograms	NONE	N/A	600 micrograms per ml	0.2 ml	120 micrograms	
1 month	90 micrograms	NONE	N/A	600 micrograms per ml	0.15 ml	90 micrograms	
Birth	60 micrograms	NONE	N/A	600 micrograms per ml	0.1 ml	60 micrograms	

Route: Intravenous/intraosseous **administer as a rapid bolus.**

300 micrograms per ml

AGE	INITIAL DOSE	REPEAT DOSE	DOSE INTERVAL	CONCENTRATION	VOLUME	MAX DOSE	NOTE
≥12 years	600 micrograms	600 micrograms	3–5 minutes	300 micrograms per ml	2 ml	3 milligrams	The adult dosage can be given as 500 or 600 micrograms to a maximum of 3 milligrams depending on presentation available.
11 years	500 micrograms	NONE	N/A	300 micrograms per ml	1.7 ml	500 micrograms	
10 years	500 micrograms	NONE	N/A	300 micrograms per ml	1.7 ml	500 micrograms	
9 years	500 micrograms	NONE	N/A	300 micrograms per ml	1.7 ml	500 micrograms	
8 years	500 micrograms	NONE	N/A	300 micrograms per ml	1.7 ml	500 micrograms	
7 years	400 micrograms	NONE	N/A	300 micrograms per ml	1.3 ml	400 micrograms	
6 years	400 micrograms	NONE	N/A	300 micrograms per ml	1.3 ml	400 micrograms	
5 years	300 micrograms	NONE	N/A	300 micrograms per ml	1 ml	300 micrograms	
4 years	300 micrograms	NONE	N/A	300 micrograms per ml	1 ml	300 micrograms	
3 years	240 micrograms	NONE	N/A	300 micrograms per ml	0.8 ml	240 micrograms	
2 years	240 micrograms	NONE	N/A	300 micrograms per ml	0.8 ml	240 micrograms	
18 months	200 micrograms	NONE	N/A	300 micrograms per ml	0.7 ml	200 micrograms	
12 months	200 micrograms	NONE	N/A	300 micrograms per ml	0.7 ml	200 micrograms	
9 months	120 micrograms	NONE	N/A	300 micrograms per ml	0.4 ml	120 micrograms	
6 months	120 micrograms	NONE	N/A	300 micrograms per ml	0.4 ml	120 micrograms	
3 months	120 micrograms	NONE	N/A	300 micrograms per ml	0.4 ml	120 micrograms	
1 month	90 micrograms	NONE	N/A	300 micrograms per ml	0.3 ml	90 micrograms	
Birth	60 micrograms	NONE	N/A	300 micrograms per ml	0.2 ml	60 micrograms	

Route: Intravenous/intraosseous **administer as a rapid bolus**.

200 micrograms per ml

AGE	INITIAL DOSE	REPEAT DOSE	DOSE INTERVAL	CONCENTRATION	VOLUME	MAX DOSE	NOTE
≥12 years	600 micrograms	600 micrograms	3–5 minutes	200 micrograms per ml	3 ml	3 milligrams	The adult dosage can be given as 500 or 600 micrograms to a maximum of 3 milligrams depending on presentation available.
11 years	500 micrograms	NONE	N/A	200 micrograms per ml	2.5 ml	500 micrograms	
10 years	500 micrograms	NONE	N/A	200 micrograms per ml	2.5 ml	500 micrograms	
9 years	500 micrograms	NONE	N/A	200 micrograms per ml	2.5 ml	500 micrograms	
8 years	500 micrograms	NONE	N/A	200 micrograms per ml	2.5 ml	500 micrograms	
7 years	400 micrograms	NONE	N/A	200 micrograms per ml	2 ml	400 micrograms	
6 years	400 micrograms	NONE	N/A	200 micrograms per ml	2 ml	400 micrograms	
5 years	300 micrograms	NONE	N/A	200 micrograms per ml	1.5 ml	300 micrograms	
4 years	300 micrograms	NONE	N/A	200 micrograms per ml	1.5 ml	300 micrograms	
3 years	240 micrograms	NONE	N/A	200 micrograms per ml	1.2 ml	240 micrograms	
2 years	240 micrograms	NONE	N/A	200 micrograms per ml	1.2 ml	240 micrograms	
18 months	200 micrograms	NONE	N/A	200 micrograms per ml	1 ml	200 micrograms	
12 months	200 micrograms	NONE	N/A	200 micrograms per ml	1 ml	200 micrograms	
9 months	120 micrograms	NONE	N/A	200 micrograms per ml	0.6 ml	120 micrograms	
6 months	120 micrograms	NONE	N/A	200 micrograms per ml	0.6 ml	120 micrograms	
3 months	120 micrograms	NONE	N/A	200 micrograms per ml	0.6 ml	120 micrograms	
1 month	100 micrograms	NONE	N/A	200 micrograms per ml	0.5 ml	100 micrograms	
Birth	80 micrograms	NONE	N/A	200 micrograms per ml	0.4 ml	80 micrograms	

Route: Intravenous/intraosseous **administer as a rapid bolus**.

100 micrograms per ml

AGE	INITIAL DOSE	REPEAT DOSE	DOSE INTERVAL	CONCENTRATION	VOLUME	MAX DOSE	NOTE
≥12 years	600 micrograms	600 micrograms	3–5 minutes	100 micrograms per ml	6 ml	3 milligrams	The adult dosage can be given as 500 or 600 micrograms to a maximum of 3 milligrams depending on presentation available.
11 years	500 micrograms	NONE	N/A	100 micrograms per ml	5 ml	500 micrograms	
10 years	500 micrograms	NONE	N/A	100 micrograms per ml	5 ml	500 micrograms	
9 years	500 micrograms	NONE	N/A	100 micrograms per ml	5 ml	500 micrograms	
8 years	500 micrograms	NONE	N/A	100 micrograms per ml	5 ml	500 micrograms	
7 years	400 micrograms	NONE	N/A	100 micrograms per ml	4 ml	400 micrograms	
6 years	400 micrograms	NONE	N/A	100 micrograms per ml	4 ml	400 micrograms	
5 years	300 micrograms	NONE	N/A	100 micrograms per ml	3 ml	300 micrograms	
4 years	300 micrograms	NONE	N/A	100 micrograms per ml	3 ml	300 micrograms	
3 years	240 micrograms	NONE	N/A	100 micrograms per ml	2.4 ml	240 micrograms	
2 years	240 micrograms	NONE	N/A	100 micrograms per ml	2.4 ml	240 micrograms	
18 months	200 micrograms	NONE	N/A	100 micrograms per ml	2 ml	200 micrograms	
12 months	200 micrograms	NONE	N/A	100 micrograms per ml	2 ml	200 micrograms	
9 months	120 micrograms	NONE	N/A	100 micrograms per ml	1.2 ml	120 micrograms	
6 months	120 micrograms	NONE	N/A	100 micrograms per ml	1.2 ml	120 micrograms	
3 months	120 micrograms	NONE	N/A	100 micrograms per ml	1.2 ml	120 micrograms	
1 month	90 micrograms	NONE	N/A	100 micrograms per ml	0.9 ml	90 micrograms	
Birth	70 micrograms	NONE	N/A	100 micrograms per ml	0.7 ml	70 micrograms	

Presentation

Injection vial containing 600 milligrams of benzylpenicillin sodium as powder for solution for injection.

Injection vial containing 1.2 gram of benzylpenicillin sodium powder for solution for injection.

Administered intravenously, intraosseously or intramuscularly.

NB Different concentrations and volumes of administration (refer to dosage and administration tables).

Indications

Suspected meningococcal disease in the presence of:

1 a non-blanching rash (the classical, haemorrhagic, non-blanching rash (may be petechial or purpuric)

and/or

2 signs/symptoms suggestive of meningococcal septicaemia (refer to **Meningococcal Meningitis and Septicaemia** for signs/symptoms).

Actions

Antibiotic: narrow-spectrum.

Contra-indications

Known severe penicillin allergy (more than a simple rash alone).

Additional Information

- Meningococcal septicaemia is commonest in children and young adults.
- It may be rapidly progressive and fatal.
- Early administration of benzylpenicillin improves outcome.
- Two sites should be used for IM injection when administering more than 2ml of volume.

Dosage and Administration

Administer en-route to hospital (unless already administered).

NB IV/IO and IM concentrations are different and have different volumes of administration.

Route: Intravenous/intraosseous – by slow injection.

AGE	INITIAL DOSE	REPEAT DOSE	DOSE INTERVAL	CONCENTRATION	VOLUME	MAX DOSE
Adult	1.2 grams	NONE	N/A	1.2 grams dissolved in 20 ml water for injection	20 ml	1.2 grams
11 years	1.2 grams	NONE	N/A	1.2 grams dissolved in 20 ml water for injection	20 ml	1.2 grams
10 years	1.2 grams	NONE	N/A	1.2 grams dissolved in 20 ml water for injection	20 ml	1.2 grams
9 years	600 milligrams	NONE	N/A	600 milligrams dissolved in 10 ml water for injection	10 ml	600 milligrams
8 years	600 milligrams	NONE	N/A	600 milligrams dissolved in 10 ml water for injection	10 ml	600 milligrams
7 years	600 milligrams	NONE	N/A	600 milligrams dissolved in 10 ml water for injection	10 ml	600 milligrams
6 years	600 milligrams	NONE	N/A	600 milligrams dissolved in 10 ml water for injection	10 ml	600 milligrams
5 years	600 milligrams	NONE	N/A	600 milligrams dissolved in 10 ml water for injection	10 ml	600 milligrams
4 years	600 milligrams	NONE	N/A	600 milligrams dissolved in 10 ml water for injection	10 ml	600 milligrams

AGE	INITIAL DOSE	REPEAT DOSE	DOSE INTERVAL	CONCENTRATION	VOLUME	MAX DOSE
3 years	600 milligrams	NONE	N/A	600 milligrams dissolved in 10 ml water for injection	10 ml	600 milligrams
2 years	600 milligrams	NONE	N/A	600 milligrams dissolved in 10 ml water for injection	10 ml	600 milligrams
18 months	600 milligrams	NONE	N/A	600 milligrams dissolved in 10 ml water for injection	10 ml	600 milligrams
12 months	600 milligrams	NONE	N/A	600 milligrams dissolved in 10 ml water for injection	10 ml	600 milligrams
9 months	300 milligrams	NONE	N/A	600 milligrams dissolved in 10 ml water for injection	5 ml	300 milligrams
6 months	300 milligrams	NONE	N/A	600 milligrams dissolved in 10 ml water for injection	5 ml	300 milligrams
3 months	300 milligrams	NONE	N/A	600 milligrams dissolved in 10 ml water for injection	5 ml	300 milligrams
1 month	300 milligrams	NONE	N/A	600 milligrams dissolved in 10 ml water for injection	5 ml	300 milligrams
Birth	300 milligrams	NONE	N/A	600 milligrams dissolved in 10 ml water for injection	5 ml	300 milligrams

Route: Intramuscular (antero-lateral aspect of thigh or upper arm – preferably in a well perfused area) if rapid intravascular access cannot be obtained.

AGE	INITIAL DOSE	REPEAT DOSE	DOSE INTERVAL	CONCENTRATION	VOLUME	MAX DOSE
Adult	1.2 grams	NONE	N/A	1.2 grams dissolved in 4 ml water for injection	4 ml	1.2 grams
11 years	1.2 grams	NONE	N/A	1.2 grams dissolved in 4 ml water for injection	4 ml	1.2 grams
10 years	1.2 grams	NONE	N/A	1.2 grams dissolved in 4 ml water for injection	4 ml	1.2 grams
9 years	600 milligrams	NONE	N/A	600 milligrams dissolved in 2 ml water for injection	2 ml	600 milligrams
8 years	600 milligrams	NONE	N/A	600 milligrams dissolved in 2 ml water for injection	2 ml	600 milligrams

Benzylpenicillin Sodium

AGE	INITIAL DOSE	REPEAT DOSE	DOSE INTERVAL	CONCENTRATION	VOLUME	MAX DOSE
7 years	600 milligrams	NONE	N/A	600 milligrams dissolved in 2 ml water for injection	2 ml	600 milligrams
6 years	600 milligrams	NONE	N/A	600 milligrams dissolved in 2 ml water for injection	2 ml	600 milligrams
5 years	600 milligrams	NONE	N/A	600 milligrams dissolved in 2 ml water for injection	2 ml	600 milligrams
4 years	600 milligrams	NONE	N/A	600 milligrams dissolved in 2 ml water for injection	2 ml	600 milligrams
3 years	600 milligrams	NONE	N/A	600 milligrams dissolved in 2 ml water for injection	2 ml	600 milligrams
2 years	600 milligrams	NONE	N/A	600 milligrams dissolved in 2 ml water for injection	2 ml	600 milligrams
18 months	600 milligrams	NONE	N/A	600 milligrams dissolved in 2 ml water for injection	2 ml	600 milligrams
12 months	600 milligrams	NONE	N/A	600 milligrams dissolved in 2 ml water for injection	2 ml	600 milligrams
9 months	300 milligrams	NONE	N/A	600 milligrams dissolved in 2 ml water for injection	1 ml	300 milligrams
6 months	300 milligrams	NONE	N/A	600 milligrams dissolved in 2 ml water for injection	1 ml	300 milligrams
3 months	300 milligrams	NONE	N/A	600 milligrams dissolved in 2 ml water for injection	1 ml	300 milligrams
1 month	300 milligrams	NONE	N/A	600 milligrams dissolved in 2 ml water for injection	1 ml	300 milligrams
Birth	300 milligrams	NONE	N/A	600 milligrams dissolved in 2 ml water for injection	1 ml	300 milligrams

Bibliography

British National Formulary. Benzylpenicillin Sodium. Available from: https://bnf.nice.org.uk/drug/benzylpenicillin-sodium.html, 2018.

Chlorphenamine

CPH

Presentation

Ampoule containing 10 milligrams of chlorphenamine maleate in 1 ml.

Tablet containing 4 milligrams of chlorphenamine maleate.

Oral solution containing 2 milligrams of chlorphenamine maleate in 5 ml.

Indications

Severe anaphylactic reactions after initial resuscitation.

Symptomatic allergic reactions falling short of anaphylaxis but causing patient distress (e.g. severe itching).

Actions

An antihistamine with anticholingergic properties that blocks the effect of histamine released during a hypersensitivity (allergic) reaction.

Contra-indications

Known hypersensitivity.

The anticholinergic properties of chlorphenamine are intensified by monoamine oxidase inhibitors (MAOIs). Chlorphenamine injection is therefore contraindicated in patients who have been treated with MAOIs within the last fourteen days.

Cautions

Pregnancy and breastfeeding.

Hypotension.

Epilepsy.

Glaucoma.

Severe liver disease.

Side Effects

Sedation.

Dry mouth.

Headache.

Blurred vision.

Urinary retention.

Psychomotor impairment.

Gastrointestinal disturbance.

Convulsions (rare).

Children and older people are more likely to suffer side effects.

Warn anyone receiving chlorphenamine against driving or undertaking any other complex psychomotor task, due to the sedative and psychomotor side effects.

With the intravenous preparation, transient hypotension, central nervous system (CNS) stimulation and irritant effects.

Dosage and Administration

Route: Intravenous/intraosseous/intramuscular. The IV route is the preferred route for anaphylaxis, given SLOWLY over 1 minute. Small doses can be diluted with sodium chloride 0.9%.

AGE	INITIAL DOSE	REPEAT DOSE	DOSE INTERVAL	CONCENTRATION	VOLUME	MAX DOSE
≥ 12 years	10 milligrams	NONE	N/A	10 milligrams in 1 ml	1 ml	10 milligrams
11 years	5 milligrams	NONE	N/A	10 milligrams in 1 ml	0.5 ml	5 milligrams
10 years	5 milligrams	NONE	N/A	10 milligrams in 1 ml	0.5 ml	5 milligrams
9 years	5 milligrams	NONE	N/A	10 milligrams in 1 ml	0.5 ml	5 milligrams
8 years	5 milligrams	NONE	N/A	10 milligrams in 1 ml	0.5 ml	5 milligrams
7 years	5 milligrams	NONE	N/A	10 milligrams in 1 ml	0.5 ml	5 milligrams
6 years	5 milligrams	NONE	N/A	10 milligrams in 1 ml	0.5 ml	5 milligrams
5 years	2.5 milligrams	NONE	N/A	10 milligrams in 1 ml	0.25 ml	2.5 milligrams
4 years	2.5 milligrams	NONE	N/A	10 milligrams in 1 ml	0.25 ml	2.5 milligrams
3 years	2.5 milligrams	NONE	N/A	10 milligrams in 1 ml	0.25 ml	2.5 milligrams
2 years	2.5 milligrams	NONE	N/A	10 milligrams in 1 ml	0.25 ml	2.5 milligrams
18 months	2.5 milligrams	NONE	N/A	10 milligrams in 1 ml	0.25 ml	2.5 milligrams
12 months	2.5 milligrams	NONE	N/A	10 milligrams in 1 ml	0.25 ml	2.5 milligrams
9 months	2.5 milligrams	NONE	N/A	10 milligrams in 1 ml	0.25 ml	2.5 milligrams
6 months	2.5 milligrams	NONE	N/A	10 milligrams in 1 ml	0.25 ml	2.5 milligrams
3 months	1 milligram	N/A	N/A	10 milligrams in 1 ml	0.1 ml	1 milligram
1 month	1 milligram	N/A	N/A	10 milligrams in 1 ml	0.1 ml	1 milligram
Birth	N/A	N/A	N/A	N/A	N/A	N/A

Route: Oral 4 milligram tablet.

AGE	INITIAL DOSE	REPEAT DOSE	DOSE INTERVAL	CONCENTRATION	VOLUME	MAX DOSE
≥ 12 years	4 milligrams	NONE	N/A	4 milligrams per tablet	1 tablet	4 milligrams
11 years	2 milligrams	NONE	N/A	4 milligrams per tablet	½ of one tablet	2 milligrams
10 years	2 milligrams	NONE	N/A	4 milligrams per tablet	½ of one tablet	2 milligrams
9 years	2 milligrams	NONE	N/A	4 milligrams per tablet	½ of one tablet	2 milligrams
8 years	2 milligrams	NONE	N/A	4 milligrams per tablet	½ of one tablet	2 milligrams
7 years	2 milligrams	NONE	N/A	4 milligrams per tablet	½ of one tablet	2 milligrams
6 years	2 milligrams	NONE	N/A	4 milligrams per tablet	½ of one tablet	2 milligrams
5 years	N/A	N/A	N/A	N/A	N/A	N/A
4 years	N/A	N/A	N/A	N/A	N/A	N/A
3 years	N/A	N/A	N/A	N/A	N/A	N/A
2 years	N/A	N/A	N/A	N/A	N/A	N/A
18 months	N/A	N/A	N/A	N/A	N/A	N/A
12 months	N/A	N/A	N/A	N/A	N/A	N/A
9 months	N/A	N/A	N/A	N/A	N/A	N/A
6 months	N/A	N/A	N/A	N/A	N/A	N/A
3 months	N/A	N/A	N/A	N/A	N/A	N/A
1 month	N/A	N/A	N/A	N/A	N/A	N/A
Birth	N/A	N/A	N/A	N/A	N/A	N/A

Route: Oral 2 milligrams in 5 ml solution.

AGE	INITIAL DOSE	REPEAT DOSE	DOSE INTERVAL	CONCENTRATION	VOLUME	MAX DOSE
≥ 12 years	4 milligrams	NONE	N/A	2 milligrams in 5 ml	10 ml	4 milligrams
11 years	2 milligrams	NONE	N/A	2 milligrams in 5 ml	5 ml	2 milligrams
10 years	2 milligrams	NONE	N/A	2 milligrams in 5 ml	5 ml	2 milligrams
9 years	2 milligrams	NONE	N/A	2 milligrams in 5 ml	5 ml	2 milligrams
8 years	2 milligrams	NONE	N/A	2 milligrams in 5 ml	5 ml	2 milligrams
7 years	2 milligrams	NONE	N/A	2 milligrams in 5 ml	5 ml	2 milligrams
6 years	2 milligrams	NONE	N/A	2 milligrams in 5 ml	5 ml	2 milligrams
5 years	1 milligram	NONE	N/A	2 milligrams in 5 ml	2.5 ml	1 milligram
4 years	1 milligram	NONE	N/A	2 milligrams in 5 ml	2.5 ml	1 milligram
3 years	1 milligram	NONE	N/A	2 milligrams in 5 ml	2.5 ml	1 milligram
2 years	1 milligram	NONE	N/A	2 milligrams in 5 ml	2.5 ml	1 milligram
18 months	1 milligram	NONE	N/A	2 milligrams in 5 ml	2.5 ml	1 milligram
12 months	1 milligram	NONE	N/A	2 milligrams in 5 ml	2.5 ml	1 milligram
9 months	1 milligram	NONE	N/A	2 milligrams in 5 ml	2.5 ml	1 milligram

Chlorphenamine

CPH

AGE	INITIAL DOSE	REPEAT DOSE	DOSE INTERVAL	CONCENTRATION	VOLUME	MAX DOSE
6 months	1 milligram	NONE	N/A	2 milligrams in 5 ml	2.5 ml	1 milligram
3 months	1 milligram	NONE	N/A	2 milligrams in 5 ml	2.5 ml	1 milligram
1 month	1 milligram	NONE	N/A	2 milligrams in 5 ml	2.5 ml	1 milligram
Birth	N/A	N/A	N/A	N/A	N/A	N/A

Bibliography

1. Children's British National Formulary. *Chlorphenamine Maleate.* Available from: https://bnfc.nice.org.uk/drug/chlorphenamine-maleate.html, 2018.
2. Resuscitation Council (UK). *Emergency treatment of anaphylactic reactions: Guidelines for healthcare providers* Available from: https://www.resus.org.uk/anaphylaxis/emergency-treatment-of-anaphylactic-reactions/, 2008.

SECTION 7 Medicines

Clopidogrel

Presentation

Tablet containing clopidogrel:

- 75 milligrams
- 300 milligrams.

Indications

Acute ST-elevation myocardial infarction (STEMI):

- In patients not already taking clopidogrel.
- In patients receiving thrombolytic treatment.
- Anticipated thrombolytic treatment.
- Anticipated primary percutaneous coronary intervention (PPCI).

Actions

Inhibits platelet aggregation.

Contra-indications

- Known allergy or hypersensitivity to clopidogrel.
- Known severe liver impairment.
- Active pathological bleeding such as peptic ulcer or intracranial haemorrhage.

Cautions

As the likely benefits of a single dose of clopidogrel outweigh the potential risks, clopidogrel may be administered in:

- Pregnancy.
- Patients taking non-steroidal anti-inflammatory drugs (NSAIDs).
- Patients with renal impairment.

Side Effects

- Dyspepsia.
- Abdominal pain.
- Diarrhoea.
- Bleeding (gastrointestinal and intracranial) – the occurrence of severe bleeding is similar to that observed with the administration of aspirin.

Dosage and Administration

Adults aged 18–75 years with acute ST-elevation myocardial infarction (STEMI) receiving thrombolysis or anticipated primary PCI, as per locally agreed STEMI care pathways.

NOTE: To be administered in conjunction with aspirin unless there is a known aspirin allergy or sensitivity (refer to **Aspirin** for administration and dosage).

Route: Oral.

Patient care pathway: Thrombolysis.

AGE	INITIAL DOSE	REPEAT DOSE	DOSE INTERVAL	CONCENTRATION	VOLUME	MAX DOSE
Adult	300 milligrams	NONE	N/A	75 milligrams per tablet	4 tablets	300 milligrams
Adult	300 milligrams	NONE	N/A	300 milligrams per tablet	1 tablet	300 milligrams

Patient care pathway: Primary percutaneous coronary intervention.

AGE	INITIAL DOSE	REPEAT DOSE	DOSE INTERVAL	CONCENTRATION	VOLUME	MAX DOSE
Adult	600 milligrams	NONE	N/A	75 milligrams per tablet	8 tablets	600 milligrams
Adult	600 milligrams	NONE	N/A	300 milligrams per tablet	2 tablets	600 milligrams

Bibliography

British National Formulary. Clopidogrel. Available from: https://bnf.nice.org.uk/drug/clopidogrel.html, 2018.

Dexamethasone

DEX

Presentation

- Dexamethasone 2 milligram soluble tablets, sugar free
- Dexamethasone 2 milligrams in 5 ml oral solution, sugar free

Indications

Mild/moderate/severe croup, refer to modified Taussid Score, refer to **Respiratory Illness in Children**.

Actions

Corticosteroid – reduces subglottic inflammation.

Contra-indications

Impending respiratory failure.

Cautions

Upper airway compromise can be worsened by any procedure distressing the child – including the administration of medication.

Side Effects

- Gastro-intestinal upset.
- Hypersensitivity anaphylactic reaction.

Additional Information

A single dose pre-hospital is advised. If you feel the child needs a second dose in the same episode of illness they must be reviewed by a senior healthcare professional; seek senior clinical advice.

If the child vomits less than 30 minutes after having a dose, the same dose can be given again.

Dosage and Administration

Route: Oral tablet. Dissolve the 2 milligram tablets in water.

AGE	INITIAL DOSE	REPEAT DOSE	DOSE INTERVAL	CONCENTRATION	VOLUME	MAX DOSE
11 years	N/A	N/A	N/A	N/A	N/A	N/A
10 years	N/A	N/A	N/A	N/A	N/A	N/A
9 years	N/A	N/A	N/A	N/A	N/A	N/A
8 years	N/A	N/A	N/A	N/A	N/A	N/A
7 years	N/A	N/A	N/A	N/A	N/A	N/A
6 years	4 milligrams	NONE	N/A	2 milligrams per tablet	2 tablets	4 milligrams
5 years	4 milligrams	NONE	N/A	2 milligrams per tablet	2 tablets	4 milligrams
4 years	4 milligrams	NONE	N/A	2 milligrams per tablet	2 tablets	4 milligrams
3 years	4 milligrams	NONE	N/A	2 milligrams per tablet	2 tablets	4 milligrams
2 years	4 milligrams	NONE	N/A	2 milligrams per tablet	2 tablets	4 milligrams
18 months	4 milligrams	NONE	N/A	2 milligrams per tablet	2 tablets	4 milligrams
12 months	2 milligrams	NONE	N/A	2 milligrams per tablet	1 tablet	2 milligrams
9 months	2 milligrams	NONE	N/A	2 milligrams per tablet	1 tablet	2 milligrams
6 months	2 milligrams	NONE	N/A	2 milligrams per tablet	1 tablet	2 milligrams
3 months	2 milligrams	NONE	N/A	2 milligrams per tablet	1 tablet	2 milligrams
1 month	2 milligrams	NONE	N/A	2 milligrams per tablet	1 tablet	2 milligrams
Birth	N/A	N/A	N/A	N/A	N/A	N/A

Oral Solution

Route: Oral solution.

AGE	INITIAL DOSE	REPEAT DOSE	DOSE INTERVAL	CONCENTRATION	VOLUME	MAX DOSE
9 years	N/A	N/A	N/A	N/A	N/A	N/A
8 years	N/A	N/A	N/A	N/A	N/A	N/A
7 years	N/A	N/A	N/A	N/A	N/A	N/A
6 years	3.2 milligrams	NONE	N/A	2 milligrams in 5 ml	8 ml	3.2 milligrams
5 years	2.9 milligrams	NONE	N/A	2 milligrams in 5 ml	7 ml	2.9 milligrams
4 years	2.4 milligrams	NONE	N/A	2 milligrams in 5 ml	6 ml	2.4 milligrams
3 years	2.1 milligrams	NONE	N/A	2 milligrams in 5 ml	5 ml	2.1 milligrams
2 years	1.8 milligrams	NONE	N/A	2 milligrams in 5 ml	5 ml	1.8 milligrams
18 months	1.7 milligrams	NONE	N/A	2 milligrams in 5 ml	4 ml	1.7 milligrams
12 months	1.5 milligrams	NONE	N/A	2 milligrams in 5 ml	4 ml	1.5 milligrams
9 months	1.4 milligrams	NONE	N/A	2 milligrams in 5 ml	3 ml	1.4 milligrams
6 months	1.2 milligrams	NONE	N/A	2 milligrams in 5 ml	3 ml	1.2 milligrams
3 months	0.9 milligrams	NONE	N/A	2 milligrams in 5 ml	2 ml	0.9 milligrams
1 month	0.67 milligrams	NONE	N/A	2 milligrams in 5 ml	2 ml	0.67 milligrams
Birth	N/A	N/A	N/A	N/A	N/A	N/A

Bibliography

1. British National Formulary. *Dexamethasone.* Available from: https://bnf.nice.org.uk/drug/dexamethasone.html, 2018.

2. Medicines for Children. *Dexamethasone for croup* Available from: https://www.medicinesforchildren.org.uk/sites/default/files/content-type/leaflet/pdf/20140822115538_0.pdf, 2017.

Diazepam

Presentation

Ampoule containing 10 milligrams diazepam in an oil-in-water emulsion making up 2 ml.

Diazepam 10mg/2ml solution for injection (only used when the emulsion is unavailable as more irritant than emulsion).

Rectal tube containing 2.5 milligrams, 5 milligrams or 10 milligrams diazepam.

Indications

Patients who have prolonged (lasting 5 minutes or more) **OR** repeated (three or more in an hour) convulsions who are **CURRENTLY CONVULSING** – not secondary to an uncorrected hypoxic or hypoglycaemic episode (see 'Additional Information' below).

Eclamptic convulsions (initiate treatment if seizure lasts over 2–3 minutes or if it is recurrent).

Symptomatic cocaine toxicity (severe hypertension, chest pain or convulsions).

Actions

Central nervous system depressant, acts as an anticonvulsant and sedative.

Cautions

Should be used with caution if alcohol, antidepressants or other CNS depressants have been taken as side effects are more likely.

A dose of buccal midazolam or rectal diazepam given by a parent or carer may be the first dose administered for this seizure. The first dose given by the paramedic may be the second dose of benzodiazepine given for the seizure and IV/IO access may be needed, refer to **Convulsions in Adults**.

Contra-indications

Patients with known hypersensitivity.

Side Effects

Respiratory depression may occur, especially in the presence of alcohol (which enhances the depressive side effect of diazepam). Opioid drugs similarly enhance diazepam's cardiac and respiratory depressive effects.

Hypotension may occur. This may be significant if the patient has to be moved from a horizontal position to allow for extrication from an address. Caution should therefore be exercised and consideration given to either removing the patient flat or, if the convulsion has stopped and it is considered safe, allowing a 10-minute recovery period prior to removal.

Other side effects include light-headedness, unsteadiness, drowsiness, confusion and amnesia.

Additional Information

If the patient is prescribed buccal midazolam and a supply is available, this may be administered according to the prescriber's instructions.

Diazepam should only be used if the patient has been convulsing for 5 minutes or more (and is still convulsing), or if convulsions recur in rapid succession without time for full recovery in between. There is no value in giving 'preventative' diazepam if the convulsion has ceased. In any clearly sick or ill child, there must be no delay at the scene while administering the drug – it can be administered en-route to hospital.

If IV access can be gained rapidly, then this is preferable to the PR route. If buccal midazolam is available, use that in preference to gaining IV access for the first dose of diazepam.

Early consideration should be given to using the buccal or PR route when IV access cannot be rapidly and safely obtained, **commonly the case in children**. In small children the buccal or PR route should be considered the first treatment option (with IV access being sought subsequently). When giving rectal medication, offer parental explanation and maintain patient dignity.

All patients who continue to convulse should receive a total of **TWO** doses of benzodiazepine (midazolam or diazepam) 10 minutes apart, the second dose should be IV/IO if possible. Only give a second rectal dose if IV/IO access cannot be obtained in the 10 minutes between the first and second doses.

Care must be taken when inserting rectal tubes. They should be inserted no more than 2.5 cm in children or 4–5 cm in adults. All tubes have an insertion marker on the nozzle.

The **full** dose should be given at the appropriate times. It is **not** appropriate to either i) gradually 'titrate the dose upwards' or ii) to only give a partial dose if the convulsion stops (once started, even if the convulsion stops, that dose must be given). If this approach is followed, convulsion recurrence is much less likely.

Dosage and Administration

Rectal

Route: Rectal

For convulsions give the full dose.

NB In recurrent or ongoing convulsions, for the second dose, IV/IO access is recommended.

AGE	INITIAL DOSE	REPEAT DOSE	DOSE INTERVAL	CONCEN-TRATION	VOLUME	MAX DOSE
Adult ≥70 years	10 milligrams	10 milligrams	10 minutes	10 milligrams in 2.5 ml	1 x 10 milligram tube	20 milligrams
Adult <70 years	20 milligrams	10 milligrams	10 minutes	10 milligrams in 2.5 ml	1 or 2 x 10 milligram tube	30 milligrams
11 years	10 milligrams	10 milligrams	10 minutes	10 milligrams in 2.5 ml	1 x 10 milligram tube	20 milligrams
10 years	10 milligrams	10 milligrams	10 minutes	10 milligrams in 2.5 ml	1 x 10 milligram tube	20 milligrams
9 years	10 milligrams	10 milligrams	10 minutes	10 milligrams in 2.5 ml	1 x 10 milligram tube	20 milligrams
8 years	10 milligrams	10 milligrams	10 minutes	10 milligrams in 2.5 ml	1 x 10 milligram tube	20 milligrams
7 years	10 milligrams	10 milligrams	10 minutes	10 milligrams in 2.5 ml	1 x 10 milligram tube	20 milligrams
6 years	10 milligrams	10 milligrams	10 minutes	10 milligrams in 2.5 ml	1 x 10 milligram tube	20 milligrams
5 years	10 milligrams	10 milligrams	10 minutes	10 milligrams in 2.5 ml	1 x 10 milligram tube	20 milligrams
4 years	5 milligrams	5 milligrams	10 minutes	5 milligrams in 2.5 ml	1 x 5 milligram tube	10 milligrams
3 years	5 milligrams	5 milligrams	10 minutes	5 milligrams in 2.5 ml	1 x 5 milligram tube	10 milligrams
2 years	5 milligrams	5 milligrams	10 minutes	5 milligrams in 2.5 ml	1 x 5 milligram tube	10 milligrams
18 months	5 milligrams	5 milligrams	10 minutes	5 milligrams in 2.5 ml	1 x 5 milligram tube	10 milligrams
12 months	5 milligrams	5 milligrams	10 minutes	5 milligrams in 2.5 ml	1 x 5 milligram tube	10 milligrams
9 months	5 milligrams	5 milligrams	10 minutes	5 milligrams in 2.5 ml	1 x 5 milligram tube	10 milligrams
6 months	5 milligrams	5 milligrams	10 minutes	5 milligrams in 2.5 ml	1 x 5 milligram tube	10 milligrams
3 months	2.5 milligrams	2.5 milligrams	10 minutes	2.5 milligrams in 1.25 ml	1 x 2.5 milligram tube	5 milligrams
1 month	2.5 milligrams	2.5 milligrams	10 minutes	2.5 milligrams in 1.25 ml	1 x 2.5 milligram tube	5 milligrams
Birth and neonatal dose, up to 1 month.	1.25 milligrams	1.25 milligrams	10 minutes	2.5 milligrams in 1.25 ml	0.5 x 2.5 milligram tube	2.5 milligram

Diazepam

Intravenous/intraosseous

Route: Intravenous/intraosseous – administer **SLOWLY** over 2 minutes for adults (3–5 minutes for children).

For convulsions give the full dose. In symptomatic cocaine toxicity titrate slowly to response.

NB The second benzodiazepine dose should be IV/IO wherever possible (i.e. IV/IO diazepam).

Be ready to support ventilations.

AGE	INITIAL DOSE	REPEAT DOSE	DOSE INTERVAL	CONCEN-TRATION	VOLUME	MAX DOSE
Adult	10 milligrams	10 milligrams	10 minutes	10 milligrams in 2 ml	2 ml	20 milligrams
11 years	10 milligrams	10 milligrams	10 minutes	10 milligrams in 2 ml	2ml	20 milligrams
10 years	10 milligrams	10 milligrams	10 minutes	10 milligrams in 2 ml	2 ml	20 milligrams
9 years	9 milligrams	9 milligrams	10 minutes	10 milligrams in 2 ml	1.8 ml	18 milligrams
8 years	8 milligrams	8 milligrams	10 minutes	10 milligrams in 2 ml	1.6 ml	16 milligrams
7 years	7 milligrams	7 milligrams	10 minutes	10 milligrams in 2 ml	1.4 ml	14 milligrams
6 years	6.5 milligrams	6.5 milligrams	10 minutes	10 milligrams in 2 ml	1.3 ml	13 milligrams
5 years	6 milligrams	6 milligrams	10 minutes	10 milligrams in 2 ml	1.2 ml	12 milligrams
4 years	5 milligrams	5 milligrams	10 minutes	10 milligrams in 2 ml	1 ml	10 milligrams
3 years	4.5 milligrams	4.5 milligrams	10 minutes	10 milligrams in 2 ml	0.9 ml	9 milligrams
2 years	4 milligrams	4 milligrams	10 minutes	10 milligrams in 2 ml	0.8ml	8 milligrams
18 months	3.5 milligrams	3.5 milligrams	10 minutes	10 milligrams in 2 ml	0.7 ml	7 milligrams
12 months	3 milligrams	3 milligrams	10 minutes	10 milligrams in 2 ml	0.6 ml	6 milligrams
9 months	3 milligrams	3 milligrams	10 minutes	10 milligrams in 2 ml	0.6 ml	6 milligrams
6 months	2.5 milligrams	2.5 milligrams	10 minutes	10 milligrams in 2 ml	0.5 ml	5 milligrams
3 months	2 milligrams	2 milligrams	10 minutes	10 milligrams in 2 ml	0.4 ml	4 milligrams
1 month	1.5 milligrams	1.5 milligrams	10 minutes	10 milligrams in 2 ml	0.3 ml	3 milligrams
Birth	1 milligram	1 milligram	10 minutes	10 milligrams in 2 ml	0.2 ml	2 milligrams

Bibliography

1. American Epilepsy Society. Available from: https://www.aesnet.org/clinical_resources/guidelines.
2. NHS Evidence. *Diazepam*. Available from: https://bnf.nice.org.uk/.
3. National Institute for Health and Care Excellence. *Epilepsies: Diagnosis and Management* (CG137), 2012. Available from: https://www.nice.org.uk/guidance/cg137.

Furosemide

Presentation

20 milligrams in 2 ml injection ampoules

50 milligrams in 5 ml injection ampoules

Indications

Consider IV furosemide for pulmonary oedema and/or respiratory distress due to acute heart failure.

Actions

Furosemide is a potent diuretic with a rapid onset (within 30 minutes) and short duration.

Contra-indications

- Reduced GCS with liver cirrhosis.
- Cardiogenic shock.
- Severe renal failure with anuria.
- Children under 18 years old.

Cautions

- Hypokalaemia (low potassium) could induce arrhythmias.
- Pregnancy.
- Hypotensive patient.

Side Effects

Hypotension.

Gastrointestinal disturbances.

Additional Information

Consider furosemide when the time to get the patient to hospital is prolonged.

Dosage and Administration

Intravenous

Route: Intravenous

Administer **SLOWLY OVER** 2 minutes in accordance with the table below.

AGE	INITIAL DOSE	REPEAT DOSE	DOSE INTERVAL	CONCENTRATION	VOLUME	MAX DOSE
Adult 18 years and over	40 milligrams	NONE	N/A	20 milligrams/2 ml	4 ml	40 milligrams
Adult 18 years and over	40 milligrams	NONE	N/A	50 milligrams/5 ml	4 ml	40 milligrams

Bibliography

1. NHS Evidence. *Furosemide*. Available from: http://www.evidence.nhs.uk/formulary/bnf/current/2-cardiovascular-system/22-diuretics/222-loop-diuretics/furosemide, 2011.
2. British Medical Association and the Royal Pharmaceutical Society. *British National Formulary 75 (BNF) March – September 2018*. London: The Pharmaceutical Press.
3. Bussmann, W. Effect of sublingual nitroglycerin in emergency treatment of severe pulmonary edema. *American Journal of Cardiology*. 1978, 41(5): 931–936.
4. Crane SD, Elliott MW, Gilligan P et al. Randomised controlled comparison of continuous positive airways pressure, bilevel non-invasive ventilation, and standard treatment in emergency department patients with acute cardiogenic pulmonary oedema. *Emergency Medicine Journal*. 2004, 21: 155–161.
5. Mebazza A, Yilmaz MB, Levy P et al. Recommendations on pre-hospital and early hospital management of acute heart failure: a consensus paper from the Heart Failure Association of the European Society of Cardiology, the European Society of Emergency Medicine and the Society of Academic Emergency Medicine – Short Version. *European Heart Journal*. 2015, 36(30): 1958–1966.
6. National Institute for Health and Care Excellence. *Acute Heart Failure: Diagnosis and management* [CG187]. Manchester: NICE, 2014. Available from: https://www.nice.org.uk/guidance/cg187

Presentation

Glucagon injection, 1 milligram of powder in vial for reconstitution with water for injection.

Indications

Hypoglycaemia, clinically suspected hypoglycaemia or unconscious patients where hypoglycaemia is considered a likely cause (blood glucose <4.0 millimoles per litre).

NB Glucagon should only be administered when oral glucose administration is not possible or is ineffective, **AND/OR** when IV access to administer 10% glucose is not possible.

Actions

Glucagon is a hormone that induces the conversion of glycogen to glucose in the liver, thereby raising blood glucose levels.

Contra-indications

- Pheochromocytoma.
- Glucagon should NOT be given by IV injection because of increased vomiting associated with IV use.

Cautions

- Low glycogen stores (e.g. recent use of glucagon or starvation).
- For hypoglycaemic seizures, glucose 10% IV is the preferred intervention.

Side Effects

- Nausea, vomiting.
- Abdominal pain in adults.
- Diarrhoea in children.
- Hypokalaemia.
- Hypotension in adults.
- Acute hypersensitivity reaction, although this is rare.

Additional Information

- Check whether glucagon has already been administered by a relative/carer.
- Glucagon should only be administered once.
- Confirm effectiveness by checking blood glucose 10 to 15 minutes after administration.
- Glucagon may take up to 15 minutes to work.
- Glucagon can be ineffective in the very young, older people, undernourished patients or those with hepatic disease. Glucagon is relatively ineffective once body glycogen stores have been exhausted, especially in hypoglycaemic, non-diabetic children.
- When treating hypoglycaemia, use all available clinical information to help decide between glucagon IM, glucose 40% oral gel, or glucose 10% IV.
- Hypoglycaemic patients who are convulsing should preferably be given glucose 10% IV.
  - If the patient is conscious, use glucose 40% gel as first line treatment. Unconscious patients will require glucose 10% IV.
  - A newborn baby's liver has very limited glycogen stores, so hypoglycaemia may not be effectively treated using intramuscular glucagon. Glucagon works by stimulating the liver to convert glycogen into glucose.
  - Glucagon may also be ineffective in some instances of alcohol-induced hypoglycaemia.

Dosage and Administration

Intramuscular

Route: Intramuscular – antero-lateral aspect of thigh or upper arm.

Intramuscular

NB If no response within 10 minutes, administer intravenous glucose – refer to **Glucose 10%**.

AGE	INITIAL DOSE	REPEAT DOSE	DOSE INTERVAL	CONCENTRATION	VOLUME	MAX DOSE
Adult ≥12 years	1 milligram	NONE	N/A	1 milligram per vial	1 vial	1 milligram
11 years	1 milligram	NONE	N/A	1 milligram per vial	1 vial	1 milligram
10 years	1 milligram	NONE	N/A	1 milligram per vial	1 vial	1 milligram
9 years	1 milligram	NONE	N/A	1 milligram per vial	1 vial	1 milligram
8 years	1 milligram	NONE	N/A	1 milligram per vial	1 vial	1 milligram
7 years	500 micrograms	NONE	N/A	1 milligram per vial	0.5 vial	500 micrograms
6 years	500 micrograms	NONE	N/A	1 milligram per vial	0.5 vial	500 micrograms

AGE	INITIAL DOSE	REPEAT DOSE	DOSE INTERVAL	CONCENTRATION	VOLUME	MAX DOSE
5 years	500 micrograms	NONE	N/A	1 milligram per vial	0.5 vial	500 micrograms
4 years	500 micrograms	NONE	N/A	1 milligram per vial	0.5 vial	500 micrograms
3 years	500 micrograms	NONE	N/A	1 milligram per vial	0.5 vial	500 micrograms
2 years	500 micrograms	NONE	N/A	1 milligram per vial	0.5 vial	500 micrograms
18 months	500 micrograms	NONE	N/A	1 milligram per vial	0.5 vial	500 micrograms
12 months	500 micrograms	NONE	N/A	1 milligram per vial	0.5 vial	500 micrograms
9 months	500 micrograms	NONE	N/A	1 milligram per vial	0.5 vial	500 micrograms
6 months	500 micrograms	NONE	N/A	1 milligram per vial	0.5 vial	500 micrograms
3 months	500 micrograms	NONE	N/A	1 milligram per vial	0.5 vial	500 micrograms
1 month	500 micrograms	NONE	N/A	1 milligram per vial	0.5 vial	500 micrograms
Birth	100 micrograms	NONE	N/A	1 milligram per vial	0.1 vial	100 micrograms

Bibliography

BNF. *Glucagon*. Available from: https://bnf.nice.org.uk/drug/glucagon.html, 2018.

Glucose 10% GLX

Presentation

500 ml pack of 10% glucose solution (50 grams).

WARNING! Glucose and saline fluid bags are commonly confused as they are both clear fluids. STOP and CHECK before administration.

Indications

Hypoglycaemia (blood glucose <4.0 millimoles per litre) or suspected hypoglycaemia when oral administration is not possible and a rapid improvement in clinical state and blood glucose level is required.

An unconscious patient, where hypoglycaemia is considered a likely cause.

Management of hypoglycaemia in patients who have not responded to the administration of IM Glucagon after 10 minutes.

Actions

Reversal of hypoglycaemia by direct delivery of glucose (sugar) to the systemic circulation.

Cautions

Flush IV line thoroughly with sodium chloride 0.9% after administration to reduce vein irritation from residual glucose injection, refer to **0.9% Sodium Chloride**.

Contra-indications

IM or subcutaneous injection.

Additional Information

When treating hypoglycaemia, use all available clinical information to help decide between Glucose 10% IV, Glucose 40% oral gel, or Glucagon IM.

The IO route of administration may be used in exceptional cases when IV access cannot be obtained and other methods are not possible/effective. There is an increased risk of osteomyelitis compared to isotonic fluids.

Dosage and Administration

IV infusion: Peripherally via secure cannula into large vein or central access as Glucose 10% is an irritant, especially if extravasation occurs.

If the patient has shown no response, the dose may be repeated after 5 minutes.

If the patient has shown a **PARTIAL** response then a further infusion may be necessary, titrated to response to restore a normal GCS.

If after the second dose there has been **NO** response, pre-alert and transport rapidly to further care. Consider an alternative diagnosis or the likelihood of a third dose en-route benefiting the patient.

Intravenous/intraosseous infusion

Route: Intravenous/intraosseous infusion.

NB Neonatal doses are intentionally larger per kilo than those used in older children.

AGE	INITIAL DOSE	REPEAT DOSE	DOSE INTERVAL	CONCENTRATION	VOLUME	MAX DOSE
Adult ≥12 years	10 grams glucose	10 grams glucose	5 minutes	50 grams in 500 ml	100 ml	300 ml (30 g glucose)
11 years	7 grams glucose	7 grams glucose	5 minutes	50 grams in 500 ml	70 ml	210 ml (21g glucose)
10 years	6.5 grams glucose	6.5 grams glucose	5 minutes	50 grams in 500 ml	65 ml	195 ml (19.5 g glucose)
9 years	6 grams glucose	6 grams glucose	5 minutes	50 grams in 500 ml	60 ml	180 ml (18 g glucose)
8 years	5 grams glucose	5 grams glucose	5 minutes	50 grams in 500 ml	50 ml	150 ml (15 g glucose)
7 years	5 grams glucose	5 grams glucose	5 minutes	50 grams in 500 ml	50 ml	150 ml (15 g glucose)
6 years	4 grams glucose	4 grams glucose	5 minutes	50 grams in 500 ml	40 ml	120 ml (12 g glucose)
5 years	4 grams glucose	4 grams glucose	5 minutes	50 grams in 500 ml	40 ml	120 ml (12 g glucose)

AGE	INITIAL DOSE	REPEAT DOSE	DOSE INTERVAL	CONCENTRATION	VOLUME	MAX DOSE
4 years	3 grams glucose	3 grams glucose	5 minutes	50 grams in 500 ml	30 ml	90 ml (9 g glucose)
3 years	3 grams glucose	3 grams glucose	5 minutes	50 grams in 500 ml	30 ml	90 ml (9 g glucose)
2 years	2.5 grams glucose	2.5 grams glucose	5 minutes	50 grams in 500 ml	25 ml	75 ml (7.5 g glucose)
18 months	2 grams glucose	2 grams glucose	5 minutes	50 grams in 500 ml	20 ml	60 ml (6 g glucose)
12 months	2 grams glucose	2 grams glucose	5 minutes	50 grams in 500 ml	20 ml	60 ml (6 g glucose)
9 months	2 grams glucose	2 grams glucose	5 minutes	50 grams in 500 ml	20 ml	60 ml (6 g glucose)
6 months	1.5 grams glucose	1.5 grams glucose	5 minutes	50 grams in 500 ml	15 ml	45 ml (4.5 g glucose)
3 months	1 gram glucose	1 gram glucose	5 minutes	50 grams in 500 ml	10 ml	30 ml (3 g glucose)
1 month	1 gram glucose	1 gram glucose	5 minutes	50 grams in 500 ml	10 ml	30 ml (3 g glucose)
Birth	900 milligrams	900 milligrams	5 minutes	50 grams in 500 ml	9 ml	27 ml (2.7 g glucose)

Bibliography

1. Injectable Medicines Guide. *Monograph for Intravenous Glucose (Treatment of Hypoglycaemia in Adults), Version 2.* Available from: http://medusa.wales.nhs.uk/IVGuidePrint.asp?Drugno=1860&format=3, 2018.
2. University College London Hospitals NHS Foundation Trust. *Injectable Medicines Administration Guide, 3rd edition.* Chichester: Wiley-Blackwell, 2010.
3. British National Formulary. *Glucose*. Available from: https://bnf.nice.org.uk/drug/glucose.html, 2018.
4. Baxter Healthcare Ltd. *Summary of Product Characteristics (SPC) Glucose 10% w/v Solution for Infusion.* Available from: http://www.medicines.org.uk/emc/medicine/30172, 2016.

Glucose 40% Oral Gel

GLG

Presentation

Plastic tube containing 25g glucose 40% oral gel.

Indications

Known or suspected hypoglycaemia in a conscious patient where there is no risk of choking or aspiration.

Actions

Rapid increase in blood glucose levels via buccal absorption.

Cautions

Altered consciousness – risk of choking or aspiration (in such circumstances glucose gel can be administered by soaking a gauze swab and placing it between the patient's lip and gum to aid absorption).

Side Effects

None.

Additional Information

Can be repeated as necessary in the hypoglycaemic patient.

Treatment failure should prompt the use of an alternative such as glucagon IM or glucose 10% IV.

Refer to **Glucagon** or **Glucose 10%**.

Contra-indications

None.

Dosage and Administration

The gel should be squeezed into the mouth between the teeth and gums.

Route: Buccal – Measure blood glucose level after each dose.

NB Assess more frequently in children who require a smaller dose for a response. This medicine should only be administered if the child has a gag reflex.

NB Consider IM glucagon or IV glucose 10% if no clinical improvement.

AGE	INITIAL DOSE	REPEAT DOSE	DOSE INTERVAL	CONCENTRATION	VOLUME	MAX DOSE
≥ 12 years	10–20 grams	10 grams	5 minutes	10 grams in 25 grams of gel	1–2 tubes	2 tubes/20 grams
11 years	10 grams	10 grams	5 minutes	10 grams in 25 grams of gel	1 tube	2 tubes/20 grams
10 years	10 grams	10 grams	5 minutes	10 grams in 25 grams of gel	1 tube	2 tubes/20 grams
9 years	10 grams	10 grams	5 minutes	10 grams in 25 grams of gel	1 tube	2 tubes/20 grams
8 years	10 grams	10 grams	5 minutes	10 grams in 25 grams of gel	1 tube	2 tubes/20 grams
7 years	10 grams	10 grams	5 minutes	10 grams in 25 grams of gel	1 tube	2 tubes/20 grams
6 years	10 grams	10 grams	5 minutes	10 grams in 25 grams of gel	1 tube	2 tubes/20 grams
5 years	10 grams	10 grams	5 minutes	10 grams in 25 grams of gel	1 tube	2 tubes/20 grams
4 years	10 grams	10 grams	5 minutes	10 grams in 25 grams of gel	1 tube	2 tubes/20 grams
3 years	10 grams	10 grams	5 minutes	10 grams in 25 grams of gel	1 tube	2 tubes/20 grams
2 years	10 grams	10 grams	5 minutes	10 grams in 25 grams of gel	1 tube	2 tubes/20 grams
Children <2 years	An appropriate amount should be administered, considering the child's size	See initial dose	5 minutes	10 grams in 25 grams of gel	1 tube	An appropriate amount should be administered, considering the child's size

Glyceryl Trinitrate (GTN)

Presentation

Sublingual spray containing 400 micrograms glyceryl trinitrate per metered dose.

Sublingual tablets containing glyceryl trinitrate 300, 500 or 600 micrograms per tablet.

Indications

Cardiac chest pain due to angina or myocardial infarction, when systolic blood pressure is greater than 90mmHg.

Breathlessness due to pulmonary oedema in acute heart failure when systolic blood pressure is greater than 110 mmHg.

Patients with suspected cocaine toxicity presenting with chest pain.

Actions

A potent vasodilator drug resulting in:

- Dilatation of coronary arteries/relief of coronary spasm.
- Dilatation of systemic veins resulting in lower pre-load.
- Reduced blood pressure.

Cautions

Patients with suspected posterior myocardial infarction or right-ventricular infarction.

Contra-Indications

Hypotension (systolic blood pressure <90mmHg in angina/myocardial infarction, or <110 mmHg in acute heart failure).

Hypovolaemia.

Head trauma.

Cerebral haemorrhage.

Sildenafil (Viagra) and other related drugs – glyceryl trinitrate must not be given to patients who have taken sildenafil or related drugs within the previous 24 hours. Profound hypotension may occur.

Unconscious patients.

Known severe aortic or mitral stenosis.

Side Effects

Headache.

Dizziness.

Hypotension.

Additional Information

GTN tablets must be discarded 8 weeks after first opening.

NB To reduce the risk of cross contamination between patients, the nozzle of the spray must not come into contact with the patient's mouth. Wipe after each use with a detergent wipe.

SECTION 7 Medicines

Dosage and Administration

The oral mucosa must be moist for GTN absorption, moisten if necessary.

ANGINA or MYOCARDIAL INFARCTION (systolic BP >90 mmHg)

Route: Sublingual tablet/spray (administer under the patient's tongue and close mouth).

NB The effect of the first dose should be assessed over 5 minutes; further doses can be administered provided the systolic blood pressure is **>90 mmHg**. Remove the tablet if side effects occur, for example, hypotension.

AGE	INITIAL DOSE	REPEAT DOSE	DOSE INTERVAL	CONCENTRATION	VOLUME	MAX DOSE
Adult ≥18 years	400–800 micrograms	400–800 micrograms	5–10 minutes	400 micrograms per dose spray	1–2 sprays	No limit
Adult ≥18 years	300 micrograms	300 micrograms	5–10 minutes	300 micrograms per tablet	1 tablet	No limit
Adult ≥18 years	500 micrograms	500 micrograms	5–10 minutes	500 micrograms per tablet	1 tablet	No limit
Adult ≥18 years	600 micrograms	600 micrograms	5–10 minutes	600 micrograms per tablet	1 tablet	No limit

Glyceryl Trinitrate (GTN)

ACUTE HEART FAILURE (systolic BP >110 mmHg)

Route: Sublingual tablet/spray (administer under the patient's tongue and close mouth).

NB The effect of the first dose should be assessed over 5 minutes; further doses can be administered provided the systolic blood pressure is **>110 mmHg**. Remove the tablet if side effects occur, for example, hypotension.

AGE	INITIAL DOSE	REPEAT DOSE	DOSE INTERVAL	CONCENTRATION	VOLUME	MAX DOSE
Adult ≥18 years	400–800 micrograms	400–800 micrograms	5–10 minutes	400 micrograms per dose spray	1–2 sprays	6 sprays (2.4 milligrams)
Adult ≥18 years	300 micrograms	300 micrograms	5–10 minutes	300 micrograms per tablet	1 tablet	6 tablets (1.8 milligrams)
Adult ≥18 years	500 micrograms	500 micrograms	5–10 minutes	500 micrograms per tablet	1 tablet	3 tablets (1.5 milligrams)
Adult ≥18 years	600 micrograms	600 micrograms	5–10 minutes	600 micrograms per tablet	1 tablet	3 tablets (1.8 milligrams)

Heparin (Unfractionated)

Presentation

An ampoule of unfractionated heparin containing 5,000 units per ml.

Indications

ST-elevation myocardial infarction (STEMI) where heparin is required as adjunctive therapy with tenecteplase to reduce the risk of re-infarction.

It is extremely important that the initial bolus dose is given at the earliest opportunity prior to administration of thrombolytic agents and a heparin infusion is commenced immediately on arrival at hospital.

A further intravenous bolus dose of 1,000 units heparin may be required if a heparin infusion **HAS NOT** commenced within 45 minutes of the original bolus of thrombolytic agent.

Actions

Anticoagulant.

Contra-indications

- **Haemophilia and other haemorrhagic disorders.**
- Thrombocytopenia.
- Recent cerebral haemorrhage.
- Severe hypertension.
- Severe liver disease.
- Oesophageal varices.
- Peptic ulcer.
- Major trauma.
- Recent surgery to eye or nervous system.
- Acute bacterial endocarditis.
- Spinal or epidural anaesthesia.

Side Effects

Haemorrhage – major or minor.

Additional Information

Analysis of MINAP data suggests inadequate anticoagulation following pre-hospital thrombolytic treatment is associated with increased risks of re-infarction.

AT HOSPITAL it is essential that the care of the patient is handed over as soon as possible to a member of hospital staff qualified to administer the second bolus (if not already given) and commence a heparin infusion.

Dosage and Administration

Heparin dosage when administered with **TENECTEPLASE.**

Route: Intravenous single bolus unfractionated heparin.

AGE	INITIAL DOSE	REPEAT DOSE	DOSE INTERVAL	CONCENTRATION	VOLUME	MAX DOSE
≥18 and <67 kg	4,000 units	A further intravenous bolus dose of 1,000 units heparin may be required if a heparin infusion HAS NOT commenced within 45 minutes of the original bolus of thrombolytic agent.	N/A	5,000 units/ml	0.8 ml	4,000 units
≥18 and ≥67 kg	5,000 units	A further intravenous bolus dose of 1,000 units heparin may be required if a heparin infusion HAS NOT commenced within 45 minutes of the original bolus of thrombolytic agent.	N/A	5,000 units/ml	1 ml	5,000 units

Bibliography

British National Formulary. Heparin (Unfractionated). Available from: https://bnf.nice.org.uk/drug/heparin-unfractionated.html, 2018.

Hydrocortisone

Presentation

Solution for injection: Hydrocortisone sodium phosphate 100mg/1ml solution for injection ampoules.

Powder for solution for injection: Hydrocortisone (as Hydrocortisone sodium succinate) 100 mg powder for reconstitution with up to 2 ml of water.

An ampoule containing 100 milligrams hydrocortisone sodium succinate for reconstitution with up to 2 ml of water.

Indications

Severe or life-threatening asthma.

Anaphylaxis.

Adrenal crisis (including Addisonian crisis) which is a time-critical medical emergency with an associated mortality.

Adrenal crisis may occur in patients on long-term steroid therapy, either:

- as replacement therapy for adrenal insufficiency from any cause
- in long-term therapy at doses of 5+mg prednisolone, e.g. for immune-suppression.

Administer hydrocortisone to:

1 Patients in an established adrenal crisis (IV administration preferable). Ensure parenteral hydrocortisone is given prior to transportation.

2 Patients with suspected adrenal insufficiency or on long-term steroid therapy who have become unwell, to prevent them having an adrenal crisis. (IM administration is usually sufficient.)

3 If in doubt about adrenal insufficiency, it is better to administer hydrocortisone.

Actions

Glucocorticoid drug that restores blood pressure, blood sugar, cardiac synchronicity and volume. High levels are important to survive shock. Therapeutic actions include suppression of inflammation and immune response.

Contra-indications

Known allergy to the product/excipients.

Where a patient has adrenal crisis it is preferable to give whatever preparation is available.

Cautions

None relevant to a single dose.

Avoid intramuscular administration if patient likely to require thrombolysis.

Side Effects

Both sodium phosphate and sodium succinate solutions contain significant amounts of phosphate preservative and may cause stinging or burning sensations.

Dosage and Administration

1. Severe or life-threatening asthma and adrenal crisis. NB If there is any doubt about previous steroid administration, it is better to administer further hydrocortisone. There is no toxic dose for hydrocortisone, but advanced hypocortisolaemia may rapidly prove fatal.

Route: Preferably: intravenous (**SLOW** injection over a minimum of 2 minutes to avoid side effects).

Otherwise: intramuscular (upper arm or thigh) where IV access is not possible.

Note that patients with a larger BMI will need a longer IM needle.

AGE	INITIAL DOSE	REPEAT DOSE	DOSE INTERVAL	CONCENTRATION	VOLUME	MAX DOSE
Adult	100 milligrams	NONE	N/A	100 milligrams in 1 ml	1 ml	100 milligrams
11 years	100 milligrams	NONE	N/A	100 milligrams in 1 ml	1 ml	100 milligrams
10 years	100 milligrams	NONE	N/A	100 milligrams in 1 ml	1 ml	100 milligrams
9 years	100 milligrams	NONE	N/A	100 milligrams in 1 ml	1 ml	100 milligrams
8 years	100 milligrams	NONE	N/A	100 milligrams in 1 ml	1 ml	100 milligrams
7 years	100 milligrams	NONE	N/A	100 milligrams in 1 ml	1 ml	100 milligrams
6 years	100 milligrams	NONE	N/A	100 milligrams in 1 ml	1 ml	100 milligrams
5 years	50 milligrams	NONE	N/A	100 milligrams in 1 ml	0.5 ml	50 milligrams

AGE	INITIAL DOSE	REPEAT DOSE	DOSE INTERVAL	CONCENTRATION	VOLUME	MAX DOSE
4 years	50 milligrams	NONE	N/A	100 milligrams in 1 ml	0.5 ml	50 milligrams
3 years	50 milligrams	NONE	N/A	100 milligrams in 1 ml	0.5 ml	50 milligrams
2 years	50 milligrams	NONE	N/A	100 milligrams in 1 ml	0.5 ml	50 milligrams
18 months	50 milligrams	NONE	N/A	100 milligrams in 1 ml	0.5 ml	50 milligrams
12 months	50 milligrams	NONE	N/A	100 milligrams in 1 ml	0.5 ml	50 milligrams
9 months	50 milligrams	NONE	N/A	100 milligrams in 1 ml	0.5 ml	50 milligrams
6 months	50 milligrams	NONE	N/A	100 milligrams in 1 ml	0.5 ml	50 milligrams
3 months	25 milligrams	NONE	N/A	100 milligrams in 1 ml	0.25 ml	25 milligrams
1 month	25 milligrams	NONE	N/A	100 milligrams in 1 ml	0.25 ml	25 milligrams
Birth	10 milligrams	NONE	N/A	100 milligrams in 1 ml	0.1 ml	10 milligrams

Route: Intravenous (**SLOW** injection over a minimum of 2 minutes to avoid side effects)/intraosseous OR intramuscular (when IV access is impossible).

AGE	INITIAL DOSE	REPEAT DOSE	DOSE INTERVAL	CONCENTRATION	VOLUME	MAX DOSE
Adult	100 milligrams	NONE	N/A	100 milligrams in 2 ml	2 ml	100 milligrams
11 years	100 milligrams	NONE	N/A	100 milligrams in 2 ml	2 ml	100 milligrams
10 years	100 milligrams	NONE	N/A	100 milligrams in 2 ml	2 ml	100 milligrams
9 years	100 milligrams	NONE	N/A	100 milligrams in 2 ml	2 ml	100 milligrams
8 years	100 milligrams	NONE	N/A	100 milligrams in 2 ml	2 ml	100 milligrams
7 years	100 milligrams	NONE	N/A	100 milligrams in 2 ml	2 ml	100 milligrams
6 years	100 milligrams	NONE	N/A	100 milligrams in 2 ml	2 ml	100 milligrams
5 years	50 milligrams	NONE	N/A	100 milligrams in 2 ml	1 ml	50 milligrams
4 years	50 milligrams	NONE	N/A	100 milligrams in 2 ml	1 ml	50 milligrams
3 years	50 milligrams	NONE	N/A	100 milligrams in 2 ml	1 ml	50 milligrams
2 years	50 milligrams	NONE	N/A	100 milligrams in 2 ml	1 ml	50 milligrams
18 months	50 milligrams	NONE	N/A	100 milligrams in 2 ml	1 ml	50 milligrams

AGE	INITIAL DOSE	REPEAT DOSE	DOSE INTERVAL	CONCENTRATION	VOLUME	MAX DOSE
12 months	50 milligrams	NONE	N/A	100 milligrams in 2 ml	1 ml	50 milligrams
9 months	50 milligrams	NONE	N/A	100 milligrams in 2 ml	1 ml	50 milligrams
6 months	50 milligrams	NONE	N/A	100 milligrams in 2 ml	1 ml	50 milligrams
3 months	25 milligrams	NONE	N/A	100 milligrams in 2 ml	0.5 ml	25 milligrams
1 month	25 milligrams	NONE	N/A	100 milligrams in 2 ml	0.5 ml	25 milligrams
Birth	10 milligrams	NONE	N/A	100 milligrams in 2 ml	0.2 ml	10 milligrams

2. **Anaphylaxis**

Route: Intravenous (**SLOW** injection over a minimum of 2 minutes to avoid side effects)/intraosseous OR intramuscular (when IV access is impossible).

AGE	INITIAL DOSE	REPEAT DOSE	DOSE INTERVAL	CONCENTRATION	VOLUME	MAX DOSE
Adult	200 milligrams	NONE	N/A	100 milligrams in 1 ml	2 ml	200 milligrams
11 years	100 milligrams	NONE	N/A	100 milligrams in 1 ml	1 ml	100 milligrams
10 years	100 milligrams	NONE	N/A	100 milligrams in 1 ml	1 ml	100 milligrams
9 years	100 milligrams	NONE	N/A	100 milligrams in 1 ml	1 ml	100 milligrams
8 years	100 milligrams	NONE	N/A	100 milligrams in 1 ml	1 ml	100 milligrams
7 years	100 milligrams	NONE	N/A	100 milligrams in 1 ml	1 ml	100 milligrams
6 years	100 milligrams	NONE	N/A	100 milligrams in 1 ml	1 ml	100 milligrams
5 years	50 milligrams	NONE	N/A	100 milligrams in 1 ml	0.5 ml	50 milligrams
4 years	50 milligrams	NONE	N/A	100 milligrams in 1 ml	0.5 ml	50 milligrams
3 years	50 milligrams	NONE	N/A	100 milligrams in 1 ml	0.5 ml	50 milligrams
2 years	50 milligrams	NONE	N/A	100 milligrams in 1 ml	0.5 ml	50 milligrams
18 months	50 milligrams	NONE	N/A	100 milligrams in 1 ml	0.5 ml	50 milligrams
12 months	50 milligrams	NONE	N/A	100 milligrams in 1 ml	0.5 ml	50 milligrams
9 months	50 milligrams	NONE	N/A	100 milligrams in 1 ml	0.5 ml	50 milligrams
6 months	50 milligrams	NONE	N/A	100 milligrams in 1 ml	0.5 ml	50 milligrams

AGE	INITIAL DOSE	REPEAT DOSE	DOSE INTERVAL	CONCENTRATION	VOLUME	MAX DOSE
3 months	25 milligrams	NONE	N/A	100 milligrams in 1 ml	0.25 ml	25 milligrams
1 month	25 milligrams	NONE	N/A	100 milligrams in 1 ml	0.25 ml	25 milligrams
Birth	10 milligrams	NONE	N/A	100 milligrams in 1 ml	0.1 ml	10 milligrams

Route: Intravenous (**SLOW** injection over a minimum of 2 minutes to avoid side effects)/intraosseous OR intramuscular (when IV access is impossible).

AGE	INITIAL DOSE	REPEAT DOSE	DOSE INTERVAL	CONCENTRATION	VOLUME	MAX DOSE
Adult	200 milligrams	NONE	N/A	100 milligrams in 2 ml	4 ml	200 milligrams
11 years	100 milligrams	NONE	N/A	100 milligrams in 2 ml	2 ml	100 milligrams
10 years	100 milligrams	NONE	N/A	100 milligrams in 2 ml	2 ml	100 milligrams
9 years	100 milligrams	NONE	N/A	100 milligrams in 2 ml	2 ml	100 milligrams
8 years	100 milligrams	NONE	N/A	100 milligrams in 2 ml	2 ml	100 milligrams
7 years	100 milligrams	NONE	N/A	100 milligrams in 2 ml	2 ml	100 milligrams
6 years	100 milligrams	NONE	N/A	100 milligrams in 2 ml	2 ml	100 milligrams
5 years	50 milligrams	NONE	N/A	100 milligrams in 2 ml	1 ml	50 milligrams
4 years	50 milligrams	NONE	N/A	100 milligrams in 2 ml	1 ml	50 milligrams
3 years	50 milligrams	NONE	N/A	100 milligrams in 2 ml	1 ml	50 milligrams
2 years	50 milligrams	NONE	N/A	100 milligrams in 2 ml	1 ml	50 milligrams
18 months	50 milligrams	NONE	N/A	100 milligrams in 2 ml	1 ml	50 milligrams
12 months	50 milligrams	NONE	N/A	100 milligrams in 2 ml	1 ml	50 milligrams
9 months	50 milligrams	NONE	N/A	100 milligrams in 2 ml	1 ml	50 milligrams
6 months	50 milligrams	NONE	N/A	100 milligrams in 2 ml	1 ml	50 milligrams
3 months	25 milligrams	NONE	N/A	100 milligrams in 2 ml	0.5 ml	25 milligrams
1 month	25 milligrams	NONE	N/A	100 milligrams in 2 ml	0.5 ml	25 milligrams
Birth	10 milligrams	NONE	N/A	100 milligrams in 2 ml	0.2 ml	10 milligrams

Bibliography

British National Formulary. Hydrocortisone. Available from: https://bnf.nice.org.uk/drug/hydrocortisone.html, 2018.

Presentation

Solution or suspension containing ibuprofen 100 milligrams in 5 ml (ibuprofen 20mg in 1ml).

Tablet containing 200 milligrams or 400 milligrams ibuprofen.

Indications

Relief of mild to moderate pain.

Pyrexia with discomfort (may help to relieve the misery and often unpleasant symptoms that often accompany febrile illness, e.g. aches and pains).

Soft tissue injuries.

Best when used as part of a balanced analgesic regimen.

Actions

Analgesic (relieves pain).

Antipyretic (reduces temperature).

Anti-inflammatory (reduces inflammation).

Contra-indications

Do **NOT** administer if the patient is:

- Dehydrated.
- Hypovolaemic.
- Known to have renal insufficiency.
- Patients with active upper gastrointestinal disturbance (e.g. oesophagitis, peptic ulcer, dyspepsia).
- A woman in the last trimester of pregnancy.
- A child with chickenpox.
- A patient who has previously shown hypersensitivity reactions (e.g. asthma, rhinitis, angioedema or urticaria), in response to ibuprofen, aspirin or other non-steroidal anti-inflammatory drugs.
- A patient with active peptic ulcer/haemorrhage.
- Patient with severe heart failure (NYHA Class IV), renal failure or hepatic failure.

Avoid giving further non-steroidal anti-inflammatory drugs (NSAIDs) (i.e. ibuprofen), if an NSAID containing product (e.g. diclofenac, naproxen) has been used within the previous 4 hours or if the maximum cumulative daily dose has already been given.

Cautions

- **Asthma:** Use cautiously in asthmatic patients due to the possible risk of hypersensitivity and bronchoconstriction. If an asthmatic has not used NSAIDs previously, do not use acutely in the pre-hospital setting.
- **Older people:** Exercise caution in older patients (>65 years old) that have not used and tolerated NSAIDs recently.
- Patients with coagulation defects.
- Crohn's disease and ulcerative colitis as condition may be exacerbated.
- Avoid in patients with established ischaemic heart disease, peripheral arterial disease, cerebrovascular disease, congestive heart failure.
- Hypertension.

Side Effects

May cause nausea, vomiting and tinnitus.

Dosage and Administration

Route: Oral.

NB

- Given up to 3 times a day, preferably following food.

AGE	INITIAL DOSE	REPEAT DOSE	DOSE INTERVAL	CONCEN-TRATION	VOLUME	MAX DOSE
12 years – Adult	400 milligrams	400 milligrams	8 hours	Various	Varies	1.2 grams per 24 hours
11 years	300 milligrams	300 milligrams	8 hours	100 milligrams in 5 ml	15 ml	900 milligrams per 24 hours
10 years	300 milligrams	300 milligrams	8 hours	100 milligrams in 5 ml	15 ml	900 milligrams per 24 hours
9 years	200 milligrams	200 milligrams	8 hours	100 milligrams in 5 ml	10 ml	600 milligrams per 24 hours
8 years	200 milligrams	200 milligrams	8 hours	100 milligrams in 5 ml	10 ml	600 milligrams per 24 hours

AGE	INITIAL DOSE	REPEAT DOSE	DOSE INTERVAL	CONCEN-TRATION	VOLUME	MAX DOSE
7 years	200 milligrams	200 milligrams	8 hours	100 milligrams in 5 ml	10 ml	600 milligrams per 24 hours
6 years	150 milligrams	150 milligrams	8 hours	100 milligrams in 5 ml	7.5 ml	450 milligrams per 24 hours
5 years	150 milligrams	150 milligrams	8 hours	100 milligrams in 5 ml	7.5 ml	450 milligrams per 24 hours
4 years	150 milligrams	150 milligrams	8 hours	100 milligrams in 5 ml	7.5 ml	450 milligrams per 24 hours
3 years	100 milligrams	100 milligrams	8 hours	100 milligrams in 5 ml	5 ml	300 milligrams per 24 hours
2 years	100 milligrams	100 milligrams	8 hours	100 milligrams in 5 ml	5 ml	300 milligrams per 24 hours
18 months	100 milligrams	100 milligrams	8 hours	100 milligrams in 5 ml	5 ml	300 milligrams per 24 hours
12 months	100 milligrams	100 milligrams	8 hours	100 milligrams in 5 ml	5 ml	300 milligrams per 24 hours
9 months	50 milligrams	50 milligrams	8 hours	100 milligrams in 5 ml	2.5 ml	150 milligrams per 24 hours
6 months	50 milligrams	50 milligrams	8 hours	100 milligrams in 5 ml	2.5 ml	150 milligrams per 24 hours
3 months	50 milligrams	50 milligrams	8 hours	100 milligrams in 5 ml	2.5 ml	150 milligrams per 24 hours
1 month	N/A	N/A	N/A	N/A	N/A	N/A
Birth	N/A	N/A	N/A	N/A	N/A	N/A

Bibliography

British National Formulary. *Ibuprofen*. Available from: https://bnf.nice.org.uk/drug/ibuprofen.html, 2018.

Ipratropium Bromide

Presentation

Nebuliser liquid Ipratropium bromide 250 microgram per 1 ml liquid unit dose vial.

Nebuliser liquid Ipratropium bromide 500 microgram per 2 ml liquid unit dose vial (Ipratropium bromide 250 micorgram per 1 ml).

Indications

Acute, severe or life-threatening asthma.

Acute asthma unresponsive to salbutamol.

Exacerbation of chronic obstructive pulmonary disease (COPD), unresponsive to salbutamol.

Actions

1 Ipratropium bromide is an antimuscarinic bronchodilator drug. It may provide short-term relief in acute asthma, but $beta_2$ agonists (such as salbutamol) generally work more quickly.

2 Ipratropium is considered of greater benefit in:

  a children suffering acute asthma

  b adults suffering with COPD.

Contra-indications

None in the emergency situation.

Cautions

Ipratropium should be used with care in patients with:

- Glaucoma (protect the eyes from mist).
- Pregnancy and breastfeeding.
- Prostatic hyperplasia.

If COPD is a possibility limit nebulisation with oxygen to 6 minutes.

Side Effects

Nausea.

Dry mouth (common).

Tachycardia/arrhythmia.

Paroxysmal tightness of the chest.

Allergic reaction.

Dosage and Administration

- **In life-threatening or acute severe asthma:** undertake a **TIME CRITICAL** transfer to the **NEAREST SUITABLE RECEIVING HOSPITAL** and provide nebulisation en-route.
- If COPD is a possibility limit nebulisation to 6 minutes.

Route: Nebuliser with 6–8 litres per minute oxygen (refer to **Oxygen**).

AGE	INITIAL DOSE	REPEAT DOSE	DOSE INTERVAL	CONCENTRATION	VOLUME	MAX DOSE
Adult	500 micrograms	NONE	N/A	250 micrograms in 1 ml	2 ml	500 micrograms
11 years	250 micrograms	NONE	N/A	250 micrograms in 1 ml	1 ml	250 micrograms
10 years	250 micrograms	NONE	N/A	250 micrograms in 1 ml	1 ml	250 micrograms
9 years	250 micrograms	NONE	N/A	250 micrograms in 1 ml	1 ml	250 micrograms
8 years	250 micrograms	NONE	N/A	250 micrograms in 1 ml	1 ml	250 micrograms
7 years	250 micrograms	NONE	N/A	250 micrograms in 1 ml	1 ml	250 micrograms
6 years	250 micrograms	NONE	N/A	250 micrograms in 1 ml	1 ml	250 micrograms
5 years	250 micrograms	NONE	N/A	250 micrograms in 1 ml	1 ml	250 micrograms
4 years	250 micrograms	NONE	N/A	250 micrograms in 1 ml	1 ml	250 micrograms
3 years	250 micrograms	NONE	N/A	250 micrograms in 1 ml	1 ml	250 micrograms
2 years	250 micrograms	NONE	N/A	250 micrograms in 1 ml	1 ml	250 micrograms

AGE	INITIAL DOSE	REPEAT DOSE	DOSE INTERVAL	CONCENTRATION	VOLUME	MAX DOSE
18 months	250 micrograms	NONE	N/A	250 micrograms in 1 ml	1 ml	250 micrograms
12 months	125–250 micrograms	NONE	N/A	250 micrograms in 1 ml	0.5 ml–1 ml	125–250 micrograms
9 months	125–250 micrograms	NONE	N/A	250 micrograms in 1 ml	0.5 ml–1 ml	125–250 micrograms
6 months	125–250 micrograms	NONE	N/A	250 micrograms in 1 ml	0.5 ml–1 ml	125–250 micrograms
3 months	125–250 micrograms	NONE	N/A	250 micrograms in 1 ml	0.5 ml–1 ml	125–250 micrograms
1 month	125–250 micrograms	NONE	N/A	250 micrograms in 1 ml	0.5 ml–1 ml	125–250 micrograms
Birth	N/A	N/A	N/A	N/A	N/A	N/A

Route: Nebuliser with 6–8 litres per minute oxygen (refer to **Oxygen**).

AGE	INITIAL DOSE	REPEAT DOSE	DOSE INTERVAL	CONCENTRATION	VOLUME	MAX DOSE
Adult	500 micrograms	NONE	N/A	500 micrograms in 2 ml	2 ml	500 micrograms
11 years	250 micrograms	NONE	N/A	500 micrograms in 2 ml	1 ml	250 micrograms
10 years	250 micrograms	NONE	N/A	500 micrograms in 2 ml	1 ml	250 micrograms
9 years	250 micrograms	NONE	N/A	500 micrograms in 2 ml	1 ml	250 micrograms
8 years	250 micrograms	NONE	N/A	500 micrograms in 2 ml	1 ml	250 micrograms
7 years	250 micrograms	NONE	N/A	500 micrograms in 2 ml	1 ml	250 micrograms
6 years	250 micrograms	NONE	N/A	500 micrograms in 2 ml	1 ml	250 micrograms
5 years	250 micrograms	NONE	N/A	500 micrograms in 2 ml	1 ml	250 micrograms
4 years	250 micrograms	NONE	N/A	500 micrograms in 2 ml	1 ml	250 micrograms
3 years	250 micrograms	NONE	N/A	500 micrograms in 2 ml	1 ml	250 micrograms
2 years	250 micrograms	NONE	N/A	500 micrograms in 2 ml	1 ml	250 micrograms
18 months	250 micrograms	NONE	N/A	500 micrograms in 2 ml	1 ml	250 micrograms
12 months	125–250 micrograms	NONE	N/A	500 micrograms in 2 ml	0.5 ml–1 ml	125–250 micrograms
9 months	125–250 micrograms	NONE	N/A	500 micrograms in 2 ml	0.5 ml–1 ml	125–250 micrograms
6 months	125–250 micrograms	NONE	N/A	500 micrograms in 2 ml	0.5 ml–1 ml	125–250 micrograms

AGE	INITIAL DOSE	REPEAT DOSE	DOSE INTERVAL	CONCENTRATION	VOLUME	MAX DOSE
3 months	125–250 micrograms	NONE	N/A	500 micrograms in 2 ml	0.5 ml–1 ml	125–250 micrograms
1 month	125–250 micrograms	NONE	N/A	500 micrograms in 2 ml	0.5 ml–1 ml	125–250 micrograms
Birth	N/A	N/A	N/A	N/A	N/A	N/A

Bibliography

British National Formulary. *Ipratropium Bromide.* Available from: https://bnf.nice.org.uk/drug/ipratropium-bromide.html, 2018.

Metoclopramide Hydrochloride MTC

Presentation

Metoclopramide 10 milligrams / 2 ml solution for injection ampoules (metoclopramide hydrochloride 5 mg per 1 ml).

Indications

The treatment of nausea or vomiting in adults aged 18 and over.

Prevention and treatment of nausea and vomiting following administration of morphine sulfate.

Actions

An anti-emetic which acts centrally as well as on the gastrointestinal tract.

Contra-indications

- Age less than 18 years.
- Renal failure.
- Phaeochromocytoma.
- Gastrointestinal obstruction.
- Perforation/haemorrhage/3–4 days after GI surgery.
- Cases of drug overdose.

Cautions

If patient is likely to require thrombolysis then intramuscular administration of any drug should be avoided.

Side Effects

Severe extra-pyramidal effects are more common in children and young adults.

- Drowsiness and restlessness.
- Cardiac conduction abnormalities following IV administration.
- Diarrhoea.
- Rash.

Additional Information

Metoclopramide should always be given in a separate syringe to morphine sulfate. The drugs must not be mixed.

Dosage and Administration

Route: administer by intramuscular injection or slow intravenous injection over at least 3 minutes.

NB Monitor pulse, blood pressure, respiratory rate and cardiac rhythm before, during and after administration.

AGE	INITIAL DOSE	REPEAT DOSE	DOSE INTERVAL	CONCENTRATION	VOLUME	MAX DOSE
≥18 years	10 milligrams	NONE	N/A	10 milligrams in 2 ml	2 ml	10 milligrams

Bibliography

British National Formulary. *Metoclopramide Hydrochloride.* Available from: https://bnf.nice.org.uk/drug/metoclopramide-hydrochloride.html, 2018.

Presentation

Midazolam oromucosal solution, 5 mg/ml, (pre-filled syringes containing 2.5 mg, 5 mg, 7.5 mg or 10 mg).

Indications

- Convulsion lasting 5 minutes or more and STILL FITTING or 3 or more convulsions in an hour.
- Convulsion continuing 10 minutes after first dose of medication.

A PGD is required to administer midazolam unless a patient has their own prescribed supply. If the midazolam is prescribed for the patient the clinician MUST follow the prescriber's instructions for its administration. If a PGD is being used the document will state the clinical situation in which the medicine can be administered.

Actions

Short-acting benzodiazepine with anxiolytic, sedative and anticonvulsant properties. Onset of action is dependent on the route of administration. The buccal route onset of action is usually within 5 minutes. The sedative effect decreases from 15 minutes onwards.

Cautions

Always check the dose of the midazolam presentation carefully. Administration can lead to respiratory depression leading to respiratory arrest. Susceptible patients are children, adults over 60 years and those with chronic illness (renal, hepatic or cardiac).

Enhanced side effects when alcohol or other sedative drugs are present.

Contra-Indications

None.

Side Effects

- Respiratory depression.
- Hypotension.
- Reduced level of consciousness leading to impaired airway control.
- Confusion leading to increased agitation.
- Amnesia in some patients.

Additional Information

When administered for convulsions in known epileptic patients ask/look to see if the patient has an individualised treatment plan or an Epilepsy Passport. Aim to follow patient's own treatment plan when possible and effective.

Carefully monitor vital signs for delayed respiratory or cardiovascular side effects as the effect of the midazolam and other drugs such as rectal diazepam reach a peak effect.

Dosage and Administration

Convulsions

Route: Buccal.

AGE	INITIAL DOSE	REPEAT DOSE	DOSE INTERVAL	CONCEN-TRATION	VOLUME	MAX DOSE
Adult	10 milligrams	10 milligrams	10 mins	5 milligrams in 1 ml	2 ml pre-filled syringe	20 milligrams
11 years	10 milligrams	10 milligrams	10 mins	5 milligrams in 1 ml	2 ml pre-filled syringe	20 milligrams
10 years	10 milligrams	10 milligrams	10 mins	5 milligrams in 1 ml	2 ml pre-filled syringe	20 milligrams
9 years	7.5 milligrams	7.5 milligrams	10 mins	5 milligrams in 1 ml	1.5 ml pre-filled syringe	15 milligrams
8 years	7.5 milligrams	7.5 milligrams	10 mins	5 milligrams in 1 ml	1.5 ml pre-filled syringe	15 milligrams
7 years	7.5 milligrams	7.5 milligrams	10 mins	5 milligrams in 1 ml	1.5 ml pre-filled syringe	15 milligrams
6 years	7.5 milligrams	7.5 milligrams	10 mins	5 milligrams in 1 ml	1.5 ml pre-filled syringe	15 milligrams
5 years	7.5 milligrams	7.5 milligrams	10 mins	5 milligrams in 1 ml	1.5 ml pre-filled syringe	15 milligrams
4 years	5 milligrams	5 milligrams	10 mins	5 milligrams in 1 ml	1 ml pre-filled syringe	10 milligrams

AGE	INITIAL DOSE	REPEAT DOSE	DOSE INTERVAL	CONCEN-TRATION	VOLUME	MAX DOSE
3 years	5 milligrams	5 milligrams	10 mins	5 milligrams in 1 ml	1 ml pre-filled syringe	10 milligrams
2 years	5 milligrams	5 milligrams	10 mins	5 milligrams in 1 ml	1 ml pre-filled syringe	10 milligrams
18 months	5 milligrams	5 milligrams	10 mins	5 milligrams in 1 ml	1 ml pre-filled syringe	10 milligrams
12 months	5 milligrams	5 milligrams	10 mins	5 milligrams in 1 ml	1 ml pre-filled syringe	10 milligrams
9 months	2.5 milligrams	2.5 milligrams	10 mins	5 milligrams in 1 ml	0.5 ml pre-filled syringe	5 milligrams
6 months	2.5 milligrams	2.5 milligrams	10 mins	5 milligrams in 1 ml	0.5 ml pre-filled syringe	5 milligrams
3 months	See Epilepsy Passport	See Epilepsy Passport	10 mins	5 milligrams in 1 ml	See Epilepsy Passport	See Epilepsy Passport
1 month	See Epilepsy Passport	See Epilepsy Passport	10 mins	5 milligrams in 1 ml	See Epilepsy Passport	See Epilepsy Passport
Birth	See Epilepsy Passport	See Epilepsy Passport	10 mins	5 milligrams in 1 ml	See Epilepsy Passport	See Epilepsy Passport

Presentation

Tablet containing misoprostol:

- 200 micrograms.

Indications

Post-partum haemorrhage within 24 hours of delivery of the newborn baby where bleeding from the uterus is uncontrollable by uterine massage.

Miscarriage with life-threatening bleeding and a confirmed diagnosis (e.g. where a patient has gone home with medical management and starts to bleed).

Both Oxytocin and ergometrine are contra-indicated in hypertension (BP >140/90); in this case misoprostol should be administered instead.

In all other circumstances, misoprostol should only be used if Oxytocin or other oxytocics are unavailable or if they have been ineffective at reducing haemorrhage after 15 minutes.

Actions

Stimulates contraction of the uterus.

Onset of action 7–10 minutes.

Contra-indications

- Known hypersensitivity to misoprostol.
- Active labour.
- Possible multiple pregnancy/known or suspected fetus in utero.

Side Effects

- Abdominal pain.
- Nausea and vomiting.
- Diarrhoea.
- Pyrexia.
- Shivering.

Additional Information

Oxytocin and misoprostol reduce bleeding from a pregnant uterus through different pathways; therefore, if one drug has not been effective after 15 minutes, the other may be administered in addition.

Dosage and Administration

- Administer sublingually unless the patient is unable to maintain their airway.
- The vaginal route is not appropriate in post-partum haemorrhage or for miscarriage, but the rectal route may be considered when appropriate (e.g. impaired consciousness).

Route: Sublingual.

AGE	INITIAL DOSE	REPEAT DOSE	DOSE INTERVAL	CONCENTRATION	VOLUME	MAX DOSE
Adult	800 micrograms	None	N/A	200 micrograms per tablet	4 tablets	800 micrograms

Route: Rectal.

NB At the time of publication there is no rectal preparation of misoprostol – therefore the same tablets can be administered sublingually or rectally.

AGE	INITIAL DOSE	REPEAT DOSE	DOSE INTERVAL	CONCENTRATION	VOLUME	MAX DOSE
Adult	800 micrograms	None	N/A	200 micrograms per tablet	4 tablets	800 micrograms

Bibliography

1. Woollard M, Hinshaw K, Simpson H, Wieteska S. Emergencies in early pregnancy and complications following gynaecological surgery. In *Pre-hospital Obstetric Emergency Training*. Oxford: Wiley-Blackwell, 2009: 53–61.
2. Woollard M, Hinshaw K, Simpson H, Wieteska S. Emergencies after delivery. In *Pre-hospital Obstetric Emergency Training*. Oxford: Wiley-Blackwell, 2009: 111–124.
3. Royal College of Obstetricians and Gynaecologists. *Prevention and Management of Postpartum Haemorrhage* (Green-top guideline 52). London: RCOG, 2016.
4. Mousa HA, Alfirevic Z. Treatment for primary postpartum haemorrhage. *Cochrane Database of Systematic Reviews* 2007, 1: CD003249.
5. Starrs A, Winikoff B. Misoprostol for postpartum hemorrhage: moving from evidence to practice. *International Journal of Gynaecology and Obstetrics* 2012, 116(1): 1–3.

Presentation

Solution for injection ampoules: morphine sulfate 10 mg/ml (morphine sulfate 10 mg per 1 ml).

Oral solution: morphine sulfate 10 mg/5 ml (morphine sulfate 2 mg per 1 ml).

Indications

Pain associated with suspected myocardial infarction (analgesic of first choice).

Severe pain as a component of a balanced analgesia regimen.

The decision about which analgesia and which route should be guided by clinical judgement. Refer to **Pain Management in Adults** and **Pain Management in Children**.

Actions

Morphine is a strong opioid analgesic.

Morphine produces sedation, euphoria and analgesia; it may both depress respiration and induce hypotension.

Histamine is released following morphine administration and this may contribute to its vasodilatory effects. This may also account for the urticaria and bronchoconstriction that are sometimes seen.

Contra-Indications

Do **NOT** administer morphine in the following circumstances:

- Children under 1 year of age.
- Respiratory depression (adult <10 breaths per minute, child <20 breaths per minute).
- Hypotension (actual, not estimated, systolic blood pressure <90 mmHg in adults, <80 mmHg in school children, <70 mmHg in pre-school children).
- Head injury with significantly impaired level of consciousness (e.g. below P on the AVPU scale or below 9 on the GCS).
- Known hypersensitivity to morphine.
- Severe headache.

Cautions

Known severe renal or hepatic impairment – smaller doses may be used carefully and titrated to effect.

Use with **extreme** caution (minimal doses) during pregnancy. **NOTE:** Not to be used for labour pain where Nitrous Oxide (Entonox®) is the analgesic of choice.

Use morphine **WITH GREAT CAUTION** in patients with chest injuries, particularly those with any respiratory difficulty, although if respiration is inhibited by pain, analgesia may actually improve respiratory status.

Any patients with other respiratory problems (e.g. asthma, COPD).

Head injury. Agitation following head injury may be due to acute brain injury, hypoxia or pain. The decision to administer analgesia to an agitated head injured patient is a clinical one. It is vital that if such a patient receives opioids they are closely monitored since opioids can cause disproportionate respiratory depression, which may ultimately lead to an elevated intracranial pressure through a raised arterial pCO_2.

Acute alcohol intoxication. All opioid drugs potentiate the central nervous system depressant effects of alcohol and they should therefore be used with great caution in patients who have consumed significant quantities of alcohol.

Medications. Prescribed antidepressants, sedatives or major tranquillisers may potentiate the respiratory and cardiovascular depressant effects of morphine.

Smaller doses should be considered for lightweight children over age 12 and for older patients who may be more susceptible to complications.

Side Effects

- Respiratory depression.
- Cardiovascular depression.
- Nausea and vomiting.
- Drowsiness.
- Pupillary constriction.

Additional Information

Morphine injection is a Class A controlled drug under Schedule 2 of the Misuse of Drugs Regulations 2001. It must be stored securely and its movements recorded in a controlled drug register. It may only be possessed and administered by healthcare professionals authorised in the legislation.

Morphine is not licensed for use in children but its use has been approved by the Medicines and Healthcare Products Regulatory Agency (MHRA) for 'off label' use. This means that it can legally be administered under these guidelines by paramedics.

Unused morphine in open vials or syringes must be discarded in the presence of a witness according to local policy and procedures.

Special Precautions

Naloxone can be used to reverse morphine related respiratory or cardiovascular depression. It should be carefully titrated after assessment and appropriate management of ABC for that particular patient and situation, refer to **Naloxone Hydrochloride**.

Morphine frequently induces nausea or vomiting which may be potentiated by the movement of the ambulance. Titrating to the lowest dose to achieve analgesia will reduce the risk of vomiting. The use of an anti-emetic should also be considered whenever administering any opioid analgesic, refer to **Ondansetron** and **Metoclopramide**.

Dosage and Administration

Administration must be in conjunction with pain score monitoring, refer to **Pain Management in Adults** and **Pain Management in Children**.

Intravenous morphine takes a minimum of 2–3 minutes before starting to take effect, reaching its peak between 10 and 20 minutes.

The absorption of intramuscular, subcutaneous or oral morphine is variable, particularly in patients with major trauma, shock and cardiac conditions; these routes should preferably be avoided if the circumstances favour intravenous or intraosseous administration.

Morphine **should be** diluted with sodium chloride 0.9% to make a concentration of 10 milligrams in 10 ml (1 milligram in 1 ml) unless it is being administered by the intramuscular or subcutaneous route when it should not be diluted.

ADULTS – If pain is not reduced to a tolerable level after 10 milligrams of IV/IO morphine, then further **2 milligram** doses may be administered by slow IV/IO injection every 5 minutes to **20 milligrams maximum**. The patient should be closely observed throughout the remaining treatment and transfer. Smaller doses should be considered for lightweight children over age 12 and for older patients who may be more susceptible to complications.

CHILDREN – The doses and volumes given below are for the initial and maximum doses. Administer **0.1 ml/kg** (equal to **100 micrograms/kg**) as an initial slow IV injection over 2 minutes. If pain is not reduced to a tolerable level after 5 minutes then a further dose of up to **100 micrograms/kg**, titrated to response, may be repeated (**maximum dose 200 micrograms/kg**).

NOTE: Peak effect of each dose may not occur until 10–20 minutes after administration.

Intravenous/intraosseous

Route: Intravenous/intraosseous – administer by slow IV injection (rate of approximately 2 milligrams per minute up to appropriate dose for age). Observe the patient for at least 5 minutes after completion of initial dose before repeating the dose if required.

AGE	INITIAL DOSE	REPEAT DOSE	DOSE INTERVAL	DILUTED CONCENTRATION	VOLUME	MAX DOSE
≥ 12 years and adult	10 milligrams	10 milligrams	5 minutes	10 milligrams in 10 ml	10 ml	20 milligrams
11 years	3.5 milligrams	3.5 milligrams	5 minutes	10 milligrams in 10 ml	3.5 ml	7 milligrams
10 years	3 milligrams	3 milligrams	5 minutes	10 milligrams in 10 ml	3 ml	6 milligrams
9 years	3 milligrams	3 milligrams	5 minutes	10 milligrams in 10 ml	3 ml	6 milligrams
8 years	2.5 milligrams	2.5 milligrams	5 minutes	10 milligrams in 10 ml	2.5 ml	5 milligrams
7 years	2.5 milligrams	2.5 milligrams	5 minutes	10 milligrams in 10 ml	2.5 ml	5 milligrams
6 years	2 milligrams	2 milligrams	5 minutes	10 milligrams in 10 ml	2 ml	4 milligrams
5 years	2 milligrams	2 milligrams	5 minutes	10 milligrams in 10 ml	2 ml	4 milligrams
4 years	1.5 milligrams	1.5 milligrams	5 minutes	10 milligrams in 10 ml	1.5 ml	3 milligrams
3 years	1.5 milligrams	1.5 milligrams	5 minutes	10 milligrams in 10 ml	1.5 ml	3 milligrams
2 years	1 milligram	1 milligram	5 minutes	10 milligrams in 10 ml	1 ml	2 milligrams
18 months	1 milligram	1 milligram	5 minutes	10 milligrams in 10 ml	1 ml	2 milligrams

AGE	INITIAL DOSE	REPEAT DOSE	DOSE INTERVAL	DILUTED CONCENTRATION	VOLUME	MAX DOSE
12 months	1 milligram	1 milligram	5 minutes	10 milligrams in 10 ml	1 ml	2 milligrams
9 months	N/A	N/A	N/A	N/A	N/A	N/A
6 months	N/A	N/A	N/A	N/A	N/A	N/A
3 months	N/A	N/A	N/A	N/A	N/A	N/A
1 month	N/A	N/A	N/A	N/A	N/A	N/A
Birth	N/A	N/A	N/A	N/A	N/A	N/A

Oral

Route: Oral.

NB Only administer via the oral route in patients with major trauma, shock or cardiac conditions if the IV/IO routes are not accessible.

AGE	INITIAL DOSE	REPEAT DOSE	DOSE INTERVAL	DILUTED CONCENTRATION	VOLUME	MAX DOSE
≥ 12 years and adult	20 milligrams	20 milligrams	60 minutes	10 milligrams in 5 ml	10 ml	40 milligrams
11 years	7 milligrams	NONE	N/A	10 milligrams in 5 ml	3.5 ml	7 milligrams
10 years	6 milligrams	NONE	N/A	10 milligrams in 5 ml	3 ml	6 milligrams
9 years	6 milligrams	NONE	N/A	10 milligrams in 5 ml	3 ml	6 milligrams
8 years	5 milligrams	NONE	N/A	10 milligrams in 5 ml	2.5 ml	5 milligrams
7 years	5 milligrams	NONE	N/A	10 milligrams in 5 ml	2.5 ml	5 milligrams
6 years	4 milligrams	NONE	N/A	10 milligrams in 5 ml	2 ml	4 milligrams
5 years	4 milligrams	NONE	N/A	10 milligrams in 5 ml	2 ml	4 milligrams
4 years	3 milligrams	NONE	N/A	10 milligrams in 5 ml	1.5 ml	3 milligrams
3 years	3 milligrams	NONE	N/A	10 milligrams in 5 ml	1.5 ml	3 milligrams
2 years	2 milligrams	NONE	N/A	10 milligrams in 5 ml	1 ml	2 milligrams
18 months	2 milligrams	NONE	N/A	10 milligrams in 5 ml	1 ml	2 milligrams
12 months	2 milligrams	NONE	N/A	10 milligrams in 5 ml	1 ml	2 milligrams
9 months	N/A	N/A	N/A	N/A	N/A	N/A
6 months	N/A	N/A	N/A	N/A	N/A	N/A
3 months	N/A	N/A	N/A	N/A	N/A	N/A
1 month	N/A	N/A	N/A	N/A	N/A	N/A
Birth	N/A	N/A	N/A	N/A	N/A	N/A

Intramuscular/subcutaneous

Route: Intramuscular/subcutaneous.

NB Only administer via the intramuscular or subcutaneous route in patients with major trauma, shock or cardiac conditions if the IV/IO routes are not accessible.

AGE	INITIAL DOSE	REPEAT DOSE	DOSE INTERVAL	DILUTED CONCENTRATION	VOLUME	MAX DOSE
≥ 12 years and adult	10 milligrams	10 milligrams	60 minutes	10 milligrams in 1 ml	1 ml	20 milligrams
11 years	3.5 milligrams	3.5 milligrams	60 minutes	10 milligrams in 1 ml	0.35 ml	7 milligrams
10 years	3 milligrams	3 milligrams	60 minutes	10 milligrams in 1 ml	0.30 ml	6 milligrams
9 years	3 milligrams	3 milligrams	60 minutes	10 milligrams in 1 ml	0.30 ml	6 milligrams
8 years	2.5 milligrams	2.5 milligrams	60 minutes	10 milligrams in 1 ml	0.25 ml	5 milligrams
7 years	2.5 milligrams	2.5 milligrams	60 minutes	10 milligrams in 1 ml	0.25 ml	5 milligrams
6 years	2 milligrams	2 milligrams	60 minutes	10 milligrams in 1 ml	0.20 ml	4 milligrams
5 years	2 milligrams	2 milligrams	60 minutes	10 milligrams in 1 ml	0.20 ml	4 milligrams
4 years	1.5 milligrams	1.5 milligrams	60 minutes	10 milligrams in 1 ml	0.15 ml	3 milligrams
3 years	1.5 milligrams	1.5 milligrams	60 minutes	10 milligrams in 1 ml	0.15 ml	3 milligrams
2 years	1 milligram	1 milligram	60 minutes	10 milligrams in 1 ml	0.10 ml	2 milligrams
18 months	1 milligram	1 milligram	60 minutes	10 milligrams in 1 ml	0.10 ml	2 milligrams
12 months	1 milligram	1 milligram	60 minutes	10 milligrams in 1 ml	0.10 ml	2 milligrams
9 months	N/A	N/A	N/A	N/A	N/A	N/A
6 months	N/A	N/A	N/A	N/A	N/A	N/A
3 months	N/A	N/A	N/A	N/A	N/A	N/A
1 months	N/A	N/A	N/A	N/A	N/A	N/A
Birth	N/A	N/A	N/A	N/A	N/A	N/A

Morphine Sulfate for the Management of Pain in Adults at the End of Life

AGE	INITIAL DOSE	REPEAT DOSE	DOSE INTERVAL	CONCEN-TRATION	VOLUME	MAX DOSE
Adult ≥18 years For opioid naive/patients with an unknown opioid tolerance who also have severe respiratory compromise	2.5 milligrams in 1.25 millilitres	N/A	N/A	N/A	N/A	N/A
Adult ≥18 years For patients who are on a known dose of a strong regular opioid	Administer the usual breakthrough dose or 1/6 of the total 24 hour dosage of oral morphine	N/A	N/A	N/A	N/A	N/A

Presentation

Naloxone hydrochloride 400 micrograms per 1 ml ampoule.

Indications

The reversal of acute opioid or opiate toxicity for respiratory arrest or respiratory depression.

Unconsciousness, associated with respiratory depression of unknown cause, where opioid overdose is a possibility. Refer to **Altered Level of Consciousness**.

In cardiac arrest, where opioid toxicity is considered to be the likely cause.

Patients exposed to high-potency veterinary or anaesthetic preparations should be given naloxone urgently if:

- Consciousness is impaired

OR

- Exposure occurred within the last 10 minutes, even if asymptomatic.

If an antidote is supplied with the opioid medication, such as diprenorphine (Revivon) or naloxone, it should be administered immediately.

Actions

Complete or partial reversal of the respiratory depression effects of opioid drugs.

The aim of naloxone administration is to restore adequate respirations but not necessarily to restore full consciousness.

Contra-indications

Neonates born to opioid addicted mothers can result in serious withdrawal effects. Emphasis should be on bag-valve-mask ventilation and oxygenation.

Side Effects

- In patients who are physically dependent on opioids, naloxone may precipitate violent withdrawal symptoms, including cardiac arrhythmias. It is better, in these cases, to titrate the dose of naloxone as described in the dosing charts in this guideline to effectively reverse the cardiac and respiratory depression, but still leave the patient in a 'groggy' state with regular reassessment of ventilation and circulation.
- Vomiting is a common side effect following naloxone administration, ensure access to suction.

Additional Information

When indicated, naloxone can be administered via the intravenous, intramuscular, intraosseous, subcutaneous or intranasal route. Very ill patients will require intravenous naloxone to ensure rapid absorption of the total dose.

Refer to local procedures/product instructions for the route of administration and for intranasal dose and time intervals.

For intramuscular administration, the drug should be **undiluted** (into the outer aspect of the thigh or upper arm), but absorption may be unpredictable.

All cases of opioid overdose should be transported to hospital, even if the initial response to naloxone has been good. The duration of action of naloxone is usually 30 to 90 minutes and this is shorter than some opioids such as methadone; therefore additional doses of naloxone may be necessary to maintain reversal of opioid induced respiratory depression. Patients who have ingested methadone require observation for at least 8 hours following overdose to prevent accidental death. If the patient refuses to go to hospital, consider, if the patient consents, a loading dose of **800 micrograms IM** to minimise the risk described above. For patients who refuse transfer to hospital if possible leave in the care of a responsible adult and leave an advice leaflet advising of action to be taken in the event that the symptoms return.

Some patients at risk of opiate misuse (or their carers) may have been given take home naloxone as a harm-reduction measure.

The large difference in doses between adult and children reflects the likely aetiology of the opiate ingestion and aims of treatment.

In children aged under 12, the aetiology is likely to be accidental ingestion and they are unlikely to be dependent on opiates (unless they are an end of life care patient) so the aim is to totally reverse the opiate. If you feel the child needs further doses in the same episode of illness they must be reviewed by a senior healthcare professional; seek senior clinical advice.

Adults are more likely to be dependant opiate users and may become aggressive if the opiate is reversed, so the aim is a controlled reversal.

Methadone is a long-acting synthetic opioid that is used in opioid harm reduction and substance misuse programmes. Methadone has an elimination half-life of between 15 and 60 hours, in contrast to the shorter-acting naloxone which has a half-life of 1 to 1.5 hours.

Cautions for End of Life Care Patients

The use of naloxone in palliative care is not routinely practised, as patients on regular opioids can be physically dependant. It is only indicated in circumstances where a clinician suspects opioid induced toxicity, from intentional or unintentional overdose. The aim is to reverse life-threatening respiratory depression only i.e. if the respiratory rate is <8 breaths per minute and the patient is unconscious and or cyanosed. Refer to **End of Life Care**.

Dosage and Administration: IV/IO

Respiratory arrest/respiratory depression/cardiac arrest

Route: Intravenous/intraosseous

For adults who may be opiate dependant: administer **slowly**, 1 ml at a time. Titrate to response relieving respiratory depression but maintain patient in 'groggy' state. For known or potentially aggressive adults suffering respiratory depression: dilute up to 800 micrograms (2 ml) of naloxone into 8 ml of water for injections or sodium chloride 0.9% to a total volume of 10 ml and administer **slowly**, titrating to response, 1 ml at a time.

If there is no response after the initial dose, repeat the dose, up to the maximum dose or until an effect is noted.

NB The duration of action of naloxone is short.

For children: give the full dose with the aim of totally reversing the opiate effects.

Seek advice to exceed the maximum dose as per local procedures.

In cardiac arrest, children or adults, repeat up to maximum dose until ROSC achieved.

AGE	ROUTE	INITIAL DOSE	REPEAT DOSE	DOSE INTERVAL	CONCENTRATION	VOLUME	MAX DOSE
≥12 years	IV/IO	400 micrograms	400 micrograms	3 minutes	400 micrograms in 1 ml	1 ml	4,000 micrograms
11 years	IV/IO	2,000 micrograms	Seek advice	N/A	400 micrograms in 1 ml	5 ml	2,000 micrograms
10 years	IV/IO	2,000 micrograms	Seek advice	N/A	400 micrograms in 1 ml	5 ml	2,000 micrograms
9 years	IV/IO	2,000 micrograms	Seek advice	N/A	400 micrograms in 1 ml	5 ml	2,000 micrograms
8 years	IV/IO	2,000 micrograms	Seek advice	N/A	400 micrograms in 1 ml	5 ml	2,000 micrograms
7 years	IV/IO	2,000 micrograms	Seek advice	N/A	400 micrograms in 1 ml	5 ml	2,000 micrograms
6 years	IV/IO	2,000 micrograms	Seek advice	N/A	400 micrograms in 1 ml	5 ml	2,000 micrograms
5 years	IV/IO	2,000 micrograms	Seek advice	N/A	400 micrograms in 1 ml	5 ml	2,000 micrograms
4 years	IV/IO	1,600 micrograms	400 micrograms	1 minute	400 micrograms in 1 ml	4 ml	2,000 micrograms
3 years	IV/IO	1,200 micrograms	800 micrograms	1 minute	400 micrograms in 1 ml	3 ml	2,000 micrograms
2 years	IV/IO	1,200 micrograms	800 micrograms	1 minute	400 micrograms in 1 ml	3 ml	2,000 micrograms
18 months	IV/IO	1,000 micrograms	1,000 micrograms	1 minute	400 micrograms in 1 ml	2.5 ml	2,000 micrograms
12 months	IV/IO	1,000 micrograms	1,000 micrograms	1 minute	400 micrograms in 1 ml	2.5 ml	2,000 micrograms
9 months	IV/IO	800 micrograms	800 micrograms	1 minute	400 micrograms in 1 ml	2 ml	2,000 micrograms
6 months	IV/IO	800 micrograms	800 micrograms	1 minute	400 micrograms in 1 ml	2 ml	2,000 micrograms
3 months	IV/IO	400 micrograms	400 micrograms	1 minute	400 micrograms in 1 ml	1 ml	2,000 micrograms
1 month	IV/IO	400 micrograms	400 micrograms	1 minute	400 micrograms in 1 ml	1 ml	2,000 micrograms
Birth	IV/IO	N/A	N/A	N/A	N/A	N/A	N/A

Naloxone Hydrochloride NLX

Dosage and Administration: IM

Respiratory arrest/respiratory depression where the IV/IO route is unavailable or the ambulance clinician is not trained to administer drugs via the IV/IO route.

Route: Intramuscular/subcutaneous. Only use this route if the IV/IO route is not available.

If there is no response after the initial dose, give up to the maximum dose or until an effect is noted. **NB** the half-life of naloxone is short.

For children: give the full dose with the aim of totally reversing the opiate effects.

Administering large volumes via the intramuscular route could lead to poor absorption and/or tissue damage. Therefore, divide the dose where necessary and practicable. Vary the site of injection for repeated doses.

AGE	INITIAL DOSE	REPEAT DOSE	DOSE INTERVAL	CONCENTRATION	VOLUME	MAX DOSE
≥12 years	400 micrograms	400 micrograms	3 minutes	400 micrograms in 1 ml	1 ml	4,000 micrograms
1 month – 11 years	400 micrograms	400 micrograms	3 minutes	400 micrograms in 1 ml	1 ml	2,000 micrograms
Birth	N/A	N/A	N/A	N/A	N/A	N/A

Bibliography

1. British National Formulary. *Naloxone Hydrochloride.* Available from: https://bnf.nice.org.uk/drug/naloxone-hydrochloride.html, 2019.
2. Medicines Q&As. *What naloxone doses should be used in adults to reverse urgently the effects opioids or opiates?* Available from: https://www.sps.nhs.uk/wp-content/uploads/2015/11/UKMi_QA-_Naloxone-dosing_Aug-17_FINAL.pdf, 2017.

Nitrous Oxide (Entonox®) NOO

Presentation

Nitrous Oxide (Entonox®) 1ml per 1ml medical gas is a combination of nitrous oxide 50% and oxygen 50%. It is stored in medical cylinders that have a blue body with white shoulders.

Indications

Moderate to severe pain.

Labour pains.

Actions

Inhaled analgesic agent.

Contra-indications

Nitrous oxide may have a deleterious effect if administered to patients with closed body cavities containing air since nitrous oxide diffuses into such a space with a resulting increase in pressure.

Do not give Entonox to patients with:

- Severe head injuries with impaired consciousness due to possible presence of intracranial air.
- Decompression sickness (the bends) where Entonox can cause nitrogen bubbles within the blood stream to expand, aggravating the problem further. Consider anyone that has been diving within the previous 24 hours to be at risk.
- Violently disturbed psychiatric patients.
- Intraocular injection of gas within the last four weeks.
- Abdominal pain where intestinal obstruction is suspected.

Cautions

Any patient at risk of having a pneumothorax, pneumomediastinum and/or a pneumoperitoneum (e.g. polytrauma, penetrating torso injury).

Side Effects

Minimal side effects.

Additional Information

Prolonged use for more than 24 hours, or more frequently than every four days, can lead to vitamin B12 deficiency.

Administration of Entonox should be in conjunction with pain score monitoring.

Entonox's advantages include:

- Rapid analgesic effect with minimal side effects.
- No cardiorespiratory depression.
- Self-administered.
- Analgesic effect rapidly wears off.
- The 50% oxygen concentration is valuable in many medical and trauma conditions.
- Entonox can be administered whilst preparing to deliver other analgesics.

The usual precautions must be followed with regard to caring for the Entonox equipment and the cylinder MUST be inverted several times before use to mix the gases when temperatures are low.

Dosage and Administration

Adults:

- Entonox should be self-administered via a facemask or mouthpiece, after suitable instruction. It takes about **3–5 minutes** to be effective, but it may be **5–10 minutes** before maximum effect is achieved.

Children:

- Entonox is effective in children provided they are capable of following the administration instructions and can activate the demand valve.

Ondansetron

Presentation

Ampoule containing 4 milligrams of ondansetron (as hydrochloride) in 2 ml.

Ampoule containing 8 milligrams of ondansetron (as hydrochloride) in 4 ml.

NB Both these preparations share the same concentration (2 milligrams in 1 ml).

Indications

Adults:

- Prevention and treatment of opiate-induced nausea and vomiting (e.g. morphine sulfate).
- Treatment of nausea or vomiting.

Children:

- Prevention and treatment of opiate-induced nausea and vomiting (e.g. morphine sulfate).
- For travel associated nausea or vomiting.

Actions

An anti-emetic that blocks 5HT receptors both centrally and in the gastrointestinal tract.

Contra-indications

Known sensitivity to ondansetron.

Infants <1 month old.

Cautions

QT interval prolongation (avoid concomitant administration of drugs that prolong QT interval).

Hepatic impairment.

Pregnancy.

Breastfeeding.

Side Effects

Hiccups.

Constipation.

Flushing.

Hypotension.

Chest pain.

Arrhythmias.

Bradycardia.

Headache.

Seizures.

Movement disorders.

Injection site reactions.

Additional Information

Ondansetron should always be given in a separate syringe to morphine sulfate – the drugs must **NOT** be mixed.

Ondansetron should **NOT** be routinely administered in the management of childhood gastroenteritis (refer to **Paediatric Gastroenteritis**).

Vomiting can be a symptom of a more serious problem. If a patient is sufficiently unwell that they require parenteral anti-emetics, the Paramedic must seek further advice from a specialist or a GP before making the decision to leave them on scene with Ondansetron.

Dosage and Administration

Note: Two preparations exist (4 mg in 2 ml and 8 mg in 4 ml). They share the same concentration, that is 2 milligrams in 1 ml.

Route: Intravenous (SLOW IV injection over 2 minutes)/intramuscular.

NB Monitor pulse, blood pressure, respiratory rate and cardiac rhythm before, during and after administration.

AGE	INITIAL DOSE	REPEAT DOSE	DOSE INTERVAL	CONCENTRATION	VOLUME	MAX DOSE
≥ 12 years	4 milligrams	NONE	N/A	2 milligrams in 1 ml	2 ml	4 milligrams
11 years	3 milligrams	NONE	N/A	2 milligrams in 1 ml	1.5 ml	3 milligrams
10 years	3 milligrams	NONE	N/A	2 milligrams in 1 ml	1.5 ml	3 milligrams
9 years	3 milligrams	NONE	N/A	2 milligrams in 1 ml	1.5 ml	3 milligrams
8 years	2.5 milligrams	NONE	N/A	2 milligrams in 1 ml	1.3 ml	2.5 milligrams
7 years	2.5 milligrams	NONE	N/A	2 milligrams in 1 ml	1.3 ml	2.5 milligrams
6 years	2 milligrams	NONE	N/A	2 milligrams in 1 ml	1 ml	2 milligrams
5 years	2 milligrams	NONE	N/A	2 milligrams in 1 ml	1 ml	2 milligrams
4 years	1.5 milligrams	NONE	N/A	2 milligrams in 1 ml	0.75 ml	1.5 milligrams
3 years	1.5 milligrams	NONE	N/A	2 milligrams in 1 ml	0.75 ml	1.5 milligrams

AGE	INITIAL DOSE	REPEAT DOSE	DOSE INTERVAL	CONCENTRATION	VOLUME	MAX DOSE
2 years	1 milligram	NONE	N/A	2 milligrams in 1 ml	0.5 ml	1 milligram
18 months	1 milligram	NONE	N/A	2 milligrams in 1 ml	0.5 ml	1 milligram
12 months	1 milligram	NONE	N/A	2 milligrams in 1 ml	0.5 ml	1 milligram
9 months	1 milligram	NONE	N/A	2 milligrams in 1 ml	0.5 ml	1 milligram
6 months	1 milligram	NONE	N/A	2 milligrams in 1 ml	0.5 ml	1 milligram
3 months	0.5 milligrams	NONE	N/A	2 milligrams in 1 ml	0.25 ml	0.5 milligrams
1 month	0.5 milligrams	NONE	N/A	2 milligrams in 1 ml	0.25 ml	0.5 milligrams
Birth	N/A	N/A	N/A	N/A	N/A	N/A

Bibliography

1. Salvucci AA, Squire B, Burdick M, Luoto M, Brazzel D, Vaezazizi R. Ondansetron is safe and effective for prehospital treatment of nausea and vomiting by paramedics. *Pre-hospital Emergency Care* 2011, 15(1): 34–8.
2. British National Formulary. *Ondansetron.* Available from: https://bnf.nice.org.uk/drug/ondansetron.html, 2018.
3. Warden CR, Moreno R, Daya M. Prospective evaluation of ondansetron for undifferentiated nausea and vomiting in the prehospital setting. *Pre-hospital Emergency Care* 2008, 12(1): 87–91.

Oxygen

Presentation

Oxygen (O_2) is a gas provided in compressed form in a cylinder. It is also available in liquid form, in a system adapted for ambulance use. It is fed via a regulator and flow meter to the patient by means of plastic tubing and an oxygen mask/nasal cannulae.

Indications

Children

- Significant illness and/or injury.

Adults

- Critical illnesses requiring high levels of supplemental oxygen (refer to Table 7.9).
- Serious illnesses requiring moderate levels of supplemental oxygen if the patient is hypoxaemic (refer to Table 7.10).
- COPD and other conditions requiring controlled or low-dose oxygen therapy (refer to Table 7.11).
- Conditions for which patients should be monitored closely but oxygen therapy is not required unless the patient is hypoxaemic (refer to Table 7.12).

Actions

Essential for cell metabolism. Adequate tissue oxygenation is essential for normal physiological function.

Oxygen assists in reversing hypoxia, by raising the concentration of inspired oxygen. Hypoxia will, however, only improve if respiratory effort or ventilation and tissue perfusion are adequate.

If ventilation is inadequate or absent, assisting or completely taking over the patient's ventilation is essential to reverse hypoxia.

Contra-indications

Explosive environments.

Cautions

Oxygen increases the fire hazard at the scene of an incident.

Defibrillation – ensure pads firmly applied to reduce spark hazard.

Side Effects

Non-humidified O_2 is drying and irritating to mucous membranes over a period of time.

In patients with COPD there is a risk that even moderately high doses of inspired oxygen can produce increased carbon dioxide levels which may cause respiratory depression and this may lead to respiratory arrest. Refer to Table 7.7 for guidance.

Dosage and Administration

- Measure oxygen saturation (SpO_2) in all patients using pulse oximetry.
- For the administration of **moderate** levels of supplemented oxygen nasal cannulae are recommended in preference to a simple face mask as they offer a more flexible dose range.
- Patients with tracheostomy or previous laryngectomy may require alternative appliances (e.g. tracheostomy masks).
- Entonox may be administered when required.
- Document oxygen administration.

Children

- **ALL** children with significant illness and/or injury should receive **HIGH** levels of supplementary oxygen.

Adults

- Administer the initial oxygen dose until a reliable oxygen saturation reading is obtained.
- If the desired oxygen saturation cannot be maintained with a simple face mask, change to a reservoir mask (non-rebreathe mask).
- For dosage and administration of supplemental oxygen refer to Tables 7.5–7.8.
- For conditions where **NO** supplemental oxygen is required unless the patient is hypoxaemic refer to Table 7.8.
- BTS guidance states that a sudden reduction of more than 3% in a patient's oxygen saturation within the target saturation range should prompt fuller assessment of the patient because this may be the first evidence of an acute illness.
- Some people aged above 70 years may have saturation measurements in the range of 92–94% when clinically stable. These people do not require oxygen therapy unless the oxygen saturation falls below the level that is known to be normal for the individual patient.

TABLE 7.5 – High levels of supplemental oxygen for adults with critical illnesses

Target saturation 94–98%

Administer the initial oxygen dose until the vital signs are normal, then reduce oxygen dose and aim for target saturation within the range of **94–98%** as per table below.

Condition	Initial dose	Method of administration
• Cardiac arrest or resuscitation: – basic life support – advanced life support – foreign body airway obstruction – traumatic cardiac arrest – maternal resuscitation. • Carbon monoxide poisoning **NOTE– Some oxygen saturation monitors cannot differentiate between carboxyhaemoglobin and oxyhaemoglobin owing to carbon monoxide poisoning.**	Maximum dose until the vital signs are normal	Bag-valve-mask
• Major trauma: – abdominal trauma – burns and scalds – electrocution – head trauma – limb trauma – spinal injury and spinal cord injury – pelvic trauma – the immersion incident – thoracic trauma – trauma in pregnancy. • Anaphylaxis • Decompression illness • Major pulmonary haemorrhage • Sepsis (e.g. meningococcal septicemia) • Shock • Drowning	15 litres per minute	Reservoir mask (non-rebreathe mask)
• Active convulsion • Hypothermia	Administer 15 litres per minute until a reliable SpO_2 measurement can be obtained and the adjust oxygen flow to aim for target saturation within the range of **94–98%**	Reservoir mask (non-rebreathe mask)

TABLE 7.6 – Moderate levels of supplemental oxygen for adults with serious illnesses if the patient is hypoxaemic

Target saturation 94–98%

Administer the initial oxygen dose until a reliable SpO_2 measurement is available, then adjust oxygen flow to aim for target saturation within the range of **94–98%** as per the table below.

Condition	Initial dose	Method of administration
• Acute hypoxaemia (cause not yet diagnosed) • Deterioration of lung fibrosis or other interstitial lung disease • Acute asthma • Acute heart failure • Pneumonia • Lung cancer • Postoperative breathlessness • Pulmonary embolism • Pleural effusions • Pneumothorax • Severe anaemia • Sickle cell crisis	**SpO_2 <85%** 10–15 litres per minute	Reservoir mask (non-rebreathe mask)
	SpO_2 ≥85–93% 2–6 litres per minute	Nasal cannulae
	SpO_2 ≥85–93% 5–10 litres per minute	Simple face mask

TABLE 7.7 – Controlled or low-dose supplemental oxygen for adults with COPD and other conditions requiring controlled or low-dose oxygen therapy

Target saturation 88–92%

Administer the initial oxygen dose until a reliable SpO_2 measurement is available, then adjust oxygen flow to aim for target saturation within the range of **88–92%** or **pre-specified range** detailed on the patient's alert card, as per the table below.

Condition	Initial dose	Method of administration
Chronic obstructive pulmonary disease (COPD) Exacerbation of cystic fibrosis	4 litres per minute	28% Venturi mask or patient's own mask
	NB If respiratory rate is >30 breaths/min using Venturi mask set flow rate to 50% above the minimum specified for the mask.	
Chronic neuromuscular disorders Chest wall disorders Morbid obesity (body mass index >40 kg/m^2)	4 litres per minute	28% Venturi mask or patient's own mask
NB If the oxygen saturation remains below 88% change to simple face mask.	5–10 litres per minute	Simple face mask
NB Critical illness **AND** COPD/or other risk factors for hypercapnia.	If a patient with COPD or other risk factors for hypercapnia sustains or develops critical illness/injury then a target saturation level of 94-98% should be aimed for, but if this results in decreased conscious level or decreased respiratory rate decrease the oxygen flow and aim for 88-92%	

TABLE 7.8 – No supplemental oxygen required for adults with these conditions unless the patient is hypoxaemic but patients should be monitored closely

Target saturation 94–98%

If hypoxaemic (SpO_2 <94%) administer the initial oxygen dose, then adjust oxygen flow to aim for target saturation within the range of **94–98%**, as per table below.

Condition

- Myocardial infarction and acute coronary syndromes
- Stroke
- Cardiac rhythm disturbance
- Non-traumatic chest pain/discomfort
- Implantable cardioverter defibrillator firing
- Pregnancy and obstetric emergencies:
  - birth imminent
  - haemorrhage during pregnancy
  - pregnancy induced hypertension
  - vaginal bleeding.
- Abdominal pain
- Headache
- Hyperventilation syndrome or dysfunctional breathing
- Most poisonings and drug overdoses (refer to Table 7.7 for **carbon monoxide poisoning** and special cases below for **paraquat or bleomycin** poisoning)
- Metabolic and renal disorders
- Acute and sub-acute neurological and muscular conditions producing muscle weakness (assess the need for assisted ventilation if **SpO_2 <94%**)
- Post convulsion
- Gastrointestinal bleeds
- Glycaemic emergencies
- Heat exhaustion/heat stroke

SPECIAL CASES

- Poisoning with paraquat
- Poisoning with bleomycin

NOTE – patients with **paraquat or bleomycin** poisoning may be harmed by supplemental oxygen so avoid oxygen unless the patient is hypoxaemic. Target saturation 85–88%.

Initial dose	Method of administration
SpO_2 <85% 10–15 litres per minute	Reservoir mask (non-rebreathe mask)
SpO_2 ≥85–93% 2–6 litres per minute	Nasal cannulae
SpO_2 ≥85–93% 5–10 litres per minute	Simple face mask

TABLE 7.9 – Critical illnesses in adults requiring HIGH levels of supplemental oxygen

- Cardiac arrest or resuscitation:
  - basic life support
  - advanced life support
  - foreign body airway obstruction
  - traumatic cardiac arrest
  - maternal resuscitation
- Major trauma:
  - abdominal trauma
  - burns and scalds
  - electrocution
  - head trauma
  - limb trauma
  - spinal injury and spinal cord injury
  - pelvic trauma
  - the immersion incident
  - thoracic trauma
  - trauma in pregnancy
- Active convulsion
- Anaphylaxis
- Decompression illness
- Carbon monoxide poisoning
- Hypothermia
- Major pulmonary haemorrhage
- Sepsis (e.g. meningococcal septicaemia)
- Shock
- Drowning

TABLE 7.10 – Serious illnesses in adults requiring MODERATE levels of supplemental oxygen if hypoxaemic

- Acute hypoxaemia
- Deterioration of lung fibrosis or other interstitial lung disease
- Acute asthma
- Acute heart failure
- Pneumonia
- Lung cancer
- Postoperative breathlessness
- Pulmonary embolism
- Pleural effusions
- Pneumothorax
- Severe anaemia
- Sickle cell crisis

TABLE 7.11 – COPD and other conditions in adults requiring CONTROLLED OR LOW-DOSE supplemental oxygen

- Chronic Obstructive Pulmonary Disease (COPD)
- Exacerbation of cystic fibrosis
- Chronic neuromuscular disorders
- Chest wall disorders
- Morbid obesity (body mass index >40 kg/m^2)

NB BTS guidance states that patients with COPD and other risk factors for hypercapnia should have the same initial target saturations as other critically ill patients pending the results of blood gas results after which these patients may need controlled oxygen therapy with target range 88–92 or supported ventilation and/or hypercapnia with respiratory acidosis.

Patients over 50 years of age who are long-term smokers with a history of exertional breathlessness and no other known cause of breathlessness should be treated as if having COPD.

TABLE 7.12 – Conditions in adults NOT requiring supplemental oxygen unless the patient is hypoxaemic

- Myocardial infarction and acute coronary syndromes
- Stroke
- Cardiac rhythm disturbance
- Non-traumatic chest pain/discomfort
- Implantable cardioverter defibrillator firing
- Pregnancy and obstetric emergencies:
  - birth imminent
  - haemorrhage during pregnancy
  - pregnancy induced hypertension
  - vaginal bleeding
- Abdominal pain
- Headache
- Hyperventilation syndrome or dysfunctional breathing
- Most poisonings and drug overdoses (except carbon monoxide poisoning)
- Metabolic and renal disorders
- Acute and sub-acute neurological and muscular conditions producing muscle weakness
- Post convulsion
- Gastrointestinal bleeds
- Glycaemic emergencies
- Heat exhaustion/heat stroke

Special cases:

- Paraquat poisoning
- Bleomycin poisoning

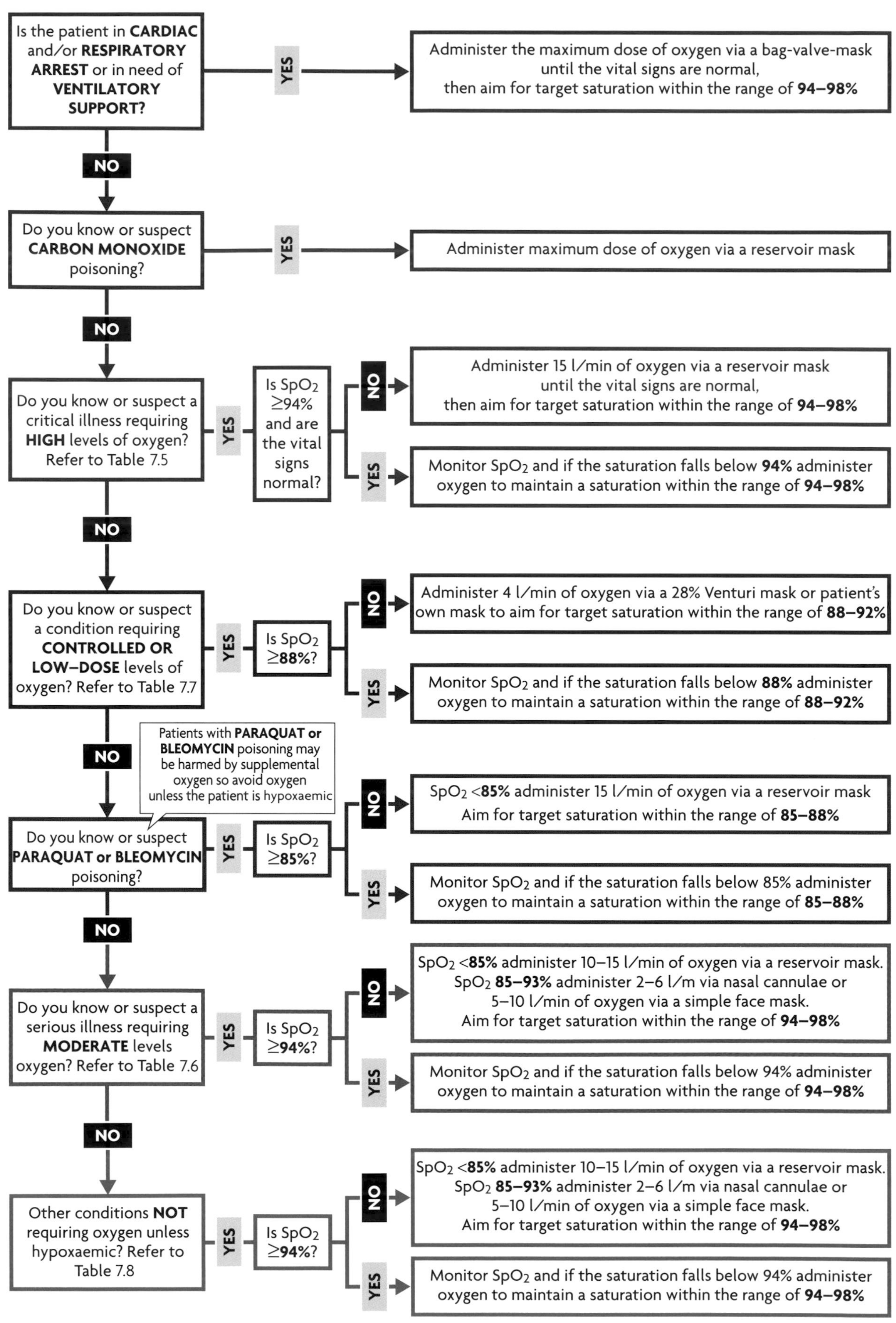

Figure 7.1 – Administration of supplemental oxygen algorithm.

Bibliography

1. O'Driscoll BR, Howard LS, Davison AG, on behalf of the British Thoracic Society. BTS guideline for emergency oxygen use in adult patients. *Thorax* 2008, 63(suppl. 6): vi1–vi68.
2. O'Driscoll BR, Howard LS, Earis J, Mak V. BTS guideline for oxgen use in adults in healthcare and emergency settings. *Thorax* 2017, 72: i1–i90.

Presentation

Both oral and intravenous preparations are available.

Oral

Paracetamol solutions/suspensions:

- **Infant paracetamol suspension** (120 milligrams in 5 ml), used from 3 months to 5 years.
- **Paracetamol 6 plus suspension** (250 milligrams in 5 ml), used from 6 years of age upwards.

Paracetamol tablets

- 500 milligram tablets (tablets may be broken in half).

Intravenous

- Bottle containing paracetamol 1 gram in 100 ml (10 mg/ml) for intravenous infusion for adults, adolescents and children weighing more than 33kg.
- Bottle containing paracetamol 500 milligrams in 50 ml (10mg/ml) for intravenous infusion for term newborn, infants, toddlers and children weighing less than 33kg.

Indications

Oral

Relief of mild to moderate pain or high temperature with discomfort (not for high temperature alone).

Intravenous

As part of a balanced analgesic regimen for severe pain paracetamol is effective in reducing opioid requirements while improving analgesic efficacy and is an alternative analgesic when morphine is contraindicated.

Actions

Analgesic (pain relieving) and antipyretic (temperature reducing) drug.

Contra-indications

Known paracetamol allergy.

Do **NOT** give further paracetamol if a paracetamol–containing product (e.g. Calpol, co-codamol) has already been given within the last 4 hours (6 hours in patients with renal impairment) or if the maximum cumulative daily dose has already been given.

Cautions

Take care when administering paracetamol injection to avoid dosing errors due to confusion between milligram (mg) and millilitre (mL), which could result in accidental overdose and death. Before administering, check when paracetamol was last administered and the cumulative paracetamol dose over the previous 24 hours.

The intravenous preparations come in different sizes, and due to the small amounts that are recommended for children from birth upwards, and for patients that weigh less than 50kg, extreme vigilance is needed. Refer to local procedure and guidance on how to administer dependant on what preparations are available to you.

Side Effects

Side effects are extremely rare; occasionally intravenous paracetamol may cause hypotension if administered too rapidly.

Additional Information

A febrile child should always be conveyed to hospital except where:

- a full assessment has been carried out,

and

- the child has no apparent serious underlying illness,

and

- the child has a defined clinical pathway for reassessment and follow up, with the full consent of the parent (or carer).

Paracetamol injection is supplied in plastic and glass containers. If a glass container is used it should be remembered that close monitoring is needed at the end of the infusion to avoid air embolism.

Paracetamol is not recommended for patients with cardiac chest pain.

Dosage and Administration

Route: Oral – infant paracetamol suspension (i.e. ages 3 months – 5 years).

Ensure that:

Paracetamol (or an alternative paracetamol-containing product) has not been taken within the previous 4 hours (6 hours in renal impairment).

The maximum cumulative daily dose has not already been taken.

When administering to children the correct paracetamol-containing solution/suspension for that patient's age is being used, i.e. 'infant paracetamol suspension' for those aged 0–5 years and 'paracetamol 6 plus suspension' for ages 6 years and over.

AGE	INITIAL DOSE	REPEAT DOSE	DOSE INTERVAL	CONCEN-TRATION	VOLUME	MAX DOSE
Adult	N/A	N/A	N/A	N/A	N/A	N/A
11 years	N/A	N/A	N/A	N/A	N/A	N/A
10 years	N/A	N/A	N/A	N/A	N/A	N/A
9 years	N/A	N/A	N/A	N/A	N/A	N/A
8 years	N/A	N/A	N/A	N/A	N/A	N/A
7 years	N/A	N/A	N/A	N/A	N/A	N/A
6 years	N/A	N/A	N/A	N/A	N/A	N/A
5 years	240 milligrams	240 milligrams	4–6 hours	120 milligrams in 5 ml	10 ml	960 milligrams in 24 hours
4 years	240 milligrams	240 milligrams	4–6 hours	120 milligrams in 5 ml	10 ml	960 milligrams in 24 hours
3 years	180 milligrams	180 milligrams	4–6 hours	120 milligrams in 5 ml	7.5 ml	720 milligrams in 24 hours
2 years	180 milligrams	180 milligrams	4–6 hours	120 milligrams in 5 ml	7.5 ml	720 milligrams in 24 hours
18 months	120 milligrams	120 milligrams	4–6 hours	120 milligrams in 5 ml	5 ml	480 milligrams in 24 hours
12 months	120 milligrams	120 milligrams	4–6 hours	120 milligrams in 5 ml	5 ml	480 milligrams in 24 hours
9 months	120 milligrams	120 milligrams	4–6 hours	120 milligrams in 5 ml	5 ml	480 milligrams in 24 hours
6 months	120 milligrams	120 milligrams	4–6 hours	120 milligrams in 5 ml	5 ml	480 milligrams in 24 hours
3 months	60 milligrams	60 milligrams	4–6 hours	120 milligrams in 5 ml	2.5 ml	240 milligrams in 24 hours
1 month	N/A	N/A	N/A	N/A	N/A	N/A
Birth	N/A	N/A	N/A	N/A	N/A	N/A

Route: Oral – paracetamol 6 plus suspension (i.e. ages 6 years and over).

Ensure that:

Paracetamol (or an alternative paracetamol-containing product) has not been taken within the previous 4 hours (6 hours in renal impairment).

The maximum cumulative daily dose has not already been taken.

When administering to children the correct paracetamol-containing solution/suspension for that patient's age is being used, i.e. 'infant paracetamol suspension' for those aged 0–5 years and 'paracetamol 6 plus suspension' for ages 6 years and over.

AGE	INITIAL DOSE	REPEAT DOSE	DOSE INTERVAL	CONCEN-TRATION	VOLUME	MAX DOSE
16 years – Adult AND **over** 50 kg	500 milligrams – 1 gram	500 milligrams – 1 gram	4–6 hours	250 milligrams in 5 ml	10–20 ml	2–4 grams in 24 hours
12 – 15 years OR 50 kg and **under**	500–750 milligrams	500–750 milligrams	4–6 hours	250 milligrams in 5 ml	10–15 ml	2–3 grams in 24 hours
11 years	500 milligrams	500 milligrams	4–6 hours	250 milligrams in 5 ml	10 ml	2 grams in 24 hours
10 years	500 milligrams	500 milligrams	4–6 hours	250 milligrams in 5 ml	10 ml	2 grams in 24 hours
9 years	375 milligrams	375 milligrams	4–6 hours	250 milligrams in 5 ml	7.5 ml	1.5 grams in 24 hours
8 years	375 milligrams	375 milligrams	4–6 hours	250 milligrams in 5 ml	7.5 ml	1.5 grams in 24 hours
7 years	250 milligrams	250 milligrams	4–6 hours	250 milligrams in 5 ml	5 ml	1 gram in 24 hours
6 years	250 milligrams	250 milligrams	4–6 hours	250 milligrams in 5 ml	5 ml	1 gram in 24 hours
5 years	N/A	N/A	N/A	N/A	N/A	N/A
4 years	N/A	N/A	N/A	N/A	N/A	N/A
3 years	N/A	N/A	N/A	N/A	N/A	N/A
2 years	N/A	N/A	N/A	N/A	N/A	N/A
18 months	N/A	N/A	N/A	N/A	N/A	N/A
12 months	N/A	N/A	N/A	N/A	N/A	N/A
9 months	N/A	N/A	N/A	N/A	N/A	N/A
6 months	N/A	N/A	N/A	N/A	N/A	N/A
3 months	N/A	N/A	N/A	N/A	N/A	N/A
1 month	N/A	N/A	N/A	N/A	N/A	N/A
Birth	N/A	N/A	N/A	N/A	N/A	N/A

Paracetamol

Route: Oral – tablet.

Ensure that:

Paracetamol (or an alternative paracetamol-containing product) has not been taken within the previous 4 hours (6 hours in renal impairment).

The maximum cumulative daily dose has not already been taken.

AGE	INITIAL DOSE	REPEAT DOSE	DOSE INTERVAL	CONCEN-TRATION	VOLUME	MAX DOSE
16 years – Adult AND **over** 50 kg	500 milligrams – 1 gram	500 milligrams – 1 gram	4–6 hours	500 milligrams per tablet	1–2 tablets	2–4 grams in 24 hours
12 years – 15 years OR 50 kg and **under**	500–750 milligrams	500–750 milligrams	4–6 hours	500 milligrams per tablet	1–1.5 tablets	2–3 grams in 24 hours

Route: Intravenous infusion; given over 15 minutes.

Ensure that:

Paracetamol (or an alternative paracetamol-containing product) has not been taken within the previous 4 hours (6 hours in renal impairment).

The maximum cumulative daily dose has not already been taken.

IV paracetamol is only used when managing **severe pain** (use an oral preparation when managing fever with discomfort).

AGE	INITIAL DOSE	REPEAT DOSE	DOSE INTERVAL	CONCEN-TRATION	VOLUME	MAX DOSE
12 years – Adult AND **over** 50 kg	1 gram	1 gram	4–6 hours	10 milligrams in 1 ml	100 ml	4 grams in 24 hours
12 years – Adult AND **under** 50 kg	750 milligrams	750 milligrams	4–6 hours	10 milligrams in 1 ml	75 ml	3 grams in 24 hours
11 years	500 milligrams	500 milligrams	4–6 hours	10 milligrams in 1 ml	50 ml	2 grams in 24 hours
10 years	500 milligrams	500 milligrams	4–6 hours	10 milligrams in 1 ml	50 ml	2 grams in 24 hours
9 years	450 milligrams	450 milligrams	4–6 hours	10 milligrams in 1 ml	45 ml	1.8 grams in 24 hours
8 years	400 milligrams	400 milligrams	4–6 hours	10 milligrams in 1 ml	40 ml	1.6 grams in 24 hours
7 years	350 milligrams	350 milligrams	4–6 hours	10 milligrams in 1 ml	35 ml	1.4 grams in 24 hours
6 years	300 milligrams	300 milligrams	4–6 hours	10 milligrams in 1 ml	30 ml	1.2 grams in 24 hours
5 years	300 milligrams	300 milligrams	4–6 hours	10 milligrams in 1 ml	30 ml	1.2 gram in 24 hours
4 years	250 milligrams	250 milligrams	4–6 hours	10 milligrams in 1 ml	25 ml	1 gram in 24 hours

AGE	INITIAL DOSE	REPEAT DOSE	DOSE INTERVAL	CONCEN-TRATION	VOLUME	MAX DOSE
3 years	200 milligrams	200 milligrams	4–6 hours	10 milligrams in 1 ml	20 ml	800 milligrams in 24 hours
2 years	200 milligrams	200 milligrams	4–6 hours	10 milligrams in 1 ml	20 ml	800 milligrams in 24 hours
18 months	150 milligrams	150 milligrams	4–6 hours	10 milligrams in 1 ml	15 ml	600 milligrams in 24 hours
12 months	150 milligrams	150 milligrams	4–6 hours	10 milligrams in 1 ml	15 ml	600 milligrams in 24 hours
9 months	90 milligrams	90 milligrams	4–6 hours	10 milligrams in 1 ml	9 ml	270 milligrams in 24 hours
6 months	80 milligrams	80 milligrams	4–6 hours	10 milligrams in 1 ml	8 ml	240 milligrams in 24 hours
3 months	60 milligrams	60 milligrams	4–6 hours	10 milligrams in 1 ml	6 ml	180 milligrams in 24 hours
1 month	45 milligrams	45 milligrams	4–6 hours	10 milligrams in 1 ml	4.5 ml	135 milligrams in 24 hours
Birth	35 milligrams	35 milligrams	4–6 hours	10 milligrams in 1 ml	3.5ml	105 milligrams in 24 hours

Salbutamol

Presentation

Nebules containing salbutamol 2.5 milligrams/ 2.5 ml or 5 milligrams/2.5 ml.

Indications

Acute asthma attack where normal inhaler therapy has failed to relieve symptoms.

Expiratory wheezing associated with allergy, anaphylaxis, smoke inhalation or other lower airway cause.

Exacerbation of chronic obstructive pulmonary disease (COPD).

Actions

Salbutamol is a selective $beta_2$ adrenoreceptor stimulant drug. This has a relaxant effect on the smooth muscle in the medium and smaller airways, which are in spasm in acute asthma attacks. If given by nebuliser, especially if oxygen powered, its smooth-muscle relaxing action, combined with the airway moistening effect of nebulisation, can relieve the attack rapidly.

Contra-indications

None in the emergency situation.

Cautions

Salbutamol should be used with care in patients with:

- Hypertension.
- Angina.
- Overactive thyroid.
- Late pregnancy (can relax uterus).
- Severe hypertension may occur in patients on beta-blockers and half doses should be used unless there is profound hypotension.

If COPD is a possibility limit nebulisation with oxygen to 6 minutes.

Side Effects

Tremor (shaking).

Tachycardia.

Palpitations.

Headache.

Feeling of tension.

Peripheral vasodilatation.

Muscle cramps.

Rash.

Additional Information

In acute severe or life-threatening asthma ipratropium should be given after the first dose of salbutamol. In acute asthma or COPD unresponsive to salbutamol alone, a single dose of ipratropium may be given after salbutamol.

Salbutamol often provides initial relief. In more severe attacks, however, the use of steroids by injection or orally and further nebuliser therapy will be required. Do not be lulled into a false sense of security by an initial improvement after salbutamol nebulisation.

Nebules should be protected from light after removal from the foil overwrap pouch. They should be disposed of after a reduced period of expiry, indicated on the pouch.

SECTION 7 Medicines

Dosage and Administration

- **In life-threatening or acute severe asthma:** undertake a **TIME CRITICAL** transfer to the **NEAREST SUITABLE RECEIVING HOSPITAL** and provide nebulisation en-route.
- If COPD is a possibility limit nebulisation with oxygen to 6 minutes.
- The pulse rate in children may exceed 140 after significant doses of salbutamol; this is not usually of any clinical significance and should not usually preclude further use of the drug.
- Repeat doses should be discontinued if the side effects are becoming significant (e.g. tremors, tachycardia >140 beats per minute in adults) – this is a clinical decision by the ambulance clinician.

Route: Nebulised with 6–8 litres per minute of oxygen.

Nebulised - 2.5 milligrams in 2.5 ml

AGE	INITIAL DOSE	REPEAT DOSE	DOSE INTERVAL	CONCENTRATION	VOLUME	MAX DOSE
Adult	5 milligrams	5 milligrams	5 minutes	2.5 milligrams in 2.5 ml	5 ml	No limit
11 years	5 milligrams	5 milligrams	5 minutes	2.5 milligrams in 2.5 ml	5 ml	No limit
10 years	5 milligrams	5 milligrams	5 minutes	2.5 milligrams in 2.5 ml	5 ml	No limit
9 years	5 milligrams	5 milligrams	5 minutes	2.5 milligrams in 2.5 ml	5 ml	No limit

AGE	INITIAL DOSE	REPEAT DOSE	DOSE INTERVAL	CONCENTRATION	VOLUME	MAX DOSE
8 years	5 milligrams	5 milligrams	5 minutes	2.5 milligrams in 2.5 ml	5 ml	No limit
7 years	5 milligrams	5 milligrams	5 minutes	2.5 milligrams in 2.5 ml	5 ml	No limit
6 years	5 milligrams	5 milligrams	5 minutes	2.5 milligrams in 2.5 ml	5 ml	No limit
5 years	2.5 milligrams	2.5 milligrams	5 minutes	2.5 milligrams in 2.5 ml	2.5 ml	No limit
4 years	2.5 milligrams	2.5 milligrams	5 minutes	2.5 milligrams in 2.5 ml	2.5 ml	No limit
3 years	2.5 milligrams	2.5 milligrams	5 minutes	2.5 milligrams in 2.5 ml	2.5 ml	No limit
2 years	2.5 milligrams	2.5 milligrams	5 minutes	2.5 milligrams in 2.5 ml	2.5 ml	No limit
18 months	2.5 milligrams	2.5 milligrams	5 minutes	2.5 milligrams in 2.5 ml	2.5 ml	No limit
12 months	2.5 milligrams	2.5 milligrams	5 minutes	2.5 milligrams in 2.5 ml	2.5 ml	No limit
9 months	2.5 milligrams	2.5 milligrams	5 minutes	2.5 milligrams in 2.5 ml	2.5 ml	No limit
6 months	2.5 milligrams	2.5 milligrams	5 minutes	2.5 milligrams in 2.5 ml	2.5 ml	No limit
3 months	2.5 milligrams	2.5 milligrams	5 minutes	2.5 milligrams in 2.5 ml	2.5 ml	No limit
1 month	2.5 milligrams	2.5 milligrams	5 minutes	2.5 milligrams in 2.5 ml	2.5 ml	No limit
Birth	N/A	N/A	N/A	N/A	N/A	N/A

Route: Nebulised with 6–8 litres per minute of oxygen.

Nebulised - 5 milligrams in 2.5 ml

AGE	INITIAL DOSE	REPEAT DOSE	DOSE INTERVAL	CONCENTRATION	VOLUME	MAX DOSE
Adult	5 milligrams	5 milligrams	5 minutes	5 milligrams in 2.5 ml	2.5 ml	No limit
11 years	5 milligrams	5 milligrams	5 minutes	5 milligrams in 2.5 ml	2.5 ml	No limit
10 years	5 milligrams	5 milligrams	5 minutes	5 milligrams in 2.5 ml	2.5 ml	No limit
9 years	5 milligrams	5 milligrams	5 minutes	5 milligrams in 2.5 ml	2.5 ml	No limit
8 years	5 milligrams	5 milligrams	5 minutes	5 milligrams in 2.5 ml	2.5 ml	No limit
7 years	5 milligrams	5 milligrams	5 minutes	5 milligrams in 2.5 ml	2.5 ml	No limit
6 years	5 milligrams	5 milligrams	5 minutes	5 milligrams in 2.5 ml	2.5 ml	No limit
5 years	2.5 milligrams	2.5 milligrams	5 minutes	5 milligrams in 2.5 ml	1.25 ml	No limit

AGE	INITIAL DOSE	REPEAT DOSE	DOSE INTERVAL	CONCENTRATION	VOLUME	MAX DOSE
4 years	2.5 milligrams	2.5 milligrams	5 minutes	5 milligrams in 2.5 ml	1.25 ml	No limit
3 years	2.5 milligrams	2.5 milligrams	5 minutes	5 milligrams in 2.5 ml	1.25 ml	No limit
2 years	2.5 milligrams	2.5 milligrams	5 minutes	5 milligrams in 2.5 ml	1.25 ml	No limit
18 months	2.5 milligrams	2.5 milligrams	5 minutes	5 milligrams in 2.5 ml	1.25 ml	No limit
12 months	2.5 milligrams	2.5 milligrams	5 minutes	5 milligrams in 2.5 ml	1.25 ml	No limit
9 months	2.5 milligrams	2.5 milligrams	5 minutes	5 milligrams in 2.5 ml	1.25 ml	No limit
6 months	2.5 milligrams	2.5 milligrams	5 minutes	5 milligrams in 2.5 ml	1.25 ml	No limit
3 months	2.5 milligrams	2.5 milligrams	5 minutes	5 milligrams in 2.5 ml	1.25 ml	No limit
1 month	2.5 milligrams	2.5 milligrams	5 minutes	5 milligrams in 2.5 ml	1.25 ml	No limit
Birth	N/A	N/A	N/A	N/A	N/A	N/A

Bibliography

NHS Evidence. *Salbutamol.* Available from: http://www.evidence.nhs.uk/formulary/bnf/current/3-respiratory-system/31-bronchodilators/311-adrenoceptor-agonists/3111-selective-beta2-agonists/salbutamol, 2011.

Sodium Chloride 0.9%

Presentation

100 ml, 250 ml, 500 ml and 1,000 ml packs of sodium chloride intravenous infusion 0.9%.

5 ml and 10 ml ampoules for use as flushes.

5 ml and 10 ml pre-loaded syringes for use as flushes.

Indications

Adult fluid therapy

- Medical conditions without haemorrhage.
- Medical conditions with haemorrhage.
- Trauma related haemorrhage.
- Burns.
- Limb crush injury.

Child fluid therapy

- Medical conditions.
- Trauma related haemorrhage.
- Burns.

Flush

- As a flush to confirm patency of an intravenous or intraosseous cannula.
- As a flush following drug administration.

Actions

Increases vascular fluid volume which consequently raises cardiac output and improves perfusion.

Contra-indications

None.

Side Effects

Over-infusion may precipitate pulmonary oedema and cause breathlessness.

Additional Information

Fluid replacement in cases of dehydration should occur over hours; rapid fluid replacement is seldom indicated; refer to **Intravascular Fluid Therapy in Adults** and **Intravascular Fluid Therapy in Children.**

Dosage and Administration

Route: Intravenous or intraosseous for **ALL** conditions.

FLUSH

AGE	INITIAL DOSE	REPEAT DOSE	DOSE INTERVAL	CONCEN-TRATION	VOLUME	MAX DOSE
Adult	2 ml – 5 ml	2 ml – 5 ml	PRN	0.9%	2 – 5 ml	N/A
Adult	10 ml – 20 ml (if infusing glucose)	10 ml – 20 ml (if infusing glucose)	PRN	0.9%	10 – 20 ml	N/A
5 – 11 years	2 ml – 5 ml	2 ml – 5 ml	PRN	0.9%	2 – 5 ml	N/A
5 – 11 years	5 ml – 10 ml (if infusing glucose)	5 ml – 10 ml (if infusing glucose)	PRN	0.9%	5 – 10 ml	N/A
Birth – <5 years	2 ml	2 ml	PRN	0.9%	2 ml	N/A
Birth – <5 years	2 ml – 5 ml (if infusing glucose)	2 ml – 5ml (if infusing glucose)	PRN	0.9%	2 – 5 ml	N/A

ADULT MEDICAL EMERGENCIES

General medical conditions without haemorrhage: Anaphylaxis, hyperglycaemic ketoacidosis, dehydration[a]

AGE	INITIAL DOSE	REPEAT DOSE	DOSE INTERVAL	CONCENTRATION	VOLUME	MAX DOSE
Adult	250 ml	250 ml	PRN	0.9%	250 ml	2 litres

Sepsis: Clinical signs of infection **AND** systolic BP<90 mmHg

AGE	INITIAL DOSE	REPEAT DOSE	DOSE INTERVAL	CONCENTRATION	VOLUME	MAX DOSE
Adult	500 ml	500 ml	15 minutes	0.9%	500 ml	2 litres

a In cases of dehydration fluid replacement should usually occur over hours.

Medical conditions with haemorrhage: Systolic BP<90 mmHg and signs of poor perfusion

AGE	INITIAL DOSE	REPEAT DOSE	DOSE INTERVAL	CONCENTRATION	VOLUME	MAX DOSE
Adult	250 ml	250 ml	PRN	0.9%	250 ml	2 litres

ADULT TRAUMA EMERGENCIES

Blunt trauma, head trauma or penetrating limb trauma: To maintain a palpable central pulse (carotid or femoral)

AGE	INITIAL DOSE	REPEAT DOSE	DOSE INTERVAL	CONCENTRATION	VOLUME	MAX DOSE
Adult	250 ml	250 ml	PRN	0.9%	250 ml	2 litres

Penetrating torso trauma: To maintain a palpable central pulse (carotid or femoral)

AGE	INITIAL DOSE	REPEAT DOSE	DOSE INTERVAL	CONCENTRATION	VOLUME	MAX DOSE
Adult	250 ml	250 ml	PRN	0.9%	250 ml	2 litres

Burns:

- Total body surface area (TBSA): between 15% and 25% and time to hospital is greater than 30 minutes
- TBSA: more than 25%

AGE	INITIAL DOSE	REPEAT DOSE	DOSE INTERVAL	CONCENTRATION	VOLUME	MAX DOSE
Adult	1 litre	NONE	N/A	0.9%	1 litre	1 litre

Limb crush injury

NB Manage crush injury of the torso as per blunt trauma.

AGE	INITIAL DOSE	REPEAT DOSE	DOSE INTERVAL	CONCENTRATION	VOLUME	MAX DOSE
Adult	2 litres	NONE	N/A	0.9%	2 litres	2 litres

MEDICAL EMERGENCIES IN CHILDREN (20 ml/kg)

NB Exceptions: cardiac failure, renal failure, diabetic ketoacidosis (see following).

AGE	INITIAL DOSE	REPEAT DOSE	DOSE INTERVAL	CONCENTRATION	VOLUME	MAX DOSE
11 years	500 ml	500 ml	PRN	0.9%	500 ml	1,000 ml
10 years	500 ml	500 ml	PRN	0.9%	500 ml	1,000 ml
9 years	500 ml	500 ml	PRN	0.9%	500 ml	1,000 ml
8 years	500 ml	500 ml	PRN	0.9%	500 ml	1,000 ml
7 years	460 ml	460 ml	PRN	0.9%	460 ml	920 ml
6 years	420 ml	420 ml	PRN	0.9%	420 ml	840 ml
5 years	380 ml	380 ml	PRN	0.9%	380 ml	760 ml
4 years	320 ml	320 ml	PRN	0.9%	320 ml	640 ml
3 years	280 ml	280 ml	PRN	0.9%	280 ml	560 ml
2 years	240 ml	240 ml	PRN	0.9%	240 ml	480 ml
18 months	220 ml	220 ml	PRN	0.9%	220 ml	440 ml

AGE	INITIAL DOSE	REPEAT DOSE	DOSE INTERVAL	CONCENTRATION	VOLUME	MAX DOSE
12 months	200 ml	200 ml	PRN	0.9%	200 ml	400 ml
9 months	180 ml	180 ml	PRN	0.9%	180 ml	360 ml
6 months	160 ml	160 ml	PRN	0.9%	160 ml	320 ml
3 months	120 ml	120 ml	PRN	0.9%	120 ml	240 ml
1 month	90 ml	90 ml	PRN	0.9%	90 ml	180 ml
Birth	70 ml	70 ml	PRN	0.9%	70 ml	140 ml

MEDICAL EMERGENCIES IN CHILDREN

Heart failure or renal failure (10 ml/kg)

AGE	INITIAL DOSE	REPEAT DOSE	DOSE INTERVAL	CONCENTRATION	VOLUME	MAX DOSE
11 years	350 ml	350 ml	PRN	0.9%	350 ml	1,000 ml
10 years	320 ml	320 ml	PRN	0.9%	320 ml	1,000 ml
9 years	290 ml	290 ml	PRN	0.9%	290 ml	1,000 ml
8 years	250 ml	250 ml	PRN	0.9%	250 ml	1,000 ml
7 years	230 ml	230 ml	PRN	0.9%	230 ml	920 ml
6 years	210 ml	210 ml	PRN	0.9%	210 ml	840 ml
5 years	190 ml	190 ml	PRN	0.9%	190 ml	760 ml
4 years	160 ml	160 ml	PRN	0.9%	160 ml	640 ml
3 years	140 ml	140 ml	PRN	0.9%	140 ml	560 ml
2 years	120 ml	120 ml	PRN	0.9%	120 ml	480 ml
18 months	110 ml	110 ml	PRN	0.9%	110 ml	440 ml
12 months	100 ml	100 ml	PRN	0.9%	100 ml	400 ml
9 months	90 ml	90 ml	PRN	0.9%	90 ml	360 ml
6 months	80 ml	80 ml	PRN	0.9%	80 ml	320 ml
3 months	60 ml	60 ml	PRN	0.9%	60 ml	240 ml
1 month	45 ml	45 ml	PRN	0.9%	45 ml	180 ml
Birth	35 ml	35 ml	PRN	0.9%	35 ml	140 ml

MEDICAL EMERGENCIES IN CHILDREN

Diabetic ketoacidosis (10 ml/kg) administer **ONCE** only over 15 minutes.

AGE	INITIAL DOSE	REPEAT DOSE	DOSE INTERVAL	CONCENTRATION	VOLUME	MAX DOSE
11 years	350 ml	NONE	NA	0.9%	350 ml	350 ml
10 years	320 ml	NONE	NA	0.9%	320 ml	320 ml
9 years	290 ml	NONE	NA	0.9%	290 ml	290 ml
8 years	250 ml	NONE	NA	0.9%	250 ml	250 ml
7 years	230 ml	NONE	NA	0.9%	230 ml	230 ml
6 years	210 ml	NONE	NA	0.9%	210 ml	210 ml
5 years	190 ml	NONE	NA	0.9%	190 ml	190 ml
4 years	160 ml	NONE	NA	0.9%	160 ml	160 ml
3 years	140 ml	NONE	NA	0.9%	140 ml	140 ml
2 years	120 ml	NONE	NA	0.9%	120 ml	120 ml

Sodium Chloride 0.9%

AGE	INITIAL DOSE	REPEAT DOSE	DOSE INTERVAL	CONCENTRATION	VOLUME	MAX DOSE
18 months	110 ml	NONE	NA	0.9%	110 ml	110 ml
12 months	100 ml	NONE	NA	0.9%	100 ml	100 ml
9 months	90 ml	NONE	NA	0.9%	90 ml	90 ml
6 months	80 ml	NONE	NA	0.9%	80 ml	80 ml
3 months	60 ml	NONE	NA	0.9%	60 ml	60 ml
1 month	45 ml	NONE	NA	0.9%	45 ml	45 ml
Birth	35 ml	NONE	NA	0.9%	35 ml	35 ml

TRAUMA EMERGENCIES IN CHILDREN (5 ml/kg)[b]

NB Exceptions: burns.

AGE	INITIAL DOSE	REPEAT DOSE	DOSE INTERVAL	CONCENTRATION	VOLUME	MAX DOSE
11 years	175 ml	175 ml	PRN	0.9%	175 ml	1,000 ml
10 years	160 ml	160 ml	PRN	0.9%	160 ml	1,000 ml
9 years	145 ml	145 ml	PRN	0.9%	145 ml	1,000 ml
8 years	130 ml	130 ml	PRN	0.9%	130 ml	1,000 ml
7 years	115 ml	115 ml	PRN	0.9%	115 ml	920 ml
6 years	105 ml	105 ml	PRN	0.9%	105 ml	840 ml
5 years	95 ml	95 ml	PRN	0.9%	95 ml	760 ml
4 years	80 ml	80 ml	PRN	0.9%	80 ml	640 ml
3 years	70 ml	70 ml	PRN	0.9%	70 ml	560 ml
2 years	60 ml	60 ml	PRN	0.9%	60 ml	480 ml
18 months	55 ml	55 ml	PRN	0.9%	55 ml	440 ml
12 months	50 ml	50 ml	PRN	0.9%	50 ml	400 ml
9 months	45 ml	45 ml	PRN	0.9%	45 ml	360 ml
6 months	40 ml	40 ml	PRN	0.9%	40 ml	320 ml
3 months	30 ml	30 ml	PRN	0.9%	30 ml	240 ml
1 month	20 ml	20 ml	PRN	0.9%	20 ml	180 ml
Birth	20 ml	20 ml	PRN	0.9%	20 ml	140 ml

Burns (10 ml/kg, given over 1 hour):

- TBSA: between 10% and 20% and time to hospital is greater than 30 minutes
- TBSA: more than 20%

AGE	INITIAL DOSE	REPEAT DOSE	DOSE INTERVAL	CONCENTRATION	VOLUME	MAX DOSE
11 years	350 ml	NONE	N/A	0.9%	350 ml	350 ml
10 years	320 ml	NONE	N/A	0.9%	320 ml	320 ml
9 years	290 ml	NONE	N/A	0.9%	290 ml	290 ml
8 years	250 ml	NONE	N/A	0.9%	250 ml	250 ml
7 years	230 ml	NONE	N/A	0.9%	230 ml	230 ml
6 years	210 ml	NONE	N/A	0.9%	210 ml	210 ml

b Seek advice to exceed maximum dose in trauma.

Sodium Chloride 0.9%

AGE	INITIAL DOSE	REPEAT DOSE	DOSE INTERVAL	CONCENTRATION	VOLUME	MAX DOSE
5 years	190 ml	NONE	N/A	0.9%	190 ml	190 ml
4 years	160 ml	NONE	N/A	0.9%	160 ml	160 ml
3 years	140 ml	NONE	N/A	0.9%	140 ml	140 ml
2 years	120 ml	NONE	N/A	0.9%	120 ml	120 ml
18 months	110 ml	NONE	N/A	0.9%	110 ml	110 ml
12 months	100 ml	NONE	N/A	0.9%	100 ml	100 ml
9 months	90 ml	NONE	N/A	0.9%	90 ml	90 ml
6 months	80 ml	NONE	N/A	0.9%	80 ml	80 ml
3 months	60 ml	NONE	N/A	0.9%	60 ml	60 ml
1 month	45 ml	NONE	N/A	0.9%	45 ml	45 ml
Birth	35 ml	NONE	N/A	0.9%	35 ml	35 ml

Sodium Lactate Compound

Presentation

250 ml, 500 ml and 1,000 ml packs of compound sodium lactate intravenous infusion (also called Hartmann's solution for injection or Ringer's lactate solution for injection).

Indications

Blood and fluid loss, to correct hypovolaemia and improve tissue perfusion if sodium chloride 0.9% is **NOT** available.

Dehydration.

Actions

Increases vascular fluid volume which consequently raises cardiac output and improves perfusion.

Contra-indications

Diabetic hyperglycaemic ketoacidotic coma, and precoma. **NB** Administer 0.9% sodium chloride intravenous infusion.

Neonates.

Cautions

Sodium lactate should not be used in limb crush injury when 0.9% sodium chloride is available.

Renal failure.

Liver failure.

Side Effects

Infusion of an excessive volume may overload the circulation and precipitate heart failure (increased breathlessness, wheezing and distended neck veins). Volume overload is unlikely if the patient is correctly assessed initially and it is very unlikely indeed if patient response is assessed after initial 250 ml infusion and then after each 250 ml of infusion. If there is evidence of this complication, the patient should be transported rapidly to nearest suitable receiving hospital whilst administering high-flow oxygen.

Do not administer further fluid.

Additional Information

Compound sodium lactate intravenous infusion contains mainly sodium, but also small amounts of potassium and lactate. It is useful for initial fluid replacement in cases of blood loss.

The volume of compound sodium lactate intravenous infusion needed is 3 times as great as the volume of blood loss. Sodium lactate has **NO** oxygen carrying capacity.

Dosage and Administration if sodium chloride 0.9% is NOT available

Route: Intravenous or intraosseous for **ALL** conditions.

ADULT MEDICAL EMERGENCIES

General medical conditions without haemorrhage: anaphylaxis, dehydration. In cases of dehydration fluid replacement should usually occur over hours.

NB Exception sodium lactate compound is contra-indicated in diabetic ketoacidosis – refer to **0.9% Sodium Chloride**.

AGE	INITIAL DOSE	REPEAT DOSE	DOSE INTERVAL	CONCENTRATION	VOLUME	MAX DOSE
Adult	250 ml	250 ml	PRN	Compound	250 ml	1 litre

Sepsis: Clinical signs of infection **AND** systolic BP<90 mmHg **AND** tachypnoea

AGE	INITIAL DOSE	REPEAT DOSE	DOSE INTERVAL	CONCENTRATION	VOLUME	MAX DOSE
Adult	1 litre	1 litre	30 minutes	Compound	1 litre	2 litres

ADULT TRAUMA EMERGENCIES

Medical conditions with haemorrhage: Systolic BP<90 mmHg and signs of poor perfusion

AGE	INITIAL DOSE	REPEAT DOSE	DOSE INTERVAL	CONCENTRATION	VOLUME	MAX DOSE
Adult	250 ml	250 ml	PRN	Compound	250 ml	2 litres

Sodium Lactate Compound

Blunt trauma, head trauma or penetrating limb trauma: Systolic BP<90 mmHg and signs of poor perfusion

AGE	INITIAL DOSE	REPEAT DOSE	DOSE INTERVAL	CONCENTRATION	VOLUME	MAX DOSE
Adult	250 ml	250 ml	PRN	Compound	250 ml	2 litres

Penetrating torso trauma: Systolic BP<60 mmHg and signs of poor perfusion

AGE	INITIAL DOSE	REPEAT DOSE	DOSE INTERVAL	CONCENTRATION	VOLUME	MAX DOSE
Adult	250 ml	250 ml	PRN	Compound	250 ml	2 litres

Burns:

- TBSA: between 15% and 25% and time to hospital is greater than 30 minutes.
- TBSA: more than 25%.

AGE	INITIAL DOSE	REPEAT DOSE	DOSE INTERVAL	CONCENTRATION	VOLUME	MAX DOSE
Adult	1 litre	N/A	N/A	Compound	1 litre	1 litre

Limb crush injury

NB Sodium chloride 0.9% is the fluid of choice in crush injury. **NB** Manage crush injury of the torso as per blunt trauma.

AGE	INITIAL DOSE	REPEAT DOSE	DOSE INTERVAL	CONCENTRATION	VOLUME	MAX DOSE
Adult	2 litres	N/A	N/A	Compound	2 litres	2 litres

MEDICAL EMERGENCIES IN CHILDREN (20 ml/kg) – NB Exceptions heart failure, renal failure, liver failure, diabetic ketoacidosis (sodium lactate compound is contra-indicated in diabetic ketoacidosis – refer to **0.9% Sodium Chloride**).

AGE	INITIAL DOSE	REPEAT DOSE	DOSE INTERVAL	CONCENTRATION	VOLUME	MAX DOSE
11 years	500 ml	500 ml	PRN	Compound	500 ml	1 litre
10 years	500 ml	500 ml	PRN	Compound	500 ml	1 litre
9 years	500 ml	500 ml	PRN	Compound	500 ml	1 litre
8 years	500 ml	500 ml	PRN	Compound	500 ml	1 litre
7 years	460 ml	460 ml	PRN	Compound	460 ml	920 ml
6 years	420 ml	420 ml	PRN	Compound	420 ml	840 ml
5 years	380 ml	380 ml	PRN	Compound	380 ml	760 ml
4 years	320 ml	320 ml	PRN	Compound	320 ml	640 ml
3 years	280 ml	280 ml	PRN	Compound	280 ml	560 ml
2 years	240 ml	240 ml	PRN	Compound	240 ml	480 ml
18 months	220 ml	220 ml	PRN	Compound	220 ml	440 ml
12 months	200 ml	200 ml	PRN	Compound	200 ml	400 ml
9 months	180 ml	180 ml	PRN	Compound	180 ml	360 ml
6 months	160 ml	160 ml	PRN	Compound	160 ml	320 ml
3 months	120 ml	120 ml	PRN	Compound	120 ml	240 ml
1 month	90 ml	90 ml	PRN	Compound	90 ml	180 ml
Birth	N/A	N/A	N/A	N/A	N/A	N/A

MEDICAL EMERGENCIES IN CHILDREN

Heart failure or renal failure (10 ml/kg)

AGE	INITIAL DOSE	REPEAT DOSE	DOSE INTERVAL	CONCENTRATION	VOLUME	MAX DOSE
11 years	350 ml	350 ml	PRN	Compound	350 ml	700 ml
10 years	320 ml	320 ml	PRN	Compound	320 ml	640 ml
9 years	290 ml	290 ml	PRN	Compound	290 ml	580 ml
8 years	250 ml	250 ml	PRN	Compound	250 ml	500 ml
7 years	230 ml	230 ml	PRN	Compound	230 ml	460 ml
6 years	210 ml	210 ml	PRN	Compound	210 ml	420 ml
5 years	190 ml	190 ml	PRN	Compound	190 ml	380 ml
4 years	160 ml	160 ml	PRN	Compound	160 ml	320 ml
3 years	140 ml	140 ml	PRN	Compound	140 ml	280 ml
2 years	120 ml	120 ml	PRN	Compound	120 ml	240 ml
18 months	110 ml	110 ml	PRN	Compound	110 ml	220 ml
12 months	100 ml	100 ml	PRN	Compound	100 ml	200 ml
9 months	90 ml	90 ml	PRN	Compound	90 ml	180 ml
6 months	80 ml	80 ml	PRN	Compound	80 ml	160 ml
3 months	60 ml	60 ml	PRN	Compound	60 ml	120 ml
1 month	45 ml	45 ml	PRN	Compound	45 ml	90 ml
Birth	N/A	N/A	N/A	N/A	N/A	N/A

TRAUMA EMERGENCIES IN CHILDREN (5 ml/kg)

NB Exceptions: burns.

AGE	INITIAL DOSE	REPEAT DOSE	DOSE INTERVAL	CONCENTRATION	VOLUME	MAX DOSE
11 years	175 ml	175 ml	PRN	Compound	175 ml	1 litre
10 years	160 ml	160 ml	PRN	Compound	160 ml	1 litre
9 years	145 ml	145 ml	PRN	Compound	145 ml	1 litre
8 years	130 ml	130 ml	PRN	Compound	130 ml	1 litre
7 years	115 ml	115 ml	PRN	Compound	115 ml	920 ml
6 years	105 ml	105 ml	PRN	Compound	105 ml	840 ml
5 years	95 ml	95 ml	PRN	Compound	95 ml	760 ml
4 years	80 ml	80 ml	PRN	Compound	80 ml	640 ml
3 years	70 ml	70 ml	PRN	Compound	70 ml	560 ml
2 years	60 ml	60 ml	PRN	Compound	60 ml	480 ml
18 months	55 ml	55 ml	PRN	Compound	55 ml	440 ml
12 months	50 ml	50 ml	PRN	Compound	50 ml	400 ml
9 months	45 ml	45 ml	PRN	Compound	45 ml	360 ml
6 months	40 ml	40 ml	PRN	Compound	40 ml	320 ml
3 months	30 ml	30 ml	PRN	Compound	30 ml	240 ml
1 month	20 ml	20 ml	PRN	Compound	20 ml	180 ml
Birth	N/A	N/A	N/A	N/A	N/A	N/A

Burns (10 ml/kg, given over 1 hour):

- TBSA: between 10% and 20% and time to hospital is greater than 30 minutes.
- TBSA: more than 20%.

AGE	INITIAL DOSE	REPEAT DOSE	DOSE INTERVAL	CONCENTRATION	VOLUME	MAX DOSE
11 years	350 ml	NONE	N/A	Compound	350 ml	350 ml
10 years	320 ml	NONE	N/A	Compound	320 ml	320 ml
9 years	290 ml	NONE	N/A	Compound	290 ml	290 ml
8 years	250 ml	NONE	N/A	Compound	250 ml	250 ml
7 years	230 ml	NONE	N/A	Compound	230 ml	230 ml
6 years	210 ml	NONE	N/A	Compound	210 ml	210 ml
5 years	190 ml	NONE	N/A	Compound	190 ml	190 ml
4 years	160 ml	NONE	N/A	Compound	160 ml	160 ml
3 years	140 ml	NONE	N/A	Compound	140 ml	140 ml
2 years	120 ml	NONE	N/A	Compound	120 ml	120 ml
18 months	110 ml	NONE	N/A	Compound	110 ml	110 ml
12 months	100 ml	NONE	N/A	Compound	100 ml	100 ml
9 months	90 ml	NONE	N/A	Compound	90 ml	90 ml
6 months	80 ml	NONE	N/A	Compound	80 ml	80 ml
3 months	60 ml	NONE	N/A	Compound	60 ml	60 ml
1 month	45 ml	NONE	N/A	Compound	45 ml	45 ml
Birth	N/A	N/A	N/A	N/A	N/A	N/A

Syntometrine

Presentation

An ampoule containing ergometrine 500 micrograms and oxytocin 5 units in 1 ml.

Indications

Post-partum haemorrhage within 24 hours of delivery of the infant where bleeding from the uterus is uncontrollable by uterine massage.

Miscarriage with life-threatening bleeding and a confirmed diagnosis (e.g. where a patient has gone home with medical management and starts to bleed).

Actions

Stimulates contraction of the uterus.

Onset of action 7–10 minutes.

Contra-indications

- Known hypersensitivity to syntometrine.
- Active labour.
- Severe cardiac, liver or kidney disease.
- Hypertension and severe pre-eclampsia.
- Possible multiple pregnancy/known or suspected fetus in utero.

Side Effects

- Nausea and vomiting.
- Abdominal pain.
- Headache.
- Hypertension and bradycardia.
- Chest pain and, rarely, anaphylactic reactions.

Additional Information

Syntometrine and misoprostol reduce bleeding from a pregnant uterus through different pathways; therefore if one drug has not been effective after 15 minutes, the other may be administered in addition.

Dosage and Administration

Route: Intramuscular.

AGE	INITIAL DOSE	REPEAT DOSE	DOSE INTERVAL	CONCENTRATION	VOLUME	MAX DOSE
Adult	500 micrograms of ergometrine and 5 units of oxytocin	None	N/A	500 micrograms of ergometrine and 5 units of oxytocin in 1 ml	1 ml	500 micrograms of ergometrine and 5 units of oxytocin

Bibliography

NHS Evidence. *Syntometrine*. Available from: https://www.evidence.nhs.uk/formulary/bnf/current/7-obstetrics-gynaecology-and-urinary-tract-disorders/71-drugs-used-in-obstetrics/711-prostaglandins-and-oxytocics/ergometrine-maleate/with-oxytocin/syntometrine, 2011.

Presentation

Vials of **tenecteplase** 10,000 units for reconstitution with 10 ml water for injection, or 8,000 units for reconstitution with 8 ml water for injection.

NOTE: Whilst the strength of thrombolytics is traditionally expressed in 'units' these units are unique to each particular drug and are **NOT** interchangeable.

Indications

Acute ST segment elevation MI (STEMI) within 6 hours of symptom onset where primary percutaneous coronary intervention (PPCI) is **NOT** readily available.

Ensure patient fulfils the criteria for drug administration following the model checklist (below). Variation of these criteria is justifiable at local level with agreement of appropriate key stakeholders (e.g. cardiac network, or in the context of an approved clinical trial).

Contra-indications

See checklist.

Actions

Activates the fibrinolytic system, inducing the breaking up of intravascular thrombi and emboli.

Side Effects

Bleeding:

- Major – seek medical advice and transport to hospital rapidly.
- Minor (e.g. at injection sites) – use local pressure.

Arrhythmias – these are usually benign in the form of transient idioventricular rhythms and usually require no special treatment. Treat ventricular fibrillation (VF) as a complication of myocardial infarction (MI) with standard protocols; bradycardia with atropine as required.

Anaphylaxis – extremely rare (0.1%) with third generation bolus agents.

Hypotension – often responds to laying the patient flat.

Additional Information

PPCI is now the dominant reperfusion treatment and should be used where available; patients with STEMI will be taken direct to a specialist cardiac centre instead of receiving thrombolysis (refer to **Acute Coronary Syndrome**). Local guidelines should be followed.

'Time is muscle!' Do not delay transportation to hospital if difficulties arise whilst setting up the equipment or establishing IV access. Qualified single responders should administer a thrombolytic if indicated while awaiting arrival of an ambulance.

In All Cases

Ensure a defibrillator is immediately available at all times.

Monitor conscious level, pulse, blood pressure and cardiac rhythm during and following injections. Manage complications (associated with the acute MI) as they occur using standard protocols. The main early adverse event associated with thrombolysis is bleeding, which should be managed according to standard guidelines.

AT HOSPITAL – emphasise the need to commence a heparin infusion in accordance with local guidelines – to reduce the risk of re-infarction.

Thrombolysis Checklist

Is primary PCI available?

- **YES** – undertake a **TIME CRITICAL** transfer to PPCI capable hospital.
- **NO** – ask the patient the questions listed below, to determine whether they are suitable to receive thrombolysis.

Assessment Questions	Yes	No
Has the patient suffered a haemorrhagic stroke or stroke of unknown origin at any time?	❐	❐
Has the patient suffered a transient ischaemic attack in the preceding 6 months?	❐	❐
Has the patient suffered a central nervous system trauma or neoplasm?	❐	❐
Has the patient had recent trauma, surgery, or head injury within the preceding 3 weeks?	❐	❐
Has the patient suffered from gastrointestinal bleeding (within the last month)?	❐	❐
Has the patient a known bleeding disorder?	❐	❐
Do you suspect aortic dissection?	❐	❐
Has the patient a non-compressible puncture (e.g. liver biopsy, lumbar puncture)?	❐	❐
Is the patient taking oral anticoagulant therapy (e.g. warfarin)?	❐	❐
Is the patient pregnant or within 1 week post-partum?	❐	❐
Is the patient's systolic blood pressure >180 mmHg and/or diastolic blood pressure >110 mmHg?	❐	❐
Is the patient suffering from advanced liver disease?	❐	❐
Is the patient suffering from active peptic ulcer?	❐	❐

If the patient answers **YES TO ANY** of the above questions, thrombolysis **IS NOT** indicated; seek advice.

If the patient answers **NO TO ALL** of the above questions and thrombolysis is indicated, refer to the dosage and administration table.

Dosage and Administration

1 Administer a bolus of intravenous injection of un-fractionated heparin before administration of tenecteplase (refer to **Heparin**). Flush the cannula well with saline.

2 **AT HOSPITAL** – It is essential that the care of the patient is handed over as soon as possible to a member of hospital staff qualified to administer a heparin infusion.

3 Consider halving the dose in patients aged 75 or over to reduce the risk of intracranial haemorrhage. This will be determined by local pathways.

Route: Intravenous single bolus adjusted for patient weight.

AGE	WEIGHT	INITIAL DOSE	REPEAT DOSE	DOSE INTERVAL	CONCEN-TRATION	VOLUME	MAX DOSE
≥18	<60 kg (<9st 6lbs)	6,000 units	NONE	N/A	1,000 U/ml	6 ml	6,000 units
≥18	60–69 kg (9st 6lbs–10st 13lbs)	7,000 units	NONE	N/A	1,000 U/ml	7 ml	7,000 units
≥18	70–79 kg (11st–12st 7lbs)	8,000 units	NONE	N/A	1,000 U/ml	8 ml	8,000 units
≥18	80–90 kg (12st 8lbs–14st 2lbs)	9,000 units	NONE	N/A	1,000 U/ml	9 ml	9,000 units
≥18	>90 kg (>14st 2lbs)	10,000 units	NONE	N/A	1,000 U/ml	10 ml	10,000 units

Bibliography

1. Ibanez B, James S, Agewall S, et al. 2017 ESC Guidelines for the management of acute myocardial infarction in patients presenting with ST-segment elevation: The Task Force for the management of acute myocardial infarction in patients presenting with ST-segment elevation of the European Society of Cardiology (ESC). *Eur Heart J* 2018, 29(2): 119–177.
2. The British National Formulary. Tenecteplase. *BNF 63.* Available from: https://bnf.nice.org.uk/drug/tenecteplase.html, 2019.

SECTION 7 Medicines

Presentation

Vial containing 500 mg tranexamic acid in 5 ml (100 mg/ml).

Indications

Patients with signs of actual or suspected severe haemorrhage in the following clinical scenarios:

- Injured patients triggering local network major trauma criteria.
- Patients with a time critical injury where significant internal or external haemorrhage is known or suspected.
- Post-partum haemorrhage if after administration of an uterotonic drug the patient continues to bleed.
- Bleeding due to disorders of obstetric origin.

Trauma

Treatment of known or suspected severe traumatic internal or external haemorrhage as soon as clinically possible on arrival at the scene and within 3 hours of bleeding starting in adults and children who are considered to be at risk of significant haemorrhage. This may be demonstrated by one or more of:

- Systolic blood pressure < 90mmHg or absent radial pulse or heart rate > 110 bpm believed to be due to bleeding in adults. In children this may be demonstrated by changes in the normal physiological parameters for age (see JRCALC page for age).
- Any patient where haemostatic gauze, arterial tourniquet/s, chest dressing/s or pressure dressing/s have been applied.
- Patient who has suffered a traumatic cardiac arrest.

The above would include women who have recently given birth but have suffered subsequent trauma.

Women who are pregnant and/or breastfeeding should have tranexamic acid administered in life threatening circumstances.

Post-Partum Haemorrhage

Either of the following criteria:

- Woman who has given birth within 3 hours, with post-partum haemorrhage causing haemodynamic instability (has lost 500ml or more of blood) **which has not responded to the administration of an uterotonic drug**.
- Woman with a post-partum haemorrhage when uterine trauma (rupture) is suspected.
- Woman for whom uterotonic drugs are contraindicated (i.e. patient has high blood pressure).
- Women who are breastfeeding should have tranexamic acid administered in life threatening circumstances.

Obstetric Emergencies

Life-threatening bleeding due to disorders of obstetric origin.

Women who are pregnant and/or breastfeeding should have tranexamic acid administered in life threatening circumstances.

Actions

Tranexamic acid is an anti-fibrinolytic which reduces the breakdown of a blood clot.

Contra-Indications

- Known previous anaphylactic reaction to Tranexamic Acid.
- Bleeding started more than 3 hours ago.
- Obvious resolution of haemorrhage.
- Isolated head injury.
- Post-partum haemorrhage before the administration of an uterotonic unless trauma is suspected cause.
- Critical interventions required (must only be given after critical interventions have been performed: i.e. airway managed; control or splinting of major haemorrhage etc. and if administration does not delay transfer, noting it may be administered en route).

Cautions

Contact the local senior on call clinician for advice on the below if required:

- Patients with a known history of convulsions or convulsions from any cause during the incident. High dose regimes have been associated with convulsions; however, in the low dose regime recommended here, the benefit from giving tranexamic acid for severe haemorrhage outweighs the risk of convulsions. An increase in convulsion rate may be due to the antagonistic effect of tranexamic acid on GABA receptors. Treat convulsions which may be caused by treatment with tranexamic acid as per JRCALC and Trust guidance (management not covered under this PGD).
- Patients with a known history of acute venous or arterial thrombosis. In the low dose regime recommended here, the benefit from giving tranexamic acid for severe haemorrhage outweighs the risk of thrombotic events.

This information should be passed to the receiving hospital.

- Patients with known severe renal impairment (eGFR <30 ml/min 1.73 m^2). There is a risk of accumulation of tranexamic acid. In the low dose regime recommended here, the benefit from giving tranexamic acid for severe haemorrhage outweighs the risk of accumulation. This information should be passed to the receiving hospital.
- Rapid injection may cause hypotension and loss of consciousness.
- Do not administer through the same line as blood products or penicillin antibiotics (including co-amoxiclav).

Side Effects

Common side effects (more than 1 in 100 but less than 1 in 10)

- Nausea.
- Vomiting.
- Diarrhoea.

Serious adverse effects (unknown rate of incidence)

- Hypersensitivity reactions including anaphylaxis have been reported.
- Rapid injection may cause hypotension.
- Arterial or venous embolism at any site.

Dosage and Administration

Route: Intravenous/Intraosseous – **administer SLOWLY over 10 minutes – can be given as 10 aliquots administered 1 minute apart.**

Post-partum haemorrhage in women: A second dose can be administered if bleeding continues after 30 minutes of the first dose being administered. Any further doses are not permissible within 24 hours.

AGE	INITIAL DOSE	REPEAT DOSE	DOSE INTERVAL	CONCENTRATION	VOLUME	MAX DOSE
>12 years – Adult	1 gram	NONE	N/A	100 mg/ml	10 ml	1 gram
11 years	500 mg	NONE	N/A	100 mg/ml	5 ml	500 mg
10 years	500 mg	NONE	N/A	100 mg/ml	5 ml	500 mg
9 years	450 mg	NONE	N/A	100 mg/ml	4.5 ml	450 mg
8 years	400 mg	NONE	N/A	100 mg/ml	4 ml	400 mg
7 years	350 mg	NONE	N/A	100 mg/ml	3.5 ml	350 mg
6 years	300 mg	NONE	N/A	100 mg/ml	3 ml	300 mg
5 years	300 mg	NONE	N/A	100 mg/ml	3 ml	300 mg
4 years	250 mg	NONE	N/A	100 mg/ml	2.5 ml	250 mg
3 years	200 mg	NONE	N/A	100 mg/ml	2 ml	200 mg
2 years	200 mg	NONE	N/A	100 mg/ml	2 ml	200 mg
18 months	150 mg	NONE	N/A	100 mg/ml	1.5 ml	150 mg
12 months	150 mg	NONE	N/A	100 mg/ml	1.5 ml	150 mg
9 months	150 mg	NONE	N/A	100 mg/ml	1.5 ml	150 mg
6 months	100 mg	NONE	N/A	100 mg/ml	1 ml	100 mg
3 months	100 mg	NONE	N/A	100 mg/ml	1 ml	100 mg
1 month	50 mg	NONE	N/A	100 mg/ml	0.5 ml	50 mg
Birth	50 mg	NONE	N/A	100 mg/ml	0.5 ml	50 mg

Bibliography

1. CRASH-2 trial collaborators. Effects of tranexamic acid on death, vascular occlusive events, and blood transfusion in trauma patients with significant haemorrhage (CRASH-2): a randomised, placebo-controlled trial. *The Lancet* 2010, 376(9734): 23–32.
2. CRASH-2 trial collaborators. The importance of early treatment with tranexamic acid in bleeding trauma patients: an exploratory analysis of the CRASH-2 randomised controlled trial. *The Lancet* 2011, 377(9771): 1096–101.e2.
3. Yeguiayan J-M, Rosencher N, Vivien B. Early administration of tranexamic acid in trauma patients. *The Lancet* 2011, 378(9785): 27–8.

4. Cap AP, Baer DG, Orman JA, Aden J, Ryan K, Blackbourne LH. Tranexamic acid for trauma patients: a critical review of the literature. *Journal of Trauma and Acute Care Surgery* 2011, 71(1): S9–14: doi 10.1097/TA.0b013e31822114af.

5. NHS Evidence. *Tranexamic acid.* Available from: http://www.evidence.nhs.uk/formulary/bnf/current/2-cardiovascular-system/211-antifibrinolytic-drugs-and-haemostatics/tranexamic-acid, 2011.

6. World Maternal Antifibrinolytic Trial (The WOMAN Trial). Effect of early tranexamic acid administration on mortality, hysterectomy, and other morbidities in women with post-partum haemorrhage (WOMAN): an international, randomised, double-blind, placebo-controlled trial. *The Lancet* 2017, 389(10084): 2105–2116. Available from: http://thelancet.com/journals/lancet/article/PIIS0140-6736(17)30638-4/fulltext.

7. World Health Organization. WHO recommendations for the prevention and treatment of postpartum haemorrhage. Available from: https://apps.who.int/iris/bitstream/handle/10665/75411/9789241548502_eng.pdf;jsessionid=FE21E3AB386D8541DD10B4973CA037B9?sequence=1, 2012.

Intravascular Fluid Therapy in Adults

1. Introduction[1,2,3,4,5,6,7,8]

- Despite a lack of evidence demonstrating any significant beneficial effects, pre-hospital fluid therapy has become an established practice.
- There is, however, a significant body of evidence that indicates that routine pre-hospital intravascular fluid therapy may, in fact, be detrimental.
- Adverse effects may be attributed to prolonged on-scene times delaying time to definitive surgical intervention, thrombus disruption, dilution of clotting factors and other coagulopathies.

2. Pathophysiology[3,8,9]

- The objective of fluid therapy is to improve end-organ perfusion and, as a consequence, oxygen delivery.
- By increasing the circulating volume, cardiac output and blood pressure are increased by the Bainbridge Reflex and Frank–Starling Law of the Heart.
- The speed with which a given fluid will produce its effect will largely be determined by how it is distributed throughout the body and how long it remains in the vascular space.

2.1 pH buffering

- Reduced perfusion leads to acidosis as a result of anaerobic metabolism producing lactic acid, phosphoric acids and unoxidised amino acids.
- This acidosis can depress cardiac function (negative inotropic effect) and cause arrhythmias.

2.2 Oxygen transport

- Crystalloid fluids currently used in the pre-hospital environment have no oxygen carrying capacity.
- However, the administration of fluids reduces blood viscosity which in turn may lead to improved peripheral blood flow and hence oxygen delivery.

2.3 Haemostasis

- In general, administration of fluid has a detrimental effect on haemostasis and a tendency to increase bleeding.
- The administration of fluid raises intravascular pressures and usually causes vasodilation, both of which may precipitate disruption of the primary haemostatic thrombus.
- Furthermore, supplemental administration of fluid reduces blood viscosity and dilutes clotting factors both of which can be detrimental to haemostatic mechanisms.
- Finally, in order to minimise hypothermia-induced coagulopathies, the use of cold fluids should be avoided if possible.

3. Haemorrhagic Emergencies[10,11,12,13,14,15,16,17,18,19,20,21,22]

- Haemorrhage may occur as a result of traumatic or medical aetiologies and may be classified as:
  - **apparent** (external) blood loss
  - **concealed** (internal) blood loss.
- Current thinking suggests that fluids should **ONLY** be administered when there are signs of impaired major organ perfusion (refer to Table 7.13).
- Control of external haemorrhage must be achieved before administering fluids.

3.1 Trauma

3.1.1 Penetrating trauma to the trunk

- Penetrating trauma to the trunk carries the risk of significant disruption of major vessels that, due to their location, are not amenable to compression or other methods of haemorrhage control.
- As a consequence of this inability to control further bleeding, the general aim of fluid therapy is to maintain a palpable central pulse (carotid or femoral).

3.1.2 Penetrating trauma to the limbs

- Penetrating trauma to the limbs also carries a risk of significant disruption of major vessels; however, these vessels are both fewer and more amenable to compression or other methods of haemorrhage control.
- As a consequence of this ability to control further bleeding, the general aim of fluid therapy is to maintain a palpable central pulse (carotid or femoral).

3.1.3 Blunt trauma to trunk or limbs

- Blunt trauma to the trunk carries a lower risk of major vessel disruption; consequently, the trigger point for fluid administration is different from penetrating trauma.
- In cases of blunt trauma to the trunk or limbs, the aim of fluid therapy is to maintain a palpable peripheral pulse (radial).

3.1.4 Trauma to the head (all types)

- Significant head injury results in raised intracranial pressure (ICP) as cerebral tissues

TABLE 7.13 – Early Indicators of Impaired Major Organ Perfusion

SIGNS	CAUSE
Tachypnoea	↑ Metabolic acidosis
Tachycardia	↓ Cardiac output
Hypotension	↓ Vascular volume
↓ Consciousness	↓ Cerebral perfusion

swell within the enclosed skull; to ensure adequate cerebral perfusion pressure (CPP) the body compensates and raises the mean arterial blood pressure (MAP).

CPP = MAP – ICP

- As a result of this compensatory mechanism, significant head injuries are usually associated with hypertension and **NOT** hypotension.
- Hypotension in the setting of significant head injury indicates not only significant blood loss but also **CRITICALLY IMPAIRED CEREBRAL PERFUSION.**
- In order to support cerebral perfusion the administration of fluids may be required.
- In the setting of significant head injury with hypotension, fluid therapy should be titrated to maintain a palpable central pulse (carotid or femoral).
- Hypertensive head injury does not normally require fluid therapy. Research concerning pre-hospital hypertonic saline has yet to demonstrate conclusive evidence of beneficial effect.

3.2 Medical conditions

- Principles of fluid therapy in medically related haemorrhage are fundamentally no different from those of blunt trauma.
- Generally, the aim of fluid therapy is to maintain systolic blood pressure at 90 mmHg.
- Medically related haemorrhage may also be complicated by vascular disease, coagulopathies or the presence of tumours.

3.3 Fluid therapy following haemorrhage

- **DO NOT** delay at scene to obtain vascular access or to commence fluid replacement; wherever possible obtain vascular access and administer fluid **EN-ROUTE TO HOSPITAL.**
- If the clinician determines that there is a definite need for fluid therapy they should obtain vascular access.
- Clinicians should attempt to gain intravenous access in the first instance; however, they may consider intraosseous access where intravenous access fails or is unlikely to be successful.
- Vascular access devices should be flushed with 5 ml of 0.9% sodium chloride for injection to confirm patency prior to administering large volumes of fluid.
- Once patent vascular access is confirmed, administer a single bolus of 250 ml of crystalloid (refer to Table 7.14).
- Where the need for intravascular fluid therapy is less certain, clinicians should still obtain vascular access and flush to confirm patency.

TABLE 7.14 – Dosages for Fluid Therapy – Haemorrhagic Emergencies

INITIAL DOSE	REPEAT DOSE	REPEAT INTERVAL	MAXIMUM DOSE
250 ml	250 ml	PRN	2 litres

- **Do not connect any fluids to the cannula unless intravascular fluid therapy is indicated.**

NB The slow administration of fluids to keep a vein open (TKO/TKVO) should not be practised to avoid inadvertent excess fluid administration.

4. Non-Haemorrhagic Emergencies[23,24,15,16,17,18,19,20,25,26,27,28,29,30,31,32,33,34,35]

4.1 Trauma

- The loss of bodily fluids other than blood, as a result of trauma, is rare. Burn injuries are notable exceptions (see exceptions and special circumstances below).

4.2 Medical conditions

- Patients suffering medical emergencies may experience fluid loss as a result of dehydration (e.g. heat related illness, vomiting or diarrhoea) and/or redistribution of fluid from the vascular compartment (e.g. as a result of anaphylaxis).
- The volume of fluids lost to such processes can easily be underestimated.
- Such patients may be significantly dehydrated resulting in reduced fluid volumes in both the vascular and tissue compartments which has usually taken time to develop and will take time to correct.
- Rapid fluid replacement into the vascular compartment can compromise the cardiovascular system particularly where there is pre-existing cardiovascular disease and in the elderly.
- In cases of dehydration, fluid replacement should be aimed at gradual re-hydration over many hours rather than minutes. Oral electrolyte solutions may be an appropriate consideration in some patients (e.g. heat illness).

4.3 Fluid therapy

- **DO NOT** delay at scene to obtain vascular access or to provide fluid replacement; wherever possible obtain vascular access and administer fluid **EN-ROUTE TO HOSPITAL.**
- If the clinician determines that there is a definite need for fluid therapy, they should obtain vascular access.

Intravascular Fluid Therapy in Adults

- Clinicians should attempt to gain intravenous access in the first instance; however, they may consider intraosseous access where intravenous access fails or is unlikely to be successful.
- Vascular access devices should be flushed with 5 ml of 0.9% sodium chloride for injection to confirm patency prior to administering large volumes of fluid.
- Once patent vascular access is confirmed, administer a single bolus of 250 ml of crystalloid (refer to Table 7.15).
- Where the need for intravascular fluid therapy is less certain, clinicians should still obtain vascular access and flush to confirm patency.
- **Do not connect any fluids to the cannula unless intravascular fluid therapy is indicated.**

NB The slow administration of fluids to keep a vein open (TKO/TKVO) should not be practised to avoid inadvertent excess fluid administration.

- Monitor the physiological response, re-assess perfusion, pulse, respiratory rate and blood pressure wherever possible.
- If these observations improve, suspend any further administration.
- If there is no improvement, administer further 250 ml boluses, reassessing for improvement after each fluid bolus (refer to Table 7.15).
- The maximum cumulative fluid dose is usually 2 litres (refer to Table 7.15).
- If the patient remains hypotensive despite repeated 250 ml boluses OR the patient is likely to remain on scene for a considerable time (e.g. due to extrication difficulties), request senior clinical support (according to local procedures).

4.4 Exceptions and special circumstances

4.4.1 Burns

Where burn surface area is:

- <15% do not administer fluid.
- ≥15 – <25% and time to hospital is greater than 30 minutes, then administer 1 litre sodium chloride 0.9% (refer to Table 7.16).
- ≥25% administer 1 litre sodium chloride 0.9% (refer to Table 7.16).

NB If fluid therapy is indicated **DO NOT** delay transfer to further care but continue fluid therapy en-route – stopping if practicable to insert the cannula.

- Care must be taken to ensure that elderly or heart failure patients are not over-infused.
- In order to minimise the risk of hypothermia, the use of cold fluids should be avoided if possible.

4.4.2 Sepsis

- Sepsis should be suspected in patients who:
  - present with fever/feeling unwell
  - **and** NEWS greater than or equal to 5
  - **and/or** look unwell with history of infection.
- Patients with sepsis will benefit from early fluid therapy and an appropriate hospital alert/ information call.
- Intravascular fluid should be administered in cases of suspected sepsis (refer to Table 3.90 and Table 3.91 in **Sepsis**).

4.4.3 Anaphylaxis

Large volumes of fluid may leak from the patient's circulation during an anaphylactic reaction. There will also be vasodilation, a low blood pressure and signs of shock. If there is intravenous access, infuse intravenous fluids immediately. Give a rapid IV fluid challenge (500–1000 ml) and monitor the response; give further doses as necessary. If intravenous access is delayed or impossible, the intra-osseous route can be used. Do not delay the administration of IM adrenaline attempting intra-osseous access.

5. General Exceptions

5.1 Diabetic Ketoacidosis (DKA)

Young adults (18-25 years of age) with a low BMI may be at increased risk of cerebral oedema if given IV fluids. Therefore this group of patients should not be given IV fluids unless there is significant evidence of hypovolaemic shock (as opposed to dehydration) and a maximum of 10ml/kg given. If these patients deteriorate during fluid administration, stop administering fluid immediately. If it is felt that further fluid administration cannot wait until hospital admission, senior medical advice must be sought. Caution should also be applied when considering IV fluid therapy for patients in DKA who are elderly, pregnant, suffering heart/ renal failure or who have additional co-morbidities.

TABLE 7.15 – Dosages for Fluid Therapy

INITIAL DOSE	REPEAT DOSE	REPEAT INTERVAL	MAXIMUM DOSE
250 ml	250 ml	PRN	2 litres

TABLE 7.16 – Dosages for Fluid Therapy – Burns

INITIAL DOSE	REPEAT DOSE	REPEAT INTERVAL	MAXIMUM DOSE
1 litre over 1 hour	NONE[a]	N/A	1 litre

a Seek senior clinical input for prolonged delays

SECTION 7 Medicines

Intravascular Fluid Therapy in Adults

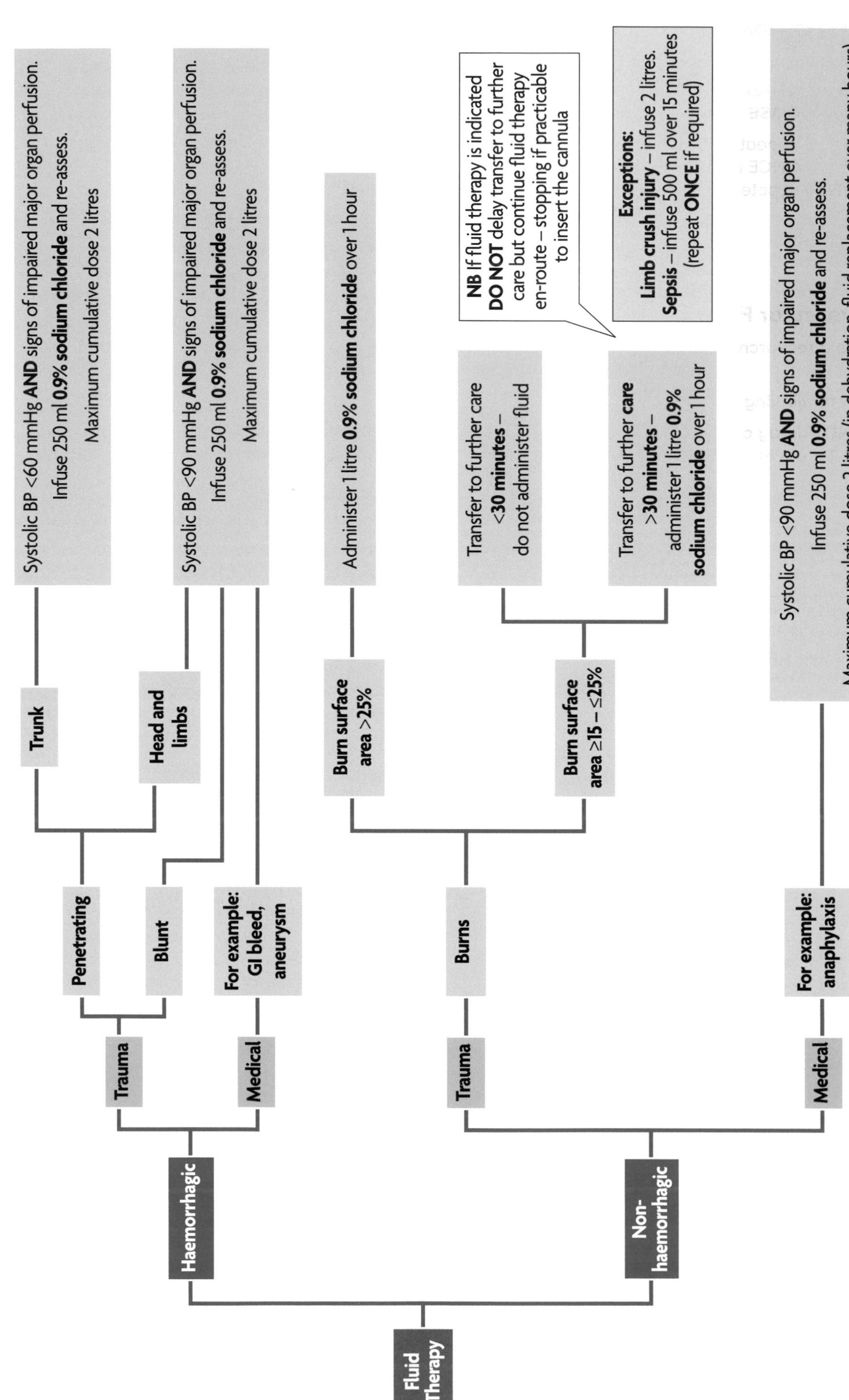

Figure 7.2 – Intravascular fluid therapy algorithm – adults

Intravascular Fluid Therapy in Adults

TABLE 7.17 – Dosages for Fluid Therapy – Sepsis

INITIAL DOSE	REPEAT DOSE	REPEAT INTERVAL	MAXIMUM DOSE
500ml over 15 minutes	Repeat ONCE if still hypotensive	PRN	2 litres

TABLE 7.18 – Dosages for Fluid Therapy – Anapylaxis

INITIAL DOSE	REPEAT DOSE	REPEAT INTERVAL	MAXIMUM DOSE
500–1000ml	500–1000ml	PRN	2 litres

KEY POINTS!

Intravascular Fluid Therapy (Adults)

- **Current research shows little evidence to support the routine use of IV fluids in adult acute blood loss.**
- **Current thinking is that fluids should only be administered when major organ perfusion is impaired.**
- **DO NOT delay on scene for vascular access or fluid replacement; wherever possible obtain vascular access and administer fluid EN-ROUTE TO HOSPITAL stopping if practicable to insert the cannula.**

Bibliography

1. Revell M, Porter K, Greaves I. Fluid resuscitation in pre-hospital trauma care: a consensus view. *Emergency Medicine Journal* 2002, 19(6): 494–498.
2. Bickell WH, Wall MJJ, Pepe PE, Martin RR, Ginger VF, Allen M K, et al. Immediate versus delayed fluid resuscitation in patients with trauma. *New England Journal of Medicine* 1994, 331: 1105–9.
3. Consensus Working Group on Pre-hospital Fluids. Fluid resuscitation in pre-hospital trauma care: a consensus view. *Journal of the Royal Army Medical Corps* 2001, 147(2): 147–52.
4. Cotton BA, Jerome R, Collier BR, Khetarpal S, Holevar M, Tucker B, et al. Guidelines for pre-hospital fluid resuscitation in the injured patient. *Journal of Trauma* 2009, 67(2): 389–402.
5. Dutton AM. Pre-hospital intravenous fluid replacement in trauma: an outmoded concept? *Journal of the Royal Society of Medicine* 1995, 88(4): 213P–216P.
6. Gausche M, Tadeo RE, Zane MC, Lewis RJ. Out-of-hospital intravenous access: unnecessary procedures and excessive cost. *Academic Emergency Medicine* 1998, 5(9): 878–82.
7. Henderson RA, Thomson DP, Bahrs BA, Norman MP. Unnecessary intravenous access in the emergency setting. *Prehospital Emergency Care* 1998, 2(4): 312–16.
8. Mitra B, Cameron PA, Mori A, Fitzgerald M. Acute coagulopathy and early deaths post major trauma. *Injury* 2012, 43(1): 22–5.
9. Roberts K, Revell M, Youssef H, Bradbury AW, Adam DJ. Hypotensive resuscitation in patients with ruptured abdominal aortic aneurysm. *European Journal of Vascular & Endovascular Surgery* 2005, 31(4): 339–44.
10. Kaweski SM, Sise MJ, Virgilio RW. The effect of pre-hospital fluids on survival in trauma patients. *Journal of Trauma* 1990, 30(10): 1215–18; discussion 1218–19.
11. Spahn D, Cerny V, Coats T, Duranteau J, Fernandez-Mondejar F, Gordini G, et al. Management of bleeding following major trauma: a European guideline. *Critical Care* 2007, 11(1): R17.
12. Eckstein M, Chan L, Schneir A, Palmer R. Effect of pre-hospital advanced life support on outcomes of major trauma patients. *Journal of Trauma* 2000, 48(4): 643–8.
13. Honigman B, Rohweder K, Moore EE, Lowenstein SR, Pons PT. Pre-hospital advanced trauma life support for penetrating cardiac wounds. *Annals of Emergency Medicine* 1990, 19(2): 145–50.
14. National Institute for Clinical Excellence. *Pre-hospital Initiation of Fluid Replacement Therapy in Trauma* (TA74). London: NICE. Available from: https://www.nice.org.uk/guidance/ta74, 2004.
15. Bulger EM, May S, Brasel KJ, Schreiber M, Kerby JD, Tisherman SA, et al. Out-of-hospital hypertonic resuscitation following severe traumatic brain injury: a randomized controlled trial. *Journal of the American Medical Association* 2010, 304(13): 1455–64.
16. Chung KK, Wolf SE, Cancio LC, Alvarado R, Jones JA, McCorcle J, et al. Resuscitation of severely burned military casualties: fluid begets more fluid. *Journal of Trauma* 2009, 67(2): 231–7; discussion 237.
17. Cooper DJ, Myles PS, McDermott FT, Murray LJ, Laidlaw J, Cooper G, et al. Pre-hospital hypertonic saline resuscitation of patients with hypotension and severe traumatic brain injury: a randomized controlled trial. *Journal of the American Medical* Association 2004, 291(11): 1350–7.
18. Holcroft JW, Vassar MJ, Turner JE, Derlet RW, Kramer GC. 3% NaCl and 7.5% NaCl/dextran 70 in the resuscitation of severely injured patients. *Annals of Surgery* 1987, 206(3): 279–88.
19. Maningas PA, Mattox KL, Pepe PE, Jones RL, Feliciano DV, Burch JM. Hypertonic saline-dextran solutions for the pre-hospital management of traumatic hypotension. *American Journal of Surgery* 1989, 157(5): 528–33; discussion 533–4.
20. Thompson R, Greaves I. Hypertonic saline-hydroxyethyl starch in trauma resuscitation. *Journal of the Royal Army Medical Corps* 2006, 152(1): 6–12.

21. Vassar MJ, Perry CA, Gannaway WL, Holcroft JW. 7.5% sodium chloride/dextran for resuscitation of trauma patients undergoing helicopter transport. *Archives of Surgery* 1991, 126(9): 1065–72.
22. Vassar MJ, Perry CA, Holcroft JW. Pre-hospital resuscitation of hypotensive trauma patients with 7.5% NaCl versus 7.5% NaCl with added dextran: a controlled trial. *Journal of Trauma* 1993, 34(5): 622–32; discussion 632–3.
23. Allison K, Porter K. Consensus on the pre-hospital approach to burns patient management. *Emergency Medicine Journal* 2004, 21(1): 112–14.
24. Williams G, Dziewulski P. Intravascular fluid therapy in burns injury. In Group. TJRCALGD, editor, 2011.
25. Greaves I, Porter K, Smith JE. Consensus statement on the early management of crush injury and prevention of crush syndrome. *Journal of the Royal Army Medical Corps* 2003, 149(4): 255–9.
26. Holcomb JB. Fluid resuscitation in modern combat casualty care: lessons learned from Somalia. *Journal of Trauma* 2003, 54(suppl.): S46–51.
27. Treharne LJ, Kay AR. The initial management of acute burns. *Journal of the Royal Army Medical Corps* 2001, 147(2): 198–205.
28. Mattox KL, Maningas PA, Moore EE, Mateer JR, Marx JA, Aprahamian C, et al. Pre-hospital hypertonic saline/dextran infusion for post-traumatic hypotension: the U.S.A. Multicenter Trial. *Annals of Surgery* 1991, 213(5): 482–91.
29. Smith JE, Hall MJ. Hypertonic saline. *Journal of the Royal Army Medical Corps* 2004, 150(4): 239–43.
30. Pons PT, Moore EE, Cusick JM, Brunko M, Antuna B, Owens L. Pre-hospital venous access in an urban paramedic system: a prospective on-scene analysis. *Journal of Trauma* 1988, 28(10): 1460–3.
31. Jones SE, Nesper TP, Alcouloumre E. Pre-hospital intravenous line placement: a prospective study. *Annals of Emergency Medicine* 1989, 18(3): 244–6.
32. Minville V, Pianezza A, Asehnoune K, Cabardis S, Smail N. Pre-hospital intravenous line placement assessment in the French emergency system: a prospective study. *European Journal of Anaesthesia* 2006, 23(7): 594–7.
33. Sampalis JS, Tamim H, Denis R, Boukas S, Ruest SA, Nikolis A, et al. Ineffectiveness of on-site intravenous lines: is pre-hospital time the culprit? *Journal of Trauma* 1997, 43(4): 608–15; discussion 615–17.
34. Daniels R. Surviving Sepsis Campaign: indications for fluid administration in patients with sepsis. Personal communication, 2011.
35. Dellinger RP, Levy MM, Cadet JM, Bion J, Parker MM, Jaeschke R, et al. Surviving Sepsis Campaign: international guidelines for management of severe sepsis and septic shock 2008. *Critical Care Medicine* 2008, 36(1): 296–327: doi 10.1097/01.CCM.0000298158.12101.41.

Intravascular Fluid Therapy in Children

1. Introduction

- There has been no significant research in paediatric fluid administration in the literature and thus advice is dependent on that of adult studies and expert consensus.

2. Pathophysiology

- Although the basic pathophysiology is similar to adults, children have one very important difference. Their relatively healthy hearts and vasculature make the compensatory mechanisms very efficient. This means that only subtle signs of circulatory failure (shock) may be evident even in children with severe intravascular fluid depletion. When compensatory mechanisms start to fail, the child is in extremis and will deteriorate very quickly.

3. Assessment

- It is crucial that children with shock are treated before decompensation occurs whenever possible. There is no one sign that reliably dictates the state of shock a child may be in and a combination of all the markers of shock, along with an assessment of the mechanism of the shock (the history) must all be taken into account when deciding how shocked a child is.
- Blood pressure drops late in children for the reasons given above, and therefore is not a good indicator of the degree of volume depletion of the child. It is therefore of limited use in the pre-hospital setting, but if it is taken and found to be low (for the age of the child), this can be regarded as a pre-terminal sign.
- The following should be assessed:
  - pulse rate and volume
  - capillary refill measured on the forehead or sternum
  - respiratory rate
  - colour (pallor etc.)
  - cold peripheries
  - conscious level (AVPU) including drowsiness.

These must be considered as a whole in the light of what is known about the mechanism (i.e. volume of blood or fluid lost).

Only when all these are taken together can a rough estimate of the degree of shock be made. Each one of these is not reliable when measured on its own.

NB Children have compensatory physiological mechanisms that maintain "normal' blood pressures even in the face of significant blood loss; as a result, 'permissive hypotension' is neither recommended or practised in paediatric trauma. Small boluses (5 ml/kg) of fluid are administered and repeated (as needed) following frequent clinical reassessment (titrated against response/improvement) – see below.

NB There is **NO** evidence that the absence of the radial pulse correlates with the blood pressure or degree of shock in a consistent manner in children. Do not monitor the need for fluids against the presence of the radial pulse.

4. Management

For the management of burns and scalds see below and refer to Figure 7.3.

4.1 Medical causes of shock

It is usually difficult to measure volumes of fluid lost in children with medical causes of shock.

- 20 ml/kg is used as standard medical fluid replacement (equates to 25% of the child's blood volume).
- This can be given intravenously or intraosseously and is given as a bolus.
- The exact volume given must be documented.
- The child must be re-assessed after each bolus.
- It may be repeated once – total 40 ml/kg.

4.2 Exceptions

Diabetic Ketoacidosos (DKA).

Children with DKA may be prone to cerebral oedema if given IV fluids. Cerebral oedema is thought to be responsible for approximately 70-80% of diabetes-related deaths of children in the UK. Therefore IV fluids should not be given unless there is significant evidence of hypovolaemic shock and an absolute maximum of 10ml/kg administered.
If these patients deteriorate during fluid administration, stop administering fluid immediately. If it is felt that further fluid administration cannot wait until hospital admission, senior medical advice must be sought.

Anaphylaxis

Large volumes of fluid may leak from the patient's circulation during an anaphylactic reaction. There will also be vasodilation, a low blood pressure and signs of shock. If there is intravenous access, infuse intravenous fluids immediately. Give a rapid IV fluid challenge (20 ml/kg) and monitor the response; give further doses as necessary. If intravenous access is delayed or impossible, the intra-osseous route can be used. Do not delay the administration of IM adrenaline attempting intra-osseous access.

4.3 Trauma: hypovolaemic shock

- Fluid overload should be avoided. For ease and because all trauma patients should not be overloaded, it is not necessary to distinguish between compressible and non compressible haemorrhage.
- 5 ml/kg aliquots of fluid should be given.
- Re-assessment should be undertaken after each 5 ml/kg dose, using the signs described above.

Intravascular Fluid Therapy in Children

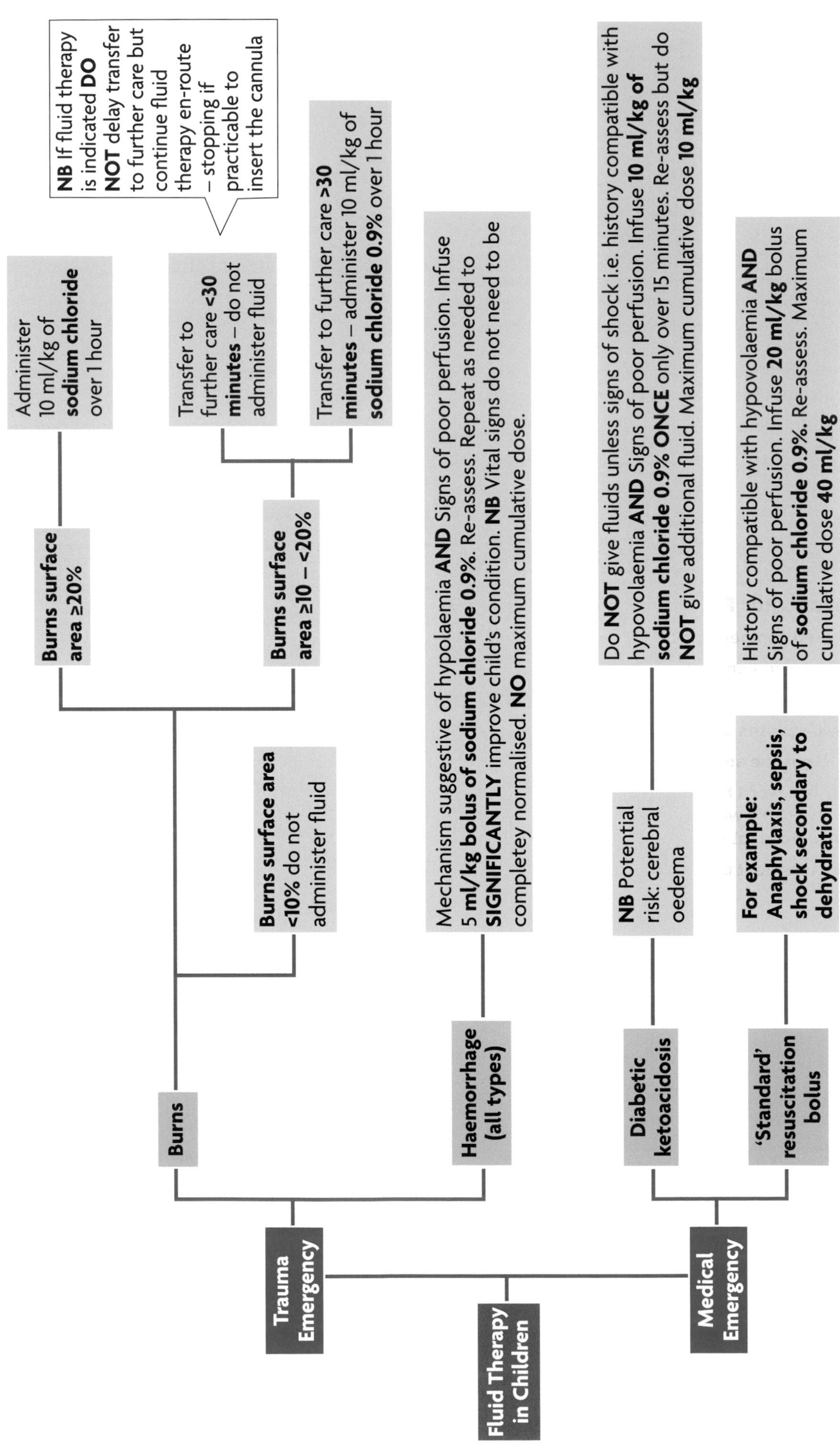

Fluid Therapy in Children
Trauma Emergency
Medical Emergency
Burns
Haemorrhage (all types)
Burns surface area <10% do not administer fluid
Burns surface area ≥20%
Burns surface area ≥10 – <20%
Administer 10 ml/kg of sodium chloride over 1 hour
Transfer to further care <30 minutes – do not administer fluid
Transfer to further care >30 minutes – administer 10 ml/kg of sodium chloride 0.9% over 1 hour
NB If fluid therapy is indicated DO NOT delay transfer to further care but continue fluid therapy en-route – stopping if practicable to insert the cannula
Mechanism suggestive of hypolaemia AND Signs of poor perfusion. Infuse 5 ml/kg bolus of sodium chloride 0.9%. Re-assess. Repeat as needed to SIGNIFICANTLY improve child's condition. NB Vital signs do not need to be completey normalised. NO maximum cumulative dose.
Diabetic ketoacidosis
NB Potential risk: cerebral oedema
Do NOT give fluids unless signs of shock i.e. history compatible with hypovolaemia AND Signs of poor perfusion. Infuse 10 ml/kg of sodium chloride 0.9% ONCE only over 15 minutes. Re-assess but do NOT give additional fluid. Maximum cumulative dose 10 ml/kg
'Standard' resuscitation bolus
For example: Anaphylaxis, sepsis, shock secondary to dehydration
History compatible with hypovolaemia AND Signs of poor perfusion. Infuse 20 ml/kg bolus of sodium chloride 0.9%. Re-assess. Maximum cumulative dose 40 ml/kg

Figure 7.3 – Assessment and management of intravascular fluid therapy in children.

Intravascular Fluid Therapy in Children

- The 5 ml/kg dose can be repeated until the child is **significantly** improved. The vital signs (e.g. pulse) need not be normalised, but the child must be obviously more stable. There is no absolute upper dose.
- The child must be constantly re-assessed during transport.
- Clinical deterioration should be addressed with further 5 ml/kg fluid bolus(es), until the child improves clinically.

4.4 Burns

- Children lose fluids rapidly from severe burns and scalds and should have intravenous sodium chloride 0.9% started early.
- If the child has a >10% but <20% burn and the hospital time is more than 30 minutes, fluids should be started, and if greater than 20% burn fluid should be given regardless of the time to hospital.

Where burn surface area is:

- <10% do not administer fluid.
- ≥10 – <20% and time to hospital is greater than 30 minutes then administer **sodium chloride 0.9%** 10ml/kg over an hour.
- ≥20% administer **sodium chloride 0.9%** 10 ml/kg over an hour.
- The total dose must be calculated and given as regular, tiny portions of this to aim to have infused the correct amount over the hour.
- If fluid therapy is indicated **DO NOT** delay transfer to further care but continue fluid therapy en-route – stopping if practicable to insert the cannula.
- Vascular access also means analgesia can be administered.

KEY POINTS!

Intravascular Fluid Therapy in Children

- **Children compensate well for shock.**
- **Once decompensated, they deteriorate very rapidly.**
- **All physiological signs must be taken in combination to diagnose shock.**
- **20 ml/kg is the standard bolus for medically caused shock.**
- **5 ml/kg is the standard bolus for traumatic shock.**
- **10 ml/kg over 1 hour should be given to children with burns ≥20% and also to children with burns of ≥10 and <20% whose journey time will be more than 30 minutes. This procedure must not delay the time to hospital admission.**
- **Re-assessment after each bolus is vital to avoid fluid overload.**
- **Fluids should be used with extreme caution in DKA, renal failure and cardiac failure.**

Page for Age: BIRTH[a]

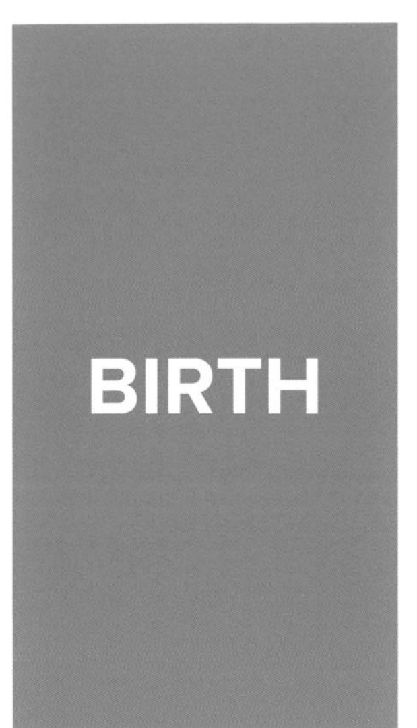

Vital Signs

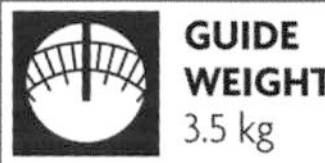

GUIDE WEIGHT	HEART RATE	RESPIRATION RATE	SYSTOLIC BLOOD PRESSURE
3.5 kg	110–160	30–40	70–90

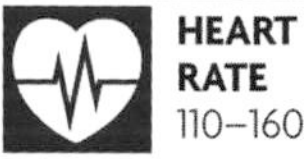
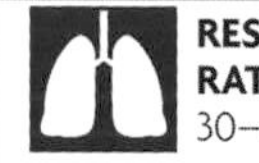
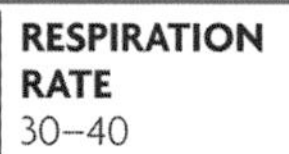
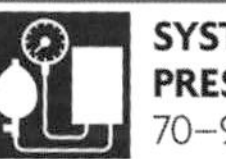

Airway Size by Type

OROPHARYNGEAL AIRWAY	LARYNGEAL MASK	I-GEL AIRWAY	ENDOTRACHEAL TUBE
000	1	1	Diameter: **3 mm**: Length: **10 cm**

Intravascular Fluid

NAME	ROUTE	INITIAL DOSE	REPEAT DOSE	DOSE INTERVAL	CONCENTRATION	VOLUME	MAX DOSE
0.9% Sodium Chloride (5 ml/kg)	IV/IO	20 ml	20 ml	PRN	0.9%	20 ml	140 ml
0.9% Sodium Chloride (10ml/kg)	IV/IO	35 ml	35 ml	PRN	0.9%	35 ml	140 ml
0.9% Sodium Chloride (20 ml/kg)	IV/IO	70 ml	70 ml	PRN	0.9%	70 ml	140 ml

Cardiac Arrest

NAME	ROUTE	INITIAL DOSE	REPEAT DOSE	DOSE INTERVAL	CONCENTRATION	VOLUME	MAX DOSE
Adrenaline	IV/IO	35 micrograms	35 micrograms	3–5 minutes	1 milligram in 10 ml (1:10,000)	0.35 ml	No limit

Quick Reference Table

NAME	ROUTE	INITIAL DOSE	REPEAT DOSE	DOSE INTERVAL	CONCEN-TRATION	VOLUME	MAX DOSE
Activated Charcoal	Oral	N/A	N/A	N/A	N/A	N/A	N/A
Adrenaline - anaphylaxis/ asthma	IM	150 micrograms	150 micrograms	5 minutes	1 milligram in 1 ml (1:1,000)	0.15 ml	No limit
Benzylpenicillin	IV/IO	300 milligrams	NONE	N/A	600 milligrams dissolved in 10 ml water for injection	5 ml	300 milligrams
Benzylpenicillin	IM	300 milligrams	NONE	N/A	600 milligrams dissolved in 2 ml water for injection	1 ml	300 milligrams
Chlorphenamine	IV/IO/IM	N/A	N/A	N/A	N/A	N/A	N/A
Chlorphenamine	Oral (tablet)	N/A	N/A	N/A	N/A	N/A	N/A
Chlorphenamine	Oral (solution)	N/A	N/A	N/A	N/A	N/A	N/A
Dexamethasone - croup	Oral	N/A	N/A	N/A	N/A	N/A	N/A

a The Page for Age is provided for ease of use and quick look purposes. It is not a substitute for the information contained in the complete drugs guidelines or for sound clinical judgement.

Page for Age: BIRTH

NAME	ROUTE	INITIAL DOSE	REPEAT DOSE	DOSE INTERVAL	CONCEN-TRATION	VOLUME	MAX DOSE
Diazepam	Rectal	1.25 milligrams	1.25 milligrams	10 minutes	2.5 milligrams in 1.25 ml	0.5 x 2.5 milligram tube	2.5 milligram
Diazepam	IV/IO	1 milligram	1 milligram	10 minutes	10 milligrams in 2 ml	0.2 ml	2 milligrams
Glucagon	IM	100 micrograms	NONE	N/A	1 milligram per vial	0.1 vial	100 micrograms
Glucose 10%	IV	900 milligrams	900 milligrams	5 minutes	50 grams in 500 ml	9 ml	27 ml (2.7 g glucose)
Glucose 40% Oral Gel	Buccal	An appropriate amount should be administered, considering the child's size	See initial dose	5 minutes	10 grams in 25 grams of gel	1 tube	An appropriate amount should be administered, considering the child's size
Hydrocortisone	IV/IO/IM	10 milligrams	NONE	N/A	100 milligrams in 1 ml	0.1 ml	10 milligrams
Hydrocortisone	IV/IO/IM	10 milligrams	NONE	N/A	100 milligrams in 2 ml	0.2 ml	10 milligrams
Ibuprofen	Oral	N/A	N/A	N/A	N/A	N/A	N/A
Ipratropium Bromide	Neb	N/A	N/A	N/A	N/A	N/A	N/A
Ipratropium Bromide	Neb	N/A	N/A	N/A	N/A	N/A	N/A
Midazolam*	Buccal	See Epilepsy Passport	See Epilepsy Passport	10 mins	5 milligrams in 1 ml	See Epilepsy Passport	See Epilepsy Passport
Morphine Sulfate	IV/IO	N/A	N/A	N/A	N/A	N/A	N/A
Morphine Sulfate	Oral	N/A	N/A	N/A	N/A	N/A	N/A
Naloxone	IM	N/A	N/A	N/A	N/A	N/A	N/A
Naloxone	IV/IO	N/A	N/A	N/A	N/A	N/A	N/A
Ondansetron	IV/IO/IM	N/A	N/A	N/A	N/A	N/A	N/A
Paracetamol - Infant suspension	Oral	N/A	N/A	N/A	N/A	N/A	N/A
Paracetamol	IV infusion/ IO	35 milligrams	35 milligrams	4–6 hours	10 milligrams in 1 ml	3.5ml	105 milligrams in 24 hours
Salbutamol	Neb	N/A	N/A	N/A	N/A	N/A	N/A
Salbutamol	Neb	N/A	N/A	N/A	N/A	N/A	N/A
Tranexamic Acid	IV	50 mg	NONE	N/A	100 mg/ml	0.5 ml	50 mg

*Give the dose as prescribed in the child's individual treatment plan/Epilepsy Passport (the dosages described above reflect the recommended dosages for a child of this age).

Page for Age: 1 MONTH

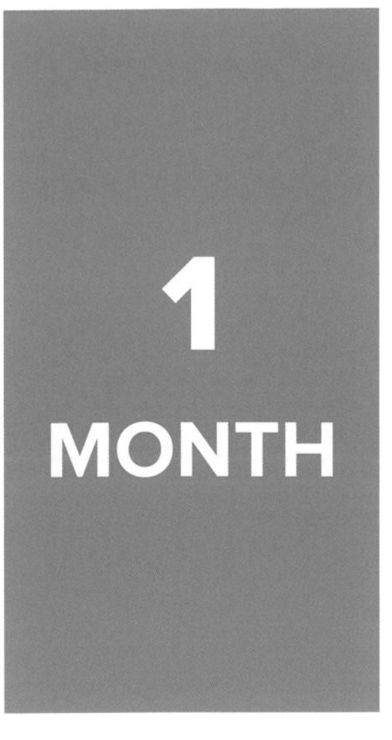

Vital Signs

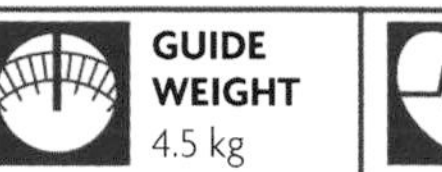 GUIDE WEIGHT	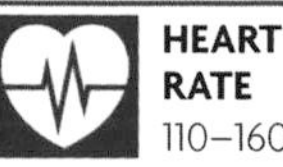 HEART RATE	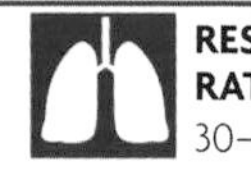 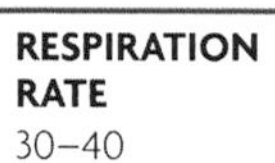 RESPIRATION RATE	 SYSTOLIC BLOOD PRESSURE
4.5 kg	110–160	30–40	70–90

Airway Size by Type

OROPHARYNGEAL AIRWAY	LARYNGEAL MASK	I-GEL AIRWAY	ENDOTRACHEAL TUBE
00	1	1	Diameter: **3 mm**; Length: **10 cm**

Defibrillation – Cardiac Arrest

MANUAL	AUTOMATED EXTERNAL DEFIBRILLATOR
20 Joules	Where possible, use a manual defibrillator. If an AED is the only defibrillator available, it should be used (preferably using paediatric attenuation pads or else in paediatric mode).

Intravascular Fluid

NAME	ROUTE	INITIAL DOSE	REPEAT DOSE	DOSE INTERVAL	CONCENTRATION	VOLUME	MAX DOSE
0.9% Sodium Chloride (5 ml/kg)	IV/IO	20 ml	20 ml	PRN	0.9%	20 ml	180 ml
0.9% Sodium Chloride (10 ml/kg)	IV/IO	45 ml	45 ml	PRN	0.9%	45 ml	180 ml
0.9% Sodium Chloride (20 ml/kg)	IV/IO	90 ml	90 ml	PRN	0.9%	90 ml	180 ml

Cardiac Arrest

NAME	ROUTE	INITIAL DOSE	REPEAT DOSE	DOSE INTERVAL	CONCEN-TRATION	VOLUME	MAX DOSE
Adrenaline	IV/IO	50 micrograms	50 micrograms	3–5 minutes	1 milligram in 10 ml (1:10,000)	0.5 ml	No limit
Amiodarone	IV/IO	25 milligrams (After 3rd shock)	25 milligrams	After 5th shock	300 milligrams in 10 ml	0.8 ml	50 milligrams

Quick Reference Table

NAME	ROUTE	INITIAL DOSE	REPEAT DOSE	DOSE INTERVAL	CONCEN-TRATION	VOLUME	MAX DOSE
Activated Charcoal	Oral	N/A	N/A	N/A	N/A	N/A	N/A
Adrenaline - anaphylaxis/ asthma	IM	150 micrograms	150 micrograms	5 minutes	1 milligram in 1 ml (1:1,000)	0.15 ml	No limit
Benzylpenicillin	IM	300 milligrams	NONE	N/A	600 milligrams dissolved in 2 ml water for injection	1 ml	300 milligrams
Benzylpenicillin	IV/IO	300 milligrams	NONE	N/A	600 milligrams dissolved in 10 ml water for injection	5 ml	300 milligrams
Chlorphenamine	IV/IO/IM	1 milligram	N/A	N/A	10 milligrams in 1 ml	0.1 ml	1 milligram
Chlorphenamine	Oral (tablet)	N/A	N/A	N/A	N/A	N/A	N/A
Chlorphenamine	Oral (solution)	1 milligram	NONE	N/A	2 milligrams in 5 ml	2.5 ml	1 milligram

Page for Age: 1 MONTH

NAME	ROUTE	INITIAL DOSE	REPEAT DOSE	DOSE INTERVAL	CONCEN-TRATION	VOLUME	MAX DOSE
Dexamethasone - croup	Oral (tablet)	2 milligrams	NONE	N/A	2 milligrams per tablet	1 tablet	2 milligrams
Dexamethasone - croup	Oral (solution)	0.67 milligrams	NONE	N/A	2 milligrams in 5 ml	2 ml	0.67 milligrams
Diazepam	Rectal	2.5 milligrams	2.5 milligrams	10 minutes	2.5 milligrams in 1.25 ml	1 x 2.5 milligram tube	5 milligrams
Diazepam	IV/IO	1.5 milligrams	1.5 milligrams	10 minutes	10 milligrams in 2 ml	0.3 ml	3 milligrams
Glucagon	IM	500 micrograms	NONE	N/A	1 milligram per vial	0.5 vial	500 micrograms
Glucose 10%	IV	1 gram glucose	1 gram glucose	5 minutes	50 grams in 500 ml	10 ml	30 ml (3 g glucose)
Glucose 40% Oral Gel	Buccal	An appropriate amount should be administered, considering the child's size	See initial dose	5 minutes	10 grams in 25 grams of gel	1 tube	An appropriate amount should be administered, considering the child's size
Hydrocortisone	IV/IO/IM	25 milligrams	NONE	N/A	100 milligrams in 1 ml	0.25 ml	25 milligrams
Hydrocortisone	IV/IO/IM	25 milligrams	NONE	N/A	100 milligrams in 2 ml	0.5 ml	25 milligrams
Ibuprofen	Oral	N/A	N/A	N/A	N/A	N/A	N/A
Ipratropium Bromide	Neb	125–250 micrograms	NONE	N/A	500 micrograms in 2 ml	0.5 ml–1 ml	125–250 micrograms
Ipratropium Bromide	Neb	125–250 micrograms	NONE	N/A	250 micrograms in 1 ml	0.5 ml–1 ml	125–250 micrograms
Midazolam*	Buccal	See Epilepsy Passport	See Epilepsy Passport	10 mins	5 milligrams in 1 ml	See Epilepsy Passport	See Epilepsy Passport
Morphine Sulfate	IV/IO	N/A	N/A	N/A	N/A	N/A	N/A
Morphine Sulfate	Oral	N/A	N/A	N/A	N/A	N/A	N/A
Naloxone IM	IM	400 micrograms	400 micrograms	3 minutes	400 micrograms in 1 ml	1 ml	2,000 micrograms
Naloxone IV/IO	IV/IO	400 micrograms	400 micrograms	1 minute	400 micrograms in 1 ml	1 ml	2,000 micrograms
Ondansetron	IV/IO/IM	0.5 milligrams	NONE	N/A	2 milligrams in 1 ml	0.25 ml	0.5 milligrams
Paracetamol - Infant suspension	Oral	N/A	N/A	N/A	N/A	N/A	N/A
Paracetamol	IV infusion/ IO	45 milligrams	45 milligrams	4–6 hours	10 milligrams in 1 ml	4.5 ml	135 milligrams in 24 hours
Salbutamol	Neb	2.5 milligrams	2.5 milligrams	5 minutes	2.5 milligrams in 2.5 ml	2.5 ml	No limit
Salbutamol	Neb	2.5 milligrams	2.5 milligrams	5 minutes	5 milligrams in 2.5 ml	1.25 ml	No limit
Tranexamic Acid	IV	50 mg	NONE	N/A	100 mg/ml	0.5 ml	50 mg

*Give the dose as prescribed in the child's individual treatment plan/Epilepsy Passport (the dosages described above reflect the recommended dosages for a child of this age).

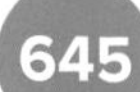

Page for Age: 3 MONTHS

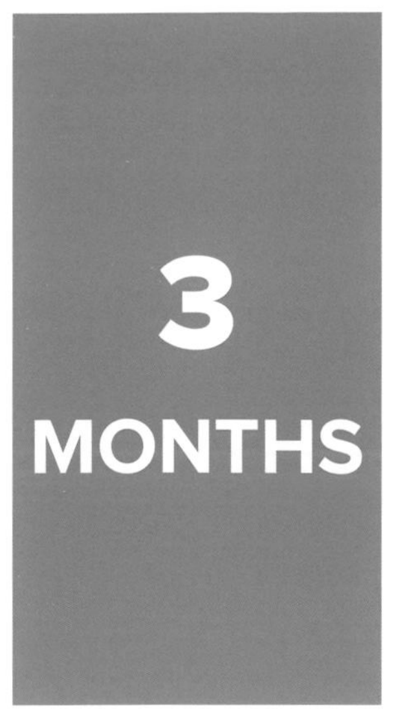

Vital Signs

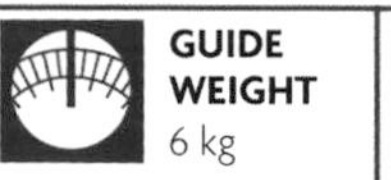 GUIDE WEIGHT	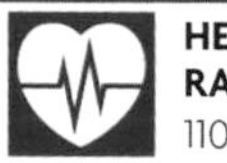 HEART RATE	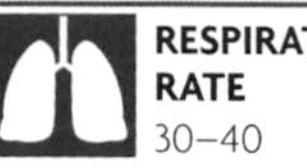 RESPIRATION RATE	 SYSTOLIC BLOOD PRESSURE
6 kg	110–160	30–40	70–90

Airway Size by Type

OROPHARYNGEAL AIRWAY	LARYNGEAL MASK	I-GEL AIRWAY	ENDOTRACHEAL TUBE
00	1.5	1.5	Diameter: **3.5 mm**; Length: **11 cm**

Defibrillation – Cardiac Arrest

MANUAL	AUTOMATED EXTERNAL DEFIBRILLATOR
25 Joules	Where possible, use a manual defibrillator. If an AED is the only defibrillator available, it should be used (preferably using paediatric attenuation pads or else in paediatric mode).

Intravascular Fluid

NAME	ROUTE	INITIAL DOSE	REPEAT DOSE	DOSE INTERVAL	CONCENTRATION	VOLUME	MAX DOSE
0.9% Sodium Chloride (5 ml/kg)	IV/IO	30 ml	30 ml	PRN	0.9%	30 ml	240 ml
0.9% Sodium Chloride (10 ml/kg)	IV/IO	60 ml	60 ml	PRN	0.9%	60 ml	240 ml
0.9% Sodium Chloride (20 ml/kg)	IV/IO	120 ml	120 ml	PRN	0.9%	120 ml	240 ml

Cardiac Arrest

NAME	ROUTE	INITIAL DOSE	REPEAT DOSE	DOSE INTERVAL	CONCEN-TRATION	VOLUME	MAX DOSE
Adrenaline	IV/IO	60 micrograms	60 micrograms	3–5 minutes	1 milligram in 10 ml (1:10,000)	0.6 ml	No limit
Amiodarone	IV/IO	30 milligrams (After 3rd shock)	30 milligrams	After 5th shock	300 milligrams in 10 ml	1 ml	60 milligrams

Quick Reference Table

NAME	ROUTE	INITIAL DOSE	REPEAT DOSE	DOSE INTERVAL	CONCENTRATION	VOLUME	MAX DOSE
Activated Charcoal	Oral	N/A	N/A	N/A	N/A	N/A	N/A
Adrenaline - anaphylaxis/ asthma	IM	150 micrograms	150 micrograms	5 minutes	1 milligram in 1 ml (1:1,000)	0.15 ml	No limit
Benzylpenicillin	IV/IO	300 milligrams	NONE	N/A	600 milligrams dissolved in 10 ml water for injection	5 ml	300 milligrams
Benzylpenicillin	IM	300 milligrams	NONE	N/A	600 milligrams dissolved in 2 ml water for injection	1 ml	300 milligrams
Chlorphenamine	IV/IO/IM	1 milligram	N/A	N/A	10 milligrams in 1 ml	0.1 ml	1 milligram
Chlorphenamine	Oral (tablet)	N/A	N/A	N/A	N/A	N/A	N/A
Chlorphenamine	Oral (solution)	1 milligram	NONE	N/A	2 milligrams in 5 ml	2.5 ml	1 milligram
Dexamethasone	Oral (solution)	0.9 milligrams	NONE	N/A	2 milligrams in 5 ml	2 ml	0.9 milligrams

Page for Age: 3 MONTHS

NAME	ROUTE	INITIAL DOSE	REPEAT DOSE	DOSE INTERVAL	CONCENTRATION	VOLUME	MAX DOSE
Dexamethasone	Oral (tablet)	2 milligrams	NONE	N/A	2 milligrams per tablet	1 tablet	2 milligrams
Diazepam	Rectal	2.5 milligrams	2.5 milligrams	10 minutes	2.5 milligrams in 1.25 ml	1 x 2.5 milligram tube	5 milligrams
Diazepam	IV/IO	2 milligrams	2 milligrams	10 minutes	10 milligrams in 2 ml	0.4 ml	4 milligrams
Glucagon	IM	500 micrograms	NONE	N/A	1 milligram per vial	0.5 vial	500 micrograms
Glucose 10%	IV	1 gram glucose	1 gram glucose	5 minutes	50 grams in 500 ml	10 ml	30 ml (3 g glucose)
Glucose 40% Oral Gel	Buccal	An appropriate amount should be administered, considering the child's size	See initial dose	5 minutes	10 grams in 25 grams of gel	1 tube	An appropriate amount should be administered, considering the child's size
Hydrocortisone	IV/IO/IM	25 milligrams	NONE	N/A	100 milligrams in 1 ml	0.25 ml	25 milligrams
Hydrocortisone	IV/IO/IM	25 milligrams	NONE	N/A	100 milligrams in 2 ml	0.5 ml	25 milligrams
Ibuprofen	Oral	50 milligrams	50 milligrams	8 hours	100 milligrams in 5 ml	2.5 ml	150 milligrams per 24 hours
Ipratropium Bromide	Neb	125–250 micrograms	NONE	N/A	250 micrograms in 1 ml	0.5 ml–1 ml	125–250 micrograms
Ipratropium Bromide	Neb	125–250 micrograms	NONE	N/A	500 micrograms in 2 ml	0.5 ml–1 ml	125–250 micrograms
Midazolam*	Buccal	See Epilepsy Passport	See Epilepsy Passport	10 mins	5 milligrams in 1 ml	See Epilepsy Passport	See Epilepsy Passport
Morphine Sulfate	IV/IO	N/A	N/A	N/A	N/A	N/A	N/A
Morphine Sulfate	Oral	N/A	N/A	N/A	N/A	N/A	N/A
Naloxone	IM	400 micrograms	400 micrograms	3 minutes	400 micrograms in 1 ml	1 ml	2,000 micrograms
Naloxone	IV/IO	400 micrograms	400 micrograms	1 minute	400 micrograms in 1 ml	1 ml	2,000 micrograms
Ondansetron	IV/IO/IM	0.5 milligrams	NONE	N/A	2 milligrams in 1 ml	0.25 ml	0.5 milligrams
Paracetamol - Infant suspension	Oral	60 milligrams	60 milligrams	4–6 hours	120 milligrams in 5 ml	2.5 ml	240 milligrams in 24 hours
Paracetamol	IV infusion/ IO	60 milligrams	60 milligrams	4–6 hours	10 milligrams in 1 ml	6 ml	180 milligrams in 24 hours
Salbutamol	Neb	2.5 milligrams	2.5 milligrams	5 minutes	2.5 milligrams in 2.5 ml	2.5 ml	No limit
Salbutamol	Neb	2.5 milligrams	2.5 milligrams	5 minutes	5 milligrams in 2.5 ml	1.25 ml	No limit
Tranexamic Acid	IV	100 mg	NONE	N/A	100 mg/ml	1 ml	100 mg

*Give the dose as prescribed in the child's individual treatment plan/Epilepsy Passport (the dosages described above reflect the recommended dosages for a child of this age).

Page for Age: 6 MONTHS

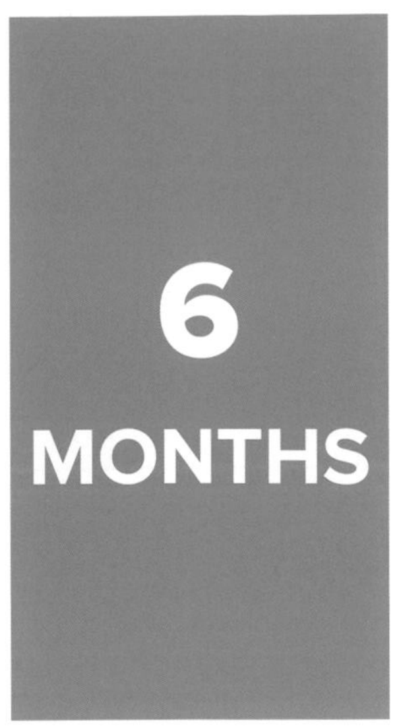

Vital Signs

 GUIDE WEIGHT 8 kg	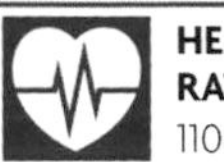 HEART RATE 110–160	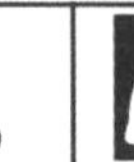 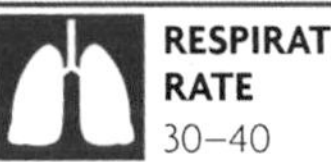 RESPIRATION RATE 30–40	 SYSTOLIC BLOOD PRESSURE 70–90

Airway Size by Type

OROPHARYNGEAL AIRWAY	LARYNGEAL MASK	I-GEL AIRWAY	ENDOTRACHEAL TUBE
00	1.5	1.5	Diameter: **4 mm**; Length: **12 cm**

Defibrillation – Cardiac Arrest

MANUAL	AUTOMATED EXTERNAL DEFIBRILLATOR
40 Joules	Where possible, use a manual defibrillator. If an AED is the only defibrillator available, it should be used (preferably using paediatric attenuation pads or else in paediatric mode).

Intravascular Fluid

NAME	ROUTE	INITIAL DOSE	REPEAT DOSE	DOSE INTERVAL	CONCENTRATION	VOLUME	MAX DOSE
0.9% Sodium Chloride (5 ml/kg)	IV/IO	40 ml	40 ml	PRN	0.9%	40 ml	320 ml
0.9% Sodium Chloride (10 ml/kg)	IV/IO	80 ml	80 ml	PRN	0.9%	80 ml	320 ml
0.9% Sodium Chloride (20 ml/kg)	IV/IO	160 ml	160 ml	PRN	0.9%	160 ml	320 ml

Cardiac Arrest

NAME	ROUTE	INITIAL DOSE	REPEAT DOSE	DOSE INTERVAL	CONCENTRATION	VOLUME	MAX DOSE
Adrenaline	IV/IO	80 micrograms	80 micrograms	3–5 minutes	1 milligram in 10 ml (1:10,000)	0.8 ml	No limit
Amiodarone	IV/IO	40 milligrams (After 3rd shock)	40 milligrams	After 5th shock	300 milligrams in 10 ml	1.3 ml	80 milligrams

Quick Reference Table

NAME	ROUTE	INITIAL DOSE	REPEAT DOSE	DOSE INTERVAL	CONCEN-TRATION	VOLUME	MAX DOSE
Activated Charcoal	Oral	N/A	N/A	N/A	N/A	N/A	N/A
Adrenaline - anaphylaxis/ asthma	IM	150 micrograms	150 micrograms	5 minutes	1 milligram in 1 ml (1:1,000)	0.15 ml	No limit
Benzylpenicillin	IV/IO	300 milligrams	NONE	N/A	600 milligrams dissolved in 10 ml water for injection	5 ml	300 milligrams
Benzylpenicillin	IM	300 milligrams	NONE	N/A	600 milligrams dissolved in 2 ml water for injection	1 ml	300 milligrams
Chlorphenamine	IV/IO/IM	2.5 milligrams	NONE	N/A	10 milligrams in 1 ml	0.25 ml	2.5 milligrams
Chlorphenamine	Oral (tablet)	N/A	N/A	N/A	N/A	N/A	N/A
Chlorphenamine	Oral (solution)	1 milligram	NONE	N/A	2 milligrams in 5 ml	2.5 ml	1 milligram

Page for Age: 6 MONTHS

NAME	ROUTE	INITIAL DOSE	REPEAT DOSE	DOSE INTERVAL	CONCEN-TRATION	VOLUME	MAX DOSE
Dexamethasone	Oral (solution)	1.2 milligrams	NONE	N/A	2 milligrams in 5 ml	3 ml	1.2 milligrams
Dexamethasone	Oral (tablet)	2 milligrams	NONE	N/A	2 milligrams per tablet	1 tablet	2 milligrams
Diazepam	Rectal	5 milligrams	5 milligrams	10 minutes	5 milligrams in 2.5 ml	1 x 5 milligram tube	10 milligrams
Diazepam	IV/IO	2.5 milligrams	2.5 milligrams	10 minutes	10 milligrams in 2 ml	0.5 ml	5 milligrams
Glucagon	IM	500 micrograms	NONE	N/A	1 milligram per vial	0.5 vial	500 micrograms
Glucose 10%	IV	1.5 grams glucose	1.5 grams glucose	5 minutes	50 grams in 500 ml	15 ml	45 ml (4.5 g glucose)
Glucose 40% Oral Gel	Buccal	An appropriate amount should be administered, considering the child's size	See initial dose	5 minutes	10 grams in 25 grams of gel	1 tube	An appropriate amount should be administered, considering the child's size
Hydrocortisone	IV/IO/IM	50 milligrams	NONE	N/A	100 milligrams in 1 ml	0.5 ml	50 milligrams
Hydrocortisone	IV/IO/IM	50 milligrams	NONE	N/A	100 milligrams in 2 ml	1 ml	50 milligrams
Ibuprofen	Oral	50 milligrams	50 milligrams	8 hours	100 milligrams in 5 ml	2.5 ml	150 milligrams per 24 hours
Ipratropium Bromide	Neb	125–250 micrograms	NONE	N/A	250 micrograms in 1 ml	0.5 ml–1 ml	125–250 micrograms
Ipratropium Bromide	Neb	125–250 micrograms	NONE	N/A	500 micrograms in 2 ml	0.5 ml–1 ml	125–250 micrograms
Midazolam*	Buccal	2.5 milligrams	2.5 milligrams	10 mins	5 milligrams in 1 ml	0.5 ml pre-filled syringe	5 milligrams
Morphine Sulfate	IV/IO	N/A	N/A	N/A	N/A	N/A	N/A
Morphine Sulfate	Oral	N/A	N/A	N/A	N/A	N/A	N/A
Naloxone	IM	400 micrograms	400 micrograms	3 minutes	400 micrograms in 1 ml	1 ml	2,000 micrograms
Naloxone	IV/IO	800 micrograms	800 micrograms	1 minute	400 micrograms in 1 ml	2 ml	2,000 micrograms
Ondansetron	IV/IO/IM	1 milligram	NONE	N/A	2 milligrams in 1 ml	0.5 ml	1 milligram
Paracetamol - Infant suspension	Oral	120 milligrams	120 milligrams	4–6 hours	120 milligrams in 5 ml	5 ml	480 milligrams in 24 hours
Paracetamol	IV infusion/IO	80 milligrams	80 milligrams	4–6 hours	10 milligrams in 1 ml	8 ml	240 milligrams in 24 hours
Salbutamol	Neb	2.5 milligrams	2.5 milligrams	5 minutes	2.5 milligrams in 2.5 ml	2.5 ml	No limit
Salbutamol	Neb	2.5 milligrams	2.5 milligrams	5 minutes	5 milligrams in 2.5 ml	1.25 ml	No limit
Tranexamic Acid	IV	100 mg	NONE	N/A	100 mg/ml	1 ml	100 mg

*Give the dose as prescribed in the child's individual treatment plan/Epilepsy Passport (the dosages described above reflect the recommended dosages for a child of this age).

Page for Age: 9 MONTHS

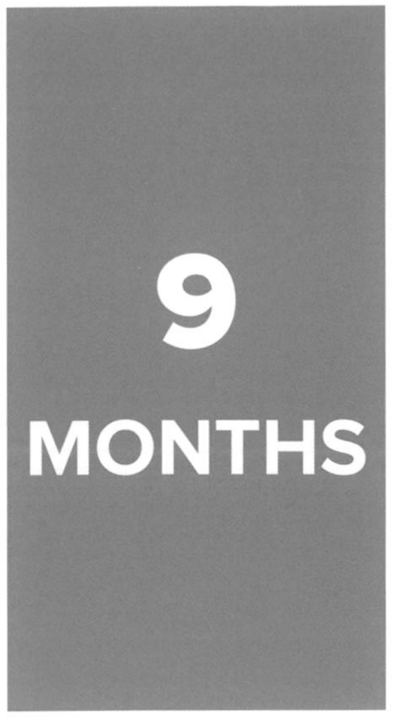

Vital Signs

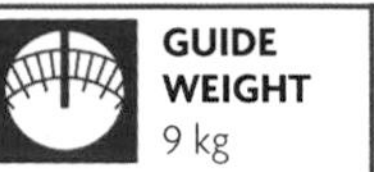 GUIDE WEIGHT 9 kg	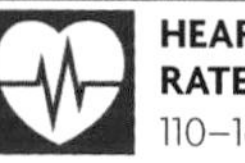 HEART RATE 110–160	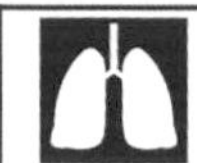 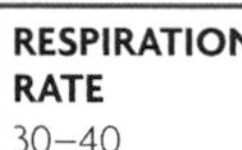 RESPIRATION RATE 30–40	 SYSTOLIC BLOOD PRESSURE 70–90

Airway Size by Type

OROPHARYNGEAL AIRWAY	LARYNGEAL MASK	I-GEL AIRWAY	ENDOTRACHEAL TUBE
00	1.5	1.5	Diameter: **4 mm**; Length: **12 cm**

Defibrillation – Cardiac Arrest

MANUAL	AUTOMATED EXTERNAL DEFIBRILLATOR
40 Joules	Where possible, use a manual defibrillator. If an AED is the only defibrillator available, it should be used (preferably using paediatric attenuation pads or else in paediatric mode).

Intravascular Fluid

NAME	ROUTE	INITIAL DOSE	REPEAT DOSE	DOSE INTERVAL	CONCENTRATION	VOLUME	MAX DOSE
0.9% Sodium Chloride (5 ml/kg)	IV/IO	45 ml	45 ml	PRN	0.9%	45 ml	360 ml
0.9% Sodium Chloride (10 ml/kg)	IV/IO	90 ml	90 ml	PRN	0.9%	90 ml	360 ml
0.9% Sodium Chloride (20 ml/kg)	IV/IO	180 ml	180 ml	PRN	0.9%	180 ml	360 ml

Cardiac Arrest

NAME	ROUTE	INITIAL DOSE	REPEAT DOSE	DOSE INTERVAL	CONCENTRATION	VOLUME	MAX DOSE
Adrenaline	IV/IO	90 micrograms	90 micrograms	3–5 minutes	1 milligram in 10 ml (1:10,000)	0.9 ml	No limit
Amiodarone	IV/IO	45 milligrams (After 3rd shock)	45 milligrams	After 5th shock	300 milligrams in 10 ml	1.5 ml	90 milligrams

Quick Reference Table

NAME	ROUTE	INITIAL DOSE	REPEAT DOSE	DOSE INTERVAL	CONCEN-TRATION	VOLUME	MAX DOSE
Activated Charcoal	Oral	N/A	N/A	N/A	N/A	N/A	N/A
Adrenaline - anaphylaxis/ asthma	IM	150 micrograms	150 micrograms	5 minutes	1 milligram in 1 ml (1:1,000)	0.15 ml	No limit
Benzylpenicillin	IV/IO	300 milligrams	NONE	N/A	600 milligrams dissolved in 10 ml water for injection	5 ml	300 milligrams
Benzylpenicillin	IM	300 milligrams	NONE	N/A	600 milligrams dissolved in 2 ml water for injection	1 ml	300 milligrams
Chlorphenamine	IV/IO	2.5 milligrams	NONE	N/A	10 milligrams in 1 ml	0.25 ml	2.5 milligrams
Chlorphenamine	Oral (tablet)	N/A	N/A	N/A	N/A	N/A	N/A
Chlorphenamine	Oral (solution)	1 milligram	NONE	N/A	2 milligrams in 5 ml	2.5 ml	1 milligram

Page for Age: 9 MONTHS

NAME	ROUTE	INITIAL DOSE	REPEAT DOSE	DOSE INTERVAL	CONCEN-TRATION	VOLUME	MAX DOSE
Dexamethasone	Oral (solution)	1.4 milligrams	NONE	N/A	2 milligrams in 5 ml	3 ml	1.4 milligrams
Dexamethasone	Oral (tablet)	2 milligrams	NONE	N/A	2 milligrams per tablet	1 tablet	2 milligrams
Diazepam	Rectal	5 milligrams	5 milligrams	10 minutes	5 milligrams in 2.5 ml	1 x 5 milligram tube	10 milligrams
Diazepam	IV/IO	3 milligrams	3 milligrams	10 minutes	10 milligrams in 2 ml	0.6 ml	6 milligrams
Glucagon	IM	500 micrograms	NONE	N/A	1 milligram per vial	0.5 vial	500 micrograms
Glucose 10%	IV	2 grams glucose	2 grams glucose	5 minutes	50 grams in 500 ml	20 ml	60 ml (6 g glucose)
Glucose 40% Oral Gel	Buccal	An appropriate amount should be administered, considering the child's size	See initial dose	5 minutes	10 grams in 25 grams of gel	1 tube	An appropriate amount should be administered, considering the child's size
Hydrocortisone	IV/IO/IM	50 milligrams	NONE	N/A	100 milligrams in 1 ml	0.5 ml	50 milligrams
Hydrocortisone	IV/IO/IM	50 milligrams	NONE	N/A	100 milligrams in 2 ml	1 ml	50 milligrams
Ibuprofen	Oral	50 milligrams	50 milligrams	8 hours	100 milligrams in 5 ml	2.5 ml	150 milligrams per 24 hours
Ipratropium Bromide	Neb	125–250 micrograms	NONE	N/A	250 micrograms in 1 ml	0.5 ml–1 ml	125–250 micrograms
Ipratropium Bromide	Neb	125–250 micrograms	NONE	N/A	500 micrograms in 2 ml	0.5 ml–1 ml	125–250 micrograms
Midazolam*	Buccal	2.5 milligrams	2.5 milligrams	10 mins	5 milligrams in 1 ml	0.5 ml pre-filled syringe	5 milligrams
Morphine Sulfate	IV/IO	N/A	N/A	N/A	N/A	N/A	N/A
Morphine Sulfate	Oral	N/A	N/A	N/A	N/A	N/A	N/A
Naloxone	IM	400 micrograms	400 micrograms	3 minutes	400 micrograms in 1 ml	1 ml	2,000 micrograms
Naloxone	IV/IO	800 micrograms	800 micrograms	1 minute	400 micrograms in 1 ml	2 ml	2,000 micrograms
Ondansetron	IV/IO/IM	1 milligram	NONE	N/A	2 milligrams in 1 ml	0.5 ml	1 milligram
Paracetamol - Infant suspension	Oral	120 milligrams	120 milligrams	4–6 hours	120 milligrams in 5 ml	5 ml	480 milligrams in 24 hours
Paracetamol	IV infusion/ IO	90 milligrams	90 milligrams	4–6 hours	10 milligrams in 1 ml	9 ml	270 milligrams in 24 hours
Salbutamol	Neb	2.5 milligrams	2.5 milligrams	5 minutes	2.5 milligrams in 2.5 ml	2.5 ml	No limit
Salbutamol	Neb	2.5 milligrams	2.5 milligrams	5 minutes	5 milligrams in 2.5 ml	1.25 ml	No limit
Tranexamic Acid	IV	150 mg	NONE	N/A	100 mg/ml	1.5 ml	150 mg

*Give the dose as prescribed in the child's individual treatment plan/Epilepsy Passport (the dosages described above reflect the recommended dosages for a child of this age).

Page for Age: 12 MONTHS

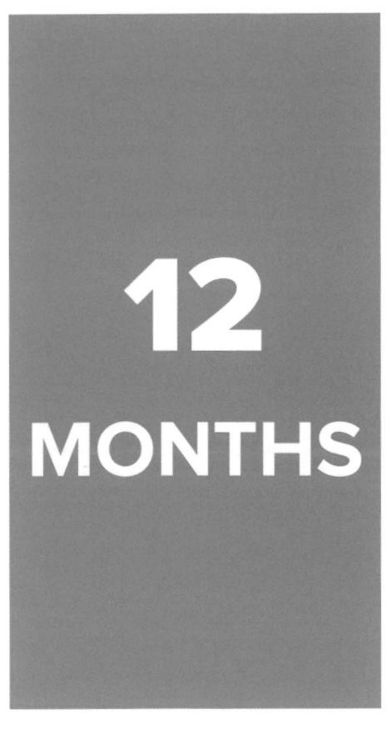

Vital Signs

GUIDE WEIGHT	HEART RATE	RESPIRATION RATE	SYSTOLIC BLOOD PRESSURE
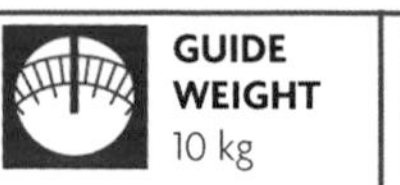 10 kg	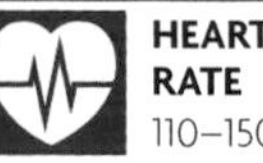 110–150	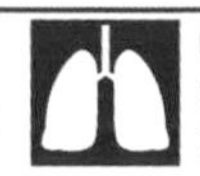 25–35	 80–95

Airway Size by Type

OROPHARYNGEAL AIRWAY	LARYNGEAL MASK	I-GEL AIRWAY	ENDOTRACHEAL TUBE
00 OR 0	1.5	1.5 OR 2	Diameter: **4.5 mm**; Length: **13 cm**

Defibrillation – Cardiac Arrest

MANUAL	AUTOMATED EXTERNAL DEFIBRILLATOR
40 Joules	A standard AED (either with paediatric attenuation pads or else in paediatric mode) can be used. If paediatric pads are not available, standard adult pads can be used (but must not overlap).

Intravascular Fluid

NAME	ROUTE	INITIAL DOSE	REPEAT DOSE	DOSE INTERVAL	CONCENTRATION	VOLUME	MAX DOSE
0.9% Sodium Chloride (5 ml/kg)	IV/IO	50 ml	50 ml	PRN	0.9%	50 ml	400 ml
0.9% Sodium Chloride (10 ml/kg)	IV/IO	100 ml	100 ml	PRN	0.9%	100 ml	400 ml
0.9% Sodium Chloride (20 ml/kg)	IV/IO	200 ml	200 ml	PRN	0.9%	200 ml	400 ml

Cardiac Arrest

NAME	ROUTE	INITIAL DOSE	REPEAT DOSE	DOSE INTERVAL	CONCENTRATION	VOLUME	MAX DOSE
Adrenaline	IV/IO	100 micrograms	100 micrograms	3–5 minutes	1 milligram in 10 ml (1:10,000)	1 ml	No limit
Amiodarone	IV/IO	50 milligrams (After 3rd shock)	50 milligrams	After 5th shock	300 milligrams in 10 ml	1.7 ml	100 milligrams

Quick Reference Table

NAME	ROUTE	INITIAL DOSE	REPEAT DOSE	DOSE INTERVAL	CONCEN-TRATION	VOLUME	MAX DOSE
Activated Charcoal*	Oral	25 g	25 g	N/A	50 grams in 250 ml	125 ml	50 grams
Adrenaline - anaphylaxis/ asthma	IM	150 micrograms	150 micrograms	5 minutes	1 milligram in 1 ml (1:1,000)	0.15 ml	No limit
Benzylpenicillin	IV/IO	600 milligrams	NONE	N/A	600 milligrams dissolved in 10 ml water for injection	10 ml	600 milligrams
Benzylpenicillin	IM	600 milligrams	NONE	N/A	600 milligrams dissolved in 2 ml water for injection	2 ml	600 milligrams
Chlorphenamine	IV/IO/IM	2.5 milligrams	NONE	N/A	10 milligrams in 1 ml	0.25 ml	2.5 milligrams
Chlorphenamine	Oral (tablet)	N/A	N/A	N/A	N/A	N/A	N/A
Chlorphenamine	Oral (solution)	1 milligram	NONE	N/A	2 milligrams in 5 ml	2.5 ml	1 milligram

Page for Age: 12 MONTHS

NAME	ROUTE	INITIAL DOSE	REPEAT DOSE	DOSE INTERVAL	CONCEN-TRATION	VOLUME	MAX DOSE
Dexamethasone	Oral (solution)	1.5 milligrams	NONE	N/A	2 milligrams in 5 ml	4 ml	1.5 milligrams
Dexamethasone	Oral	2 milligrams	NONE	N/A	2 milligrams per tablet	1 tablet	2 milligrams
Diazepam	Rectal	5 milligrams	5 milligrams	10 minutes	5 milligrams in 2.5 ml	1 x 5 milligram tube	10 milligrams
Diazepam	IV/IO	3 milligrams	3 milligrams	10 minutes	10 milligrams in 2 ml	0.6 ml	6 milligrams
Glucagon	IM	500 micrograms	NONE	N/A	1 milligram per vial	0.5 vial	500 micrograms
Glucose 10%	IV	2 grams glucose	2 grams glucose	5 minutes	50 grams in 500 ml	20 ml	60 ml (6 g glucose)
Glucose 40% Oral Gel	Buccal	An appropriate amount should be administered, considering the child's size	See initial dose	5 minutes	10 grams in 25 grams of gel	1 tube	An appropriate amount should be administered, considering the child's size
Hydrocortisone	IV/IO/IM	50 milligrams	NONE	N/A	100 milligrams in 1 ml	0.5 ml	50 milligrams
Hydrocortisone	IV/IO/IM	50 milligrams	NONE	N/A	100 milligrams in 2 ml	1 ml	50 milligrams
Ibuprofen	Oral	100 milligrams	100 milligrams	8 hours	100 milligrams in 5 ml	5 ml	300 milligrams per 24 hours
Ipratropium Bromide	Neb	125–250 micrograms	NONE	N/A	250 micrograms in 1 ml	0.5–1 ml	125–250 micrograms
Ipratropium Bromide	Neb	125–250 micrograms	NONE	N/A	500 micrograms in 2 ml	0.5–1 ml	125–250 micrograms
Midazolam**	Buccal	5 milligrams	5 milligrams	10 mins	5 milligrams in 1 ml	1 ml pre-filled syringe	10 milligrams
Morphine Sulfate	IV/IO	1 milligram	1 milligram	5 minutes	10 milligrams in 10 ml	1 ml	2 milligrams
Morphine Sulfate	Oral	2 milligrams	NONE	N/A	10 milligrams in 5 ml	1 ml	2 milligrams
Naloxone	IM	400 micrograms	400 micrograms	3 minutes	400 micrograms in 1 ml	1 ml	2,000 micrograms
Naloxone	IV/IO	1,000 micrograms	1,000 micrograms	1 minute	400 micrograms in 1 ml	2.5 ml	2,000 micrograms
Ondansetron	IV/IO/IM	1 milligram	NONE	N/A	2 milligrams in 1 ml	0.5 ml	1 milligram
Paracetamol - Infant suspension	Oral	120 milligrams	120 milligrams	4–6 hours	120 milligrams in 5 ml	5 ml	480 milligrams in 24 hours
Paracetamol	IV infusion/ IO	150 milligrams	150 milligrams	4–6 hours	10 milligrams in 1 ml	15 ml	600 milligrams in 24 hours
Salbutamol	Neb	2.5 milligrams	2.5 milligrams	5 minutes	2.5 milligrams in 2.5 ml	2.5 ml	No limit
Salbutamol	Neb	2.5 milligrams	2.5 milligrams	5 minutes	5 milligrams in 2.5 ml	1.25 ml	No limit
Tranexamic Acid	IV	150 mg	NONE	N/A	100 mg/ml	1.5 ml	150 mg

*If a large quantity of poison has been ingested, and where there is a risk to life, encourage the child to drink the full dose.

**Give the dose as prescribed in the child's individual treatment plan/Epilepsy Passport (the dosages described above reflect the recommended dosages for a child of this age).

Page for Age: 18 MONTHS

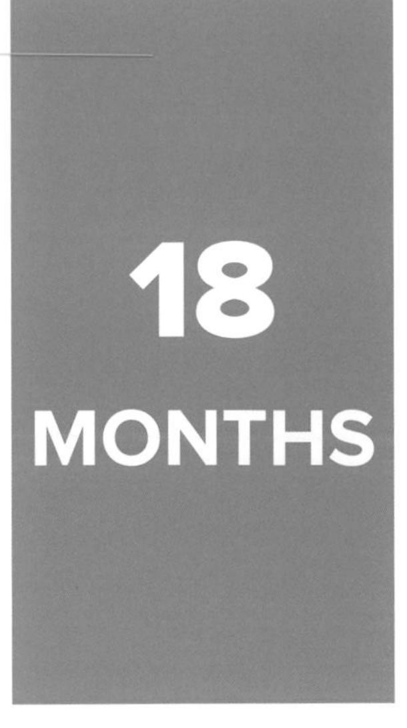

Vital Signs

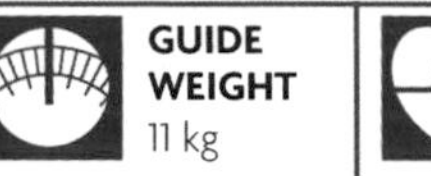 GUIDE WEIGHT 11 kg	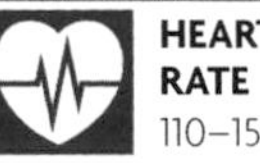 HEART RATE 110–150	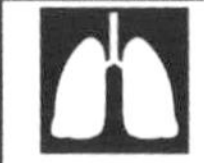 RESPIRATION RATE 25–35	 SYSTOLIC BLOOD PRESSURE 80–95

Airway Size by Type

OROPHARYNGEAL AIRWAY	LARYNGEAL MASK	I-GEL AIRWAY	ENDOTRACHEAL TUBE
00 OR 0	2	1.5 OR 2	Diameter: **4.5 mm**; Length: **13 cm**

Defibrillation – Cardiac Arrest

MANUAL	AUTOMATED EXTERNAL DEFIBRILLATOR
50 Joules	A standard AED (either with paediatric attenuation pads or else in paediatric mode) can be used. If paediatric pads are not available, standard adult pads can be used (but must not overlap).

Intravascular Fluid

NAME	ROUTE	INITIAL DOSE	REPEAT DOSE	DOSE INTERVAL	CONCENTRATION	VOLUME	MAX DOSE
0.9% Sodium Chloride (5 ml/kg)	IV/IO	55 ml	55 ml	PRN	0.9%	55 ml	440 ml
0.9% Sodium Chloride (10 ml/kg)	IV/IO	110 ml	110 ml	PRN	0.9%	110 ml	440 ml
0.9% Sodium Chloride (20 ml/kg)	IV/IO	220 ml	220 ml	PRN	0.9%	220 ml	440 ml

Cardiac Arrest

NAME	ROUTE	INITIAL DOSE	REPEAT DOSE	DOSE INTERVAL	CONCENTRATION	VOLUME	MAX DOSE
Adrenaline	IV/IO	110 micrograms	110 micrograms	3–5 minutes	1 milligram in 10 ml (1:10,000)	1.1 ml	No limit
Amiodarone	IV/IO	55 milligrams (After 3rd shock)	55 milligrams	After 5th shock	300 milligrams in 10 ml	1.8 ml	110 milligrams

Quick Reference Table

NAME	ROUTE	INITIAL DOSE	REPEAT DOSE	DOSE INTERVAL	CONCEN-TRATION	VOLUME	MAX DOSE
Activated Charcoal*	Oral	25 g	25 g	N/A	50 grams in 250 ml	125 ml	50 grams
Adrenaline - anaphylaxis/ asthma	IM	150 micrograms	150 micrograms	5 minutes	1 milligram in 1 ml (1:1,000)	0.15 ml	No limit
Benzylpenicillin	IV/IO	600 milligrams	NONE	N/A	600 milligrams dissolved in 10 ml water for injection	10 ml	600 milligrams
Benzylpenicillin	IM	600 milligrams	NONE	N/A	600 milligrams dissolved in 2 ml water for injection	2 ml	600 milligrams
Chlorphenamine	IV/IO/IM	2.5 milligrams	NONE	N/A	10 milligrams in 1 ml	0.25 ml	2.5 milligrams
Chlorphenamine	Oral (tablet)	N/A	N/A	N/A	N/A	N/A	N/A
Chlorphenamine	Oral (solution)	1 milligram	NONE	N/A	2 milligrams in 5 ml	2.5 ml	1 milligram

Page for Age: 18 MONTHS

NAME	ROUTE	INITIAL DOSE	REPEAT DOSE	DOSE INTERVAL	CONCEN-TRATION	VOLUME	MAX DOSE
Dexamethasone	Oral (solution)	1.7 milligrams	NONE	N/A	2 milligrams in 5 ml	4 ml	1.7 milligrams
Dexamethasone	Oral (tablet)	4 milligrams	NONE	N/A	2 milligrams per tablet	2 tablets	4 milligrams
Diazepam	Rectal	5 milligrams	5 milligrams	10 minutes	5 milligrams in 2.5 ml	1 x 5 milligram tube	10 milligrams
Diazepam	IV/IO	3.5 milligrams	3.5 milligrams	10 minutes	10 milligrams in 2 ml	0.7 ml	7 milligrams
Glucagon	IM	500 micrograms	NONE	N/A	1 milligram per vial	0.5 vial	500 micrograms
Glucose 10%	IV	2 grams glucose	2 grams glucose	5 minutes	50 grams in 500 ml	20 ml	60 ml (6 g glucose)
Glucose 40% Oral Gel	Buccal	An appropriate amount should be administered, considering the child's size	See initial dose	5 minutes	10 grams in 25 grams of gel	1 tube	An appropriate amount should be administered, considering the child's size
Hydrocortisone	IV/IO/IM	50 milligrams	NONE	N/A	100 milligrams in 1 ml	0.5 ml	50 milligrams
Hydrocortisone	IV/IO/IM	50 milligrams	NONE	N/A	100 milligrams in 2 ml	1 ml	50 milligrams
Ibuprofen	Oral	100 milligrams	100 milligrams	8 hours	100 milligrams in 5 ml	5 ml	300 milligrams per 24 hours
Ipratropium Bromide	Neb	250 micrograms	NONE	N/A	250 micrograms in 1 ml	1 ml	250 micrograms
Ipratropium Bromide	Neb	250 micrograms	NONE	N/A	500 micrograms in 2 ml	1 ml	250 micrograms
Midazolam**	Buccal	5 milligrams	5 milligrams	10 mins	5 milligrams in 1 ml	1 ml pre-filled syringe	10 milligrams
Morphine Sulfate	IV/IO	1 milligram	1 milligram	5 minutes	10 milligrams in 10 ml	1 ml	2 milligrams
Morphine Sulfate	Oral	2 milligrams	NONE	N/A	10 milligrams in 5 ml	1 ml	2 milligrams
Naloxone	IM	400 micrograms	400 micrograms	3 minutes	400 micrograms in 1 ml	1 ml	2,000 micrograms
Naloxone	IV/IO	1,000 micrograms	1,000 micrograms	1 minute	400 micrograms in 1 ml	2.5 ml	2,000 micrograms
Ondansetron	IV/IO/IM	1 milligram	NONE	N/A	2 milligrams in 1 ml	0.5 ml	1 milligram
Paracetamol - Infant suspension	Oral	120 milligrams	120 milligrams	4–6 hours	120 milligrams in 5 ml	5 ml	480 milligrams in 24 hours
Paracetamol	IV infusion/ IO	150 milligrams	150 milligrams	4–6 hours	10 milligrams in 1 ml	15 ml	600 milligrams in 24 hours
Salbutamol	Neb	2.5 milligrams	2.5 milligrams	5 minutes	2.5 milligrams in 2.5 ml	2.5 ml	No limit
Salbutamol	Neb	2.5 milligrams	2.5 milligrams	5 minutes	5 milligrams in 2.5 ml	1.25 ml	No limit
Tranexamic Acid	IV	150 mg	NONE	N/A	100 mg/ml	1.5 mls	150 mg

*If a large quantity of poison has been ingested, and where there is a risk to life, encourage the child to drink the full dose.

**Give the dose as prescribed in the child's individual treatment plan/Epilepsy Passport (the dosages described above reflect the recommended dosages for a child of this age).

Page for Age: 2 YEARS

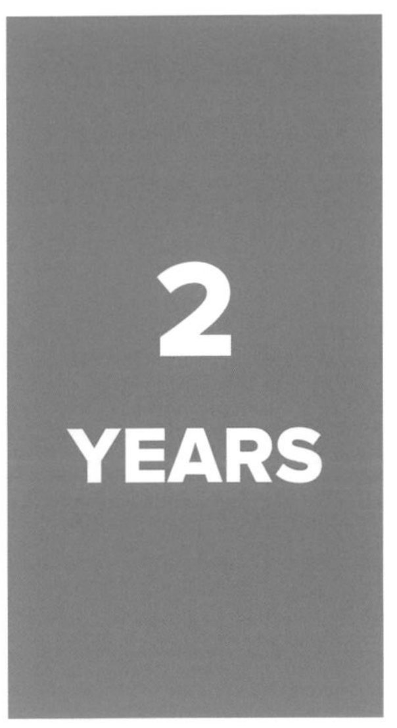

Vital Signs

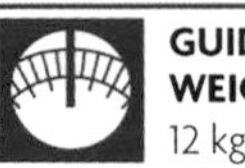 GUIDE WEIGHT 12 kg	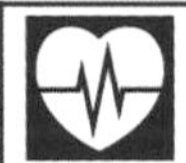 HEART RATE 95–140	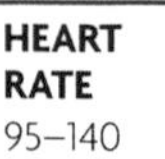 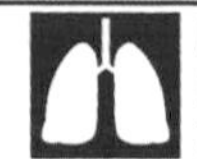 RESPIRATION RATE 25–30	 SYSTOLIC BLOOD PRESSURE 80–100

Airway Size by Type

OROPHARYNGEAL AIRWAY	LARYNGEAL MASK	I-GEL AIRWAY	ENDOTRACHEAL TUBE
0 OR 1	2	1.5 OR 2	Diameter: **5 mm**; Length: **14 cm**

Defibrillation – Cardiac Arrest

MANUAL	AUTOMATED EXTERNAL DEFIBRILLATOR
50 Joules	A standard AED (either with paediatric attenuation pads or else in paediatric mode) can be used. If paediatric pads are not available, standard adult pads can be used (but must not overlap).

Intravascular Fluid

NAME	ROUTE	INITIAL DOSE	REPEAT DOSE	DOSE INTERVAL	CONCENTRATION	VOLUME	MAX DOSE
0.9% Sodium Chloride (5 ml/kg)	IV/IO	60 ml	60 ml	PRN	0.9%	60 ml	480 ml
0.9% Sodium Chloride (10 ml/kg)	IV/IO	120 ml	120 ml	PRN	0.9%	120 ml	480 ml
0.9% Sodium Chloride (20 ml/kg)	IV/IO	240 ml	240 ml	PRN	0.9%	240 ml	480 ml

Cardiac Arrest

NAME	ROUTE	INITIAL DOSE	REPEAT DOSE	DOSE INTERVAL	CONCENTRATION	VOLUME	MAX DOSE
Adrenaline	IV/IO	120 micrograms	120 micrograms	3–5 minutes	1 milligram in 10 ml (1:10,000)	1.2 ml	No limit
Amiodarone	IV/IO	60 milligrams (After 3rd shock)	60 milligrams	After 5th shock	300 milligrams in 10 ml	2 ml	120 milligrams

Quick Reference Table

NAME	ROUTE	INITIAL DOSE	REPEAT DOSE	DOSE INTERVAL	CONCEN-TRATION	VOLUME	MAX DOSE
Activated Charcoal*	Oral	25 g	25 g	N/A	50 grams in 250 ml	125 ml	50 grams
Adrenaline - anaphylaxis/ asthma	IM	150 micrograms	150 micrograms	5 minutes	1 milligram in 1 ml (1:1,000)	0.15 ml	No limit
Benzylpenicillin	IM	600 milligrams	NONE	N/A	600 milligrams dissolved in 2 ml water for injection	2 ml	600 milligrams
Benzylpenicillin	IV/IO	600 milligrams	NONE	N/A	600 milligrams dissolved in 10 ml water for injection	10 ml	600 milligrams
Chlorphenamine	IV/IO/IM	2.5 milligrams	NONE	N/A	10 milligrams in 1 ml	0.25 ml	2.5 milligrams
Chlorphenamine	Oral (tablet)	N/A	N/A	N/A	N/A	N/A	N/A
Chlorphenamine	Oral (solution)	1 milligram	NONE	N/A	2 milligrams in 5 ml	2.5 ml	1 milligram

Page for Age: 2 YEARS

NAME	ROUTE	INITIAL DOSE	REPEAT DOSE	DOSE INTERVAL	CONCEN-TRATION	VOLUME	MAX DOSE
Dexamethasone	Oral (solution)	1.8 milligrams	NONE	N/A	2 milligrams in 5 ml	5 ml	1.8 milligrams
Dexamethasone	Oral (tablet)	4 milligrams	NONE	N/A	2 milligrams per tablet	2 tablets	4 milligrams
Diazepam	Rectal	5 milligrams	5 milligrams	10 minutes	5 milligrams in 2.5 ml	1 x 5 milligram tube	10 milligrams
Diazepam	IV/IO	4 milligrams	4 milligrams	10 minutes	10 milligrams in 2 ml	0.8ml	8 milligrams
Glucagon	IM	500 micrograms	NONE	N/A	1 milligram per vial	0.5 vial	500 micrograms
Glucose 10%	IV	2.5 grams glucose	2.5 grams glucose	5 minutes	50 grams in 500 ml	25 ml	75 ml (7.5 g glucose)
Glucose 40% Oral Gel	Buccal	10 grams	10 grams	5 minutes	10 grams in 25 grams of gel	1 tube	2 tubes/20 grams
Hydrocortisone	IV/IO/IM	50 milligrams	NONE	N/A	100 milligrams in 1 ml	0.5 ml	50 milligrams
Hydrocortisone	IV/IO/IM	50 milligrams	NONE	N/A	100 milligrams in 2 ml	1 ml	50 milligrams
Ibuprofen	Oral	100 milligrams	100 milligrams	8 hours	100 milligrams in 5 ml	5 ml	300 milligrams per 24 hours
Ipratropium Bromide	Neb	250 micrograms	NONE	N/A	250 micrograms in 1 ml	1 ml	250 micrograms
Ipratropium Bromide	Neb	250 micrograms	NONE	N/A	500 micrograms in 2 ml	1 ml	250 micrograms
Midazolam**	Buccal	5 milligrams	5 milligrams	10 mins	5 milligrams in 1 ml	1 ml pre-filled syringe	10 milligrams
Morphine Sulfate	IV/IO	1 milligram	1 milligram	5 minutes	10 milligrams in 10 ml	1 ml	2 milligrams
Morphine Sulfate	Oral	2 milligrams	NONE	N/A	10 milligrams in 5 ml	1 ml	2 milligrams
Naloxone	IM	400 micrograms	400 micrograms	3 minutes	400 micrograms in 1 ml	1 ml	2,000 micrograms
Naloxone	IV/IO	1,200 micrograms	800 micrograms	1 minute	400 micrograms in 1 ml	3 ml	2,000 micrograms
Ondansetron	IV/IO/IM	1 milligram	NONE	N/A	2 milligrams in 1 ml	0.5 ml	1 milligram
Paracetamol - Infant suspension	Oral	180 milligrams	180 milligrams	4–6 hours	120 milligrams in 5 ml	7.5 ml	720 milligrams in 24 hours
Paracetamol	IV infusion/ IO	200 milligrams	200 milligrams	4–6 hours	10 milligrams in 1 ml	20 ml	800 milligrams in 24 hours
Salbutamol	Neb	2.5 milligrams	2.5 milligrams	5 minutes	2.5 milligrams in 2.5 ml	2.5 ml	No limit
Salbutamol	Neb	2.5 milligrams	2.5 milligrams	5 minutes	5 milligrams in 2.5 ml	1.25 ml	No limit
Tranexamic Acid	IV	200 mg	NONE	N/A	100 mg/ml	2 ml	200 mg

*If a large quantity of poison has been ingested, and where there is a risk to life, encourage the child to drink the full dose.

**Give the dose as prescribed in the child's individual treatment plan/Epilepsy Passport (the dosages described above reflect the recommended dosages for a child of this age).

Page for Age: 3 YEARS

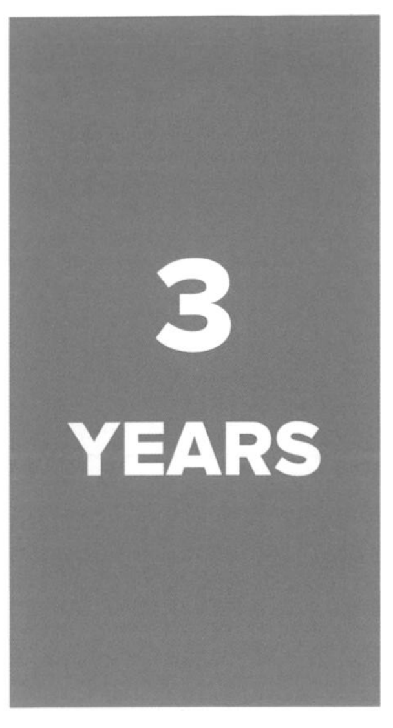

Vital Signs

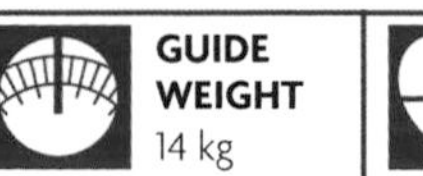 GUIDE WEIGHT 14 kg	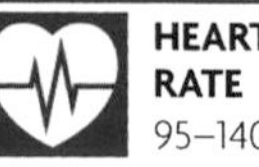 HEART RATE 95–140	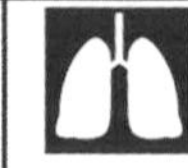 RESPIRATION RATE 25–30	 SYSTOLIC BLOOD PRESSURE 80–100

Airway Size by Type

OROPHARYNGEAL AIRWAY	LARYNGEAL MASK	I-GEL AIRWAY	ENDOTRACHEAL TUBE
1	2	2	Diameter: **5 mm**; Length: **14 cm**

Defibrillation – Cardiac Arrest

MANUAL	AUTOMATED EXTERNAL DEFIBRILLATOR
60 Joules	A standard AED (either with paediatric attenuation pads or else in paediatric mode) can be used. If paediatric pads are not available, standard adult pads can be used (but must not overlap).

Intravascular Fluid

NAME	ROUTE	INITIAL DOSE	REPEAT DOSE	DOSE INTERVAL	CONCENTRATION	VOLUME	MAX DOSE
0.9% Sodium Chloride (5 ml/kg)	IV/IO	70 ml	70 ml	PRN	0.9%	70 ml	560 ml
0.9% Sodium Chloride (10 ml/kg)	IV/IO	140 ml	140 ml	PRN	0.9%	140 ml	560 ml
0.9% Sodium Chloride (20 ml/kg)	IV/IO	280 ml	280 ml	PRN	0.9%	280 ml	560 ml

Cardiac Arrest

NAME	ROUTE	INITIAL DOSE	REPEAT DOSE	DOSE INTERVAL	CONCENTRATION	VOLUME	MAX DOSE
Adrenaline	IV/IO	140 micrograms	140 micrograms	3–5 minutes	1 milligram in 10 ml (1:10,000)	1.4 ml	No limit
Amiodarone	IV/IO	70 milligrams (After 3rd shock)	70 milligrams	After 5th shock	300 milligrams in 10 ml	2.3 ml	140 milligrams

Quick Reference Table

NAME	ROUTE	INITIAL DOSE	REPEAT DOSE	DOSE INTERVAL	CONCEN-TRATION	VOLUME	MAX DOSE
Activated Charcoal*	Oral	25 g	25 g	N/A	50 grams in 250 ml	125 ml	50 grams
Adrenaline - anaphylaxis/ asthma	IM	150 micrograms	150 micrograms	5 minutes	1 milligram in 1 ml (1:1,000)	0.15 ml	No limit
Benzylpenicillin	IV/IO	600 milligrams	NONE	N/A	600 milligrams dissolved in 10 ml water for injection	10 ml	600 milligrams
Benzylpenicillin	IM	600 milligrams	NONE	N/A	600 milligrams dissolved in 2 ml water for injection	2 ml	600 milligrams
Chlorphenamine	IV/IO/IM	2.5 milligrams	NONE	N/A	10 milligrams in 1 ml	0.25 ml	2.5 milligrams
Chlorphenamine	Oral (tablet)	N/A	N/A	N/A	N/A	N/A	N/A

Page for Age: 3 YEARS

NAME	ROUTE	INITIAL DOSE	REPEAT DOSE	DOSE INTERVAL	CONCEN-TRATION	VOLUME	MAX DOSE
Chlorphenamine	Oral (solution)	1 milligram	NONE	N/A	2 milligrams in 5 ml	2.5 ml	1 milligram
Dexamethasone	Oral (solution)	2.1 milligrams	NONE	N/A	2 milligrams in 5 ml	5 ml	2.1 milligrams
Dexamethasone	Oral (tablet)	4 milligrams	NONE	N/A	2 milligrams per tablet	2 tablets	4 milligrams
Diazepam	Rectal	5 milligrams	5 milligrams	10 minutes	5 milligrams in 2.5 ml	1 x 5 milligram tube	10 milligrams
Diazepam	IV/IO	4.5 milligrams	4.5 milligrams	10 minutes	10 milligrams in 2 ml	0.9 ml	9 milligrams
Glucagon	IM	500 micrograms	NONE	N/A	1 milligram per vial	0.5 vial	500 micrograms
Glucose 10%	IV	3 grams glucose	3 grams glucose	5 minutes	50 grams in 500 ml	30 ml	90 ml (9 g glucose)
Glucose 40% Oral Gel	Buccal	10 grams	10 grams	5 minutes	10 grams in 25 grams of gel	1 tube	2 tubes/20 grams
Hydrocortisone	IV/IO/IM	50 milligrams	NONE	N/A	100 milligrams in 1 ml	0.5 ml	50 milligrams
Hydrocortisone	IV/IO/IM	50 milligrams	NONE	N/A	100 milligrams in 2 ml	1 ml	50 milligrams
Ibuprofen	Oral	100 milligrams	100 milligrams	8 hours	100 milligrams in 5 ml	5 ml	300 milligrams per 24 hours
Ipratropium Bromide	Neb	250 micrograms	NONE	N/A	250 micrograms in 1 ml	1 ml	250 micrograms
Ipratropium Bromide	Neb	250 micrograms	NONE	N/A	500 micrograms in 2 ml	1 ml	250 micrograms
Midazolam**	Buccal	5 milligrams	5 milligrams	10 mins	5 milligrams in 1 ml	1 ml pre-filled syringe	10 milligrams
Morphine Sulfate	IV/IO	1.5 milligrams	1.5 milligrams	5 minutes	10 milligrams in 10 ml	1.5 ml	3 milligrams
Morphine Sulfate	Oral	3 milligrams	NONE	N/A	10 milligrams in 5 ml	1.5 ml	3 milligrams
Naloxone	IM	400 micrograms	400 micrograms	3 minutes	400 micrograms in 1 ml	1 ml	2,000 micrograms
Naloxone	IV/IO	1,200 micrograms	800 micrograms	1 minute	400 micrograms in 1 ml	3 ml	2,000 micrograms
Ondansetron	IV/IO/IM	1.5 milligrams	NONE	N/A	2 milligrams in 1 ml	0.75 ml	1.5 milligrams
Paracetamol - Infant suspension	Oral	180 milligrams	180 milligrams	4–6 hours	120 milligrams in 5 ml	7.5 ml	720 milligrams in 24 hours
Paracetamol	IV infusion/ IO	200 milligrams	200 milligrams	4–6 hours	10 milligrams in 1 ml	20 ml	800 milligrams in 24 hours
Salbutamol	Neb	2.5 milligrams	2.5 milligrams	5 minutes	2.5 milligrams in 2.5 ml	2.5 ml	No limit
Salbutamol	Neb	2.5 milligrams	2.5 milligrams	5 minutes	5 milligrams in 2.5 ml	1.25 ml	No limit
Tranexamic Acid	IV	200 mg	NONE	N/A	100 mg/ml	2 ml	200 mg

*If a large quantity of poison has been ingested, and where there is a risk to life, encourage the child to drink the full dose.

**Give the dose as prescribed in the child's individual treatment plan/Epilepsy Passport (the dosages described above reflect the recommended dosages for a child of this age).

Page for Age: 4 YEARS

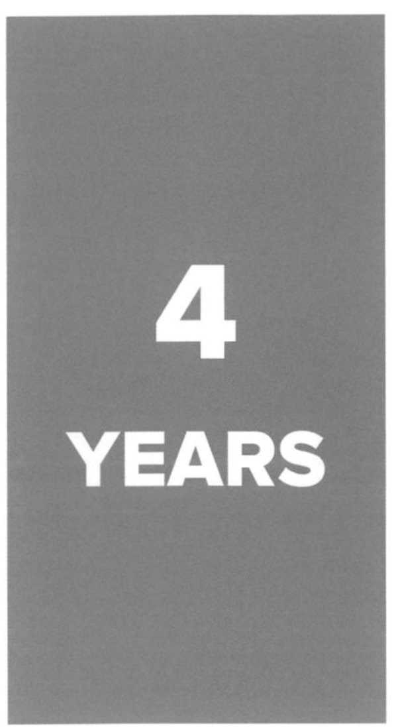

Vital Signs

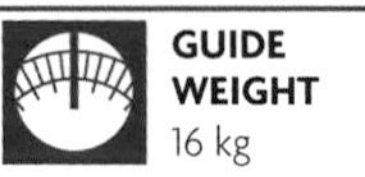 GUIDE WEIGHT	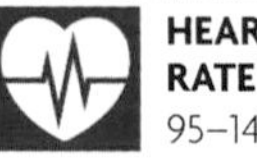 HEART RATE	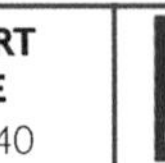 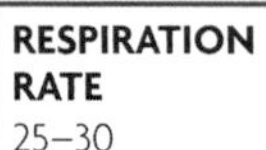 RESPIRATION RATE	 SYSTOLIC BLOOD PRESSURE
16 kg	95–140	25–30	80–100

Airway Size by Type

OROPHARYNGEAL AIRWAY	LARYNGEAL MASK	I-GEL AIRWAY	ENDOTRACHEAL TUBE
1	2	2	Diameter: **5 mm**; Length: **15 cm**

Defibrillation – Cardiac Arrest

MANUAL	AUTOMATED EXTERNAL DEFIBRILLATOR
70 Joules	A standard AED (either with paediatric attenuation pads or else in paediatric mode) can be used. If paediatric pads are not available, standard adult pads can be used (but must not overlap).

Intravascular Fluid

NAME	ROUTE	INITIAL DOSE	REPEAT DOSE	DOSE INTERVAL	CONCENTRATION	VOLUME	MAX DOSE
0.9% Sodium Chloride (5 ml/kg)	IV/IO	80 ml	80 ml	PRN	0.9%	80 ml	640 ml
0.9% Sodium Chloride (10 ml/kg)	IV/IO	160 ml	160 ml	PRN	0.9%	160 ml	640 ml
0.9% Sodium Chloride (20 ml/kg)	IV/IO	320 ml	320 ml	PRN	0.9%	320 ml	640 ml

Cardiac Arrest

NAME	ROUTE	INITIAL DOSE	REPEAT DOSE	DOSE INTERVAL	CONCENTRATION	VOLUME	MAX DOSE
Adrenaline	IV/IO	160 micrograms	160 micrograms	3–5 minutes	1 milligram in 10 ml (1:10,000)	1.6 ml	No limit
Amiodarone	IV/IO	80 milligrams (After 3rd shock)	80 milligrams	After 5th shock	300 milligrams in 10 ml	2.7 ml	160 milligrams

Quick Reference Table

NAME	ROUTE	INITIAL DOSE	REPEAT DOSE	DOSE INTERVAL	CONCEN-TRATION	VOLUME	MAX DOSE
Activated Charcoal*	Oral	25 g	25 g	N/A	50 grams in 250 ml	125 ml	50 grams
Adrenaline - anaphylaxis/ asthma	IM	150 micrograms	150 micrograms	5 minutes	1 milligram in 1 ml (1:1,000)	0.15 ml	No limit
Benzylpenicillin	IV/IO	600 milligrams	NONE	N/A	600 milligrams dissolved in 10 ml water for injection	10 ml	600 milligrams
Benzylpenicillin	IM	600 milligrams	NONE	N/A	600 milligrams dissolved in 2 ml water for injection	2 ml	600 milligrams
Chlorphenamine	IV/IO/IM	2.5 milligrams	NONE	N/A	10 milligrams in 1 ml	0.25 ml	2.5 milligrams
Chlorphenamine	Oral (tablet)	N/A	N/A	N/A	N/A	N/A	N/A

Page for Age: 4 YEARS

NAME	ROUTE	INITIAL DOSE	REPEAT DOSE	DOSE INTERVAL	CONCEN-TRATION	VOLUME	MAX DOSE
Chlorphenamine	Oral (solution)	1 milligram	NONE	N/A	2 milligrams in 5 ml	2.5 ml	1 milligram
Dexamethasone	Oral (solution)	2.4 milligrams	NONE	N/A	2 milligrams in 5 ml	6 ml	2.4 milligrams
Dexamethasone	Oral (tablet)	4 milligrams	NONE	N/A	2 milligrams per tablet	2 tablets	4 milligrams
Diazepam	Rectal	5 milligrams	5 milligrams	10 minutes	5 milligrams in 2.5 ml	1 x 5 milligram tube	10 milligrams
Diazepam	IV/IO	5 milligrams	5 milligrams	10 minutes	10 milligrams in 2 ml	1 ml	10 milligrams
Glucagon	IM	500 micrograms	NONE	N/A	1 milligram per vial	0.5 vial	500 micrograms
Glucose 10%	IV	3 grams glucose	3 grams glucose	5 minutes	50 grams in 500 ml	30 ml	90 ml (9 g glucose)
Glucose 40% Oral Gel	Buccal	10 grams	10 grams	5 minutes	10 grams in 25 grams of gel	1 tube	2 tubes/20 grams
Hydrocortisone	IV/IO/IM	50 milligrams	NONE	N/A	100 milligrams in 1 ml	0.5 ml	50 milligrams
Hydrocortisone	IV/IO/IM	50 milligrams	NONE	N/A	100 milligrams in 2 ml	1 ml	50 milligrams
Ibuprofen	Oral	150 milligrams	150 milligrams	8 hours	100 milligrams in 5 ml	7.5 ml	450 milligrams per 24 hours
Ipratropium Bromide	Neb	250 micrograms	NONE	N/A	250 micrograms in 1 ml	1 ml	250 micrograms
Ipratropium Bromide	Neb	250 micrograms	NONE	N/A	500 micrograms in 2 ml	1 ml	250 micrograms
Midazolam**	Buccal	5 milligrams	5 milligrams	10 mins	5 milligrams in 1 ml	1 ml pre-filled syringe	10 milligrams
Morphine Sulfate	IV/IO	1.5 milligrams	1.5 milligrams	5 minutes	10 milligrams in 10 ml	1.5 ml	3 milligrams
Morphine Sulfate	Oral	3 milligrams	NONE	N/A	10 milligrams in 5 ml	1.5 ml	3 milligrams
Naloxone	IM	400 micrograms	400 micrograms	3 minutes	400 micrograms in 1 ml	1 ml	2,000 micrograms
Naloxone	IV/IO	1,600 micrograms	400 micrograms	1 minute	400 micrograms in 1 ml	4 ml	2,000 micrograms
Ondansetron	IV/IO/IM	1.5 milligrams	NONE	N/A	2 milligrams in 1 ml	0.75 ml	1.5 milligrams
Paracetamol - Infant suspension	Oral	240 milligrams	240 milligrams	4–6 hours	120 milligrams in 5 ml	10 ml	960 milligrams in 24 hours
Paracetamol	IV infusion/ IO	250 milligrams	250 milligrams	4–6 hours	10 milligrams in 1 ml	25 ml	1 gram in 24 hours
Salbutamol	Neb	2.5 milligrams	2.5 milligrams	5 minutes	2.5 milligrams in 2.5 ml	2.5 ml	No limit
Salbutamol	Neb	2.5 milligrams	2.5 milligrams	5 minutes	5 milligrams in 2.5 ml	1.25 ml	No limit
Tranexamic Acid	IV	250 mg	NONE	N/A	100 mg/ml	2.5 ml	250 mg

*If a large quantity of poison has been ingested, and where there is a risk to life, encourage the child to drink the full dose.

*Give the dose as prescribed in the child's individual treatment plan/Epilepsy Passport (the dosages described above reflect the recommended dosages for a child of this age).

Page for Age: 5 YEARS

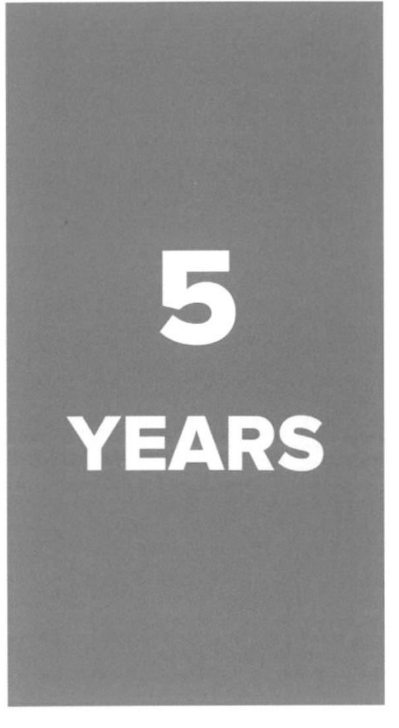

Vital Signs

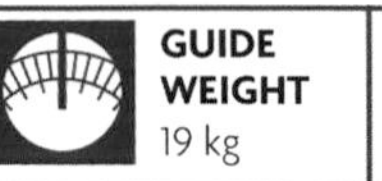 GUIDE WEIGHT 19 kg	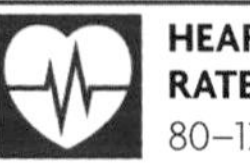 HEART RATE 80–120	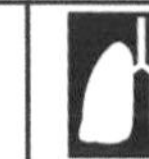 RESPIRATION RATE 20–25	 SYSTOLIC BLOOD PRESSURE 90–100

Airway Size by Type

OROPHARYNGEAL AIRWAY	LARYNGEAL MASK	I-GEL AIRWAY	ENDOTRACHEAL TUBE
1	2	2	Diameter: **5.5 mm**; Length: **15 cm**

Defibrillation – Cardiac Arrest

MANUAL	AUTOMATED EXTERNAL DEFIBRILLATOR
80 Joules	A standard AED (either with paediatric attenuation pads or else in paediatric mode) can be used. If paediatric pads are not available, standard adult pads can be used (but must not overlap).

Intravascular Fluid

NAME	ROUTE	INITIAL DOSE	REPEAT DOSE	DOSE INTERVAL	CONCENTRATION	VOLUME	MAX DOSE
0.9% Sodium Chloride (5 ml/kg)	IV/IO	95 ml	95 ml	PRN	0.9%	95 ml	760 ml
0.9% Sodium Chloride (10 ml/kg)	IV/IO	190 ml	190 ml	PRN	0.9%	190 ml	760 ml
0.9% Sodium Chloride (20 ml/kg)	IV/IO	380 ml	380 ml	PRN	0.9%	380 ml	760 ml

Cardiac Arrest

NAME	ROUTE	INITIAL DOSE	REPEAT DOSE	DOSE INTERVAL	CONCENTRATION	VOLUME	MAX DOSE
Adrenaline	IV/IO	190 micrograms	190 micrograms	3–5 minutes	1 milligram in 10 ml (1:10,000)	1.9 ml	No limit
Amiodarone	IV/IO	100 milligrams (After 3rd shock)	100 milligrams	After 5th shock	300 milligrams in 10 ml	3.3 ml	200 milligrams

Quick Reference Table

NAME	ROUTE	INITIAL DOSE	REPEAT DOSE	DOSE INTERVAL	CONCEN-TRATION	VOLUME	MAX DOSE
Activated Charcoal*	Oral	25 g	25 g	N/A	50 grams in 250 ml	125 ml	50 grams
Adrenaline - anaphylaxis/ asthma	IM	150 micrograms	150 micrograms	5 minutes	1 milligram in 1 ml (1:1,000)	0.15 ml	No limit
Benzylpenicillin	IV/IO	600 milligrams	NONE	N/A	600 milligrams dissolved in 10 ml water for injection	10 ml	600 milligrams
Benzylpenicillin	IM	600 milligrams	NONE	N/A	600 milligrams dissolved in 2 ml water for injection	2 ml	600 milligrams
Chlorphenamine	IV/IO/IM	2.5 milligrams	NONE	N/A	10 milligrams in 1 ml	0.25 ml	2.5 milligrams
Chlorphenamine	Oral (tablet)	N/A	N/A	N/A	N/A	N/A	N/A

Page for Age: 5 YEARS

NAME	ROUTE	INITIAL DOSE	REPEAT DOSE	DOSE INTERVAL	CONCEN-TRATION	VOLUME	MAX DOSE
Chlorphenamine	Oral (solution)	1 milligram	NONE	N/A	2 milligrams in 5 ml	2.5 ml	1 milligram
Dexamethasone	Oral (solution)	2.9 milligrams	NONE	N/A	2 milligrams in 5 ml	7 ml	2.9 milligrams
Dexamethasone	Oral (tablet)	4 milligrams	NONE	N/A	2 milligrams per tablet	2 tablets	4 milligrams
Diazepam	Rectal	10 milligrams	10 milligrams	10 minutes	10 milligrams in 2.5 ml	1 x 10 milligram tube	20 milligrams
Diazepam	IV/IO	6 milligrams	6 milligrams	10 minutes	10 milligrams in 2 ml	1.2 ml	12 milligrams
Glucagon	IM	500 micrograms	NONE	N/A	1 milligram per vial	0.5 vial	500 micrograms
Glucose 10%	IV	4 grams glucose	4 grams glucose	5 minutes	50 grams in 500 ml	40 ml	120 ml (12 g glucose)
Glucose 40% Oral Gel	Buccal	10 grams	10 grams	5 minutes	10 grams in 25 grams of gel	1 tube	2 tubes/20 grams
Hydrocortisone	IV/IO/IM	50 milligrams	NONE	N/A	100 milligrams in 1 ml	0.5 ml	50 milligrams
Hydrocortisone	IV/IO/IM	50 milligrams	NONE	N/A	100 milligrams in 2 ml	1 ml	50 milligrams
Ibuprofen	Oral	150 milligrams	150 milligrams	8 hours	100 milligrams in 5 ml	7.5 ml	450 milligrams per 24 hours
Ipratropium Bromide	Neb	250 micrograms	NONE	N/A	250 micrograms in 1 ml	1 ml	250 micrograms
Ipratropium Bromide	Neb	250 micrograms	NONE	N/A	500 micrograms in 2 ml	1 ml	250 micrograms
Midazolam**	Buccal	7.5 milligrams	7.5 milligrams	10 mins	5 milligrams in 1 ml	1.5 ml pre-filled syringe	15 milligrams
Morphine Sulfate	IV/IO	2 milligrams	2 milligrams	5 minutes	10 milligrams in 10 ml	2 ml	4 milligrams
Morphine Sulfate	Oral	4 milligrams	NONE	N/A	10 milligrams in 5 ml	2 ml	4 milligrams
Naloxone	IM	400 micrograms	400 micrograms	3 minutes	400 micrograms in 1 ml	1 ml	2,000 micrograms
Naloxone	IV/IO	2,000 micrograms	Seek advice	N/A	400 micrograms in 1 ml	5 ml	2,000 micrograms
Ondansetron	IV/IO/IM	2 milligrams	NONE	N/A	2 milligrams in 1 ml	1 ml	2 milligrams
Paracetamol - Infant suspension	Oral	240 milligrams	240 milligrams	4–6 hours	120 milligrams in 5 ml	10 ml	960 milligrams in 24 hours
Paracetamol	IV infusion/ IO	300 milligrams	300 milligrams	4–6 hours	10 milligrams in 1 ml	30 ml	1.2 gram in 24 hours
Salbutamol	Neb	2.5 milligrams	2.5 milligrams	5 minutes	2.5 milligrams in 2.5 ml	2.5 ml	No limit
Salbutamol	Neb	2.5 milligrams	2.5 milligrams	5 minutes	5 milligrams in 2.5 ml	1.25 ml	No limit
Tranexamic Acid	IV	300 mg	NONE	N/A	100 mg/ml	3 ml	300 mg

*If a large quantity of poison has been ingested, and where there is a risk to life, encourage the child to drink the full dose.

**Give the dose as prescribed in the child's individual treatment plan/Epilepsy Passport (the dosages described above reflect the recommended dosages for a child of this age).

Page for Age: 6 YEARS

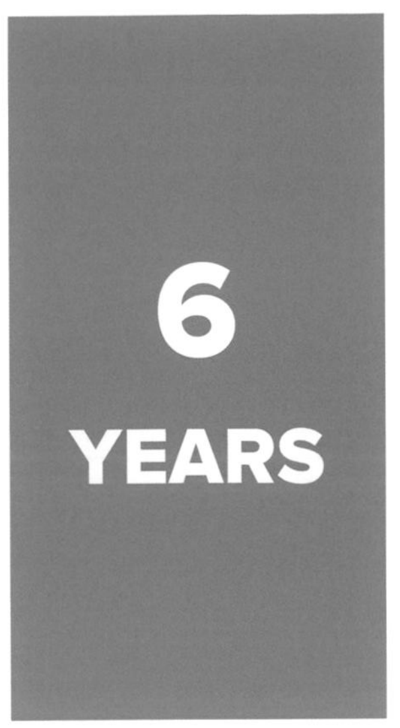

Vital Signs

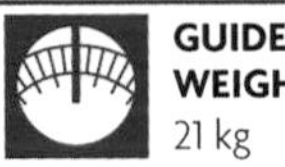 GUIDE WEIGHT 21 kg	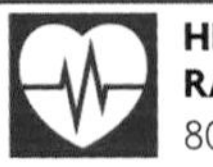 HEART RATE 80–120	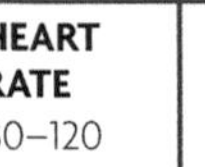 RESPIRATION RATE 20–25	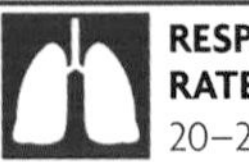  SYSTOLIC BLOOD PRESSURE 80–110

Airway Size by Type

OROPHARYNGEAL AIRWAY	LARYNGEAL MASK	I-GEL AIRWAY	ENDOTRACHEAL TUBE
1	2.5	2	Diameter: **6 mm**; Length: **16 cm**

Defibrillation – Cardiac Arrest

MANUAL	AUTOMATED EXTERNAL DEFIBRILLATOR
80 Joules	A standard AED (either with paediatric attenuation pads or else in paediatric mode) can be used. If paediatric pads are not available, standard adult pads can be used (but must not overlap).

Intravascular Fluid

NAME	ROUTE	INITIAL DOSE	REPEAT DOSE	DOSE INTERVAL	CONCENTRATION	VOLUME	MAX DOSE
0.9% Sodium Chloride (5 ml/kg)	IV/IO	105 ml	105 ml	PRN	0.9%	105 ml	840 ml
0.9% Sodium Chloride (10 ml/kg)	IV/IO	210 ml	210 ml	PRN	0.9%	210 ml	840 ml
0.9% Sodium Chloride (20 ml/kg)	IV/IO	420 ml	420 ml	PRN	0.9%	420 ml	840 ml

Cardiac Arrest

NAME	ROUTE	INITIAL DOSE	REPEAT DOSE	DOSE INTERVAL	CONCENTRATION	VOLUME	MAX DOSE
Adrenaline	IV/IO	210 micrograms	210 micrograms	3–5 minutes	1 milligram in 10 ml (1:10,000)	2.1 ml	No limit
Amiodarone	IV/IO	100 milligrams (After 3rd shock)	100 milligrams	After 5th shock	300 milligrams in 10 ml	3.3 ml	200 milligrams

Quick Reference Table

NAME	ROUTE	INITIAL DOSE	REPEAT DOSE	DOSE INTERVAL	CONCEN-TRATION	VOLUME	MAX DOSE
Activated Charcoal*	Oral	25 g	25 g	N/A	50 grams in 250 ml	125 ml	50 grams
Adrenaline - anaphylaxis/ asthma	IM	300 micrograms	300 micrograms	5 minutes	1 milligram in 1 ml (1:1,000)	0.3 ml	No limit
Benzylpenicillin	IV/IO	600 milligrams	NONE	N/A	600 milligrams dissolved in 10 ml water for injection	10 ml	600 milligrams
Benzylpenicillin	IM	600 milligrams	NONE	N/A	600 milligrams dissolved in 2 ml water for injection	2 ml	600 milligrams
Chlorphenamine	IV/IO/IM	5 milligrams	NONE	N/A	10 milligrams in 1 ml	0.5 ml	5 milligrams
Chlorphenamine	Oral (tablet)	2 milligrams	NONE	N/A	4 milligrams per tablet	½ of one tablet	2 milligrams
Chlorphenamine	Oral (solution)	2 milligrams	NONE	N/A	2 milligrams in 5 ml	5 ml	2 milligrams

Page for Age: 6 YEARS

NAME	ROUTE	INITIAL DOSE	REPEAT DOSE	DOSE INTERVAL	CONCEN-TRATION	VOLUME	MAX DOSE
Dexamethasone	Oral (solution)	3.2 milligrams	NONE	N/A	2 milligrams in 5 ml	8 ml	3.2 milligrams
Dexamethasone	Oral (tablet)	4 milligrams	NONE	N/A	2 milligrams per tablet	2 tablets	4 milligrams
Diazepam	Rectal	10 milligrams	10 milligrams	10 minutes	10 milligrams in 2.5 ml	1 x 10 milligram tube	20 milligrams
Diazepam	IV/IO	6.5 milligrams	6.5 milligrams	10 minutes	10 milligrams in 2 ml	1.3 ml	13 milligrams
Glucagon	IM	500 micrograms	NONE	N/A	1 milligram per vial	0.5 vial	500 micrograms
Glucose 10%	IV	4 grams glucose	4 grams glucose	5 minutes	50 grams in 500 ml	40 ml	120 ml (12 g glucose)
Glucose 40% Oral Gel	Buccal	10 grams	10 grams	5 minutes	10 grams in 25 grams of gel	1 tube	2 tubes/20 grams
Hydrocortisone	IV/IO/IM	100 milligrams	NONE	N/A	100 milligrams in 1 ml	1 ml	100 milligrams
Hydrocortisone	IV/IO/IM	100 milligrams	NONE	N/A	100 milligrams in 2 ml	2 ml	100 milligrams
Ibuprofen	Oral	150 milligrams	150 milligrams	8 hours	100 milligrams in 5 ml	7.5 ml	450 milligrams per 24 hours
Ipratropium Bromide	Neb	250 micrograms	NONE	N/A	250 micrograms in 1 ml	1 ml	250 micrograms
Ipratropium Bromide	Neb	250 micrograms	NONE	N/A	500 micrograms in 2 ml	1 ml	250 micrograms
Midazolam**	Buccal	7.5 milligrams	7.5 milligrams	10 mins	5 milligrams in 1 ml	1.5 ml pre-filled syringe	15 milligrams
Morphine Sulfate	IV/IO	2 milligrams	2 milligrams	5 minutes	10 milligrams in 10 ml	2 ml	4 milligrams
Morphine Sulfate	Oral	4 milligrams	NONE	N/A	10 milligrams in 5 ml	2 ml	4 milligrams
Naloxone	IM	400 micrograms	400 micrograms	3 minutes	400 micrograms in 1 ml	1 ml	2,000 micrograms
Naloxone	IV/IO	2,000 micrograms	Seek advice	N/A	400 micrograms in 1 ml	5 ml	2,000 micrograms
Ondansetron	IV/IO/IM	2 milligrams	NONE	N/A	2 milligrams in 1 ml	1 ml	2 milligrams
Paracetamol - Six Plus suspension	Oral	250 milligrams	250 milligrams	4–6 hours	250 milligrams in 5 ml	5 ml	1 gram in 24 hours
Paracetamol	IV infusion/ IO	300 milligrams	300 milligrams	4–6 hours	10 milligrams in 1 ml	30 ml	1.2 grams in 24 hours
Salbutamol	Neb	5 milligrams	5 milligrams	5 minutes	2.5 milligrams in 2.5 ml	5 ml	No limit
Salbutamol	Neb	5 milligrams	5 milligrams	5 minutes	5 milligrams in 2.5 ml	2.5 ml	No limit
Tranexamic Acid	IV	300 mg	NONE	N/A	100 mg/ml	3 ml	300 mg

*If a large quantity of poison has been ingested, and where there is a risk to life, encourage the child to drink the full dose.

*Give the dose as prescribed in the child's individual treatment plan/Epilepsy Passport (the dosages described above reflect the recommended dosages for a child of this age).

Page for Age: 7 YEARS

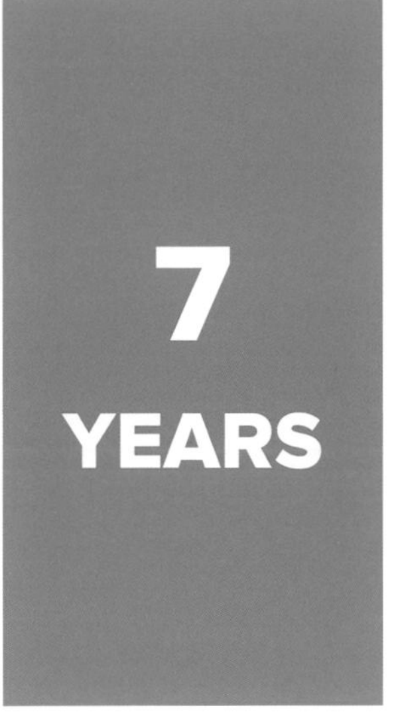

Vital Signs

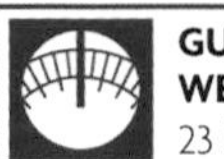 GUIDE WEIGHT 23 kg	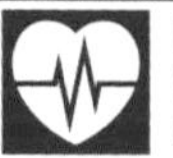 HEART RATE 80–120	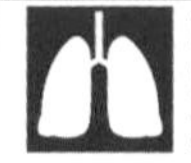 RESPIRATION RATE 20–25	 SYSTOLIC BLOOD PRESSURE 90–110

Airway Size by Type

OROPHARYNGEAL AIRWAY	LARYNGEAL MASK	I-GEL AIRWAY	ENDOTRACHEAL TUBE
1 OR 2	2.5	2	Diameter: **6 mm**; Length: **16 cm**

Defibrillation – Cardiac Arrest

MANUAL	AUTOMATED EXTERNAL DEFIBRILLATOR
100 Joules	A standard AED (either with paediatric attenuation pads or else in paediatric mode) can be used. If paediatric pads are not available, standard adult pads can be used (but must not overlap).

Intravascular Fluid

NAME	ROUTE	INITIAL DOSE	REPEAT DOSE	DOSE INTERVAL	CONCENTRATION	VOLUME	MAX DOSE
0.9% Sodium Chloride (5 ml/kg)	IV/IO	115 ml	115 ml	PRN	0.9%	115 ml	920 ml
0.9% Sodium Chloride (10 ml/kg)	IV/IO	230 ml	230 ml	PRN	0.9%	230 ml	920 ml
0.9% Sodium Chloride (20 ml/kg)	IV/IO	460 ml	460 ml	PRN	0.9%	460 ml	920 ml

Cardiac Arrest

NAME	ROUTE	INITIAL DOSE	REPEAT DOSE	DOSE INTERVAL	CONCENTRATION	VOLUME	MAX DOSE
Adrenaline	IV/IO	230 micrograms	230 micrograms	3–5 minutes	1 milligram in 10 ml (1:10,000)	2.3 ml	No limit
Amiodarone	IV/IO	120 milligrams (After 3rd shock)	120 milligrams	After 5th shock	300 milligrams in 10 ml	4 ml	240 milligrams

Quick Reference Table

NAME	ROUTE	INITIAL DOSE	REPEAT DOSE	DOSE INTERVAL	CONCEN-TRATION	VOLUME	MAX DOSE
Activated Charcoal*	Oral	25 g	25 g	N/A	50 grams in 250 ml	125 ml	50 grams
Adrenaline - anaphylaxis/ asthma	IM	300 micrograms	300 micrograms	5 minutes	1 milligram in 1 ml (1:1,000)	0.3 ml	No limit
Benzylpenicillin	IV/IO	600 milligrams	NONE	N/A	600 milligrams dissolved in 10 ml water for injection	10 ml	600 milligrams
Benzylpenicillin	IM	600 milligrams	NONE	N/A	600 milligrams dissolved in 2 ml water for injection	2 ml	600 milligrams
Chlorphenamine	IV/IO/IM	5 milligrams	NONE	N/A	10 milligrams in 1 ml	0.5 ml	5 milligrams
Chlorphenamine	Oral (tablet)	2 milligrams	NONE	N/A	4 milligrams per tablet	½ of one tablet	2 milligrams
Chlorphenamine	Oral (solution)	2 milligrams	NONE	N/A	2 milligrams in 5 ml	5 ml	2 milligrams

Page for Age: 7 YEARS

NAME	ROUTE	INITIAL DOSE	REPEAT DOSE	DOSE INTERVAL	CONCEN-TRATION	VOLUME	MAX DOSE
Dexamethasone	Oral (solution)	N/A	N/A	N/A	N/A	N/A	N/A
Dexamethasone	Oral (tablet)	N/A	N/A	N/A	N/A	N/A	N/A
Diazepam	Rectal	10 milligrams	10 milligrams	10 minutes	10 milligrams in 2.5 ml	1 x 10 milligram tube	20 milligrams
Diazepam	IV/IO	7 milligrams	7 milligrams	10 minutes	10 milligrams in 2 ml	1.4 ml	14 milligrams
Glucagon	IM	500 micrograms	NONE	N/A	1 milligram per vial	0.5 vial	500 micrograms
Glucose 10%	IV	5 grams glucose	5 grams glucose	5 minutes	50 grams in 500 ml	50 ml	150 ml (15 g glucose)
Glucose 40% Oral Gel	Buccal	10 grams	10 grams	5 minutes	10 grams in 25 grams of gel	1 tube	2 tubes/20 grams
Hydrocortisone	IV/IO/IM	100 milligrams	NONE	N/A	100 milligrams in 1 ml	1 ml	100 milligrams
Hydrocortisone	IV/IO/IM	100 milligrams	NONE	N/A	100 milligrams in 2 ml	2 ml	100 milligrams
Ibuprofen	Oral	200 milligrams	200 milligrams	8 hours	100 milligrams in 5 ml	10 ml	600 milligrams per 24 hours
Ipratropium Bromide	Neb	250 micrograms	NONE	N/A	250 micrograms in 1 ml	1 ml	250 micrograms
Ipratropium Bromide	Neb	250 micrograms	NONE	N/A	500 micrograms in 2 ml	1 ml	250 micrograms
Midazolam**	Buccal	7.5 milligrams	7.5 milligrams	10 mins	5 milligrams in 1 ml	1.5 ml pre-filled syringe	15 milligrams
Morphine Sulfate	IV/IO	2.5 milligrams	2.5 milligrams	5 minutes	10 milligrams in 10 ml	2.5 ml	5 milligrams
Morphine Sulfate	Oral	5 milligrams	NONE	N/A	10 milligrams in 5 ml	2.5 ml	5 milligrams
Naloxone	IM	400 micrograms	400 micrograms	3 minutes	400 micrograms in 1 ml	1 ml	2,000 micrograms
Naloxone	IV/IO	2,000 micrograms	Seek advice	N/A	400 micrograms in 1 ml	5 ml	2,000 micrograms
Ondansetron	IV/IO/IM	2.5 milligrams	NONE	N/A	2 milligrams in 1 ml	1.3 ml	2.5 milligrams
Paracetamol - Six Plus suspension	Oral	250 milligrams	250 milligrams	4–6 hours	250 milligrams in 5 ml	5 ml	1 gram in 24 hours
Paracetamol	IV infusion/ IO	350 milligrams	350 milligrams	4–6 hours	10 milligrams in 1 ml	35 ml	1.4 grams in 24 hours
Salbutamol	Neb	5 milligrams	5 milligrams	5 minutes	2.5 milligrams in 2.5 ml	5 ml	No limit
Salbutamol	Neb	5 milligrams	5 milligrams	5 minutes	5 milligrams in 2.5 ml	2.5 ml	No limit
Tranexamic Acid	IV	350 mg	NONE	N/A	100 mg/ml	3.5 ml	350 mg

*If a large quantity of poison has been ingested, and where there is a risk to life, encourage the child to drink the full dose.

**Give the dose as prescribed in the child's individual treatment plan/Epilepsy Passport (the dosages described above reflect the recommended dosages for a child of this age).

Page for Age: 8 YEARS

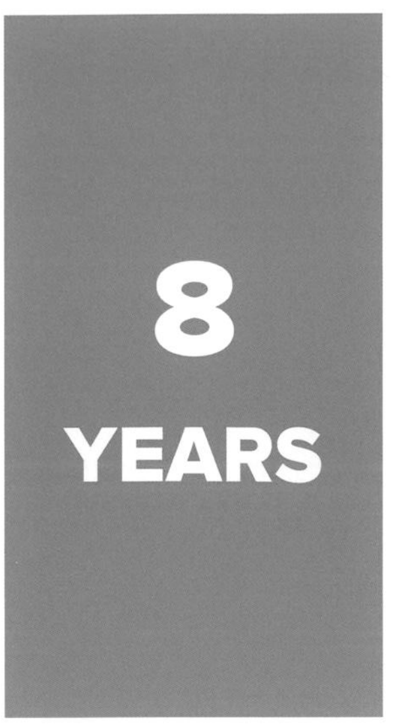

Vital Signs

 GUIDE WEIGHT	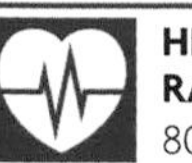 HEART RATE	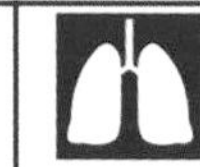 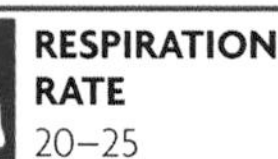 RESPIRATION RATE	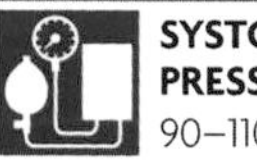 SYSTOLIC BLOOD PRESSURE
26 kg	80–120	20–25	90–110

Airway Size by Type

OROPHARYNGEAL AIRWAY	LARYNGEAL MASK	I-GEL AIRWAY	ENDOTRACHEAL TUBE
1 OR 2	2.5	2.5	Diameter: **6.5 mm**; Length: **17 cm**

Defibrillation – Cardiac Arrest

MANUAL	AUTOMATED EXTERNAL DEFIBRILLATOR
100 Joules	A standard AED (either with paediatric attenuation pads or else in paediatric mode) can be used. If paediatric pads are not available, standard adult pads can be used (but must not overlap).

Intravascular Fluid

NAME	ROUTE	INITIAL DOSE	REPEAT DOSE	DOSE INTERVAL	CONCENTRATION	VOLUME	MAX DOSE
0.9% Sodium Chloride (5 ml/kg)	IV/IO	130 ml	130 ml	PRN	0.9%	130 ml	1,000 ml
0.9% Sodium Chloride (10 ml/kg)	IV/IO	250 ml	250 ml	PRN	0.9%	250 ml	1,000 ml
0.9% Sodium Chloride (20 ml/kg)	IV/IO	500 ml	500 ml	PRN	0.9%	500 ml	1,000 ml

Cardiac Arrest

NAME	ROUTE	INITIAL DOSE	REPEAT DOSE	DOSE INTERVAL	CONCENTRATION	VOLUME	MAX DOSE
Adrenaline	IV/IO	260 micrograms	260 micrograms	3–5 minutes	1 milligram in 10 ml (1:10,000)	2.6 ml	No limit
Amiodarone	IV/IO	130 milligrams (After 3rd shock)	130 milligrams	After 5th shock	300 milligrams in 10 ml	4.3 ml	260 milligrams

Quick Reference Table

NAME	ROUTE	INITIAL DOSE	REPEAT DOSE	DOSE INTERVAL	CONCEN-TRATION	VOLUME	MAX DOSE
Activated Charcoal*	Oral	25 g	25 g	N/A	50 grams in 250 ml	125 ml	50 grams
Adrenaline - anaphylaxis/ asthma	IM	300 micrograms	300 micrograms	5 minutes	1 milligram in 1 ml (1:1,000)	0.3 ml	No limit
Benzylpenicillin	IV/IO	600 milligrams	NONE	N/A	600 milligrams dissolved in 10 ml water for injection	10 ml	600 milligrams
Benzylpenicillin	IM	600 milligrams	NONE	N/A	600 milligrams dissolved in 2 ml water for injection	2 ml	600 milligrams
Chlorphenamine	IV/IO/IM	5 milligrams	NONE	N/A	10 milligrams in 1 ml	0.5 ml	5 milligrams
Chlorphenamine	Oral (tablet)	2 milligrams	NONE	N/A	4 milligrams per tablet	½ of one tablet	2 milligrams

Page for Age: 8 YEARS

NAME	ROUTE	INITIAL DOSE	REPEAT DOSE	DOSE INTERVAL	CONCEN-TRATION	VOLUME	MAX DOSE
Chlorphenamine	Oral (solution)	2 milligrams	NONE	N/A	2 milligrams in 5 ml	5 ml	2 milligrams
Dexamethasone	Oral	N/A	N/A	N/A	N/A	N/A	N/A
Diazepam	Rectal	10 milligrams	10 milligrams	10 minutes	10 milligrams in 2.5 ml	1 x 10 milligram tube	20 milligrams
Diazepam	IV/IO	8 milligrams	8 milligrams	10 minutes	10 milligrams in 2 ml	1.6 ml	16 milligrams
Glucagon	IM	1 milligram	NONE	N/A	1 milligram per vial	1 vial	1 milligram
Glucose 10%	IV	5 grams glucose	5 grams glucose	5 minutes	50 grams in 500 ml	50 ml	150 ml (15 g glucose)
Glucose 40% Oral Gel	Buccal	10 grams	10 grams	5 minutes	10 grams in 25 grams of gel	1 tube	2 tubes/20 grams
Hydrocortisone	IV/IO/IM	100 milligrams	NONE	N/A	100 milligrams in 1 ml	1 ml	100 milligrams
Hydrocortisone	IV/IO/IM	100 milligrams	NONE	N/A	100 milligrams in 2 ml	2 ml	100 milligrams
Ibuprofen	Oral	200 milligrams	200 milligrams	8 hours	100 milligrams in 5 ml	10 ml	600 milligrams per 24 hours
Ipratropium Bromide	Neb	250 micrograms	NONE	N/A	250 micrograms in 1 ml	1 ml	250 micrograms
Ipratropium Bromide	Neb	250 micrograms	NONE	N/A	500 micrograms in 2 ml	1 ml	250 micrograms
Midazolam**	Buccal	7.5 milligrams	7.5 milligrams	10 mins	5 milligrams in 1 ml	1.5 ml pre-filled syringe	15 milligrams
Morphine Sulfate	IV/IO	2.5 milligrams	2.5 milligrams	5 minutes	10 milligrams in 10 ml	2.5 ml	5 milligrams
Morphine Sulfate	Oral	5 milligrams	NONE	N/A	10 milligrams in 5 ml	2.5 ml	5 milligrams
Naloxone	IM	400 micrograms	400 micrograms	3 minutes	400 micrograms in 1 ml	1 ml	2,000 micrograms
Naloxone	IV/IO	2,000 micrograms	Seek advice	N/A	400 micrograms in 1 ml	5 ml	2,000 micrograms
Ondansetron	IV/IO/IM	2.5 milligrams	NONE	N/A	2 milligrams in 1 ml	1.3 ml	2.5 milligrams
Paracetamol - Six Plus suspension	Oral	375 milligrams	375 milligrams	4–6 hours	250 milligrams in 5 ml	7.5 ml	1.5 grams in 24 hours
Paracetamol	IV infusion/ IO	400 milligrams	400 milligrams	4–6 hours	10 milligrams in 1 ml	40 ml	1.6 grams in 24 hours
Salbutamol	Neb	5 milligrams	5 milligrams	5 minutes	2.5 milligrams in 2.5 ml	5 ml	No limit
Salbutamol	Neb	5 milligrams	5 milligrams	5 minutes	5 milligrams in 2.5 ml	2.5 ml	No limit
Tranexamic Acid	IV	400 mg	NONE	N/A	100 mg/ml	4 ml	400 mg

*If a large quantity of poison has been ingested, and where there is a risk to life, encourage the child to drink the full dose.

**Give the dose as prescribed in the child's individual treatment plan/Epilepsy Passport (the dosages described above reflect the recommended dosages for a child of this age).

Page for Age: 10 YEARS

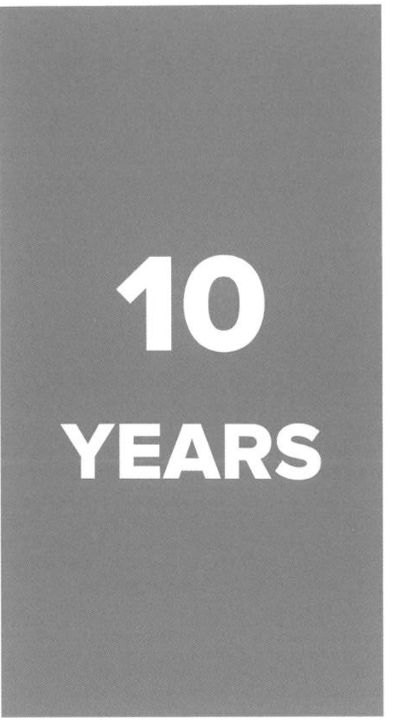

Vital Signs

 GUIDE WEIGHT 32 kg	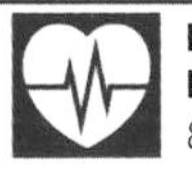 HEART RATE 80–120	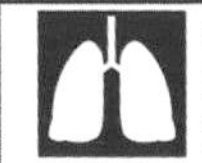 RESPIRATION RATE 20–25	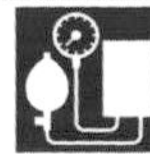 SYSTOLIC BLOOD PRESSURE 90–110

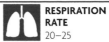

Airway Size by Type

OROPHARYNGEAL AIRWAY	LARYNGEAL MASK	I-GEL AIRWAY	ENDOTRACHEAL TUBE
2 OR 3	3	2.5 OR 3	Diameter: **7 mm**; Length: **18 cm**

Defibrillation – Cardiac Arrest

MANUAL	AUTOMATED EXTERNAL DEFIBRILLATOR
130 Joules	A standard AED can be used (without the need for paediatric attenuation pads).

Intravascular Fluid

NAME	ROUTE	INITIAL DOSE	REPEAT DOSE	DOSE INTERVAL	CONCENTRATION	VOLUME	MAX DOSE
0.9% Sodium Chloride (5 ml/kg)	IV/IO	160 ml	160 ml	PRN	0.9%	160 ml	1,000 ml
0.9% Sodium Chloride (10 ml/kg)	IV/IO	320 ml	320 ml	PRN	0.9%	320 ml	1,000 ml
0.9% Sodium Chloride (20 ml/kg)	IV/IO	500 ml	500 ml	PRN	0.9%	500 ml	1,000 ml

Cardiac Arrest

NAME	ROUTE	INITIAL DOSE	REPEAT DOSE	DOSE INTERVAL	CONCENTRATION	VOLUME	MAX DOSE
Adrenaline	IV/IO	320 micrograms	320 micrograms	3–5 minutes	1 milligram in 10 ml (1:10,000)	3.2 ml	No limit
Amiodarone	IV/IO	160 milligrams (After 3rd shock)	160 milligrams	After 5th shock	300 milligrams in 10 ml	5.3 ml	320 milligrams

Quick Reference Table

NAME	ROUTE	INITIAL DOSE	REPEAT DOSE	DOSE INTERVAL	CONCEN-TRATION	VOLUME	MAX DOSE
Activated Charcoal*	Oral	25 g	25 g	N/A	50 grams in 250 ml	125 ml	50 grams
Adrenaline - anaphylaxis/ asthma	IM	300 micrograms	300 micrograms	5 minutes	1 milligram in 1 ml (1:1,000)	0.3 ml	No limit
Benzylpenicillin	IV/IO	1.2 grams	NONE	N/A	1.2 grams dissolved in 20 ml water for injection	20 ml	1.2 grams
Benzylpenicillin	IM	1.2 grams	NONE	N/A	1.2 grams dissolved in 4 ml water for injection	4 ml	1.2 grams
Chlorphenamine	IV/IO/IM	5 milligrams	NONE	N/A	10 milligrams in 1 ml	0.5 ml	5 milligrams
Chlorphenamine	Oral (tablet)	2 milligrams	NONE	N/A	4 milligrams per tablet	½ of one tablet	2 milligrams

Page for Age: 10 YEARS

NAME	ROUTE	INITIAL DOSE	REPEAT DOSE	DOSE INTERVAL	CONCEN-TRATION	VOLUME	MAX DOSE
Chlorphenamine	Oral (solution)	2 milligrams	NONE	N/A	2 milligrams in 5 ml	5 ml	2 milligrams
Dexamethasone - croup	Oral	N/A	N/A	N/A	N/A	N/A	N/A
Diazepam	Rectal	10 milligrams	10 milligrams	10 minutes	10 milligrams in 2.5 ml	1 x 10 milligram tube	20 milligrams
Diazepam	IV/IO	10 milligrams	10 milligrams	10 minutes	10 milligrams in 2 ml	2 ml	20 milligrams
Glucagon	IM	1 milligram	NONE	N/A	1 milligram per vial	1 vial	1 milligram
Glucose 10%	IV	6.5 grams glucose	6.5 grams glucose	5 minutes	50 grams in 500 ml	65 ml	195 ml (19.5 g glucose)
Glucose 40% Oral Gel	Buccal	10 grams	10 grams	5 minutes	10 grams in 25 grams of gel	1 tube	2 tubes/20 grams
Hydrocortisone	IV/IO/IM	100 milligrams	NONE	N/A	100 milligrams in 1 ml	1 ml	100 milligrams
Hydrocortisone	IV/IO/IM	100 milligrams	NONE	N/A	100 milligrams in 2 ml	2 ml	100 milligrams
Ibuprofen	Oral	300 milligrams	300 milligrams	8 hours	100 milligrams in 5 ml	15 ml	900 milligrams per 24 hours
Ipratropium Bromide	Neb	250 micrograms	NONE	N/A	500 micrograms in 2 ml	1 ml	250 micrograms
Ipratropium Bromide	Neb	250 micrograms	NONE	N/A	250 micrograms in 1 ml	1 ml	250 micrograms
Midazolam**	Buccal	10 milligrams	10 milligrams	10 mins	5 milligrams in 1 ml	2 ml pre-filled syringe	20 milligrams
Morphine Sulfate	IV/IO	3 milligrams	3 milligrams	5 minutes	10 milligrams in 10 ml	3 ml	6 milligrams
Morphine Sulfate	Oral	6 milligrams	NONE	N/A	10 milligrams in 5 ml	3 ml	6 milligrams
Naloxone	IM	400 micrograms	400 micrograms	3 minutes	400 micrograms in 1 ml	1 ml	2,000 micrograms
Naloxone	IV/IO	2,000 micrograms	Seek advice	N/A	400 micrograms in 1 ml	5 ml	2,000 micrograms
Ondansetron	IV/IO/IM	3 milligrams	NONE	N/A	2 milligrams in 1 ml	1.5 ml	3 milligrams
Paracetamol - Six Plus suspension	Oral	500 milligrams	500 milligrams	4–6 hours	250 milligrams in 5 ml	10 ml	2 grams in 24 hours
Paracetamol	IV infusion/ IO	500 milligrams	500 milligrams	4–6 hours	10 milligrams in 1 ml	50 ml	2 grams in 24 hours
Salbutamol	Neb	5 milligrams	5 milligrams	5 minutes	2.5 milligrams in 2.5 ml	5 ml	No limit
Salbutamol	Neb	5 milligrams	5 milligrams	5 minutes	5 milligrams in 2.5 ml	2.5 ml	No limit
Tranexamic Acid	IV	500 mg	NONE	N/A	100 mg/ml	5 ml	500 mg

*If a large quantity of poison has been ingested, and where there is a risk to life, encourage the child to drink the full dose.

**Give the dose as prescribed in the child's individual treatment plan/Epilepsy Passport (the dosages described above reflect the recommended dosages for a child of this age).

Page for Age: 11 YEARS

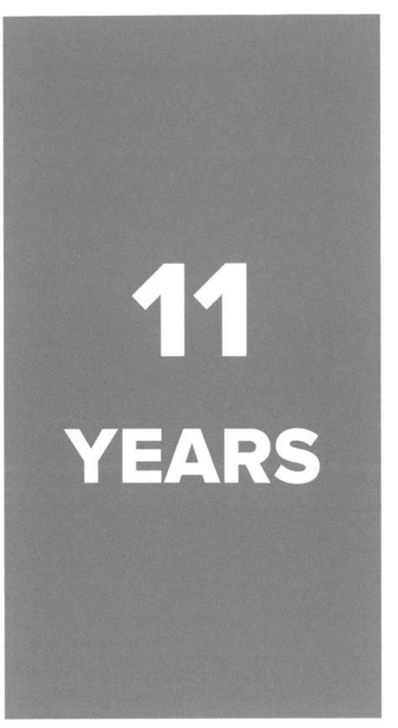

Vital Signs

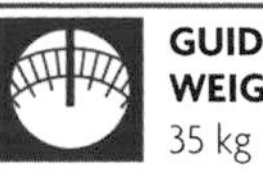 GUIDE WEIGHT 35 kg	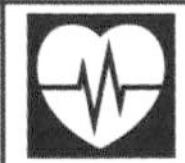 HEART RATE 80–120	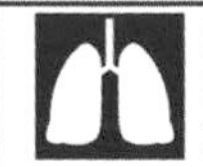 RESPIRATION RATE 20–25	 SYSTOLIC BLOOD PRESSURE 90–110

Airway Size by Type

OROPHARYNGEAL AIRWAY	LARYNGEAL MASK	I-GEL AIRWAY	ENDOTRACHEAL TUBE
2 OR 3	3	2.5 OR 3	Diameter: **7 mm**; Length: **18 cm**

Defibrillation – Cardiac Arrest

MANUAL	AUTOMATED EXTERNAL DEFIBRILLATOR
140 Joules	A standard AED can be used (without the need for paediatric attenuation pads).

Intravascular Fluid

NAME	ROUTE	INITIAL DOSE	REPEAT DOSE	DOSE INTERVAL	CONCENTRATION	VOLUME	MAX DOSE
0.9% Sodium Chloride (5 ml/kg)	IV/IO	175 ml	175 ml	PRN	0.9%	175 ml	1,000 ml
0.9% Sodium Chloride (10 ml/kg)	IV/IO	350 ml	350 ml	PRN	0.9%	350 ml	1,000 ml
0.9% Sodium Chloride (20 ml/kg)	IV/IO	500 ml	500 ml	PRN	0.9%	500 ml	1,000 ml

Cardiac Arrest

NAME	ROUTE	INITIAL DOSE	REPEAT DOSE	DOSE INTERVAL	CONCENTRATION	VOLUME	MAX DOSE
Adrenaline	IV/IO	350 micrograms	350 micrograms	3–5 minutes	1 milligram in 10 ml (1:10,000)	3.5 ml	No limit
Amiodarone	IV/IO	180 milligrams (After 3rd shock)	180 milligrams	After 5th shock	300 milligrams in 10 ml	6 ml	360 milligrams

Quick Reference Table

NAME	ROUTE	INITIAL DOSE	REPEAT DOSE	DOSE INTERVAL	CONCEN-TRATION	VOLUME	MAX DOSE
Activated Charcoal*	Oral	25 g	25 g	N/A	50 grams in 250 ml	125 ml	50 grams
Adrenaline - anaphylaxis/ asthma	IM	300 micrograms	300 micrograms	5 minutes	1 milligram in 1 ml (1:1,000)	0.3 ml	No limit
Benzylpenicillin	IV/IO	1.2 grams	NONE	N/A	1.2 grams dissolved in 20 ml water for injection	20 ml	1.2 grams
Benzylpenicillin	IM	1.2 grams	NONE	N/A	1.2 grams dissolved in 4 ml water for injection	4 ml	1.2 grams
Chlorphenamine	IV/IO/IM	5 milligrams	NONE	N/A	10 milligrams in 1 ml	0.5 ml	5 milligrams
Chlorphenamine	Oral (tablet)	2 milligrams	NONE	N/A	4 milligrams per tablet	½ of one tablet	2 milligrams

Page for Age: 11 YEARS

NAME	ROUTE	INITIAL DOSE	REPEAT DOSE	DOSE INTERVAL	CONCEN-TRATION	VOLUME	MAX DOSE
Chlorphenamine	Oral (solution)	2 milligrams	NONE	N/A	2 milligrams in 5 ml	5 ml	2 milligrams
Dexamethasone	Oral	N/A	N/A	N/A	N/A	N/A	N/A
Diazepam	Rectal	10 milligrams	10 milligrams	10 minutes	10 milligrams in 2.5 ml	1 x 10 milligram tube	20 milligrams
Diazepam	IV/IO	10 milligrams	10 milligrams	10 minutes	10 milligrams in 2 ml	2ml	20 milligrams
Glucagon	IM	1 milligram	NONE	N/A	1 milligram per vial	1 vial	1 milligram
Glucose 10%	IV	7 grams glucose	7 grams glucose	5 minutes	50 grams in 500 ml	70 ml	210 ml (21g glucose)
Glucose 40% Oral Gel	Buccal	10 grams	10 grams	5 minutes	10 grams in 25 grams of gel	1 tube	2 tubes/20 grams
Hydrocortisone	IV/IO/IM	100 milligrams	NONE	N/A	100 milligrams in 1 ml	1 ml	100 milligrams
Hydrocortisone	IV/IO/IM	100 milligrams	NONE	N/A	100 milligrams in 2 ml	2 ml	100 milligrams
Ibuprofen	Oral	300 milligrams	300 milligrams	8 hours	100 milligrams in 5 ml	15 ml	900 milligrams per 24 hours
Ipratropium Bromide	Neb	250 micrograms	NONE	N/A	250 micrograms in 1 ml	1 ml	250 micrograms
Ipratropium Bromide	Neb	250 micrograms	NONE	N/A	500 micrograms in 2 ml	1 ml	250 micrograms
Midazolam**	Buccal	10 milligrams	10 milligrams	10 mins	5 milligrams in 1 ml	2 ml pre-filled syringe	20 milligrams
Morphine Sulfate	IV/IO	3.5 milligrams	3.5 milligrams	5 minutes	10 milligrams in 10 ml	3.5 ml	7 milligrams
Morphine Sulfate	Oral	7 milligrams	NONE	N/A	10 milligrams in 5 ml	3.5 ml	7 milligrams
Naloxone	IM	400 micrograms	400 micrograms	3 minutes	400 micrograms in 1 ml	1 ml	2,000 micrograms
Naloxone	IV/IO	2,000 micrograms	Seek advice	N/A	400 micrograms in 1 ml	5 ml	2,000 micrograms
Ondansetron	IV/IO/IM	3 milligrams	NONE	N/A	2 milligrams in 1 ml	1.5 ml	3 milligrams
Paracetamol - Six Plus suspension	Oral	500 milligrams	500 milligrams	4–6 hours	250 milligrams in 5 ml	10 ml	2 grams in 24 hours
Paracetamol	IV	500 milligrams	500 milligrams	4–6 hours	10 milligrams in 1 ml	50 ml	2 grams in 24 hours
Salbutamol	Neb	5 milligrams	5 milligrams	5 minutes	5 milligrams in 2.5 ml	2.5 ml	No limit
Salbutamol	Neb	5 milligrams	5 milligrams	5 minutes	2.5 milligrams in 2.5 ml	5 ml	No limit
Tranexamic Acid	IV	500 mg	NONE	N/A	100 mg/ml	5 ml	500 mg

*If a large quantity of poison has been ingested, and where there is a risk to life, encourage the child to drink the full dose.

**Give the dose as prescribed in the child's individual treatment plan/Epilepsy Passport (the dosages described above reflect the recommended dosages for a child of this age).

Index

Index

Index

Index

Index

Index

Index

Index

Index

Index

Index

Index

Index